MAGNETIC

RESONANCE

IMAGING OF

CNS DISEASE

• A Teaching File •

MAGNETIC

RESONANCE

IMAGING OF

CNS DISEASE

• **A Teaching File** •

• **Douglas H. Yock, Jr., M.D.** •

Departments of Neuroscience and Radiology
Abbott Northwestern Hospital
Minneapolis, Minnesota

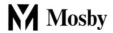 Mosby

St. Louis Baltimore Berlin Boston Carlsbad Chicago London Madrid
Naples New York Philadelphia Sydney Tokyo Toronto

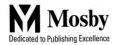
Mosby
Dedicated to Publishing Excellence

Publisher: Anne S. Patterson
Executive Editor: Susan M. Gay
Developmental Editors: Sandra Clark Brown and Maura K. Leib
Project Manager: Carol Sullivan Weis
Manufacturing Supervisor: Kathy Grone
Book Designer: Sheilah Barrett

Great care has been used in compiling and checking the information in this book to ensure its accuracy and accordance with the accepted standards and practice at the time of publication. However, as research and regulations are constantly changing, neither the publisher nor the author shall be responsible for errors or consequences arising from the use of the information contained herein.

Printed in the United States of America
Composition by the Clarinda Company
Printing/binding by Maple-Vail Manufacturing Group, York

Mosby–Year Book, Inc.
11830 Westline Industrial Drive
St. Louis, MO 63146

International Standard Book Number 0-8016-8098-0

94 95 96 97 98 / 9 8 7 6 5 4 3 2 1

PREFACE

The following chapters present a broad range of cranial and spinal MR images within a structured format. Each page features a pair of related scans. The images on facing pages often illustrate comparisons or variations. A large number of cross references is included in the text, and about 25 percent of the volume is devoted specifically to differential diagnosis.

Illustrations are limited to selected projections and pulse sequences in order to include a wide spectrum of neuropathology within a book of reasonable length. Discussions concentrate on the interpretation of MR scans, with secondary emphasis on clinical correlation and pathophysiology.

Cases in this collection offer a survey of CNS disease but do not constitute an all-inclusive atlas. Anatomical variants and technical artifacts are demonstrated only if they mimic pathology, and ENT disorders are largely omitted. The chapter on orbital lesions is an overview rather than a complete summary.

Short-term obsolescence has been minimized by updating of images, text, and references until the last possible moment before publication. Minor irregularities in the numbering of scattered cases reflect late additions.

In summary, this teaching file is intended to be integrated, practical, and efficient. I hope that the goals are realized and the result is enjoyable.

Douglas H. Yock, Jr., M.D.

ACKNOWLEDGMENTS

Most of the MR studies in this volume were performed at Abbott Northwestern Hospital by an outstanding group of skilled technologists. Several scans from Centennial Lakes MRI Center and the Minnesota Diagnostic Center in Minneapolis have also been included. Additional cases were generously contributed by Drs. William Ford, Lanning Houston, Brian Larkin, Richard Latchaw, Daniel Loes, Mary Jo Nelson, and Saul Taylor of Minneapolis, David Kispert of St. Paul, Robert McGeachie of Duluth, Mel Aguilar of Bismarck, N.D., and W. Michael Hensley of Parkersburg, W. Va.

Drs. Anthony Cook, Stephen Fry, David Larson, Mark Myers, John Steely and David Tubman shared in the daily supervision of MR procedures and in the selection of teaching material. Drs. McGeachie and Myers reviewed the manuscript; their careful attention to this time-consuming task is sincerely appreciated.

John Messerschmidt worked long hours to optimally re-photograph images from magnetic tape and optical discs. Gisela Sime processed the entire manuscript, managing as usual to maintain excellence and cheerfulness despite the heavy load and constant time pressure.

Gordon Sprenger, Robert Spinner, and Donald Brunn of Abbott Northwestern Hospital have encouraged this specific project and supported the development of a strong neuroscience program, from which the following cases have been drawn. The neurologists and neurosurgeons at Abbott Northwestern have contributed directly and indirectly to this book through active practices and collegial exchange.

Anne Patterson, Susan Gay, Maura Leib, Sandy Clark Brown, Carol Sullivan Weis, and their associates at Mosby provided expert guidance throughout the many stages of production. Gene Melander, Tim Preston, Elise Noetzel, and Brent McEwen of Clarinda Color skillfully managed the digital processing of the illustrations.

I remain grateful to the outstanding neuroradiologists who introduced me to their field: William Marshall, William Scott, and Barton Lane at Stanford University, and T. Hans Newton and David Norman at the University of California in San Francisco.

My family deserves recognition for exceptional patience and understanding during this project.

Finally, I thank the readers of the previous teaching file books who have offered encouragement.

D.H.Y.

CONTENTS

TABLE OF ILLUSTRATED
DIFFERENTIAL DIAGNOSES

SUPRATENTORIAL COMPARTMENT

MASSES AND NODULES

WHITE MATTER

TEMPORAL LOBES

BASAL GANGLIA AND PINEAL REGION

SELLA, PARASELLAR AND SUPRASELLAR REGIONS

VENTRICLES

POSTERIOR FOSSA

CEREBELLOPONTINE ANGLE AND EXTRAAXIAL LESIONS

ORBITS

SPINAL CANAL

VERTEBRAL BODIES

MASSES

OTHER EXTRADURAL LESIONS

SPINAL CORD AND INTRADURAL PATHOLOGY

1. Unless otherwise specified, axial and coronal scans are displayed with the patient's right on the reader's left.

2. All scans were performed at 1.0T or 1.5T.

3. Abbreviations used for scan techniques are:

   SE = spin echo (conventional spin echo)
   RSE = rapid spin echo (fast spin echo, turbo spin echo)
   GRE = gradient echo (gradient recalled echo, gradient refocused echo)

4. Scan parameters are given as TR/TE (repetition time/ echo time).

MAGNETIC

RESONANCE

IMAGING OF

CNS DISEASE

• A Teaching File •

CHAPTER 1

Metastases

Case 1

39-year-old man complaining of headaches.
(sagittal, noncontrast scan; SE 600/20)

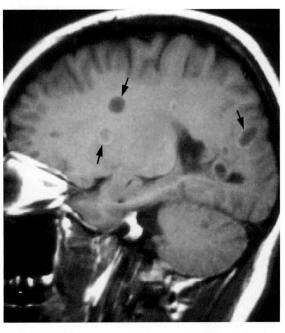

Metastatic Adenocarcinoma of Unknown Origin

Case 2

56-year-old man presenting with confusion
and seizures.
(sagittal, noncontrast scan; SE 600/17)

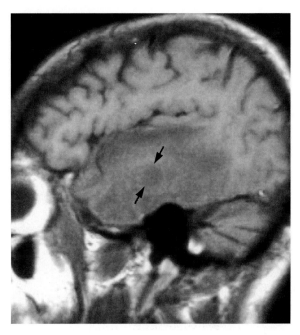

Metastatic Carcinoma of the Lung

Metastases are the most common adult intracranial neoplasms. Carcinomas of the breast and lung cause the greatest number of these lesions, although melanoma and hypernephroma metastasize to the brain with higher frequency. An intracranial mass accounts for the initial presentation of carcinoma in up to 10% of cases.

Nonhemorrhagic cerebral metastases are usually seen on T1-weighted MR scans as lesions of low signal intensity. The metastases themselves are typically well defined, as in Case 1 *(arrows)*. There is often surprisingly little reactive edema to obscure the interface between metastatic tissue and adjacent cerebral parenchyma. The appearance of multiple, sharply demarcated or "punched out" metastases may mimic multifocal inflammatory lesions.

Alternatively, extensive cerebral edema may surround and obscure an inciting metastatic nodule. In Case 2, the central metastasis is only faintly visible *(arrows)* within a large zone of T1 prolongation due to edema. As a result, the overall appearance in this case mimics that of a larger temporal lobe neoplasm, such as a primary glioma (compare to Cases 81 and 84). Contrast enhancement is useful in this situation to (1) clearly define the enhancing metastasis within the larger area of abnormal signal and (2) disclose additional lesions to confirm multiplicity and favor a metastatic process.

Case 3

58-year-old man with no cerebral symptoms.
(axial, noncontrast scan; SE 2800/90)

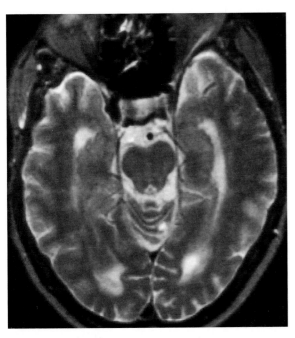

Metastatic Carcinoma of the Lung

Case 4

77-year-old man presenting with seizures.
(axial, noncontrast scan; SE 2800/90)

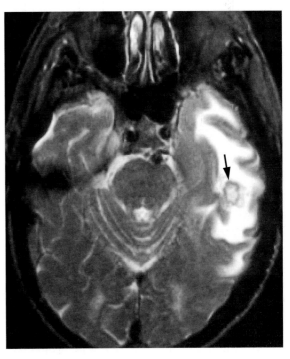

Metastatic Carcinoma of the Lung

The detection of nonhemorrhagic cerebral metastases on T2-weighted images depends on the presence of abnormal signal intensity within the lesion and/or the occurrence of surrounding edema. A small metastatic nodule with little edema may be inconspicuous and unimpressive, as in Case 3 *(arrow)*. Multiple small metastases should be included in the differential diagnosis of focal lesions of high signal intensity on T2-weighted scans (see Cases 433-436). The tiny vermian lesion in Case 3 enhanced intensely after contrast was administered and subsequently grew rapidly.

Case 4 represents the T2-weighted equivalent of Case 2. A central metastasis is largely isointense but is clearly outlined by a surrounding sea of edema. In other cases, a metastasis with long T2 values may be completely obscured by the increase in water content within adjacent white matter.

The edema provoked by some cerebral metastases is often more responsible for symptoms than the tumor itself.

Case 5

41-year-old man presenting with ataxia.
(axial, noncontrast scan; SE 2800/90)

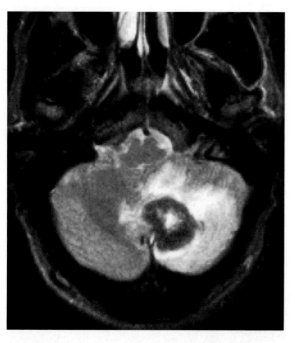

Metastatic Adenocarcinoma of the Colon

Case 6

58-year-old woman presenting with a seizure.
(axial, noncontrast scan; SE 2500/90)

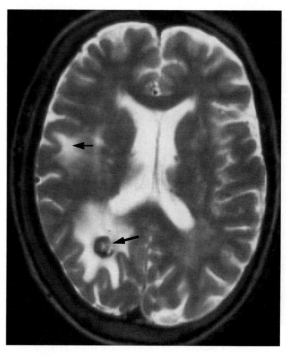

Metastatic Adenocarcinoma of the Colon

Most cerebral metastases demonstrate high signal intensity or isointensity on T2-weighted scans, as seen in Cases 3 and 4. The minority of metastatic lesions are associated with T2-shortening, causing low signal intensity on long TR, long TE spin echo images.

Such T2-shortening may be due to hemorrhage within the metastasis (see Cases 10 and 11) or to the presence of paramagnetic material (e.g., melanin; see Case 7). Other metastases demonstrate low signal intensity on T2-weighted scans in the absence of blood products or paramagnetic molecules.

Metastases from adenocarcinoma of the colon are particularly likely to present this appearance. Short T2 values in such cases reflect some intrinsic property of the tumor tissue, possibly the presence of thickly proteinaceous material within the cells. This characteristic MR finding often correlates with increased attenuation values of the lesions on precontrast CT scans.

The cerebellum is a favorite site for intracranial metastasis, as in Case 5. In fact, metastatic disease is the most common cause of a cerebellar mass in an adult (see Cases 9, 20, 22, 410, and 414 for other examples).

Some small metastases are themselves invisible on noncontrast scans but are localized by the focal edema that they incite. The small patch of subcortical edema in the right posterior frontal lobe of Case 6 *(short arrow)* is an example. By itself, this area of signal abnormality is nonspecific (compare to the appearance of progressive multifocal leukoencephalopathy in Cases 369-371). However, metastasis should be included in the differential diagnosis when this appearance is encountered.

Cerebral metastases are often found near the junction of gray and white matter. The superficial location reflects the high perfusion of cerebral cortex and is comparable to the distribution of hematogeneous cerebral infection.

Case 7A

46-year-old man presenting with headaches
and seizures.
(axial, noncontrast scan; SE 600/15)

Case 7B

Same patient.
(axial, noncontrast scan; SE 2800/90)

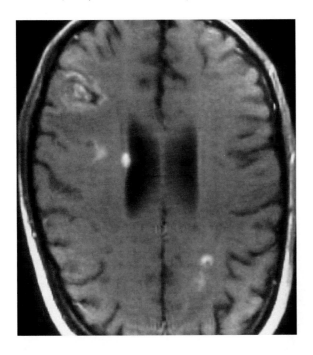

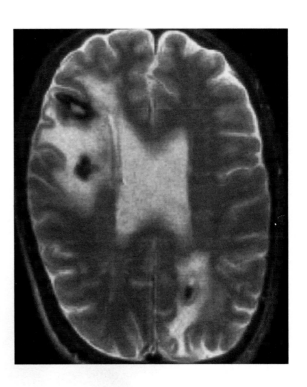

Melanoma is among the primary tumors associated with hemorrhagic cerebral metastases (see Cases 8-11). However, even in the absence of hemorrhage, cerebral metastases from melanoma often demonstrate T1-shortening and mild T2-shortening.

The presence of the melanin molecule with its unpaired electrons is believed to account for the observed paramagnetic effects on signal intensity. Amelanotic metastases from primary melanomas are not associated with shortening of T1 or T2 values in the absence of hemorrhage.

The above scans illustrate that T2-weighted images are much more sensitive to edema surrounding cerebral lesions than T1-weighted scans. The degree of hypointensity within the metastatic nodules in Case 7B would be unusual for nonhemorrhagic melanoma, which is often nearly isointense on T2-weighted images. Compare Case 7 to the small, hemorrhagic metastases in Cases 569 and 634.

Melanoma ranks as the third most common cause of cerebral metastases, after carcinomas of the breast and lung.

Case 8

63-year-old man presenting with right leg paresis.
(sagittal, noncontrast scan; SE 600/20)

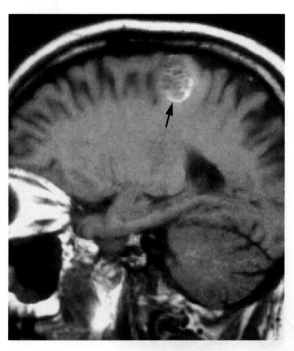

Metastatic Carcinoma of the Lung

Case 9

61-year-old woman presenting with ataxia that
became acutely worse ten days prior to admission.
(coronal, noncontrast scan; SE 600/20)

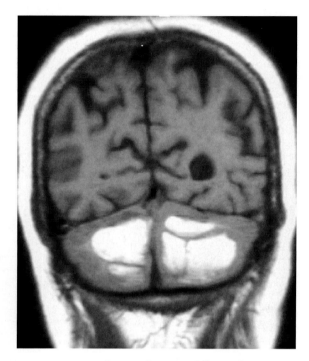

Metastatic Carcinoma of the Colon

The subcortical location and sharply defined margins of the lesion in Case 8 raise the possibility of metastatic disease. The high signal intensity on the T1-weighted image further suggests the presence of subacute or chronic hemorrhage within the lesion. (See Cases 555-558 for discussion of alterations in signal intensity caused by blood products of various ages.)

This feature narrows the likely diagnoses to those primary tumors that cause vascular metastases: melanoma, choriocarcinoma, hypernephroma, bronchogenic carcinoma, and occasionally breast carcinoma. Although hemorrhage into cerebral metastasis is often the presenting event in metastatic melanoma, a renal or pulmonary neoplasm would be more common in a 63-year-old man.

Hemorrhagic metastases such as the mass in Case 8 may simulate the appearance of cavernous angiomas or other "occult" vascular malformations (see Cases 627-630). Occasionally a hemorrhagic glioma presents in a similar manner.

In Case 9, large areas of T1-shortening suggesting subacute hemorrhage are present in both cerebellar hemispheres. Spontaneous cerebellar hemorrhage is rarely bilateral. The presence of hemorrhagic masses on both sides of midline should raise the possibility of underlying structural lesions. This case is another example of the spectrum of presentations of cerebellar metastases in adults.

Hemorrhage into a cerebral or cerebellar neoplasm is one mechanism by which such subacute or chronic lesions may cause acute symptoms. Other mechanisms include the sudden triggering of reactive cerebral edema, ventricular obstruction causing acute hydrocephalus, and critical vascular compression by an enlarging mass. Between 1% and 5% of "strokes" are found to be the result of an underlying neoplasm.

Case 10

66-year-old man presenting with personality
changes and right hemiparesis.
(axial, noncontrast scan; SE 2700/45)

Case 11

63-year-old man presenting with right leg paresis.
(axial, noncontrast scan; SE 2800/90)

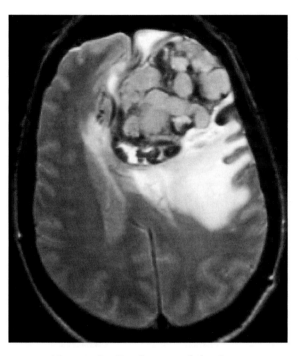

Metastatic Carcinoma of the Lung

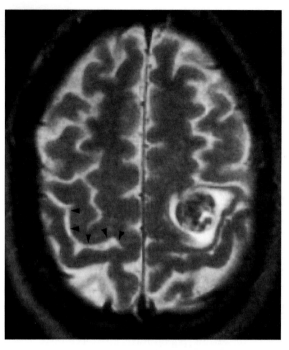

Metastatic Carcinoma of the Lung
(same patient as Case 8)

Case 10 is an example of the large size and complex architecture of some cerebral metastases. The combination of these features in a solitary lesion may mimic a primary glial neoplasm.

A multinodular or "botryoid" configuration is somewhat unusual for metastatic disease (but see Cases 22 and 23 for similar morphologies). Further complexity is caused by the areas of T2-shortening scattered throughout the tumor, which were pathologically proved to represent subacute hemorrhage. A giant cavernous angioma or thrombosed AVM is occasionally encountered with morphology resembling Case 10 (see Case 615).

Case 11 illustrates the same lesion as Case 8. The combination of T1-shortening and T2-shortening suggests a hemorrhagic mass, with the differential diagnosis including a nonhemorrhagic metastasis from melanoma. The lesion is located within the precentral gyrus, explaining the patient's lower extremity paresis. The central sulcus is compressed at the posterior margin of the mass. (Compare to the normal anatomy of the central sulcus marked by arrowheads on the opposite side.)

Cases 569 and 634 present examples of smaller hemorrhagic cerebral metastases on long TR spin echo scans. MR detection of such lesions can be enhanced by the use of gradient echo sequences that are sensitive to the local field inhomogeneities associated with blood products.

Case 10 illustrates subfalcial herniation. The combination of the metastasis and surrounding edema causes prominent frontal mass effect with a large midline shift.

Case 12

84-year-old man presenting with confusion and
mild hemiparesis.
(sagittal, noncontrast scan; SE 600/17)

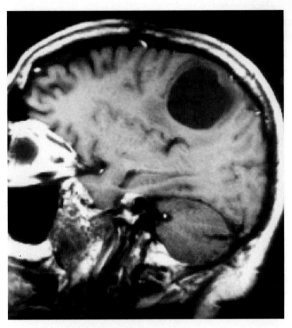

**Metastatic Squamous Cell Carcinoma
of the Lung**

Case 13

42-year-old woman presenting with headaches.
(axial, noncontrast scan; SE 2500/45)

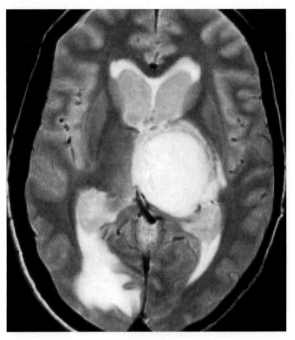

**Metastatic Squamous Cell Carcinoma
of the Lung**

Large metastases may contain cystic or necrotic areas that are apparent even on noncontrast scans. The rim of tumor tissue surrounding the cyst may be surprisingly thin and uniform, as in Cases 12 and 13 (see also Cases 410 and 414). In such instances, the alternative diagnoses of benign cyst or abscess may be considered. Solitary cystic metastases may also resemble malignant gliomas (see Cases 99 and 100), and the two tumors should be grouped together in the differential diagnosis.

A cystic appearance is often associated with metastatic squamous cell carcinomas but is also seen in metastatic adenocarcinomas. Up to 50% of cerebral metastases from pulmonary squamous cell tumors are solitary (compared with about 30% of all intracranial metastases).

The thalamic mass in Case 13 compresses the third ventricle, causing obstructive hydrocephalus with periventricular edema (see Cases 652 and 653).

Case 14

50-year-old woman presenting with seizures.
(axial, postcontrast scan; SE 600/15)

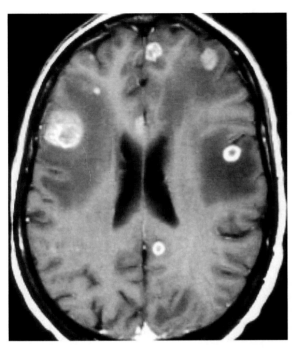

Metastatic Carcinoma of the Breast

Case 15

84-year-old man presenting with confusion.
(coronal, postcontrast scan; SE 600/15)

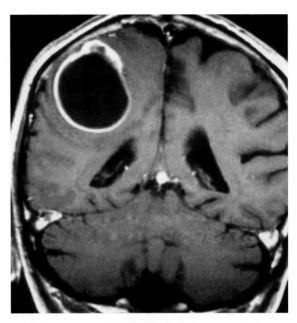

**Metastatic Squamous Cell Carcinoma
of the Lung**
(same patient as Case 12)

Multiplicity is a hallmark of metastatic disease. The size, shape, enhancement pattern, and edema of individual lesions may vary substantially, as demonstrated in Case 14.

Small cerebral metastases are often inapparent on noncontrast scans because they are nearly isointense and have not incited reactive edema. Contrast enhancement may be the only clue to the presence of such lesions. The detection of small metastases can be of clinical importance in determining the nature of an accompanying larger mass and/or judging the appropriateness of surgery for a "solitary" lesion. Postcontrast scans using magnetization transfer suppression techniques are currently the most sensitive method to demonstrate enhancing metastases.

Large cerebral metastases may retain the well-defined, homogeneously enhancing character of small lesions. When such masses are located near a dural surface, the appearance can mimic a meningioma (see Case 173).

Other metastases demonstrate peripheral enhancement surrounding a central, nonenhancing zone. The central area of little or no enhancement may represent a cyst, necrosis, or a slowly equilibrating compartment that accumulates contrast on later scans. Several lesions in Case 14 illustrate central areas of nonenhancement, while the mass in Case 15 appears to contain a large cyst. The enhancing margin of a metastatic lesion may be quite smooth and regular as in Case 15, but an irregular appearance of variable thickness is more characteristic (see Cases 21 and 99).

Occasionally, small cerebral metastases are remarkably numerous and uniform in size and morphology. Diffuse, tiny hematogeneous metastases may not enhance prominently and may be appreciated only as a finely granular texture of increased signal intensity within cortex and basal ganglia on T2-weighted scans. Alternatively, the "miliary" enhancement pattern of "carcinomatous encephalitis" (see Case 388-2) may resemble disseminated infection, noninfectious inflammatory processes, primary CNS lymphoma, subacute multifocal infarction, or vasculitis.

DIFFERENTIAL DIAGNOSIS:
SMALL PARENCHYMAL NODULE OF HIGH SIGNAL INTENSITY ON A POSTCONTRAST SCAN

Case 16

51-year-old man scanned as part of a metastatic
work-up.
(axial, postcontrast scan; SE 720/17)

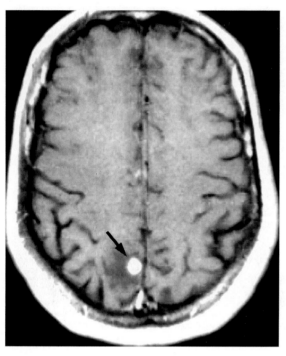

Metastatic Melanoma

Case 17

6-year-old girl presenting with headaches.
(axial, postcontrast scan; SE 600/15)

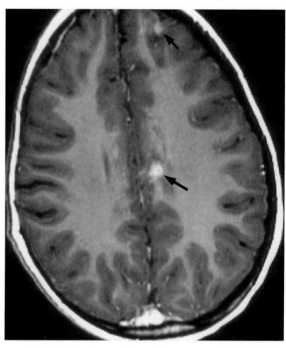

Artifact
(phase mismapping from the torcular herophili)

As discussed on the preceding page, focal, intense contrast enhancement is commonly seen in small metastatic nodules. Case 16 is a typical example, with superficial location and surrounding edema supporting the diagnosis of metastasis. A focal inflammatory lesion (of hematogeneous origin or secondary to CSF seeding) could have a similar appearance (see Cases 422-425).

Case 17 is an example of phase misregistration artifact that could be mistaken for focal pathology. Signal intensity that "belongs" within the torcular has been mismapped along the phase-encoding axis because of phase changes accumulated by protons in the blood as they flow across magnetic field gradients. This artifact is most prominent on postcontrast scans, since intravascular contrast material increases the signal intensity within venous structures.

A clue to proper interpretation of the finding in Case 17 is its location within a band or "zipper" of artifact leading back to the vascular source of the phase dispersion. Occasionally the background band of artifact is quite subtle, and the nature of the focal pseudolesion is suggested by (1) its colinear position along the phase axis with a potential source of vascular artifact and (2) the absence of confirmatory edema or direct visualization on noncontrast images.

Often other, less intense pseudolesions will occur along the same phase line as the most prominent artifact. A second pseudonodule is present anteriorly in Case 17 *(small arrow)*. Low window levels and/or wide window widths may demonstrate additional artifacts outside the head, establishing the nature of suspicious intracranial abnormalities.

Case 18

76-year-old man presenting with left hemiparesis.
(coronal, postcontrast scan; SE 600/15)

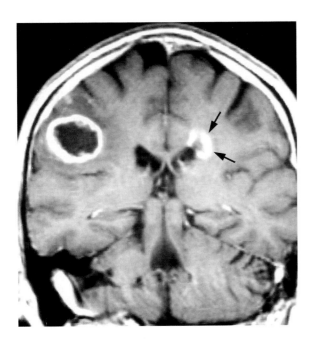

Metastatic Carcinoma of the Lung

Case 19

58-year-old man presenting with seizures.
(axial, postcontrast scan; SE 600/15)

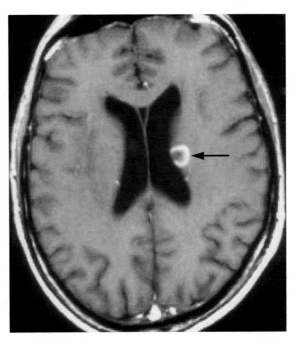

Metastatic Carcinoma of the Lung

Although superficial location is characteristic of hematogeneous metastases, deep hemisphere lesions are also encountered. The periventricular region is a common location for metastatic involvement by systemic lymphomas and carcinomas. Tumor cells can arrive at this site hematogeneously, through CSF seeding from a metastasis near the cerebral surface, or as a result of hematogeneous seeding of the highly vascular choroid plexus.

Metastases along the ventricular margin may be focal (as in these cases), multifocal, or diffuse. Small periventricular lesions as seen in Cases 18 and 19 may mimic the enhancement pattern of demyelinating plaques in multiple sclerosis (see Cases 349 and 351). The differential diagnosis of

larger subependymal masses includes primary CNS neoplasms such as glioma or ependymoma, lymphoma, and giant cell astrocytoma associated with tuberous sclerosis.

Uniform enhancement of metastatic disease lining ventricular margins may be seen with systemic lymphoma, metastatic melanoma, and metastatic carcinomas of the breast and lung (especially small cell). The differential diagnosis of enhancing ventricular margins also includes ependymal seeding or subependymal spread of gliomas and other primary CNS tumors (see Cases 104, 105, and 391), primary CNS lymphoma, and inflammatory ventriculitis (see Case 389).

Case 20

39-year-old man complaining of headaches.
(axial, noncontrast scan; SE 3000/90)

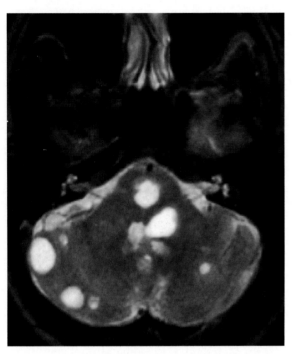

Metastatic Adenocarcinoma of Unknown Origin
(same patient as Case 1)

Case 21

54-year-old woman presenting with left facial pain.
(axial, postcontrast scan; SE 800/20)

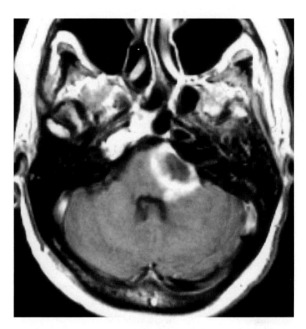

Metastatic Carcinoma of the Breast

The posterior fossa is a frequent site of intraaxial and extraaxial metastatic disease. Experience with CT scanning has previously established a high incidence of cerebellar metastases. More recently, MR has documented that intramedullary metastases involving the brainstem (and spinal cord) are also common.

Case 20 illustrates multiple "punched out" lesions within the pons and cerebellum. In a young adult, this appearance could be confused with inflammatory disease of parasitic or demyelinating origin. Metastatic disease should be considered in the differential diagnosis of unusual posterior fossa lesions, even in 30- or 40-year-old patients (see Case 173 for another example).

The region of the mid pons and brachium pontis is a common location for brain metastases, as illustrated in Case 21 (and in Case 638). A large intraaxial metastasis at this site can bulge exophytically into the cerebellopontine angle cistern, mimicking an extraaxial mass (see Cases 23 and 173).

Case 22

58-year-old woman presenting with abnormal gait.
(axial, postcontrast scan; SE 800/20)

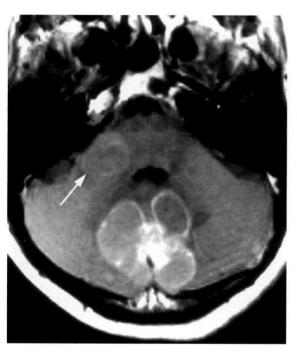

Metastatic Carcinoma of the Breast

Case 23

77-year-old man presenting with dizziness and right
facial numbness.
(coronal, postcontrast scan; SE 600/15)

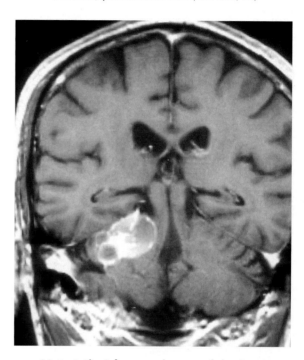

Metastatic Adenocarcinoma of the Lung

The strikingly lobulated morphology of the cerebellar mass in Case 22 is unusual but within the spectrum of metastatic disease (compare to Case 10). The correct diagnosis is supported by the presence of a second lesion in the right brachium pontis *(arrow)*.

The multinodular metastasis in Case 23 is superficial in location, abutting the tentorium. This lesion proved to be intraaxial in origin, with secondary invasion of the dura. Dural-based metastases with subsequent parenchymal invasion can produce a similar appearance.

As demonstrated in Cases 21 and 23, metastatic disease involving the lateral pons should be considered along with benign disorders in patients with facial pain or numbness indicating dysfunction of the trigeminal nerve.

Case 24

59-year-old woman scanned to exclude
cerebral metastases.
(sagittal, noncontrast scan; SE 600/15)

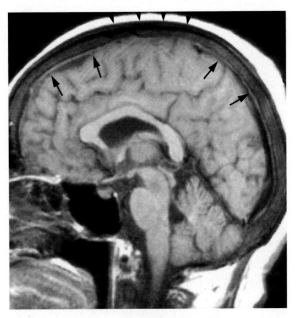

Metastatic Carcinoma of the Breast

Case 25

25-year-old man presenting with an enlarging
scalp mass.
(sagittal, noncontrast scan; SE 600/17)

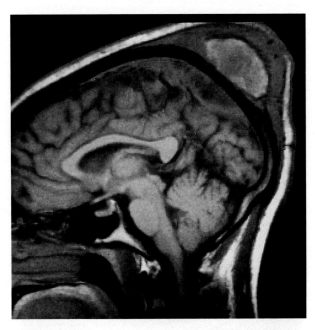

Systemic Lymphoma

Calvarial involvement by metastatic disease may be confined to bone or associated with adjacent soft tissue masses. In Case 24, the normal high signal intensity of fatty marrow in the diploic space of the skull on T1-weighted images has been uniformly replaced. This abnormally low signal intensity of the calvarium predominantly represents metastatic cellular infiltration, although reactive sclerosis may contribute in some cases (especially in metastatic carcinoma of the prostate). Only mild thickening of the underlying dura *(arrows)* and overlying scalp soft tissue *(arrowsheads)* is present.

By contrast, Case 25 demonstrates large intracranial and extracranial soft tissue masses accompanying calvarial involvement by lymphoma. Dural-based metastases may also occur without overlying calvarial lesions, as seen in Cases 26, 28, and 29.

Occasional meningiomas present as transcranial masses similar to Case 25. Such tumors may involve the skull base (e.g., with extension into the infratemporal fossa), as well as the convexity.

DIFFERENTIAL DIAGNOSIS:
DIFFUSE DURAL THICKENING AND ENHANCEMENT

Case 26

68-year-old man presenting with headaches.
(axial, postcontrast scan; SE 600/15)

Case 27

51-year-old man presenting with confusion.
(coronal, postcontrast scan; SE 600/15)

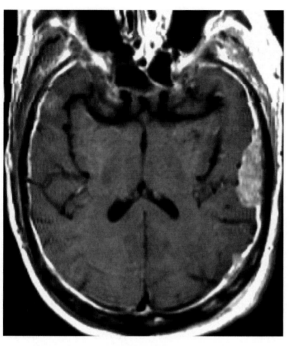

**Dural Metastases from Carcinoma
of the Prostate**

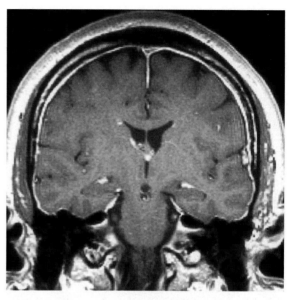

Intracranial Hypotension
(due to multiple lumbar punctures)

In Case 26, thickened rinds of enhancing dura surround both cerebral hemispheres. Superimposed mass-like nodularity is present on the left. Patchy sclerosis within the overlying calvarium helps to establish the correct diagnosis.

Dural metastatic disease is occasionally associated with subdural hemorrhage. This condition, termed "pachymeningitis interna hemorrhagica," is particularly frequent in patients with metastatic carcinoma of the breast.

Inflammatory disease can also result in meningeal thickening and enhancement. Granulomatous disorders such as tuberculosis, sarcoidosis, and meningovascular syphilis may present an appearance similar to Cases 26 and 27, with uniform and/or nodular dural thickening. Other rare causes of diffuse dural thickening include Wegener's granulomatosis, rheumatoid arthritis, granulomatous angiitis, Erdheim Chester disease (lipid granulomatosis), and idiopathic hypertrophic pachymeningitis.

Dural thickening and enhancement may also represent a benign, reactive phenomenon, unassociated with either neoplastic or inflammatory infiltration. Hyperemia of the dura (with increased blood volume) is a probable contribution to this phenomenon. Uniform dural thickening and enhancement is commonly observed as an incidental finding after craniotomy or burr holes. It is important to recognize that this finding does not necessarily imply meningeal recurrence of neoplasm in postoperative tumor cases.

Diffuse dural enhancement may also occur in cases of intracranial hypotension unassociated with calvarial surgery. An occasional clinical antecedent is lumbar puncture with removal and/or presumed leakage of CSF from the spinal dural sac. Associated reduction of intracranial pressure may allow or incite an increase in blood volume within the dura, which is manifested on MR scans as thickening and abnormally prominent enhancement. The sagittal scan in such cases usually demonstrates confirmatory inferior sagging of posterior fossa structures (see Case 463).

Case 28

53-year-old man presenting with headaches.
(axial, postcontrast scan; SE 600/16)

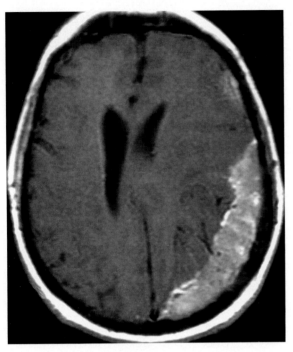

Metastatic Carcinoma of the Prostate

Case 29

57-year-old woman presenting with right
homonymous hemianopia.
(coronal, postcontrast scan; SE 600/15)

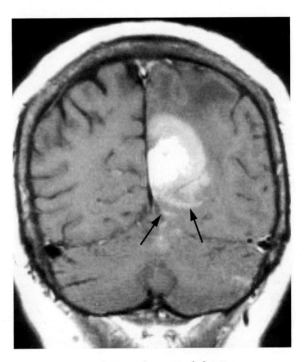

Metastatic Carcinoma of the Breast

Metastatic involvement of the dura may be an isolated primary process or may reflect extension from either calvarial or cerebral lesions.

The dural-based metastasis in Case 28 is sharply demarcated from underlying cerebral tissue. This feature, together with homogeneous contrast enhancement, resembles a meningioma. Like meningiomas, dural-based metastases may be associated with reactive changes in adjacent bone and vascular supply from dural arteries. The most common primary tumors to present in this manner are carcinomas of the prostate and breast.

The metastasis in Case 29 is based against the falx. Abnormal enhancement within the subarachnoid space at the inferior margin of the mass *(arrows)* and in vermian sulci is a clue to the presence of metastatic seeding of the leptomeninges (see Case 30). This finding usually implies intraaxial origin of a superficial metastasis (rather than leptomeningeal extension of a dural-based lesion).

Case 577 presents a noncontrast scan of the patient in Case 28.

Case 30

57-year-old woman presenting with right
homonymous hemianopia.
(sagittal, postcontrast scan; SE 600/15)

Case 31

35-year-old woman presenting with headaches.
(axial, postcontrast scan; SE 700/15).

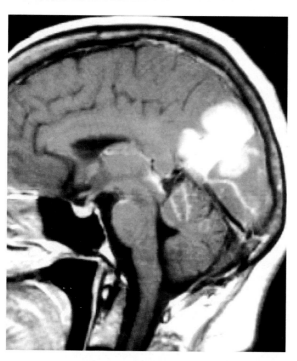

Metastatic Carcinoma of the Breast
(same patient as Case 29)

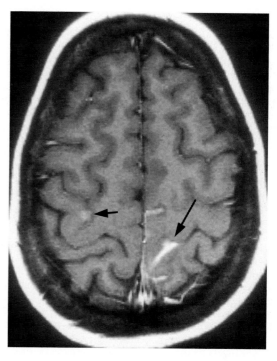

Metastatic Carcinoma of the Breast

Metastatic disease can involve the leptomeninges together with or separate from dural invasion. Enhancing meningeal tumor may occupy sulci focally or diffusely with nodular or linear patterns.

Case 31 illustrates nodular involvement limited to the depth of a sulcus in the posterior right frontal region *(short arrow)*. A linear pattern of enhancing tumor filling sulci is present at the medial left hemisphere vertex *(long arrow)*.

Case 30 demonstrates more extensive leptomeningeal carcinomatosis (or "carcinomatous meningitis") within the calcarine fissure and superior vermian sulci. The superior surface of the cerebellum is a particularly common location for meningeal seeding of a neoplasm, whether the source is a primary intracranial tumor or a systemic carcinoma (see Cases 160-162).

Leptomeningeal carcinomatosis may also present as a layer of abnormally enhancing tissue coating the surface of neural structures. In Case 30, this finding is noted in the interpeduncular and quadrigeminal regions. Cases 182 and 183 present examples of leptomeningeal neoplasm coating cranial nerves, and Cases 905 and 906 demonstrate similar findings in the spinal canal.

The differential diagnosis of sulcal enhancement includes meningeal tumor, meningitis (see Case 386), contrast enhancement occurring after subarachnoid hemorrhage, meningeal angioma (as in Sturge-Weber syndrome; see Case 770), superficial enhancement in acute/subacute infarction (see Cases 484 and 485), and congestion secondary to dural sinus thrombosis (see Case 386-2).

Communicating hydrocephalus may develop in association with meningeal carcinomatosis, as with other meningeal pathologies. Conversely, benign leptomeningeal enhancement has been reported in cases of chronic or severe obstructive hydrocephalus, possibly reflecting vascular stasis due to increased intracranial pressure.

REFERENCES

Ahmadi J, Hinton DR, Segall HD, et al: Dural invasion by craniofacial and calvarial neoplasms: MR imaging and histopathologic evaluation. *Radiology* 188:747-750, 1993.

Ahmadi J, Hinton DR, Segall HD, et al: Surgical implications of magnetic resonance-enhanced dura. *Neurosurgery* 35:370-377, 1994.

Atlas SW, Grossman RI, Gomori JM, et al: Hemorrhagic intracranial malignant neoplasms: spin echo MR imaging. *Radiology* 164:71-78, 1987.

Atlas SW, Grossman RI, Gomori JM, et al: MR imaging of intracranial metastatic melanoma. *J Comput Assist Tomogr* 11:577-582, 1987.

Bentson JR, Steckel RJ, Kagan AR: Diagnostic imaging in clinical cancer management: brain metastases. *Invest Radiol* 23:335-341, 1988.

Boorstein JM, Wong KT, Grossman RI, et al: Metastatic lesions of the brain: imaging with magnetization transfer. *Radiology* 191:799-803, 1994.

Carrier DA, Mawad ME, Kirkpatrick JB, Schmid MF: Metastatic adenocarcinoma to the brain: MR with pathologic correlation. *AJNR* 15:155-160, 1994.

Claussen C, Laniado M, Schorner W, et al: Gadolinium-DTPA in MR imaging of glioblastomas and intracranial metastases. *AJNR* 6:669-674, 1985.

Davis PC, Friedman NC, Fry SM, et al: Leptomeningeal metastasis: MR imaging. *Radiology* 163:449-454, 1987.

Davis PC, Hudgins PA, Peterman SB, Hoffman JC Jr: Diagnosis of cerebral metastases: double-dose delayed CT vs contrast-enhanced MR imaging. *AJNR* 12:293-300, 1991.

Destian S, Sze G, Krol G, et al: MR imaging of hemorrhagic intracranial neoplasms. *AJNR* 9:1115-1122, 1988.

Egelhoff JC, Ross JS, Modic MT, et al: MR imaging of metastatic GI adenocarcinoma in brain. *AJNR* 13:1221-1224, 1992.

Elster AD, MYM Chen: Can nonenhancing white matter lesions in cancer patients be disregarded? *AJNR* 13:1309-1315, 1992.

Healy ME, Hesselink JR, Press GA, Middleton MS: Increased detection of intracranial metastases with intravenous Gd-DTPA. *Radiology* 165:619-624, 1987.

Krol G, Sze G, Malkin M, Walker R: MR of cranial and spinal meningeal carcinomatosis: comparison with CT and myelography. *AJNR* 9:709-714, 1988.

Laine FJ, Braun IF, Jensen ME, et al: Perineural tumor extension through the foramen ovale: evaluation with MR imaging. *Radiology* 174:65-72, 1990.

Lee Y-Y, Tien RD, Bruner JM, et al: Loculated intracranial leptomeningeal metastases: CT and MR characteristics. *AJNR* 10:1171-1180, 1989.

Nemzek W, Poirier V, Salamat MS, Yu T: Carcinomatous encephalitis (miliary metastases): lack of contrast enhancement. *AJNR* 14:540-542, 1993.

Olsen WL, Winkler ML, Ross DA: Carcinomatous encephalitis: CT and MR findings. *AJNR* 8:553-554, 1987.

Paako E, Patronas NJ, Schellinger D: Meningeal Gd-DTPA enhancement in patients with malignancies. *J Comput Assist Tomogr* 14:542-546, 1990.

Phillips ME, Ryals TJ, Kambhu SA, et al: Neoplastic vs. inflammatory meningeal enhancement with Gd-DTPA. *J Comput Assist Tomogr* 14:536-541, 1990.

Rippe DJ, Boyko OB, Friedman HS, et al: Gd-DTPA enhanced MR imaging of leptomeningeal spread of intracranial CNS tumor in children. *AJNR* 11:329, 1990.

Rodesch G, Van Bogaert P, Mavroudakis N, et al: Neuroradiologic findings in leptomeningeal carcinomatosis: the value interest of gadolinium-enhanced MRI. *Neuroradiol* 32:26-32, 1990.

Russell EJ, Geremia GK, Johnson CE, et al: Multiple cerebral metastases: detectability with Gd-DTPA-enhanced Mr imaging. *Radiology* 165:609-618, 1987.

Schubiger O, Haller D: Metastases to the pituitary-hypothalamic axis. *Neuroradiol* 34:131-134, 1992.

Smalley SR, Laws ER Jr, O'Fallon JR, et al: Resection for solitary brain metastasis. Role of adjuvant radiation and prognostic variables in 229 patients. *J Neurosurg* 77:531-540, 1992.

Sze G, Milano E, Johnson C, et al: Detection of brain metastases: comparison of contrast-enhanced MR with unenhanced MR and enhanced CT. *AJNR* 11:785-792, 1990.

Sze G, Shin J, Krol G, et al: Intraparenchymal brain metastases: MR imaging versus contrast-enhanced CT. *Radiology* 168:187-194, 1988.

Sze G, Soletsky S, Bronen R, Krol G: MR imaging of the cranial meninges with emphasis on contrast enhancement and meningeal carcinomatosis. *AJNR* 10:965-975, 1989.

Tyrrell RL, Bundschuh CV, Modic MT: Dural carcinomatosis: MR demonstration. *J Comput Assist Tomogr* 11:329-332, 1987.

Watanabe M, Tanaka R, Takeda N: Correlation of MRI and clinical features in meningeal carcinomatosis. *Neuroradiol* 35:512-515, 1993.

West MS, Russell EJ, Breit R, et al: Calvarial and skull based metastases: comparison of nonenhanced and Gd-DTPA-enhanced MR images. *Radiology* 174:85-92, 1990.

Woodruff WW Jr, Djang WT, Mc Lendon RE, et al: Intracerebral malignant melanoma: high-field-strength MR imaging. *Radiology* 165:209-213, 1987.

Yousem DM, Patrone PM, Grossman RI: Leptomeningeal metastasis: MR evaluation. *J Comput Assist Tomogr* 14:255-261, 1990.

Yuh WTC, Engelken JD, Muhonen MG, et al: Experience with high-dose gadolinium MR imaging in the evaluation of brain metastases. *AJNR* 13:335-345, 1992.

Yuh WTC, Mayr-Yuh NA, Koci TM, et al: Metastatic lesions involving the cerebellopontine angle. *AJNR* 14:99-106, 1993.

CHAPTER 2

Meningiomas

Case 32

55-year-old man presenting with headaches.
(sagittal, noncontrast scan; SE 600/20)

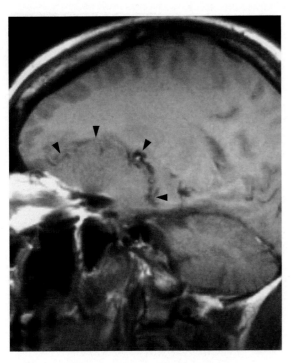

Sphenoid Wing Meningioma

Case 33

80-year-old man presenting with hemiparesis.
(sagittal, noncontrast scan; SE 600/17)

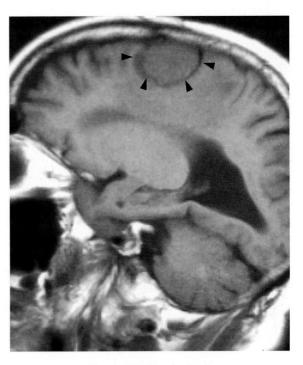

Convexity Meningioma

Meningiomas are typically homogeneous lesions with well-defined margins. Even large tumors may cause relatively little edema and mass effect. This quiescent appearance implies slow growth, with gradual invagination into adjacent parenchyma.

The signal intensity of meningiomas is usually homogeneous on all pulse sequences, analogous to their characteristically uniform CT attenuation. Margins of the tumor may be very smooth (as in Case 33) or distinctly lobulated (as in Case 32).

Many meningiomas are nearly isointense with adjacent cerebral cortex on T1-weighted images. Small, isointense tumors may be inapparent on scans performed without contrast material. Larger isointense meningiomas are de-

fined by distortions of anatomy. In Cases 32 and 33, the tumor disrupts the normal pattern of cortical convolutions in the affected area.

The margin of a meningioma on T1-weighted images is often highlighted by a zone of low signal intensity. Flow-voids within vessels (usually veins) at the perimeter of the tumor may contribute to this definition, as in Case 32 (*arrowheads*). More commonly, a "pseudocapsule" or rim of low signal intensity demarcating an otherwise isointense meningioma is due to a collar of displaced subarachnoid space. Case 33 is an example of such a "CSF cleft" (*arrowheads*; see also Case 52).

Less than 10% of intracranial meningiomas cause specific symptoms.

Case 34

51-year-old woman presenting with homonymous hemianopsia.
(sagittal, noncontrast scan; SE 600/15)

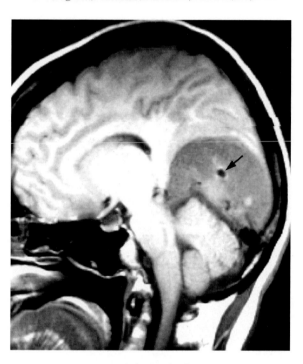

Tentorial Meningioma

Case 35

69-year-old woman presenting with a seizure.
(sagittal, noncontrast scan; SE 600/20)

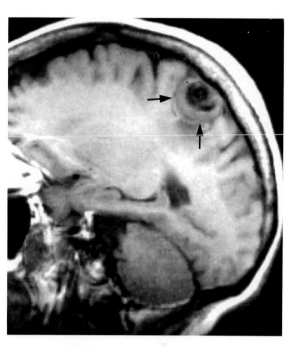

Calcified Convexity Meningioma

Some meningiomas are clearly defined on T1-weighted images by low signal intensity. The low intensity is often uniform throughout the mass, reflecting homogeneous tissue. Other meningiomas demonstrate a mixture of isointense and low intensity regions, as in Case 34.

Small foci of very low signal intensity within meningiomas (*arrow*, Case 34) may represent dense calcifications and/or "flow voids" in large vascular channels. Occasional meningiomas demonstrate calcification that is sufficiently dense and extensive to cause large areas of low signal intensity, as in Case 35. The fine, psammomatous calcification characteristic of meningimas on CT scans is rarely detected on MR studies.

Meningiomas may exhibit a faint fan-like pattern of linear striation radiating through the tissue from a central point at its base. This characteristic feature, which may be related to the pattern of dural vascular supply, is subtly suggested as a background texture in Case 34. (See Case 57 for another example.)

Meningiomas account for 15% to 20% of intracranial tumors, with a peak age incidence at 45 years and a moderate predominance in women.

Case 36

70-year-old woman presenting with dementia.
(axial, noncontrast scan; SE 2500/90)

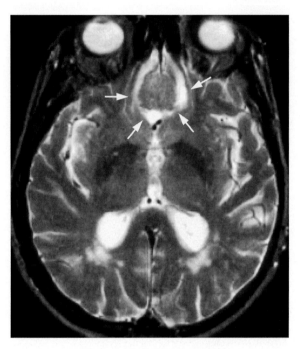

Subfrontal Meningioma

Case 37

55-year-old man presenting with worsening
aphasia.
(axial, noncontrast scan; SE 2500/90)

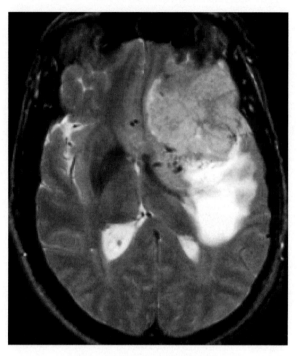

Sphenoid Wing Meningioma

Many meningiomas are nearly isointense with cerebral cortex on T2-weighted images. This isointensity may obscure small lesions on noncontrast scans. A collar of edema and/or a ring of prominent CSF surrounding the tumor may help to define it, as in Case 36 *(arrows)*.

Large, nearly isointense meningiomas are usually apparent due to distortions of anatomy and associated edema, as in Case 37. The tumor is typically homogeneous, with smooth or mildly lobulated margins.

Case 37 is an example of the extensive edema often found posterior to a sphenoid wing meningioma. If the meningioma itself is small and isointense, the adjacent edema may be misinterpreted as a primary intraaxial lesion (see Cases 83 and 84). A contrast-enhanced study clarifies the pathology in such instances.

Occasional meningiomas demonstrate lower signal intensity than gray matter on T2-weighted images (see Case 62 for an example). This appearance may reflect calcification and/or a dense, fibrous stroma with little water content.

Case 38

42-year-old woman presenting with decreased hearing.
(axial, noncontrast scan; SE 2500/90)

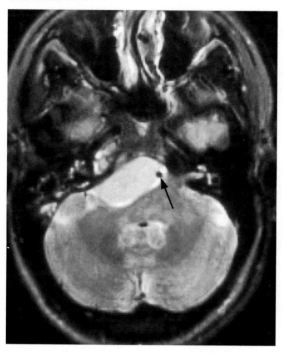

Cerebellopontine Angle Meningioma

Case 39

71-year-old man presenting with headaches.
(axial, noncontrast scan; SE 3000/80)

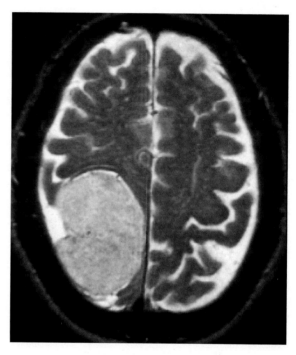

Convexity Meningioma

The spectrum of meningiomas on T2-weighted scans includes tumors with high signal intensity. Such masses are usually homogeneous and well defined, as seen in these cases.

Meningiomas demonstrating high signal intensity on T2-weighted scans are often syncytial or angioblastic in histology. Tumors that are more nearly isointense on T2-weighted images tend to represent fibroblastic or transitional varieties.

The mass in Case 38 has displaced the basilar artery *(arrow)* and has grown posteriorly to reach the region of the internal auditory meatus, correlating with the patient's hearing loss.

The very large tumor in Case 39 illustrates the size that can be attained by a slowly growing mass. The surrounding brain gradually accomodates the expanding tumor, with symptoms remaining mild and nonspecific until the lesion is very large. The absence of reactive edema also attests to slow growth.

In both of the above cases, a thin collar of displaced subarachnoid space helps to define the margin of the tumor.

Case 40

20-year-old man presenting with blurred vision.
(coronal, noncontrast scan; SE 3000/28)

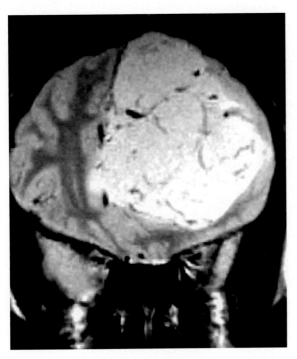

Falx Meningioma

Case 41

24-year-old man presenting with lightheadedness
and slurred speech.
(coronal, noncontrast scan; SE 600/17)

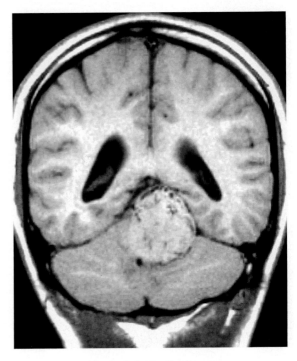

Tentorial Meningioma

Large vessels surrounding or within a meningioma may be a prominent feature of the CT or MR presentation. In Case 40, tubular channels of low signal intensity representing "flow void" are seen throughout the mass. (Contrast this appearance with Case 39.)

The impressive vascularity of some meningiomas may cause diagnostic confusion. In Case 41, the posterior fossa mass containing multiple vascular channels in a young adult could be assumed to represent a hemangioblastoma (see Cases 136-140). The tumor proved to be a meningioma arising from the tentorium.

Case 88 presents an additional example of large vessels within a meningioma.

Case 42

70-year-old woman presenting with diplopia.
(axial, noncontrast scan; SE 2500/28)

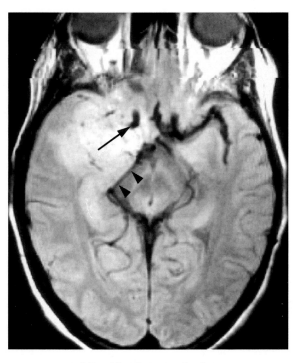

Sphenoid Wing Meningioma

Case 43

57-year-old woman presenting with bilateral
leg weakness.
(coronal, noncontrast scan; SE 2500/30)

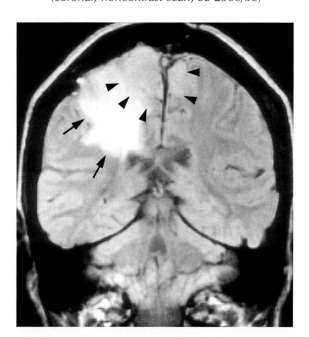

Falx Meningioma
(recurrent)

The absence of signal or "flow void" within cerebral arteries on routine spin echo MR sequences helps to define the status of vessels adjacent to tumors. In Case 42 a parasellar meningioma surrounds the supraclinoid internal carotid artery *(arrow)*. The mass crosses the tentorial margin to flatten the right side of the midbrain *(arrowheads)*.

Encasement of adjacent arteries is a characteristic feature of meningiomas in the sphenoid region. However, this finding is not histologically specific; pituitary adenomas may present a similar appearance (see Cases 215 and 216).

Case 43 demonstrates that the coronal plane is useful for evaluating lesions involving the falx or tentorium. In this instance, the relatively isointense signal of meningioma tissue is seen on both sides of the falx *(arrowheads)*. In addition, the expected "flow void" within the lumen of the superior sagittal sinus has been replaced by tissue with signal intensity matching the adjacent meningioma (compare

to Case 55). Tumor invasion and/or occlusion of a dural sinus can be confirmed by venographic MR techniques (see Cases 188C and 188D).

The meningioma in Case 43 has triggered marked edema on one side of the falx *(arrows)*, with no edema contralaterally. The mechanisms by which meningiomas incite reactive edema are unclear. Relevant factors probably include the thickness of cortex separating a tumor from underlying white matter and the presence or absence of venous compression. Edema is often a major cause of mass effect and symptomatology.

Paresis of the lower extremities may lead to initial clinical suspicion of spinal cord dysfunction in patients like Case 43. It is important to remember that parasagittal lesions near the cerebral vertex can also produce bilateral leg symptoms (through compression or invasion of the motor and sensory tracts from the medial portion of the precentral and postcentral gyri).

Case 44

43-year-old woman presenting with impaired vision.
(sagittal, noncontrast scan; SE 600/15)

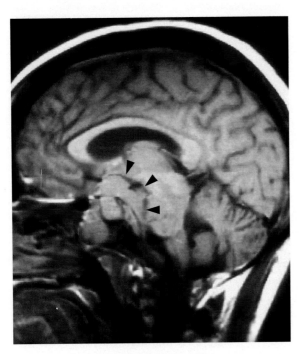

Parasellar Meningioma

Case 45

72-year-old woman presenting with right-sided proptosis.
(axial, noncontrast scan; SE 2700/45)

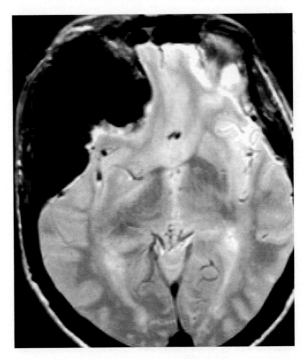

Sphenoid Wing Meningioma

Hyperostosis frequently develops at the base of intracranial meningiomas. The sclerosis may accompany calvarial invasion or be an independent reaction to adjacent tumor.

In Case 44, isointense meningioma tissue fills the sella turcica. Tumor components occupy the suprasellar cistern and sphenoid sinus. The basisphenoid bone and clivus demonstrate very low signal intensity, reflecting dense reactive hyperostosis.

A similar appearance is occasionally caused by an inflammatory lesion at the skull base. For example, aspergillosis originating in the sphenoid sinus (typically in a diabetic patient) may provoke a sclerotic bone reaction (and encase parasellar vessels) to closely resemble a basal meningioma.

Case 45 illustrates marked thickening of bone due to a meningioma permeating the sphenoid wing ("intraosseous

meningioma"). Sphenoid involvement by sclerosing meningiomas may have both cerebral and orbital consequences, with proptosis resulting from bone deformity. Associated soft tissue components of tumor may be found in the middle cranial fossa, the orbit, and extracranially in the infratemporal fossa.

Fibrous dysplasia may also cause prominent thickening of bone of the skull base or face. However, fibrous dysplasia usually demonstrates a homogeneous, intermediate signal intensity on MR scans (correlating with the characteristic "ground-glass" texture on x-rays and CT scans), rather than the markedly low signal of hyperostotic meningioma bone. Furthermore, fibrous dysplasia usually presents in the first decade of life, although the disorder is occasionally discovered in older adults (see Case 193).

Case 46

48-year-old man presenting with anosmia.
(sagittal, noncontrast scan; SE 1000/16)

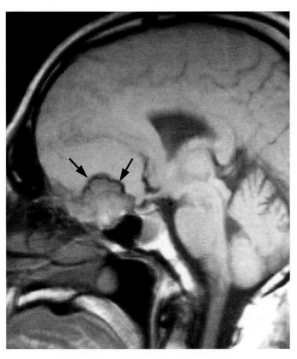

Planum Sphenoidale Meningioma

Case 47

49-year-old woman presenting with decreased vision.
(sagittal, noncontrast scan; SE 700/17)

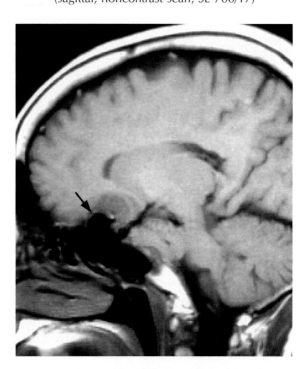

Planum Sphenoidale and Parasellar Meningioma

Meningiomas arising from the anterior skull base are often associated with characteristic bone changes. The planum sphenoidale may become markedly thickened, as in Case 46 *(arrows)*. Dense hyperostosis often produces lower signal intensity in the thickened bone than is seen here (compare to Cases 44 and 45).

A more unique and highly typical change is tumor-induced remodelling of the planum sphenoidale, so that the sphenoid sinus is expanded along the base of an overlying meningioma. Case 47 demonstrates this "blistering" or elevation of the roof of the sinus toward the meningioma *(arrow)*. The seemingly paradoxical expansion of a sinus in the direction of an overlying mass is analogous to excessive pneumatization of the sphenoid wing adjacent to an arachnoid cyst (see Case 681).

Case 48

26-year-old woman complaining of dizziness.
(coronal, postcontrast scan; SE 900/15)

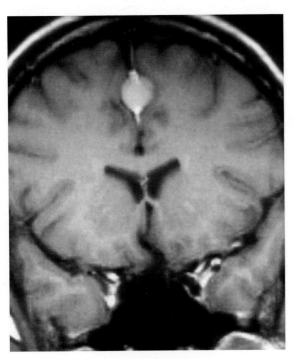

Falx Meningioma

Case 49

31-year-old woman presenting with headaches.
(sagittal, postcontrast scan; SE 600/20)

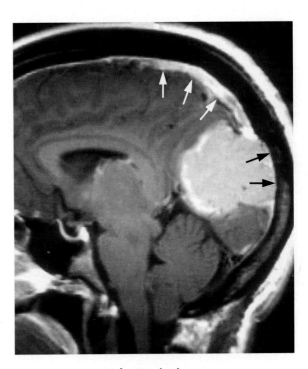

Falx Meningioma

Contrast enhancement within meningiomas is usually intense and uniform, regardless of tumor size. Case 48 illustrates a small tumor that was inconspicuous on noncontrast scans but is sharply defined by contrast enhancement.

The meningioma in Case 49 is much larger but still demonstrates typically homogeneous enhancement. In this case, axial CT scans had suggested a tentorial origin for the tumor. Coronal and sagittal MR scans corrected this impression by demonstrating a broad tumor base along the occipital inner table *(black arrows)*.

Contrast enhancement extending superiorly from the mass in Case 49 *(white arrows)* represents stasis in the superior sagittal sinus, which is compressed and/or invaded by the meningioma (see Case 43). Waves or ripples of compressed gray and white matter are seen in the cerebral hemisphere anterior to the tumor. This accordion-like morphology (including a band of displaced cortex between the superficial mass and underlying white matter) helps to establish the lesion as extraaxial.

Pediatric meningiomas may present unusual appearances and be more aggressive than adult tumors. Occasional meningiomas in children are not attached to a dural surface. Such parenchymal lesions presumably arise from rests of meningeal cells. (Rare intracerebral fibromas and schwannomas can also present as round, uniformly enhancing intracerebral masses in children.)

DIFFERENTIAL DIAGNOSIS:
INTENSELY ENHANCING EXTRAAXIAL CONVEXITY MASS

Case 50

71-year-old woman presenting with dementia.
(coronal, postcontrast scan; SE 600/15)

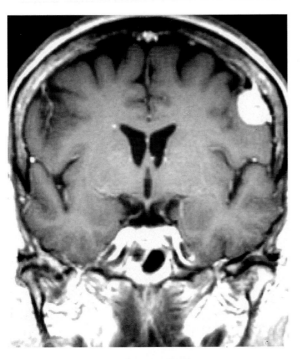

Convexity Meningioma

Case 51

50-year-old woman complaining of headaches.
(coronal, postcontrast scan; SE 600/15)

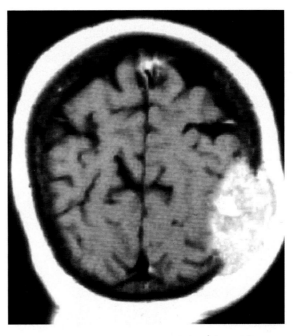

Metastatic Carcinoma of the Thyroid

As discussed in Chapter 1, metastases should be considered along with meningiomas in the differential diagnosis of dural-based tumors. Both pathologies are characteristically well defined with uniform contrast enhancement. Both may be associated with adjacent dural thickening, reactive bone changes, and angiographic supply by dural arteries.

The meningioma in Case 50 is typical in morphology. The tumor is not associated with underlying edema or significant mass effect and is probably unrelated to the patient's symptoms.

The epidural metastasis in Case 51 is accompanied by calvarial destruction and an extracranial component, strongly suggesting expansion of a skull lesion. Myeloma or solitary plasmacytoma could present an identical appearance. Other homogeneous, well-defined extraaxial malignancies may arise solely from the dura (see Cases 26 and 28) or represent invasion of neoplasm through the skull base (see Cases 197 and 199).

Case 52

44-year-old woman presenting with signs of increased intracranial pressure.
(sagittal, postcontrast scan; SE 700/15)

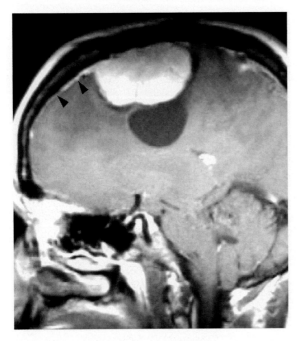

Convexity Meningioma

Case 53

51-year-old woman presenting with right homonymous hemianopsia.
(coronal, postcontrast scan; GRE sequence)

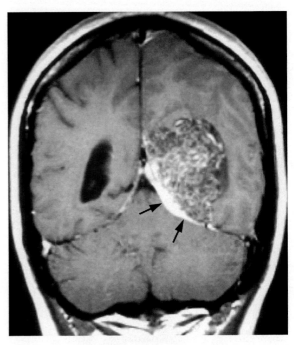

Tentorial Meningioma
(same patient as Case 34)

Because the typical appearance of meningiomas is one of the most reliable stereotypes on CT and MR scans, atypical appearances can be confusing. A small number of meningiomas contain or are associated with nonenhancing areas. These may be due to necrosis, old hemorrhage, cyst formation, or fat within the meningioma tissue or reflect loculation of adjacent CSF.

In Case 52, a large cyst is present deep to the enhancing tumor. A more laminar "halo" of CSF-like intensity values is seen along the remainder of the tissue margin, comparable to Case 33. This finding and the eccentric morphology of the cyst suggest that it represents a loculation of fluid adjacent to the meningioma, rather than an intratumoral cavity. A small, enhancing dural "tail" extends anteriorly from the main mass *(arrowheads; see Cases 54 and 55)*.

Case 53 demonstrates heterogeneous, nonenhancing areas that are clearly within the substance of the tumor. The correct diagnosis depends on the typical dural-based morphology, including localized thickening of the tentorium

(arrows). Compare Case 53 to the homogeneously enhancing tentorial meningioma in Case 143. Other tentorial meningiomas demonstrate plaque-like morphology, resembling the dural thickening seen in meningial carcinomatosis, chronic meningitis, or vascular engorgement.

In some cases, inhomogeneous enhancement of a meningioma may combine with irregular margins and prominent edema to mimic a malignant glioma or metastasis. Coronal scans can help to correctly identify such tumors by demonstrating that the mass arises from a dural base. However, superficial gliomas may invade the dura, and dural-based metastases must also be considered.

There is little correlation between atypical MR features and aggressive growth or recurrence of meningiomas (discussed in Cases 66 and 67). Most inhomogeneous tumors have expectedly benign courses, and most "malignant" meningiomas originally demonstrate conventional homogeneity.

Case 54

72-year-old woman presenting with
right-sided proptosis.
(axial, postcontrast scan; SE 600/15)

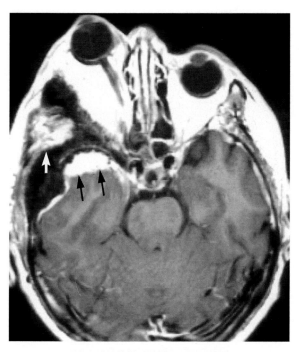

Sphenoid Wing Meningioma
(same patient as Case 45)

Case 55

74-year-old man complaining of headaches.
(coronal, postcontrast scan; SE 600/15)

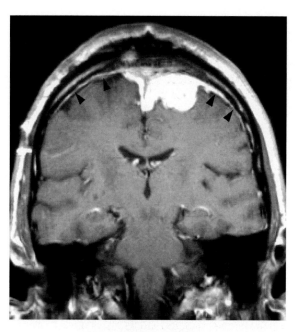

Convexity Meningioma

Some meningiomas spread along the inner table as relatively flat sheets of tissue. This "en plaque" morphology may be seen alone or in association with spherical or osseous components. The superficial location, homogeneous signal intensity, and marked contrast enhancement of such tumors remain characteristic.

Case 54 presents a postcontrast scan of the meningioma illustrated in Case 45. A plaque-like layer of enhancing tumor tissue is well defined along the anterior margin of the middle cranial fossa *(black arrows)*. Enhancing meningioma is also present within the infratemporal fossa *(white arrow)* and within the orbit (where it is difficult to distinguish from retrobulbar fat without fat suppression). Note the marked thickening of the right sphenoid bone and the prominent right-sided proptosis.

A layer of mildly thickened dural enhancement extending away from the base of a mengioma is a common MR feature, as seen in Case 55 *(arrowheads)*. In some cases, such thickening correlates with either "en plaque" extension of tumor or the presence of meningiomatous islands surrounding the main lesion. In many cases, the "tail" of dural enhancement near the base of the meningioma represents reactive thickening, without tumor involvement.

Although an enhancing dural "tail" is commonly seen at the base of meningiomas, the finding is not specific. Metastases, acoustic schwannomas, and other miscellaneous masses may also be associated with adjacent dural thickening.

The meningioma in Case 55 has grown along the falx and appears to have invaded the lumen of the superior sagittal sinus (compare to Case 43). An MR venogram or phase study could be used to assess residual blood flow in the sinus.

Case 53 illustrates another meningioma with an "en plaque" component. Additional examples of dural "tails" adjacent to meningiomas are seen in Cases 50 and 52.

Case 56

54-year-old woman presenting with decreased
vision in the right eye.
(sagittal, noncontrast scan; SE 600/15)

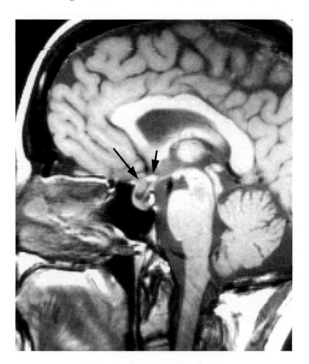

Tuberculum Meningioma

Case 57

55-year-old man presenting with headaches.
(coronal, postcontrast scan; SE 700/15)

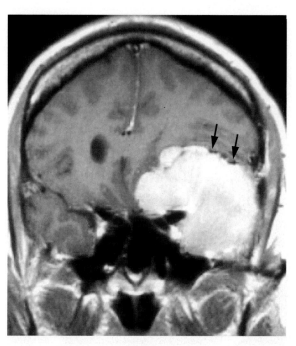

Sphenoid Wing Meningioma
(same patient as Case 32)

Along with the typical dural base, tissue homogeneity, sharp demarcation, and intense contrast enhancement of meningiomas, several characteristic locations of these tumors can help to support the diagnosis. One common area of origin is the sphenoid ridge, either in the midline (i.e., tuberculum sella region) or laterally (along the sphenoid wing).

Sagittal MR scans provide excellent definition of even small lesions affecting the optic chiasm or pituitary infundibulum. In Case 56, a focal mound of homogeneous soft tissue *(long arrow)* is perched on the tuberculum sella, immediately anterior to the optic chiasm *(short arrow)*. This

tiny meningioma was symptomatic by virtue of its critical location. (Contrast this early presentation with the late manifestation of the large convexity meningioma in Case 39.)

Case 57 illustrates a typical meningioma of the sphenoid wing. The large mass crosses the sphenoid ridge to involve both the middle cranial fossa and the anterior cranial fossa. Prominent vessels at its superior margin *(arrows)* may include displaced branches of the middle cerebral artery, as well as large veins on the surface of the tumor. Contrast enhancement is characteristically intense and uniform. A hint of radial striation is present within the tumor (compare to Case 34).

Case 58

24-year-old man studied in follow-up of prior
acoustic schwannoma.
(axial, postcontrast scan; SE 600/17)

Case 59

84-year-old man presenting with confusion.
(axial, postcontrast scan; SE 600/20)

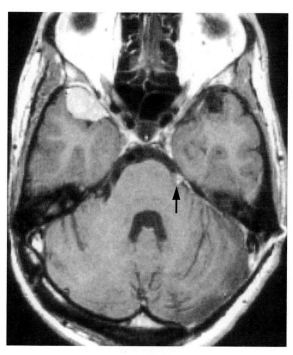

Meningioma
(in type 2 neurofibromatosis)

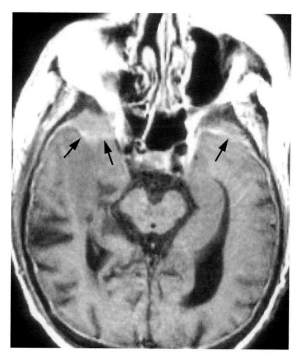

Metastatic Carcinoma of the Prostate
(dural based)

As discussed in Chapter 1, metastases to the skull or dura may produce focal extraaxial masses. Such lesions may closely resemble meningiomas in location, definition, and contrast enhancement. The two types of epidural masses may also be indistinguishable at angiography, with similar dural arterial supply and tumor stains.

The most common tumor to mimic meningioma in this manner is metastatic prostate carcinoma, particularly along the sphenoid wing, as in Case 59. Melanoma, breast carcinoma, and renal carcinoma can cause similar appearances.

Superficial gliomas may invade the dura and occasionally mimic meningiomas in other respects as well. Intracranial lymphoma is often dural based (see Case 25) and should be included in the differential diagnosis of meningioma-like lesions.

Neurofibromatosis type 2 is discussed in Case 168. In Case 58, an area of enhancement along the cisternal segment of the trigeminal nerve on the left *(arrow)* suggests a small schwannoma at this site.

Case 60

45-year-old woman presenting with diplopia.
(axial, postcontrast scan; SE 600/15)

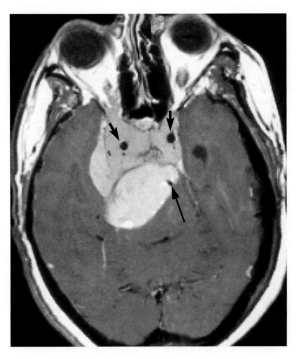

Prepontine and Parasellar Meningioma

Case 61

68-year-old man.
(sagittal, postcontrast scan; SE 850/20)

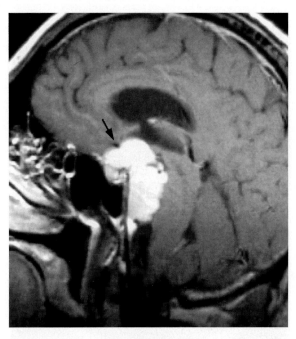

Clivus Meningioma

Meningiomas commonly extend across the tentorial hiatus from origins in either the parasellar region or the cerebellopontine angle. The morphology of transtentorial meningiomas may be plaque-like or lobular. The posterior fossa components of such tumors may occupy the prepontine or cerebellopontine angle cisterns, or both. The middle fossa components of transtentorial meningiomas commonly involve the cavernous sinus and may grow further laterally to displace the temporal lobe.

The meningioma in Case 60 expands the cavernous sinus bilaterally. The parasellar portions of the internal carotid arteries are encased on both sides *(short arrows).* The prepontine component of the mass displaces and surrounds the basilar artery *(long arrow; see Case 196 for a sagittal view of this lesion.)*

In Case 61, a mildly lobulated meningioma is based against the clivus, dorsum sella, and diaphragm sella. The suprasellar component of such a lesion may cause visual or endocrine symptoms, while the interpeduncular and prepontine components may cause cranial neuropathies. Major arterial channels *(arrow)* are seen at the rostral pole of the tumor, partially restraining its growth and contributing to a lobulated morphology.

Trigeminal schwannomas can closely mimic the appearance of parasellar or transtentorial meningiomas. The contrast enhancement pattern of large trigeminal schwannomas is often more patchy or inhomogeneous than that of meningiomas (see Case 178), resembling the typical tumor stain at angiography. The differential diagnosis of an enhancing, extraaxial mass spanning the petrous apex in an adult also includes metastasis and lymphoma.

Some meningiomas are transtentorial by virtue of tentorial origin or invasion (see Case 53). Such tumors may extend along the superior and/or inferior surface of the tentorium and are not confined by the tentorial hiatus.

Case 62

86-year-old man presenting with dizziness.
(axial, noncontrast scan; SE 2800/90)

Case 63

48-year-old woman presenting with neck pain,
bilateral hand numbness, and right leg weakness.
(sagittal, postcontrast scan; SE 600/15)

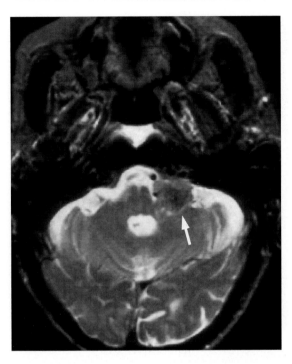

Meningioma near the Jugular Foramen

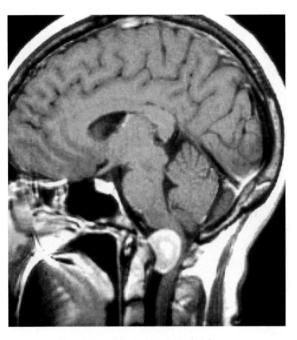

Foramen Magnum Meningioma

Meningiomas may occur at all levels within the cerebellopontine angle. Superiorly located tumors frequently cross the tentorial hiatus to involve the parasellar region, as seen in Case 60. Meningiomas occupying the midportion of the cerebellopontine angle cistern may mimic acoustic schwannomas (see Case 172). Finally, meningiomas may be found at the inferior margin of the cerebellopontine angle, as in Case 62. Such tumors may distort lower cranial nerves and/or compromise the foramen magnum.

Schwannomas and glomus jugulare tumors (see Cases 185 and 186) would be included in the differential diagnosis of a mass near the jugular foramen. The low signal in-

tensity of the lesion in Case 62 and the lack of associated expansion of the jugular foramen on adjacent scans make these alternative diagnoses unlikely.

The meningioma in Case 63 occupies a strategic location *within* the foramen magnum. Slow growth of this tumor has caused gradual thinning of the cervicomedullary junction, which can be remarkably attenuated before symptoms are manifest. (Compare to long-standing bony compromise of the craniocervical junction, as in Cases 876 and 1046.) Within the homogeneous enhancement of the tumor, a concentric circular texture or architecture can be appreciated, an occasional finding in meningiomas.

Case 64

76-year-old woman.
(axial, postcontrast scan; SE 600/15)

Case 65

45-year-old woman presenting with decreased memory and numbness of the right arm and leg.
(coronal, postcontrast scan; SE 750/20)

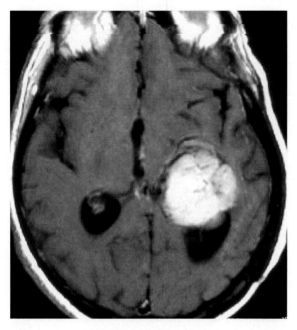

Trigone Meningioma

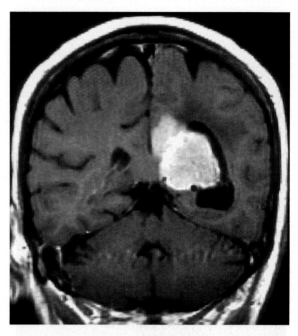

Trigone Meningioma

Intraventricular meningiomas account for about 2% of intracranial meningiomas. They most commonly occur within the atrium of the lateral ventricle, with greater frequency on the left side. Cases 64 and 65 are typical examples.

The differential diagnosis for a uniformly enhancing mass in this location would include choroid plexus papilloma (more commonly seen in children; see Case 299), ependymoma (see Case 115), choroid plexus metastasis, and vascular malformation (including an angioma in Sturge-Weber syndrome; see Case 770).

Intraventricular tumors may displace CSF as they grow, causing relatively little parenchymal mass effect. However, trigone lesions frequently "trap" the ipsilateral temporal horn, which enlarges due to continuing CSF production by choroid plexus within the obstructed segment.

Case 267 presents an unusual intraventricular meningioma located at the foramen of Monro.

Case 66

28-year-old woman
(with neurofibromatosis type 2).
(axial, noncontrast scan; SE 3000/90)

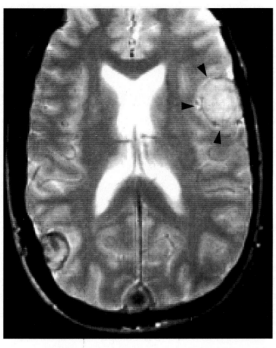

Multiple Convexity Meningiomas

Case 67

41-year-old man
(with neurofibromatosis type 2).
(axial, postcontrast scan; SE 600/15)

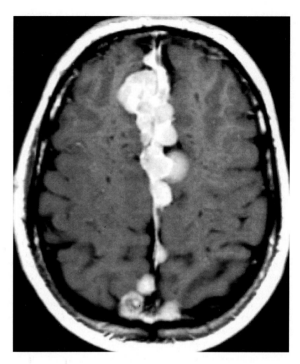

Meningiomatosis of the Falx

Multiple intracranial meningiomas may be seen sporadically, but they are more commonly encountered in association with type 2 neurofibromatosis ("bilateral acoustic neurofibromatosis"). The syndrome, previously identified as "central" neurofibromatosis, is caused by a mutation on chromosome 22 and is genetically distinct from neurofibromatosis type 1 (see Cases 764-767).

Apart from their multiplicity, the meningiomas in the above scans are typical in appearance. The lesions in Case 66 differ slightly from each other in homogeneity and internal architecture but fall within the range of appearances illustrated earlier in this chapter. The homogeneous, intense enhancement of the dural-based masses in Case 67 is characteristic.

Multifocal recurrence of aggressive meningiomas may be encountered after resection of an initially solitary lesion. Sarcomatous transformation can occur in originally benign tumors. Some histological varieties (e.g., papillary and angioblastic meningiomas) are themselves associated with the tendency toward recurrence and parenchymal invasion. Morphological features correlated with subsequent aggressive behavior of meningiomas include a plaque-like component extending over the cerebral surface from the main mass, abnormally prominent deep venous drainage from the tumor region (suggesting cortical invasion), and frond-like margins invaginating into underlying cerebral parenchyma.

Induction of meningiomas has been reported after both high and low doses of radiation. The latency period in such cases may be as long as 20 years, correlating inversely with radiation dose and directly with patient age at the time of exposure. Radiation-induced meningiomas are typically rapidly growing and aggressive tumors, with frequent multiplicity.

REFERENCES

Ahmadi J, Hinton DR, Segall HD, Couldwell WT, et al: Dural invasion by craniofacial and calvarial neoplasms: MR imaging and histopathologic evaluation. *Radiology* 188:747-749, 1993.

Ahmadi J, Hinton DR, Segall HD, et al: Surgical implications of magnetic resonance-enhances dura. *Neurosurgery* 35:370-377, 1994.

Aoki S, Barkovich AJ, Nishimura K, et al: Neurofibromatosis types 1 and 2: cranial MR findings. *Radiology* 172:527-534, 1989.

Aoki S, Sasaki Y, Machida T, Tanioka H: Contrast enhanced MR images in patients with meningiomas: importance of enhancement of the dura adjacent to the tumor. *AJNR* 11:935-938, 1990.

Black PMcL: Meningiomas. *Neurosurgery* 32:643-657, 1993.

Berry I, Brant-Zawadzki M, Osaki L, et al: Gadolinium-DTPA in clinical MR of the brain: 2. Extraaxial lesions and normal structures. *AJNR* 7:789-793, 1986.

Bradac GB, RA Schorner W, et al: Cavernous sinus meningiomas: an MRI study. *Neuroradiology* 29:578-581, 1987.

Breger RK, Papke RA, Pojunas KW, et al: Benign extraaxial tumors: contrast enhancement with Gd-DTPA. *Radiology* 163:427-430, 1987.

Buetow MP, Burton PC, Smirniotopoulos JG: Typical, atypical, and misleading features in meningioma. *Radiographics* 11:1087-1100, 1991.

Bydder GM, Kingsley DPE, Brown J, et al: MR imaging of meningiomas including studies with and without gadolinium-DTPA. *J Comput Assist Tomogr* 9:690-697, 1985.

Carpeggiani P, Crisi G, Trevisan C: MRI of intracranial meningiomas: correlations with histology and physical consistency. *Neuroradiology* 35:532-536, 1993.

Castillo M, Davis PC, Ross WK, Hoffman JC Jr: Meningioma of the chiasm and optic nerves: CT and MR findings. *J Comput Assist Tomogr* 13:679-681, 1989.

Chen TC, Zee CS, Miller CA, et al: Magnetic resonance imaging and pathological correlates of meningiomas. *Neurosurgery* 31:1015-1022, 1992.

Curnes JT: MR imaging of peripheral intracranial neoplasms: extra-axial versus intra-axial masses. *J Comput Assist Tomogr* 11:932-937, 1987.

Daemerel P, Wilms G, Lammeus M, et al: Intracranial meningiomas: correlation between MR imaging and histology in fifty patients. *J Comput Assist Tomogr* 15:45-51, 1991.

Darling CF, Byrd SE, Reyes-Mugica M, et al: MR of pediatric intracranial meningiomas. *AJNR* 15:435-444, 1994.

Elster AD, Challa VR, Gilbert TH, et al: Meningiomas: MR and histopathologic features. *Radiology* 170:857-862, 1989.

Fujii K, Fujita N, Hirabuki N, et al: Neuromas and meningiomas: evaluation of early enhancement with dynamic MR imaging. *AJNR* 13:1215-1220, 1992.

George AE, Russell EJ, Kricheff II: White matter buckling: CT sign of extraaxial mass. *AJNR* 1:425-430, 1980.

Germano IM, Edwards MSB, Davis RL, Schiffer, D: Intracranial meningiomas of the first two decades of life. *J Neurosurg* 80:447-453, 1994.

Glasier CM, Husain MM, Chadduck W, Boop FA: Meningiomas in children: MR and histopathologic findings. *AJNR* 14:237-241, 1993.

Goldsher D, Litt AW, Pinto RS, et al: Dural "tail" associated with meningiomas on Gd-DTPA-enhanced MR images: characteristics, differential diagnostic value, and possible implications of treatment. *Radiology* 176:447-450, 1990.

Haughton VM, Rimm AA, Czervionke LF, et al: Sensitivity of Gd-DTPA-enhanced MR imaging of benign extraaxial tumors. *Radiology* 166:829-834, 1988.

Hirsch WL, Sekhar LN, Lanzino G, et al: Meningiomas involving the cavernous sinus: value of imaging for predicting surgical complications. *AJR* 160:1083-1088, 1993.

Hope JKA, Armstrong DA, Babyn PS, et al: Primary meningeal tumors in children: correlation of clinical and CT findings with histologic type and prognosis. *AJNR* 13:1353-1364, 1992.

Jaaskelainen J, Haltia M, Servo A: Atypical and anaplastic meningiomas: radiology, surgery, radiotherapy and outcome. *Surg Neurol* 25:233-242, 1986.

Kaplan RD, Coon S, Drayer BP, et al: MR characteristics of meningioma subtypes at 1.5 Tesla. *J Comput Assist Tomogr* 16:366-371, 1992.

Katayama Y, Tsubokawa T, Tanaka A, Koshinaga M, et al: Magnetic resonance imaging of xanthomatous meningioma. *Neuroradiology* 35:187-189, 1992.

Kulali A, Ilcayto R, Fiskeci C: Cystic meningiomas. *Acta Neurochir (Wien)* 111:108-113, 1991.

Mack EE, Wilson CB: Meningiomas induced by high-dose cranial irradiation. *J Neurosurg* 79:28-31, 1993.

Mahmood A, Caccamo DV, Tomecek FJ, Malik GM: Atypical and malignant meningiomas: a clinicopathological review. *Neurosurgery* 33:955-963, 1993.

Mamourian AC, Lewandowski AE, Towfighi J: Cystic intraparenchymal meningioma in a child: case report. *AJNR* 12:366-367, 1991.

Mawhinney RR, Buckley JH, Holloand IM, Worthington BS: The value of magnetic resonance imaging in the diagnosis of intracranial meningiomas. *Clin Radiol* 37:429-439, 1986.

Moss R, Roskwald G, Chou S, et al: Radiation-induced meninguomas in pediatric patients. *Neurosurgery* 22:758, 1988.

Naul LG, Hise JH, Bauserman SC, Todd FD: CT and MR of meningeal melanocytoma. *AJNR* 12:315-316, 1991.

Odake G: Cystic meningiomas report of three patients. *Neurosurgery* 30:935-940, 1992.

Perry RD, Parker GD, Hallinan JH: CT and MR imaging of fourth ventricular meningiomas. *J Comput Assist Tomogr* 14:276:280, 1990.

Roda JM, Bencosme JA, Perez-Higueias A, Fraile M: Simultaneous multiple intracranial and spinal meningiomas. *Neurochirurgie* 35:92-94, 1992.

Salibi SS, Nauta HJW, Brem H, et al: Lipomeningioma: report of three cases and review of the literature. *Neurosurgery* 25:122-125, 1989.

Sheporaitis L, Osborn AG, Smirniotopoulos JG, Clunie DA, et al: Radiologic-pathologic correlation intracranial meningioma. *AJNR* 13:29-37, 1992.

Siegelman ES, Mishkin MM, Taveras JT: Past, present, and future of radiology of meningioma. *Radiographics* 11:899-910, 1991.

Spagnoli MV, Goldberg HI, Grossman RI, et al: Intracranial meningiomas high-field MR imaging. *Radiology* 161:369-375, 1986.

Sze G, Soletsky S, Bronen R, et al: MR imaging of the cranial meninges. *AJNR* 10:965, 1989.

Taylor SL, Barakos JA, Harsh GR IV, Wilson CB: Magnetic resonance imaging of tuberculum sellae meningiomas: preventing preoperative misdiagnosis as pituitary adenoma. *Neurosurgery* 31:621-627, 1992.

Terasaki KK, Zee C-S: Evolution of central necrosis in a meningioma: CT and MR features. *J Comput Assist Tomogr* 14:464-466, 1990.

Terstegge K, Schörner W, Henkes H, Heye N, et al: Hyperostosis in meningiomas: MR findings in patients with recurrent meningioma of the sphenoid wings. *AJNR* 15:555-560, 1994.

Tokumaru A, O'uchi T, Eguchi T, et al: Prominent meningeal enhancement adjacent to meningioma on Gd-DTPA-enhanced MR images: histopathologic correlation. *Radiology* 175:431-433, 1990.

Wagle VG, Villemure JG, Melanson D, et al: Diagnostic potential of magnetic resonance in cases of foramen magnum meningiomas. *Neurosurgery* 21:622-626, 1987.

Watabe T, Azuma T: T1 and T2 measurements of meningiomas and neuromas before and after Gd-DTPA. *AJNR* 10:463-470, 1989.

Wilms G, Lammens M, Marchal G, et al: Prominent dural enhancement adjacent to nonmeningiomatous malignant lesions on contrast-enhanced MR images. *AJNR* 12:761-764, 1991.

Wilms G, Lammens M, Marchal G, et al: Thickening of dura surrounding meningiomas: MR features. *J Comput Assist Tomogr* 13:763-768, 1989.

Yeakley JW, Kulkarni M, McArdle CB, et al: High-resolution MR imaging of juxtasellar meningiomas with CT and angiographic correlation. *AJNR* 9:279-285, 1988.

Young SC, Grossman RI, Goldberg HI, et al: MR of vascular encasement in parasellar masses: comparison with angiography and CT. *AJNR* 9:35-38, 1988.

Zagzag D, Gomori JN, Rappaport ZH, Shalet MN: Cystic meningiomas presenting as a ring lesion. *AJNR* 7:911-912, 1986.

Zee CS, Chin T, Segall HD, et al: Magnetic resonance imaging of meningiomas. *Semin US CT MR* 13:154-169, 1992.

Zimmerman RD, Fleming CA, Saint-Louis LA, et al: Magnetic resonance imaging of meningiomas. *AJNR* 6:149-157, 1985.

CHAPTER 3

Gliomas

Case 68

30-year-old woman presenting with seizures,
beginning with lip twitching and mouth opening.
(sagittal, noncontrast scan; SE 600/17)

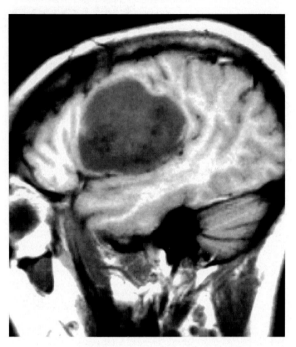

Low Grade Astrocytoma

Case 69

4-year-old boy presenting with seizures.
(coronal, postcontrast scan; SE 700/15)

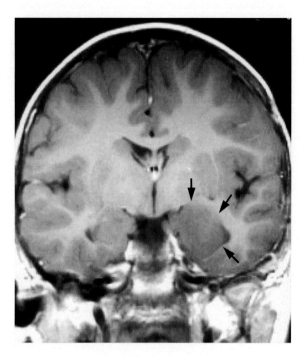

Low Grade Astrocytoma

In the absence of hemorrhage or dense calcification, the signal intensity of low grade astrocytomas on T1-weighted images is usually homogeneous and comparable to or lower than that of gray matter. Cases 68 and 69 are typical examples.

The margins of gliomas such as Case 68 may be surprisingly distinct and smooth on MR scans as compared to their poor definition on CT studies. In other patients, low grade glial neoplasms present as amorphous thickening of cortical gray matter, illustrated in Case 69 (*arrows*; see also Case 74).

Case 69 demonstrates that the coronal plane is helpful in assessing temporal lobe pathology. The deep temporal lobe is a common location for low grade tumors in children and young adults, and the history of seizures is typical for these patients (see Cases 452 and 453 for additional examples). The absence of abnormal contrast enhancement in Case 69 is common in low grade astrocytomas (see Cases 95 and 96).

An appearance comparable to Case 69 in an adult could be caused by herpes encephalitis or limbic encephalitis, an unusual paraneoplastic disorder most commonly associated with oat cell carcinoma of the lung (see Cases 397-400).

Case 70

26-year-old woman presenting with seizures.
(coronal, noncontrast scan; SE 2500/90)

Case 71

7-year-old girl presenting with seizures.
(axial, noncontrast scan; SE 2600/90)

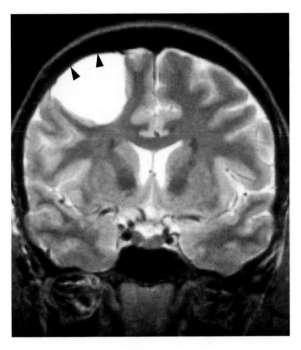

Low Grade Astrocytoma

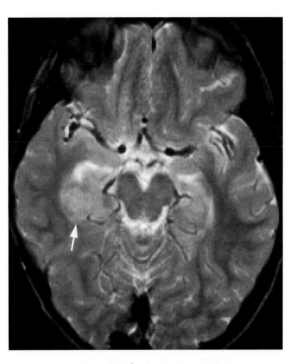

Low Grade Astrocytoma

The signal intensity of low grade gliomas on long TR spin echo images may range from isointensity to very high values. High intensity (as in Case 70) is more common, reflecting high water content in the tumor region.

The glioma in Case 70 demonstrates little mass effect for its size, suggesting a long-standing, slowly growing lesion. The absence of reactive cerebral edema also supports a chronic, low grade process. Subtle erosion of the overlying calvarium is equivocally present *(arrowheads)*, again favoring a long history of gradual evolution (compare to Case 649).

The peripheral base and sharply defined margins of a superficial glioma can resemble a localized cerebral infarct. Clues to the correct diagnosis include rounded rather than linear borders and the absence of an acute neurological deficit. MR scans typically demonstrate a characteristic gyriform morphology within subacute infarcts, illustrated in Cases 468 and 473.

Occasional gliomas (both low and high grade) remain nearly isointense to gray matter on T2-weighted scans. This appearance, seen in the medial right temporal lobe of Case 71 *(arrow)*, often correlates with precontrast high attenuation on CT scans. Both features suggest dense cellularity with little cytoplasmic or extracellular water. Other tumors that can present a similar appearance are germinomas (see Case 272) and primary cerebral lymphomas (see Cases 313 to 315).

Case 72

6-year-old boy presenting with seizures.
(axial, postcontrast scan; SE 600/15)

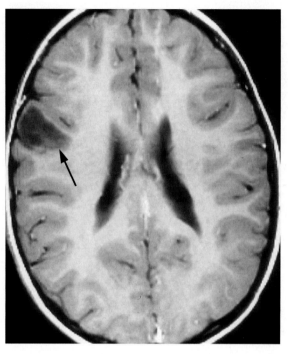

Low Grade Astrocytoma

Case 73

2-year-old girl presenting with seizures.
(axial, noncontrast scan; SE 2500/90)

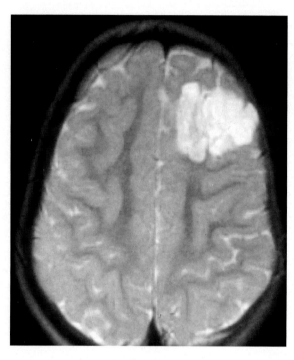

Low Grade Astrocytoma

Many low grade gliomas are superficial lesions, involving cerebral cortex and commonly presenting with seizures. Such lesions are frequently encountered in children. The tumors are typically well defined and can often be resected with good long-term survival.

As illustrated in Cases 72 and 73, these "cortical" gliomas of childhood usually demonstrate long T1 and T2 values. Contrast enhancement is typically minimal or absent. The slow growth of the tumors may cause erosion of the adjacent inner table.

If the lesion is small, as in Case 72, a cortical/subcortical hamartoma of tuberous sclerosis might be considered in the differential diagnosis (see Cases 754 and 755). A search for associated lesions, particularly subependymal nodules, is important is assessing this possibility.

The moderate lobulation of the superficial glioma in Case 73 is intermediate between the smoothly rounded margins of Case 70 and the gyriform infiltration in Case 75.

Dysembryoplastic neuroepithelial tumors (DNET) may similarly present as superficial lesions causing cortical thickening in young patients. These masses most commonly occur in the temporal or frontal lobes, often demonstrating a "mega-gyric" and/or multinodular morphology. A history of seizures, associated calvarial erosion, and a lack of contrast enhancement may closely resemble the presentation of a low grade glioma.

Case 74

41-year-old man presenting with seizures,
(coronal, postcontrast scan; SE 600/17)

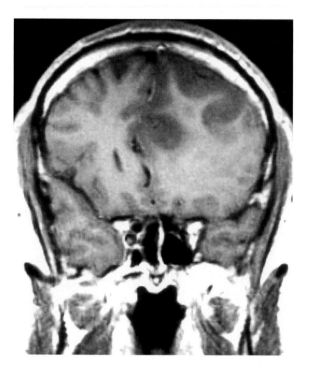

Low Grade Astrocytoma

Case 75

37-year-old man presenting with the sudden onset
of disorientation.
(axial, noncontrast scan; SE 2500/90)

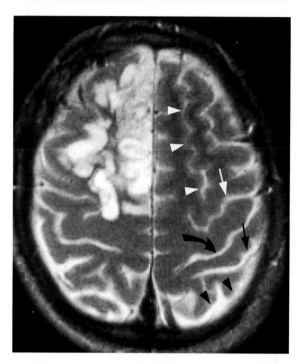

Low Grade Astrocytoma
(recurrent)

Low grade gliomas sometimes infiltrate cortex rather than developing into a centralized mass. The resulting gyriform pattern of signal abnormality (with long T1 and T2 values) may resemble cortical edema from other etiologies, such as subacute infarction or meningitis. The clinical setting usually distinguishes among these diagnostic possibilities, but occasional gliomas present with stroke-like suddenness in the reported onset of symptoms.

The glioma in Case 74 has thickened cortex of the left frontal lobe both medially and laterally. There is no evidence of laminar T1-shortening within the involved gyri, a common finding in subacute infarcts (see Cases 478 and 479). Furthermore, the zone of abnormality affects two major vascular distributions (the anterior and middle cerebral arteries), an unusual occurrence in cerebral infarction.

In Case 75, the possibility of cortical infarction could be considered. However, this lesion also crosses the watershed between the anterior and middle cerebral artery distribu-

tions. This fact, together with the observation that the lateral involvement is mainly *sub*cortical, favors a diagnosis of infiltrating neoplasm rather than infarction.

As mentioned on the preceding page, dysembryoplastic neuroepithelial tumors should be considered in the differential diagnosis of a gyriform mass involving cortex of the frontal or temporal lobes.

The normal sulcal anatomy in the rolandic region is well seen on the left side in Case 75. The superior frontal sulcus *(white arrowheads)* follows a parasagittal course before intersecting posteriorly (at a right angle) with the precentral sulcus *(white arrow)*. The intraparietal sulcus *(black arrowheads)* angles obliquely across the posterior parietal vertex before merging anteriorly with the postcentral sulcus *(black arrow)*. The central sulcus *(large curved arrow)* lies between the precentral and the postcentral sulci as the middle member of the three major laterally directed sulci.

Case 76A

7-year-old girl presenting with seizures.
(sagittal, noncontrast scan; SE 600/17)

Case 76B

Same patient.
(axial, noncontrast scan; SE 2500/28)

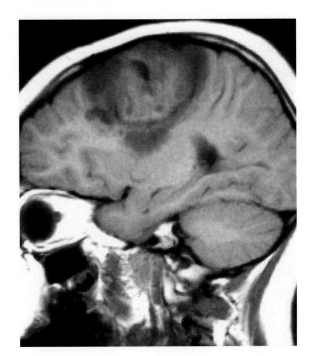
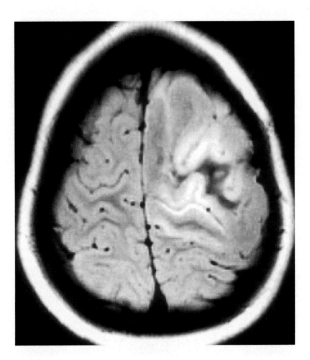

Low Grade Astrocytoma

The homogeneous signal intensity of most low grade gliomas as demonstrated in Cases 68 through 75 may be altered by calcification and/or hemorrhage. Hemorrhage is unusual in low grade astrocytomas (in contrast to oligodendrogliomas; see Cases 111 and 114). Calcification is more common, demonstrated by CT scans in 10% to 20% of low grade astrocytomas.

Small amounts of intratumoral calcification are usually inapparent on spin echo studies. (Gradient echo scans emphasizing susceptibility effects can improve the detection of parenchymal calcification.) Dense calcifications usually result in zones of low signal intensity on all pulse sequences

due to the associated low concentration of imageable protons. In Case 76, the stellate area of low signal intensity near the center of the mass on both short and long TR images correlated with dense calcification on a preceding CT scan. In other cases, heavily calcified areas within a tumor may have a more nodular morphology (see Case 631).

Oligodendrogliomas are more frequently calcified than any other glial tumors, with a large majority demonstrating this finding. Despite a lower incidence of calcification in astrocytomas, the much greater frequency of this histology makes astrocytoma the most common calcified glial neoplasm.

Case 77

33-year-old man presenting with a first seizure.
(sagittal, noncontrast scan; SE 600/17)

Case 78

1-year-old boy with a history of infantile spasms.
(coronal, noncontrast scan; SE 2800/90)

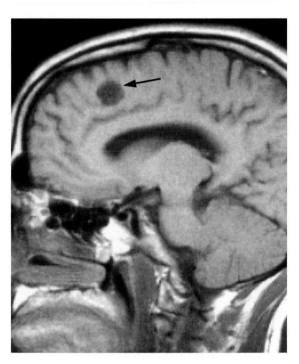

Low Grade Astrocytoma

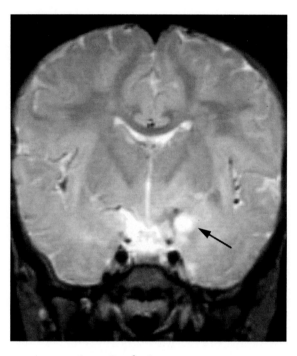

Low Grade Astrocytoma

The usually well-defined margins of low grade gliomas on MR scans may result in the demonstration of very small tumors. The masses in Cases 77 and 78 *(arrows)* are only one centimeter in diameter, but their long T1 and T2 values clearly demarcate them as foci of abnormal tissue. The appearance of these lesions is not specific, but focal glioma should be considered in the differential diagnosis, particularly in these clinical contexts.

The onset of seizures in an adult is a worrisome event. Cerebral masses are detected in approximately 20% of such cases. Seizures are a particularly common symptom of low grade neoplasms; up to 50% of oligodendrogliomas present in this manner.

Lesions in or near the hippocampal formation (as in Case 78) commonly cause seizures because of the low excitation threshold of neurons in this region. The medial temporal lobe can be difficult to assess on CT scans, and coronal MR studies are appropriate as an initial examination or following a negative CT study in such patients. See Cases 452, 453, 629, and 630 for other examples of small structural lesions within the temporal lobes of patients with seizures.

Case 79

4-year-old boy presenting with headaches
and hemiparesis.
(sagittal, noncontrast scan; SE 600/15)

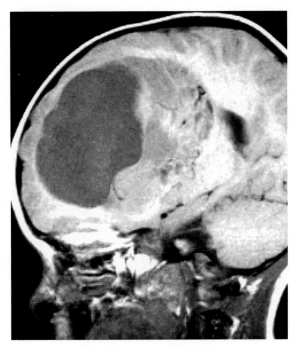

Grade III Astrocytoma

Case 80

38-year-old woman presenting with
auditory disturbance.
(coronal, noncontrast scan; SE 900/22)

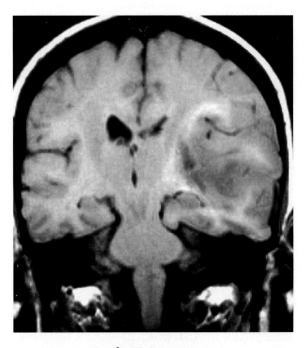

Grade III Astrocytoma

Anaplastic astrocytoma (grade III astrocytoma) and glioblastoma multiforme (grade IV astrocytoma) are often described together as "malignant" or "high grade" gliomas.

The MR spectrum of malignant gliomas overlaps that of low grade neoplasms, and occasional tumors have intermediate characteristics. However, the features of most high grade tumors are different from those of the lower grade lesions illustrated on the previous pages.

Most high grade gliomas demonstrate heterogeneous tissue texture and signal intensity on T1-weighted images. This complex architecture reflects variable cellularity as well as the common presence of necrosis, hemorrhage, and cyst formation.

The anterior half of the large frontal lobe mass in Case 79 is grossly cystic. The solid posterior portion demonstrates mixed tissue components and several low intensity foci, which may represent large vessels or dense calcifications.

Case 80 illustrates a more infiltrating morphology of a high grade glioma. The size of the mass and the variable tissue components suggest malignant histology.

Case 81

38-year-old woman presenting with
auditory disturbance.
(axial, noncontrast scan; SE 3000/30)

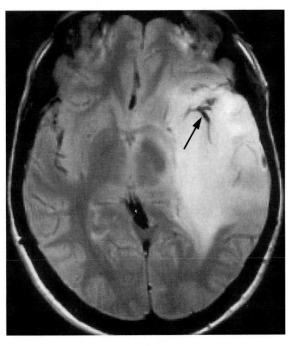

Grade III Astrocytoma
(same patient as Case 80)

Case 82

61-year-old woman presenting with
severe headaches.
(axial, noncontrast scan; SE 2600/45)

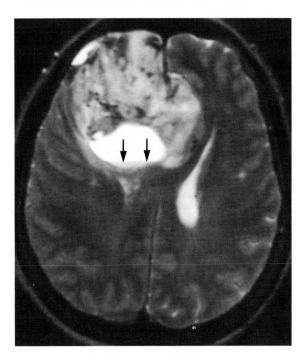

Glioblastoma Multiforme

On long TR spin echo scans, the appearance of malignant gliomas is usually dominated by high signal intensity. This prolongation of T2 values (and increased proton density) is attributable to both the tumor tissue and reactive "edema." Pathological studies have shown that tumor cells are actually present within (and beyond) the "edema" surrounding even well-defined masses.

The tumor in Case 81 is homogeneous, extending throughout an area that approximates the distribution of the middle cerebral artery. Many gliomas are found in the perisylvian region, where they may mimic recent infarction. The clinical context and predominant white matter involvement of a glioma usually allow distinction from ischemic lesions (see Cases 472 and 473). Note the displaced "flow void" of the patent middle cerebral artery near its genu *(arrow)*.

In Case 82, a much more heterogeneous glioma has grown to and around the dural margin of the anterior falx. The area of greatest signal intensity within the lesion is a fluid-filled cyst, which demonstrates a sedimentation level posteriorly *(arrows)*. Small, dark areas within the remainder of the mass represent hemorrhagic foci, which were seen as high intensity zones on a T1-weighted scan. (Compare to the appearance of calcification within the oligodendroglioma in Case 112.)

An aggressive meningioma or meningeal sarcoma arising from the falx and invading cerebral parenchyma could be considered in the differential diagnosis of Case 82. A post contrast scan may help to distinguish between these possibilities.

Case 83

74-year-old man.
(axial, noncontrast scan; SE 3000/90)

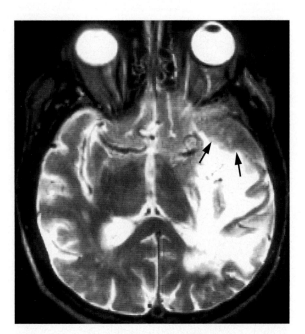

Sphenoid Wing Meningioma

Case 84

56-year-old man.
(axial, noncontrast scan; SE 2500/28)

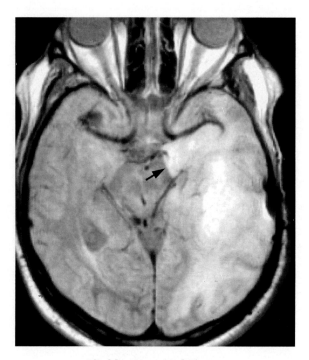

Glioblastoma Multiforme

As discussed in Case 37, meningiomas of the sphenoid wing may incite extensive edema within the temporal lobe and adjacent hemisphere. Case 83 is an example of this occurrence. The widespread cerebral edema is secondary to a relatively small, isointense meningioma at the anterior margin of the middle cranial fossa *(arrows)*. A postcontrast scan would demonstrate the enhancing meningioma and eliminate confusion with a primary intraaxial process.

The glioblastoma in Case 84 is diffusely infiltrating, resembling Case 81. Uncal herniation is present *(arrow)* causing rotation and displacement of the midbrain with deformity of the left cerebral peduncle.

CYSTIC GLIOMAS

Case 85

6-year-old boy with a history of seizures.
(sagittal, noncontrast scan; SE 600/15)

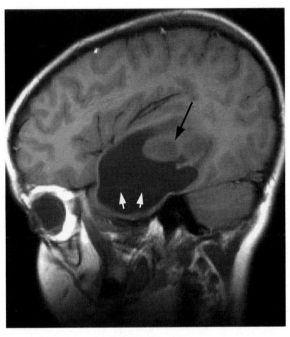

Grade III Astrocytoma

Case 86

56-year-old woman presenting with hemiparesis.
(axial, noncontrast scan; SE 3000/80)

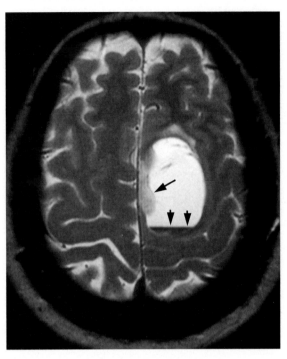

Glioblastoma Multiforme

Many low and high grade gliomas contain one or more cysts. When a tumor cyst is large and unilocular, palliative drainage may provide symptomatic improvement by reducing mass effect. Repeated aspiration or continuous drainage may be necessary due to rapid reaccumulation of fluid.

The most reliable MR (or CT) indication of a truly cystic tumor is a sedimentation level within the lesion, as demonstrated in Case 86 *(short arrows)*. The dense material settling in the dependent portion of a cyst may be cellular debris, hemorrhage, or accumulated contrast material (see also Cases 82, 129, 214, and 562). The very low signal intensity of the sedimentation layer in Case 86 suggests blood products, as discussed in Chapter 10.

In the absence of a sedimentation level, a cyst can be suspected when the content of the lesion remains completely homogeneous on all pulse sequences. Some solid tumors (particularly astrocytomas with gelatinous consistency) are remarkably uniform (see Cases 126 and 149), so

care must be taken before a mass is labeled as "cystic." Phase contrast studies and diffusion imaging may help to establish the cystic nature of an indeterminate lesion.

In Case 85, a complex mural nodule of tumor tissue is found along the posterior wall of the cyst *(black arrow)*. A thin septum is faintly visible within the cyst *(white arrows)*. Such partitions are better seen on MR scans than on CT studies but are difficult to resolve and can be missed entirely.

The malignant glioma in Case 86 demonstrates an elongated mural nodule medially *(long arrow)*. Septations cross the anterior portion of the cyst, and a small amount of edema is present anterior to the mass. Since the medial margin of the tumor is adjacent to the falx, the possibility of an atypical extraaxial lesion (e.g., meningioma) might be considered. Angiography demonstrated pial rather than dural arterial supply, and a cystic glioblastoma was confirmed at surgery.

Case 87

62-year-old woman presenting with
left hemiparesis.
(axial, noncontrast scan; SE 3000/25)

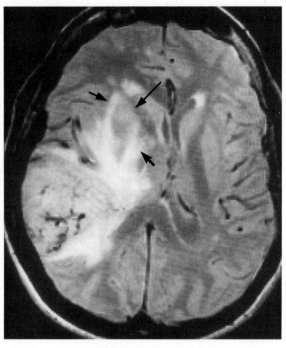

Glioblastoma Multiforme

Case 88

55-year-old man presenting with headaches.
(axial, noncontrast scan; SE 2500/45)

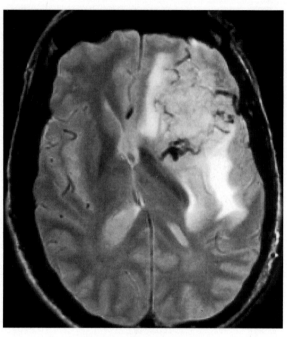

Spenoid Wing Meningioma
(same patient as Case 32)

Large, bizarre vessels within a glial neoplasm are a strong indication of malignant histology. The irregular caliber, course, and branching pattern of the "flow voids" in Case 87 represent the MR equivalent of "tumor vascularity" as previously defined by cerebral angiography.

The tumor vessels in Case 88 are equally large, but they are less irregular than in Case 87. Compare this appearance to the falx meningioma in Case 40.

Both of these tumors demonstrate moderately high signal intensity with surrounding edema. The edema in Case 87 tracks anteriorly to involve the internal *(short thick arrow)* and external *(short thin arrow)* capsules, surrounding the displaced lenticular nucleus *(long arrow)*. Both cases illustrate subfalcial herniation, with contralateral shift of the pericallosal arteries.

Case 89

13-year-old boy presenting with a seizure.
(sagittal, noncontrast scan; SE 600/15)

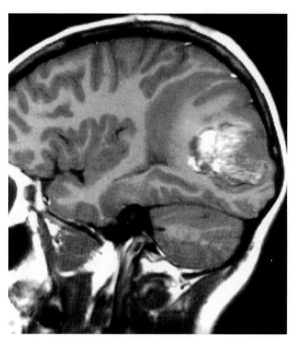

Gliomastoma Multiforme

Case 90

70-year-old woman presenting with confusion.
(axial, noncontrast scan; SE 2500/90)

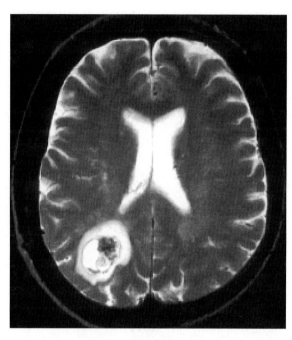

Grade III Astrocytoma

Macroscopic hemorrhage is relatively uncommon in gliomas, occurring in about 5%. Among low grade gliomas, oligodendrogliomas make up a disproportionate share of lesions presenting with gross hemorrhage. Malignant gliomas are characterized angiographically by neovascularity, which represents a likely source of bleeding (see Case 87).

Patchy T1-shortening is present throughout the occipital mass in Case 89, reflecting the presence of methemoglobin and implying subacute hemorrhage (see discussion of Cases 555-558). The texture or architecture of the lesion is more complex than the usual laminated morphology of a benign hematoma (compare to Case 557). This feature combines with the prominent surrounding edema to suggest that the hemorrhage is superimposed on an underlying structural lesion.

On T2-weighted images, recent hemorrhage demonstrates low signal intensity. The tumor in Case 90 contains blood products along with additional heterogeneous texture, suggesting hemorrhage in a neoplasm. (Case 562 presents a similar example.) The collar of surrounding

edema supports this interpretation, although benign hematomas may also present with a similar halo (see Case 556).

It is sometimes difficult to determine on initial studies whether a focal hemorrhage is benign or malignant. Clues to the latter etiology on subsequent scans include (1) unusually slow evolution/degradation of blood products; (2) discontinuity or irregularity of the hemosiderin ring formed at the perimeter of the lesion; and (3) persistent or increasing perilesional edema.

Although the morphology in Case 90 is strongly suggestive of hemorrhage within a tumor, the appearance is not histologically specific. A hemorrhagic metastasis could present identically (see Cases 8 and 11).

Microscopic hemorrhage is a common pathological feature within high grade gliomas. In fact, hemorrhage is one of the four histological parameters (along with necrosis, endothelial proliferation, and nuclear atypia) that are summed by many pathologists to establish the grade of a glial neoplasm.

Case 91

50-year-old woman presenting with confusion.
(sagittal, noncontrast scan; SE 600/15)

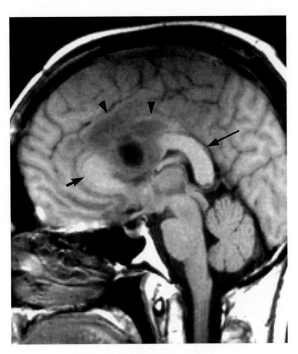

Grade II-III Astrocytoma

Case 92

29-year-old woman presenting with seizures.
(sagittal, noncontrast scan; SE 600/17)

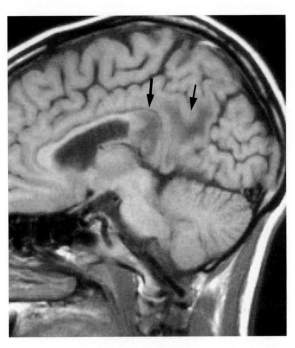

Grade III Astrocytoma

The corpus callosum is commonly involved by glial tumors, which may arise within it or grow medially from hemispheric origins. These tumors are well demonstrated by the sagittal plane of MR scans.

The mass in Case 91 occupies the anterior body of the corpus callosum, with sparing of the genu *(short arrow)* and splenium *(long arrow)*. The tumor is centrally necrotic or cystic. There is associated infiltration of the cingulate gyrus *(arrowheads)*.

In Case 92, the splenium is expanded *(thick arrow)* by a "U"-shaped glioma that traversed the corpus callosum to involve the parietal lobes bilaterally *(thin arrow)*. The small size of the remainder of the corpus callosum correlates with the prominent sulci in this young patient. The cause of this apparent atrophy was not known (see discussion of Cases 457 and 458).

In both of these cases, the tumors demonstrate abnormally low signal intensity, as is typical of gliomas on T1-weighted images.

Case 93

33-year-old woman presenting with headaches.
(axial, noncontrast scan; SE 2500/28)

Case 94

62-year-old woman presenting with rapidly
worsening vision.
(axial, noncontrast scan; SE 2500/90)

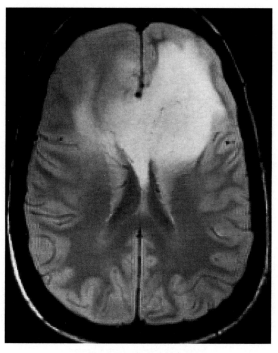

Glioblastoma Multiforme

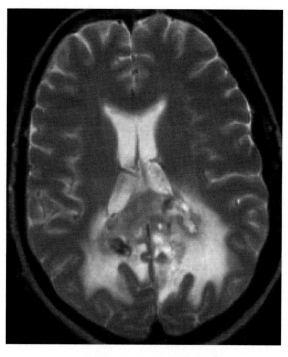

Glioblastoma Multiforme

Callosal gliomas often have "wings" extending symmetrically or asymmetrically into both cerebral hemispheres. The resulting "butterfly" morphology is well demonstrated on axial or coronal views.

The glioma in Case 93 crosses the genu of the corpus callosum and thickens the minor forceps. The tumor in Case 94 traverses the splenium of the corpus callosum and infiltrates the major forceps. The signal intensity of the tumor in Case 93 is uniformly high, while Case 94 demonstrates heterogeneous isointensity suggesting dense cellularity with a high nuclear to cytoplasmic ratio. Primary CNS lymphoma frequently involves the corpus callosum (see Case 317) and would be a diagnostic consideration in Case 94.

A number of non-neoplastic disorders can cause abnormal signal intensity and expansion of the corpus callosum resembling a tumor. Among these are multiple sclerosis, acute disseminated encephalomyelitis, and progressive multifocal leukoencephalopathy. HIV encephalitis may extend into the corpus callosum. Machiafava Bignami syndrome is a rare demyelinating disorder associated with alcohol consumption that frequently involves the corpus callosum.

Both of the above tumors infiltrate the septum pellucidum. Septal involvement is often a clue to the glial origin of smaller tumors near the foramen of Monro.

Case 95

63-year-old woman presenting with confusion.
(coronal, postcontrast scan; SE 650/20)

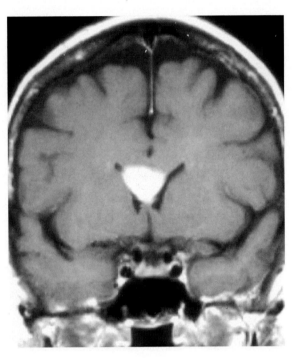

Grade II Astrocytoma of the Corpus Callosum

Case 96

1-year-old boy with a history of infantile spasms.
(coronal, postcontrast scan; SE 600/15)

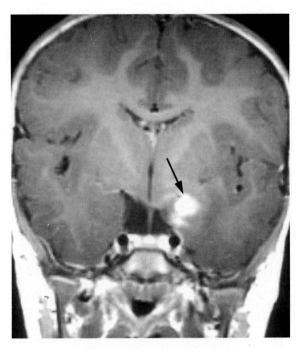

Low Grade Astrocytoma
(same patient as Case 78)

Many low grade gliomas demonstrate little or no contrast enhancement (see Cases 69 and 72 for examples). In other cases, low grade glial neoplasms enhance intensely, as illustrated above. The presence of abnormal contrast enhancement does not necessarily imply high grade malignancy. (Conversely, the absence of contrast enhancement does not exclude malignant histology; see Cases 101 and 102.) MR has proved to be more sensitive than CT to small amounts of contrast enhancement; enhancement of low grade lesions may be correspondingly more impressive on MR studies than on CT scans.

The morphology of prominent enhancement in low grade gliomas is often solid and smoothly marginated, as seen in these cases. Malignant gliomas typically present a more irregular pattern (see Cases 97 and 98, and compare Case 95 to Case 104).

Localized contrast enhancement is a nonspecific finding with a broad differential diagnosis. For example, an appearance very similar to Case 96 could be encountered in an adult with herpes encephalitis involving the uncus.

Case 97

50-year-old woman presenting with apathy.
(coronal, postcontrast scan; SE 600/15)

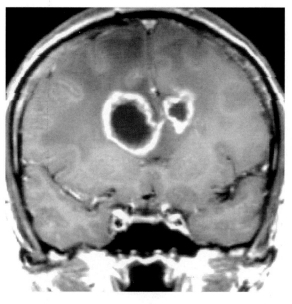

Glioblastoma Multiforme

Case 98

4-year-old boy presenting with headaches.
(axial, postcontrast scan; SE 600/15)

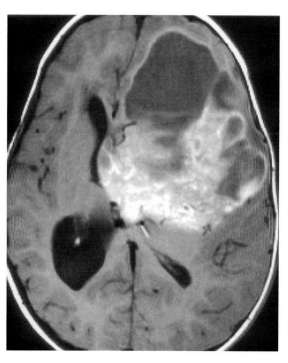

Grade III Astrocytoma
(same patient as Case 79)

Most malignant gliomas demonstrate definite contrast enhancement. However, the pattern of abnormal enhancement can be quite variable.

In some anaplastic astrocytomas, contrast enhancement is surprisingly circumscribed and homogeneous. A nodular morphology may predominate, resembling Cases 95 and 96 (see Case 106).

More characteristic of malignant gliomas is the irregular, thick-walled peripheral enhancement, illustrated in Case 97 (see also Case 711). The nonenhancing center of the tumor may gradually fill in with contrast material on delayed scans.

Complex mixed cystic and solid patterns are also common, as in Case 98 (see also Cases 104 and 105). Areas of intense nodular enhancement are often combined with rim-enhancing zones to give a coarsely heterogeneous appearance.

A contrast-enhanced scan performed within days after surgery for a malignant glioma is useful (1) to assess completeness of resection and (2) as a baseline to evaluate subsequent tumor recurrence. Benign, reactive enhancement at the margins of resection is usually minimal until late in the first week after surgery. As a result, prominent nodules of abnormal enhancement on early postoperative scans suggest residual tumor (which in turn correlates with early local recurrence and poor prognosis). Once developed, benign enhancement at the borders of tumor resection may normally persist for several months.

Case 99

37-year-old woman presenting with a seizure.
(axial, postcontrast scan; SE 1000/20)

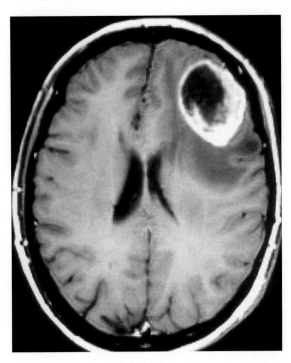

Metastatic Melanoma

Case 100

80-year-old woman being evaluated for
a possible stroke.
(axial, postcontrast scan; SE 600/15)

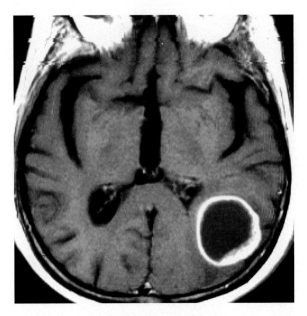

Glioblastoma Multiforme

A thick rim of contrast enhancement is not specific for malignant glial neoplasms. Metastases, as in Case 99, and CNS lymphoma (especially in immunocompromised patients; see Cases 323 and 324) may present a similar appearance.

When a lesion's rim of enhancement is relatively uniform in thickness and contour, inflammatory masses (e.g., abscess or toxoplasmosis) should be included in the differential diagnosis (see Cases 411, 412, and 421).

Both frontal lobe lesions and posterior parietal masses may become quite large without causing specific neurological deficits. A gradual change in alertness or orientation of an elderly patient may reach a threshold of detection that mimics the clinical presentation of a cerebrovascular accident.

Case 101

12-year-old boy presenting with headaches.
(coronal, postcontrast scan; SE 600/15)

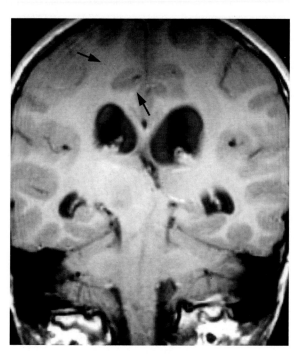

Grade III Astrocytoma

Case 102

54-year-old man presenting with seizures.
(axial, postcontrast scan; SE 600/20)

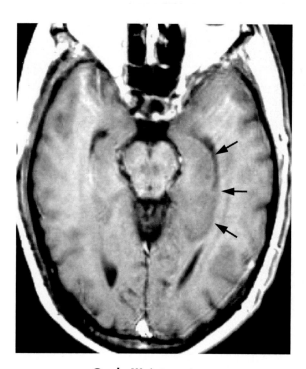

Grade III Astrocytoma

Occasional high grade gliomas do not demonstrate significant contrast enhancement. This behavior is most frequently associated with deep hemisphere lesions of dense cellularity. Specific locations where poorly enhancing malignant gliomas may be seen include the thalamus (as in Case 101) and the medial temporal lobe (as in Case 102).

The thalamic mass in Case 101 has obstructed the posterior third ventricle and aqueduct causing hydrocephalus. The glioma in Case 102 widens the left parahippocampal gyrus.

The medial temporal lobe may be involved by low or high grade gliomas in children or adults. (Cases 69, 71 and 78 present other examples.) Astrocytomas in this location tend to be relatively isointense to adjacent cortex on T1- and T2-weighted scans, with little contrast enhancement. As a result, their diagnosis may depend on careful observation of subtle mass effect in the region of the uncus and parahippocampal gyrus.

Case 103

5-year-old boy.
(coronal, noncontrast scan; SE 800/16)

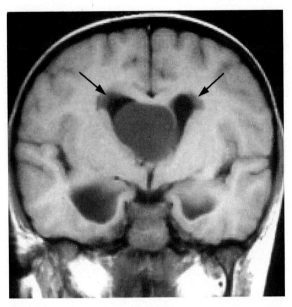

Cystic Astrocytoma
(grade II)

Case 104

66-year-old man.
(coronal, postcontrast scan; SE 800/15)

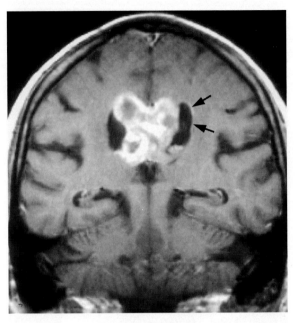

Glioblastoma Multiforme

As illustrated in Cases 93 and 94, gliomas of the corpus callosum frequently extend into the septum pellucidum. Less commonly, gliomas arise from or are centered in this structure.

The midline cystic glioma in Case 103 could be confused with a number of other lesions. Benign cysts of the septum pellucidum occur but usually demonstrate intensity values comparable to CSF. Colloid cysts of the third ventricle may reach this size and have long T1 values (see Cases 256-261), but the mass in Case 103 is centered above the roof of the third ventricle. Similarly, the location of the lesion as demonstrated by the coronal MR plane is superior to the normal range of cranipharyngiomas (which are occasionally found within the third ventricle but not above it).

Functionally, the cystic septal glioma in Case 103 has acted like a colloid cyst, obstructing the foramina of Monro to cause bilateral hydrocpehalus. A small amount of periventricular edema caps the frontal horns bilaterally *(arrows)*.

In Case 104, a solid glioma expands the posterior portion of the septum pellucidum. The pattern of thick, heterogeneous contrast enhancement is typical for a malignant glial neoplasm. (Compare to the homogeneous enhancement of the low grade callosal/septal astrocytoma in Case 95.) The tumor invades the corpus callosum, and there is subtle evidence of subependymal extension on the left *(arrows)*.

Central neurocytomas (see Case 308) are commonly attached to the septum pellucidum and should be considered in the differential diagnosis of a septal mass.

Additional septal gliomas are presented in Cases 310 and 759.

Case 105

26-year-old man presenting with seizures.
(axial, postcontrast scan; SE 700/15)

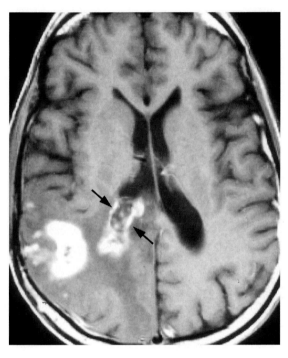

Glioblastoma Multiforme
(recurrent)

Case 106

32-year-old woman presenting with left arm
numbness and blurred vision.
(coronal, postcontrast scan; SE 600/15)

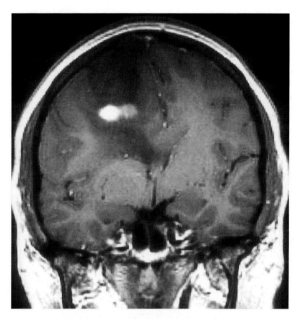

Grade III Astrocytoma

Gliomas may extend from the cerebral surface to the ventricular margin. In Case 105, mass-like areas of abnormal contrast enhancement within hemispheric tissue are accompanied by subependymal extension of enhancing tumor *(arrows)*.

Enhancement along ventricular margins may be due to inflammatory ventriculitis (see Case 389) or to subependymal neoplasm. Gliomas and ependymomas are primary considerations in the latter category because of their frequent periventricular location. Metastases from systemic solid tumors (especially oat cell carcinoma of the lung, melanoma, and breast carcinoma) can also cause a periventricular cast of tumor. Primary CNS lymphoma (see Cases 319 and 320) or secondary brain involvement by systemic lymphoma (see Case 390) may present a similar appearance.

Case 106 demonstrates a broad band of abnormal tissue extending from the vertex to the lateral ventricle. The nodules of contrast enhancement near the center of the lesion occupy only a small portion of the infiltrating neoplasm.

Case 107

36-year-old man presenting with increasing
confusion and seizures.
(coronal, noncontrast scan; SE 3000/90)

Case 108

57-year-old woman presenting with agitation
and aphasia.
(axial, noncontrast scan; SE 3000/45)

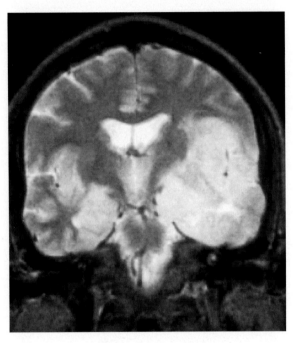

Gliomatosis Cerebri

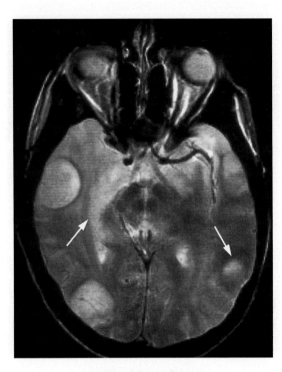

Multicentric Glioma

Occasional patients present with extensive, bihemispheral involvement by gliomatous infiltration. In most of these cases, there is microscopic continuity of tumor linking the affected areas, and the widespread process may be called "gliomatosis cerebri." In other instances, the multiple sites of tumor involvement appear to be radiographically and pathologically distinct. Cases of such "multicentric glioma" are probably rare, reflecting a generalized neoplastic susceptibility rather than extensive infiltration from a single source.

Patients with gliomatosis cerebri are often clinically problematic, with vague and generalized symptoms. In this uncertain context the widespread involvement apparent on imaging studies such as Case 107 may raise consideration of encephalitis or other inflammatory disorders (compare to Cases 387, 396, and 432). The lesions of gliomatosis cerebri often enhance minimally if at all, compounding the diagnostic confusion.

In Case 108, the multiple masses are widely separated and appear discontinuous. They are also better defined than most cases of gliomatosis cerebri.

Primary CNS lymphoma should be considered in the differential diagnosis of bihemispheral infiltrating disease (see Cases 311 and 318).

DIFFERENTIAL DIAGNOSIS:
MULTIPLE SUPERFICIAL INTRACRANIAL MASSES

Case 109

57-year-old woman presenting with confusion.
(axial, postcontrast scan; SE 700/17)

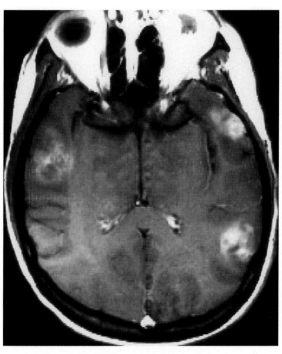

Multicentric Glioma
(same patient as Case 108)

Case 110

28-year-old woman presenting with headaches.
(axial, postcontrast scan; SE 1000/15)

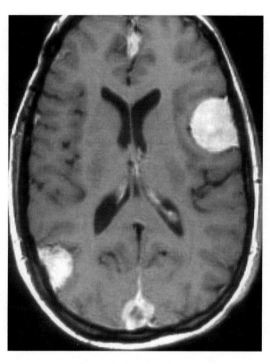

Meningiomas
(in neurofibromatosis type 2)

Although metastatic and inflammatory diseases are more common causes of multiple intracranial masses, meningiomas and gliomas should be considered in the differential diagnosis. Primary CNS lymphoma may also present in this manner (see Cases 311 and 318).

The gliomas in Case 109 are similar in location and definition to the meningiomas in Case 110. Differences in the pattern and intensity of contrast enhancement usually help to distinguish superficial intraaxial lesions from invaginating extraaxial masses.

Case 111

26-year-old woman presenting with seizures.
(sagittal, noncontrast scan; SE 600/17)

Case 112

53-year-old man presenting with severe headaches.
(axial, noncontrast scan; SE 2800/45)

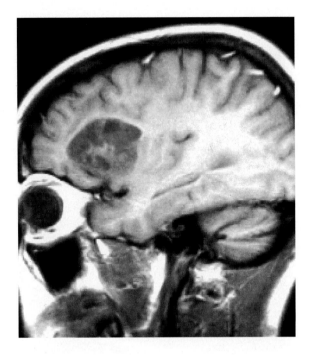

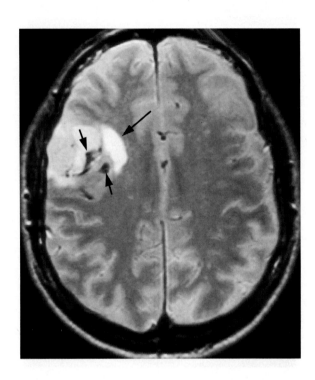

Oligodendrogliomas are much less common than astrocytomas, accounting for about 5% of primary gliomas. The frontal lobe is a characteristic location for these lesions. Up to 50% of patients with oligodendrogliomas present with seizures.

The typical MR appearance of oligodendrogliomas is coarsely heterogeneous, as illustrated in Cases 111 and 112. Both calcification and hemorrhage are more common in oligodendrogliomas than in astrocytomas, often accompanied by focal necrosis and cyst formation. These pathological features correlate with the characteristically mixed signal in-

tensity of the lesions on MR studies. The margins of the tumor are usually well defined, with variable surrounding edema.

Small zones of low signal intensity within the mass in Case 112 *(short arrows)* matched dense calcifications on a preceding CT scan. The high intensity region at the medial border of the tumor *(long arrow)* was cystic at surgery.

Compare Case 112 to the equally complex and more aggressive-looking glioblastoma in Case 82 and to the hemorrhagic infarct in Case 481.

Case 113

34-year-old woman presenting with headaches.
(axial, postcontrast scan; SE 800/15)

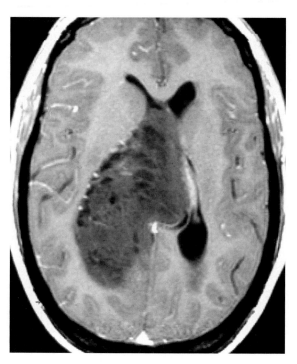

Grade III Astrocytoma

Case 114

61-year-old woman presenting with incoordination
of the left arm and leg.
(axial, noncontrast scan; SE 700/17)

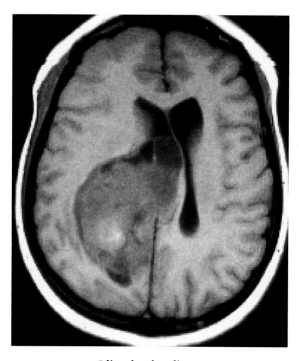

Oligodendroglioma

Several members of the glioma family can give rise to periventricular and intraventricular masses. As illustrated previously in this chapter, astrocytomas may be encountered at any depth within the cerebral hemisphere. The intraventricular mass in Case 113 is another example of a minimally enhancing high grade glioma. Multiple small cysts within the tumor were confirmed at surgery.

The oligodendroglioma in Case 114 has grown into the body of the lateral ventricle. Cystic zones are seen within the anterior portion of the mass. Vague T1-shortening is present posteriorly, probably reflecting hemorrhage and/or fine calcification. The overall appearance is very similar to Case 113.

Ependymomas may also arise within or in proximity to the ventricular system, as seen in Case 115. The differential diagnosis of intraventricular tumors should additionally include giant cell astrocytoma (see Cases 756 and 757) and central neurocytoma (see Case 308). Choroid plexus papillomas are rarely encountered in the lateral ventricles of adults (see Cases 299-303). Intraventricular meningiomas are usually more homogeneous masses (see Cases 64 and 65). Periventricular lymphomas might be considered in the differential diagnosis but would be expected to demonstrate prominent contrast enhancement (see Cases 319 and 320).

An intraventricular location allows a tumor to enlarge by displacing CSF, with relatively little mass effect on adjacent parenchyma. However, eventual ventricular obstruction can lead to rapidly increasing intracranial pressure.

Case 115A

22-year-old woman presenting with headaches, nausea, and episodic diplopia.
(sagittal, noncontrast scan; SE 600/20)

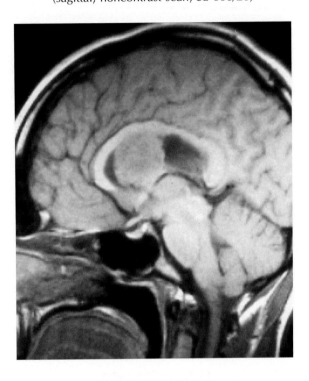

Case 115B

Same patient.
(axial, noncontrast scan; SE 2500/45)

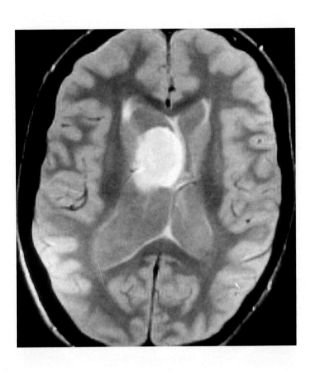

About one third of intracranial ependymomas occur in the supratentorial compartment. Supratentorial ependymomas may be found in children or adults, adjacent to the ventricular system or within cerebral parenchyma. (See Cases 152-157 for examples of the more common fourth ventricular ependymomas in children.)

In Case 115 the mass is entirely intraventricular, occupying the anterior body and frontal horn of the right lateral ventricle. This tumor is unusually homogeneous; many ependymomas contain cysts and calcification. Such heterogeneous intraventricular ependymomas mimic the appearance of oligodendrogliomas or central neurocytomas, as in Cases 114 and 308.

Subependymomas may also present as masses within the lateral ventricles and are typically well defined and homogeneous. A subependymoma of the lateral ventricle would be somewhat unusual in a 27-year-old woman (but see Case 118). Most subependymomas involve the fourth ventricle in older patients (especially men).

Contrast enhancement within ependymomas is variable. Case 309 presents a postcontrast scan of the above lesion.

High signal intensity in the region of parietal cortex bilaterally in Case 115B is artifactual.

Case 116

4-year-old girl presenting with a seizure.
(axial, noncontrast scan; SE 2000/90)

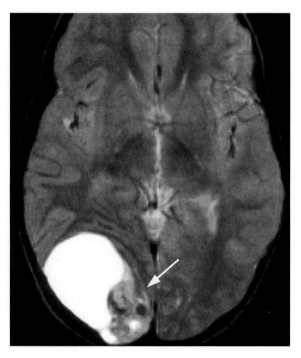

Cystic Ependymoma

Case 117

2-year-old girl presenting with nausea
and vomiting.
(axial, noncontrast scan; SE 2500/25)

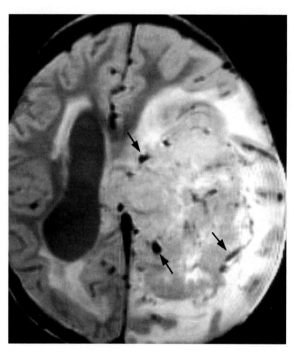

Malignant Ependymoma

Unlike posterior fossa ependymomas, supratentorial ependymomas are often parenchyma (i.e., not related to the ventricular system) and may be grossly cystic, as seen in Case 116. A mural nodule *(arrow)* is present at the posterior margin of the tumor cyst. Tissue within the nodule is heterogeneous, with areas of low signal intensity suggesting hemorrhage or calcification. The lesion is not adjacent to the ventricular system, having presumably arisen from an ependymal rest within the hemisphere. Both the occipital lobe location and the cystic nature of this mass are common for parenchymal supratentorial ependymomas in children.

In Case 117, an aggressive-looking mass fills and expands the left lateral ventricle. Extensive hemispheric edema suggests parenchymal invasion. Large "flow voids" within the tumor *(arrows)* imply that it is highly vascular.

The combination of these features favors a malignant lesion. In a 2-year-old child, the leading diagnostic possibilities would include a choroid plexus neoplasm (carcinoma or aggressive papilloma; see Case 299) and malignant ependymoma.

Periventricular edema is present along the margins of the hydrocephalic right lateral ventricle in Case 117.

Case 118A

42-year-old woman presenting with headaches.
(sagittal, noncontrast scan; SE 600/15)

Case 118B

Same patient.
(axial, noncontrast scan; SE 2600/45)

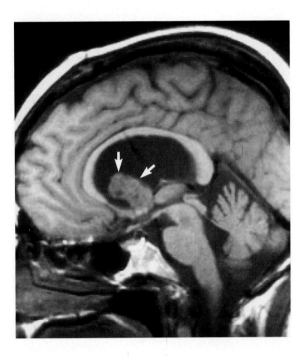

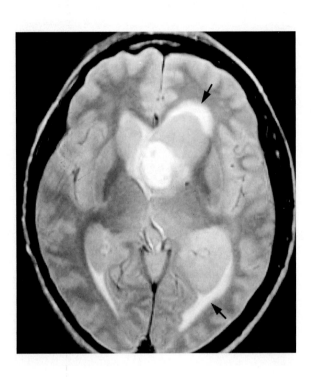

Subependymomas are low grade glial neoplasms arising along the ventricular margins. Histological examination often demonstrates a mixture of ependymal and astrocytic cell types. Most subependymomas are incidental masses found by imaging or autopsy. They most commonly involve the fourth ventricle in older patients, with a male predominance.

The tumors are rarely symptomatic unless they grow to obstruct CSF pathways. In this case, the mass has blocked the foramen of Monro, presenting like a colloid cyst (compare to Cases 256-259). Periventricular edema is present *(arrows,* Case 118B) due to hydrocephalus.

The mildly lobulated contour of the mass in Case 118A is typical of subependymomas, but choroid plexus papillomas or subependymal giant cell astrocytomas can have a similar appearance (compare to Cases 302 and 756). Relatively homogeneous high signal intensity is common on long TR images. Occasional subependymomas contain cysts and calcification causing more heterogeneity. Such tumors may resemble ependymomas or central neurocytomas (see Case 308).

Contrast enhancement within subependymomas is usually mild or absent. Case 673 presents a postcontrast scan of the above lesion.

PLEOMORPHIC XANTHOASTROCYTOMAS

Case 119A

16-year-old boy presenting with seizures.
(axial, noncontrast scan; SE 2500/90)

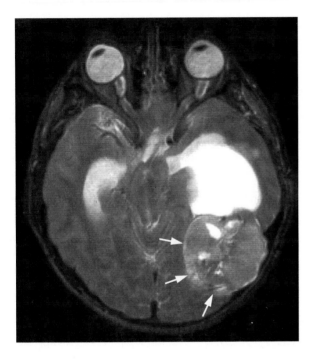

Case 119B

Same patient.
(sagittal, postcontrast scan; SE 600/20)

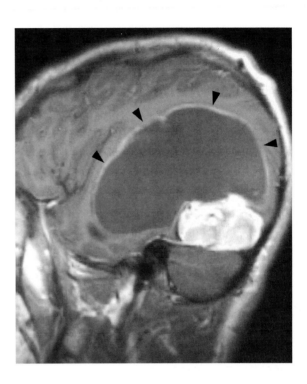

Pleomorphic xanthoastrocytoma is a glioma subtype that occurs in young patients and is usually associated with a good prognosis. The clinical picture is typically one of seizures in an adolescent or young adult. Characteristic imaging features include a superficial location in the temporal lobe, calcification, and cyst formation. Histological examination demonstrates lipid-laden cytoplasm within tumor cells.

Case 119 is a good example of a cystic tumor with a mural nodule. Note that both the nodule and the perimeter of the cyst *(arrowheads)* demonstrate contrast enhancement.

Two other unusual primary tumors may present similar clinical and imaging features. Gangliogliomas contain a mixture of glial and neuronal cells. These tumors may occur in any location above or below the tentorium (see Case 135) but are most commonly encountered in the temporal lobes of young adults. Cyst formation and calcification are common. The prognosis is usually good following tumor resection.

Dysembryoplastic neuroepithelial tumors (DNET) have recently been recognized as another neoplasm often affecting the temporal lobe in young patients and carrying a relatively good prognosis. These masses probably originate from subpial granular cells of the cortex. They commonly present as superficial lesions with long T1 and T2 values and little contrast enhancement in children or adolescents with seizures. Calcification and cysts have been reported in some cases. Recurrence after surgery is infrequent, and radiation therapy is usually not indicated.

REFERENCES

Albert FK, Forsting M, Sartor, K, et al: Early postoperative magnetic resonance imaging after resection of malignant glioma: objective evaluation of residual tumor and its influence on regrowth and prognosis. *Neurosurgery* 34:45-61, 1994.

Altman NR: MR and CT characteristics of gangliocytoma: a rare cause of epilepsy in children. *AJNR* 9:917-921, 1988.

Artico M, Bardella L, Ciapetta P, Raco A: Surgical treatment of subependymomas of the central nervous system. *Acta Neurochir (Wien)* 98:25-31, 1989.

Atlas SW: Adult supratentorial tumors. *Semin Roentgenol* 25:130-154, 1990.

Atlas SW, Grossman RI, Gomori JM, et al: Hemorrhagic intracranial malignant neoplasms: spin-echo MR imaging. *Radiology* 164:71-77, 1987.

Barnard RO, Geddes JF: The incidence of multifocal gliomas: a histologic study of large hemisphere sections. *Cancer* 60:1519-1531, 1987.

Benitez WI, Glasier CM, Husain M, et al: MR findings in childhood gangliogliomas. *J Comput Assist Tomogr* 14:712-716, 1990.

Bird C, Drayer B, Medina M, et al: Gd-DTPA enhanced MR imaging in pediatric patients after brain tumor resection. *Radiology* 169:123, 1988.

Castillo C, Davis PC, Takei Y, Hoffman JC Jr: Intracranial gangliomas: MR, CT, and clinical findings in 18 patients. *AJNR* 11:109-114, 1990.

Castillo M, Scatliff JH, Bouldin TW, Sowki K: Radiologic-pathologic correlation: intracranial astrocytoma. *AJNR* 13:1609-1616, 1992.

Claussen C, Laniado M, Schorner W, et al: Gadolinium-DTPA in Mr imaging of glioblastoma and intracranial metastases. *AJNR* 6:669-674, 1985.

Dean BL, Drayer BP, Bird CR, et al: Gliomas: classification with MR imaging. *Radiology* 174:411-415, 1990.

Destian S, Sze G, Krol G, et al: MR imaging of hemorrhagic intracranial neoplasms. *AJNR* 9:1115-1122, 1988.

Dolinskas CA, Simeone FA: CT characteristics of intraventricular oligodendrogliomas. *AJNR* 8:1077-1082, 1987.

Earnest F IV, Kelly PI, Scheithauer BW, et al: Cerebral astrocytomas: histopathologic correlation of MR and CT contrast enhancement with stereotactic biopsy. *Radiology* 166:823-827, 1988.

Elster AD, DiPersio DA: Cranial postoperative site: assessment with contrast-enhanced MR imaging. *Radiology* 174:93-98, 1990.

Forsting M, Albert FK, Kunze S, et al: Extirpation of glioblastomas: MR and CT follow-up of residual tumor and regrowth patterns. *AJNR* 14:77-87, 1993.

Graff PA, Albright AL, Pang D: Dissemination of supratentorial malignant gliomas via the cerebrospinal fluid in children. *Neurosurgery* 30:64-71, 1992.

Graif M, Bydder GM, Steiner RE, et al: Contrast-enhanced MR imaging of malignant brain tumors. *AJNR* 6:855-862, 1985.

Hashimoto M, Fujimoto K, Shinoda S, Masuzawa T: Magnetic resonance imaging of glanglion cell tumors. *Neuroradiology* 35:181-184, 1993.

Haustain J, Laniado M, Niendorf H-P, et al: Administration of Gadopentetate Dimeglumine in MR imaging of intracranial tumors: dosage and field strength. *AJNR* 13:1199-1206, 1992.

Heinz ER, Crain BJ, Radtke RA, et al: MR imaging in patients with temporal lobe seizures: correlation of results with pathologic findings. *AJNR* 11:827-832, 1990.

Johnson PC, Hunt SJ, Drayer BP: Human cerebral gliomas: correlation of postmortem MR imaging and neuropathologic findings. *Radiology* 170:211-218.

Kepes JJ: Pleomorphic xanthoastrocytoma: the birth of a diagnosis and a concept. *Brain Pathol* 3:269-274, 1993.

Kim DG, Han MH, Lee SH, et al: MRI of intracranial subependymoma: report of a case. *Neuroradiology* 35:185-186, 1993.

Kondziolka D, Lunsford LD, Martinez AJ: Unreliability of contemporary neurodiagnostic imaging in evaluating suspected adult supratentorial (low-grade) astrocytoma. *J Neurosurg* 79:533-536, 1993.

Koslow SA, Claassen D, Hirsch WL, Jungreis CA: Gliomatosis cerebri: a case report with autopsy correlation. *Neuroradiology* 34:331-333, 1992.

Lee BCP, Kneeland JB, Cahill PT, Deck MDF: MR recognition of supratentorial tumors. *AJNR* 6:871-878, 1985.

Lee Y-Y, Van Tassel P: Intracranial oligodendrogliomas: imaging findings in 35 untreated cases. *AJNR* 10:119-127, 1989.

Lee Y-Y, Van Tassel P, Bruner JM, et al: Juvenile pilocytic astrocytomas: CT and MR characteristics. *AJNR* 10:363-370, 1989.

Lipper MH, Eberhard DA, Phillips CD, Vezina L-G, et al: *AJNR* 14:1397-1404, 1993.

Lunsford LD, Martinez AJ, Latchaw RE: Magnetic resonance imaging does not define tumor boundaries. *Acta Radiol [Suppl]* 369:154-156, 1986.

MacKay IM, Bydder GM, Young IR: MR imaging of central nervous system tumors that do not display increase in T1 or T2. *J Comput Assist Tomogr* 9:1055-1061, 1985.

Madison MT, Hall WA, Latchaw RE, Loes DJ: Radiologic diagnosis, staging, and follow-up of adult central nervous system primary malignant glioma. *Radiol Clin North Am* 32:183-196, 1994.

Margetts JC, Kalyan-Raman VP: Giant-celled glioblastomas of brain: a clinical pathological and radiological study of ten cases (including immunohistochemistry and ultrastructure). *Cancer* 63:524-531, 1989.

Palma L, Guidetti B: Cystic pilocytic astrocytomas of the cerebral hemispheres. *J Neurosurg* 62:811-815, 1985.

Palma L, Celli P, Cantore G: Supratentorial ependymomas of the first two decades of life: long-term follow-up of 20 cases (including two subependymomas). *Neurosurgery* 32:169-175, 1993.

Partlow GD, del Carpio-O-Donovan R, Melanson D, Peters, TM: Bilateral thalamic glioma: review of eight cases with personality change and mental deterioration. *AJNR* 13:1225-1230, 1992.

Rippe DJ, Boyko OB, Fuller GN, et al: Gadopentetate-dimiglumine-enhanced MR imaging of gliomatosis cerebri: appearance mimicking leptomeningeal tumor dissemination. *AJNR* 11:800-801, 1990.

Ross IB, Robitaille Y, Villemure J-G, Tampieri D: Diagnosis and management of gliomatosis cerebri: recent trends. *Surg Neurol* 36:431-440, 1991.

Shaw EG, Scheithauer BW, O'Fallon JR, et al: Oligodendrogliomas: the Mayo clinic experience. *J Neurosurg* 76:428-434, 1992.

Shin YM, Chang KH, Han MH, Myung NH, et al: Gliomatosis cerebri: comparison of MR and CT features. *AJR* 161:859-862, 1993.

Spagnoli MV, Grossman RI, Packer RJ, et al: Magnetic resonance determination of gliomatosis cerebri. *Neuroradiology* 29:15-18, 1987.

Spoto GP, Press GA, Hesselink JR, Solomon M: Intracranial ependymoma and subependymoma: MR manifestations. *AJNR* 11:83-91, 1990.

Strong JA, Hatten HP Jr, Brown MT, et al: Pilocytic astrocytoma: correlation between the initial imaging features and clinical aggressiveness. *AJR* 161:369-372, 1993.

Tampieri D, Moumdjian R, Melanson D, Ethier R: Intracerebral gangliogliomas in patients with partial complex seizures, CT and MR findings. *AJNR* 12:749-755, 1991.

Tervonen O, Forbes G, Scheithauer BW, Dietz MJ: Diffuse "fibrillary" astrocytomas: correlation of MRI features with histopathologic parameters and tumor grade. *Neuroradiology* 34:173-178, 1992.

Tice H, Barnes PD, Goumnerova L, Scott RM, et al: *AJNR* 14:1293-1300, 1993.

Tien RD, Cardenas CA, Rajagopalan S: Pleomorphic xanthoastrocytoma of the brain: MR findings in six patients. *AJR* 159:1287-1290, 1992.

Tien RD, Felsberg GJ, Friedman H, et al: MR imaging of high grade cerebral gliomas: value of diffusion-weighted echoplanar pulse sequences. *AJR* 162:671-677, 1994.

Tsuchiya K, Makita K, Furui S, Nitta K: MRI appearance of calcified regions within intracranial tumors. *Neuroradiology* 35:341-344, 1993.

Watanabe M, Tanaka R, Takeda N: Magnetic resonance imaging and histopathology of cerebral gliomas. *Neuroradiology* 35:463-469, 1992.

Yanaka K, Kamozaki T, Kobayashi E, et al: MR imaging of diffuse glioma. *AJNR* 13:349-351, 1992.

Yoshino MT, Lucio R: Pleomorphic xanthoastrocytoma. *AJNR* 13:1330-1332, 1992.

Yuh WTC, Nguyen HD, Tali ET, et al: Delineation of gliomas with various doses of MR contrast material. *AJNR* 15:983-989, 1994.

CHAPTER 4

Tumors of the Posterior Fossa

Case 120

9-year-old boy presenting with diplopia.
(sagittal, noncontrast scan; SE 600/17)

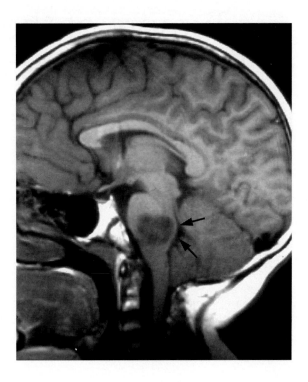

Case 121

9-year-old girl presenting with headaches
and dysphagia.
(sagittal, noncontrast scan; SE 600/17)

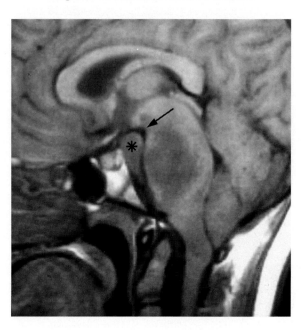

Gliomas cause the great majority of brainstem masses in children. Metastases, vascular malformations, and inflammatory disorders are more common in adults.

Brainstem gliomas in children are heterogeneous clinically and radiographically. The margins of the tumors may be well defined or indistinct. In Case 120, the pons is expanded in anteroposterior diameter by a sharply demarcated mass of low signal intensity. The normally linear floor of the fourth ventricle is convex posteriorly *(arrows)*.

Case 121 demonstrates expansion of the entire brainstem with compression and displacement of the fourth ventricle. Poorly defined low signal intensity continues caudally through the foramen magnum to involve the cervical spinal cord. In addition, exophytic tumor extends ventrally in the prepontine region *(*)*, projecting anterior to the "flow void" of the basilar artery *(arrow)*. Bilateral anterior exophytic extension of pontine gliomas may surround and encase the basilar artery (see Case 123).

Although many brainstem gliomas demonstrate prolongation of T1 as seen above, other tumors may be isointense on short TR images. High signal intensity within the brainstem on noncontrast T1-weighted scans suggests hemorrhage within a tumor or the alternative diagnosis of a vascular malformation (especially cavernous hemangioma; see Case 637).

The location of childhood gliomas within the brainstem correlates with prognosis. Focal tumors of the midbrain and medulla are associated with longer average survival than pontine or diffuse gliomas.

The cerebellar tonsils in Cases 120 and 121 are peg-shaped as they extend below the plane of the foramen magnum *(arrows)*, possibly representing Chiari I malformations rather than herniation (compare to Cases 128 and 130).

Case 122

3-year-old boy presenting with gait abnormality.
(axial, noncontrast scan; SE 2500/30)

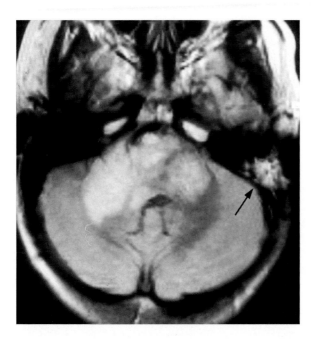

Case 123

15-year-old girl presenting with diplopia, facial
weakness, nausea, and vomiting.
(axial, noncontrast scan; SE 3000/75)

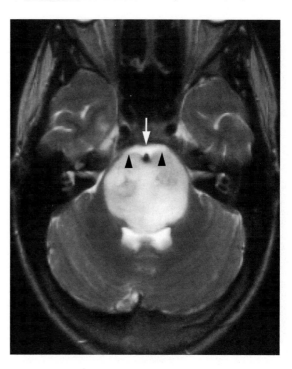

Most brainstem gliomas are readily detected on long TR spin echo images due to prominent high signal intensity. The pattern may be patchy, as in Case 122, or confluent, as in Case 123. Expansion of the pons is apparent in both cases. Case 123 illustrates bilateral anterior, exophytic extension of the glioma into the prepontine cistern *(arrowheads);* the basilar artery *(arrow)* is partially surrounded by tumor.

Occasionally, a demyelinating process involves the brainstem in young patients, causing multifocal or diffuse edema that can mimic a glioma. Multiple sclerosis and acute disseminated encephalomyelitis may both present in this manner. Relatively rapid onset of symptoms, accompanying cerebral lesions, and an inflammatory CSF profile help to distinguish such cases from brainstem neoplasms.

Neurofibromatosis type 1 may be associated with patchy areas of high signal intensity within the brainstem and cerebellar peduncles on T2-weighted images (see Cases 766 and 767). These lesions usually represent immature or disorganized tissue rather than true neoplasms. They generally do not demonstrate mass effect or abnormal contrast enhancement.

Left mastoid air cells are opacified by fluid and/or mucosal thickening in Case 122 *(arrow).*

Case 124

10-year-old boy shunted for hydrocephalus,
previously attributed to benign aqueductal stenosis.
(sagittal, noncontrast scan; SE 600/17)

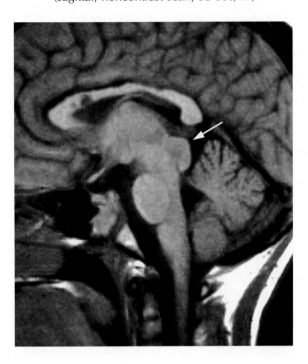

Case 125

15-year-old girl presenting with headaches
and papilledema.
(axial, noncontrast scan; SE 3000/90)

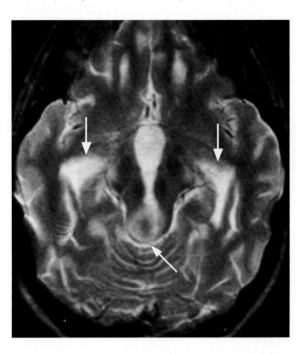

Some brainstem gliomas are focal, low grade lesions. Many of these tumors are relatively isodense on CT scans and isointense on T1-weighted MR images. Their detection is based on distortion of anatomy and/or abnormal signal intensity on T2-weighted scans.

In Case 124, a small glioma expands the midbrain tectum *(arrow)*, bulging into the quadrigeminal cistern. (Compare the diameter and morphology of the dorsal midbrain to Case 126.) The localized mass effect of the tumor effaces the aqueduct and accounts for the history of hydrocephalus. "Benign" aqueductal stenosis (see Cases 659 and 660) should be a diagnosis of exclusion after careful examination of the midbrain, best performed by MR.

Case 125 illustrates another focal glioma involving the midbrain tectum, a common location for these low grade tumors. The dorsal midbrain is expanded, with mass effect obstructing the junction of the aqueduct and third ventricle. (Compare to the appearance of pineal masses in Cases 272-280.)

Other pathologies may present as focal brainstem lesions. Cavernous hemangiomas usually demonstrate complex signal intensity with components of short T1 and short T2 (see Case 637), distinguishing them from most brainstem gliomas. Metastases to the brainstem are often accompanied by edema and typically enhance more intensely than brainstem gliomas (see Cases 21 and 638). Demyelinating disease most frequently involves the pons or middle cerebellar peduncles (see Cases 355 to 358), and is often multifocal with a suggestive clinical context. Pineal lesions occupying the quadrigeminal cistern may resemble a dorsal midbrain mass (see Cases 270 and 271).

A small area of low signal within the anterior body of the corpus callosum in Case 124 is related to prior shunting. Hydrocephalic expansion of the temporal horns is apparent in Case 125 *(upper arrows)*.

Case 126

2-year-old girl whose parents reported
a stumbling gait.
(sagittal, noncontrast scan; SE 700/17)

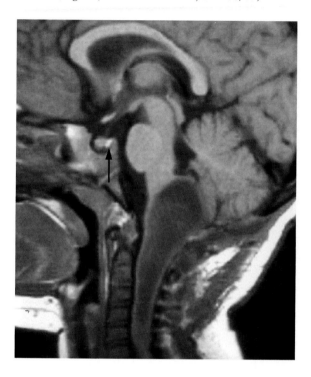

Case 127

7-year-old girl presenting with a right sixth nerve
palsy and asymmetrical reflexes.
(axial, postcontrast scan; SE 700/15)

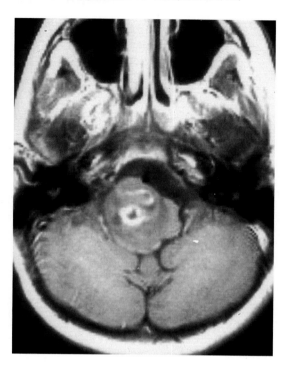

Gliomas may involve the medulla with sparing of the more rostral brainstem. Such tumors are often dorsally exophytic, as illustrated in Case 126. The decussation of fiber tracts at the pontomedullary junction is a relative barrier to the superior growth of a low grade tumor, which may instead bulge posteriorly into the vallecula, deforming the caudal fourth ventricle. The mass in Case 126 extends well into the cervical spinal cord, a common feature of medullary gliomas.

Despite the homogeneously low signal intensity of the tumor in Case 126, it was found to be solid at surgery. Many astrocytomas of the posterior fossa and cerebral hemispheres demonstrate uniform regions of long T1 and long T2 values that represent homogeneously hydrated tissue rather than true cysts (see also Cases 132 and 149). The diagnosis of a cystic neoplasm can be made when a sedi-

mentation level is observed but should not be otherwise presumed.

Case 127 illustrates a ventrally exophytic glioma of the medulla. Such tumors can accumulate in the prepontine or cerebellopontine angle cisterns, mimicking an extraaxial mass (see Case 158).

Contrast enhancement of brainstem gliomas is variable in extent and morphology. Both peripheral and solid zones of enhancement can be seen, while other tumor areas may demonstrate no accumulation of contrast material. Case 127 is a typical example of moderate, heterogeneous enhancement within a brainstem tumor.

Case 126 illustrates the normal "bright spot" in the posterior portion of the sella turcica representing the neurophypophysis (*arrow*; see Cases 221 and 222).

Case 128

4-year-old girl presenting with clumsiness
and headaches
(sagittal, noncontrast scan; SE 700/17)

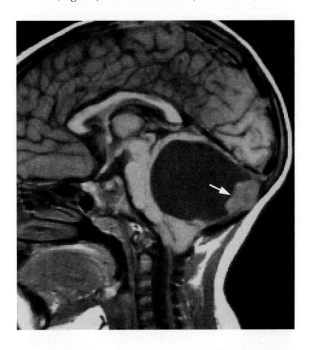

Case 129

14-year-old boy presenting with headaches and
blurred vision.
(axial, noncontrast scan; SE 3000/90)

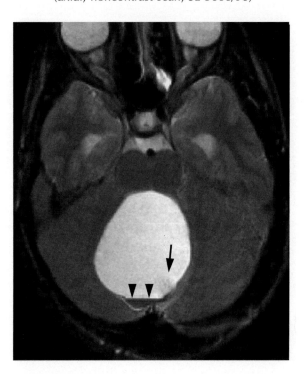

Gliomas of the cerebellum are among the most common posterior fossa tumors in children. Most of these "juvenile cerebellar astrocytomas" are histologically "pilocytic," correlating with benign behavior and a relatively good prognosis.

The majority of such cerebellar astrocytomas are cystic. A discrete mural nodule of tumor tissue is often present at the margin of the cyst, as seen clearly in Case 128 and faintly in Case 129 *(arrows)*. In other cases, the entire perimeter of the cyst is lined by a layer of tumor (see Cases 130 and 131). Mural nodules at the margin of cystic cerebellar astrocytomas typically enhance, sometimes mimicking the appearance of hemangioblastomas (see Cases 138 and 140). A small sedimentation level is present at the posterior margin of the mass in Case 129 *(arrowheads),* confirming its cystic nature.

The tumor cyst in Case 128 was centered in the midline and was mistaken for an enlarged fourth ventricle on an outside CT scan. When hydrocephalus is found on CT studies, it is important to carefully examine the third and fourth ventricles to distinguish possible enlargement from an obstructing, low attenuation lesion (see also Cases 663 and 664). The multiplanar display of MR is valuable for this purpose.

In both of the above cases the large cerebellar masses have caused anterior displacement and compression of the brainstem. Case 128 demonstrates associated kinking and occlusion of the aqueduct and herniation of the cerebellar tonsils.

A ventriculostomy had been performed prior to the MRI scan in Case 128.

Case 130

7-year-old girl presenting with papilledema.
(sagittal, postcontrast scan; SE 600/20)

Case 131

5-year-old boy presenting with ataxia.
(coronal, postcontrast scan; SE 700/20)

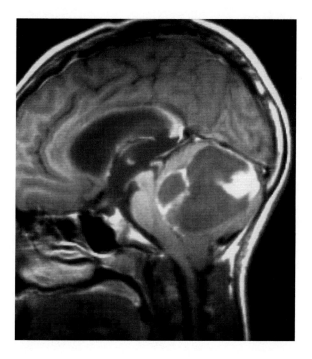

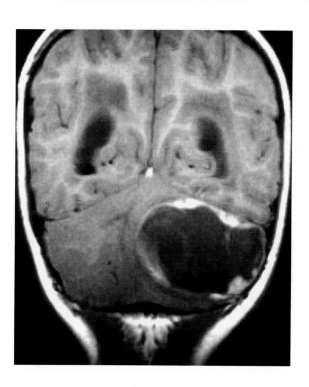

Intense enhancement is often seen along the margins of "benign" cystic cerebellar astrocytomas on MR scans in children. This enhancement is often more impressive than previously demonstrated by CT scanning. The presence of complex peripheral enhancement in these cases does not imply high grade malignancy or poor prognosis, as is more generally true in supratentorial gliomas (see Cases 95 to 98).

Postcontrast scans may also demonstrate otherwise inapparent septations or bands of tumor tissue traversing a large cyst. The two cases above illustrate multilocular cysts, in contrast to the unilocular lesions on the previous page.

The mass in Case 130 causes comparable deformities to Case 128: the posterior fossa is "tight," with flattening of the brainstem against the clivus, displacement and occlusion of the aqueduct, and herniation of the cerebellar tonsils. Associated hydrocephalus causes stretching and thinning of the corpus callosum and inferior bowing of the floor of the third ventricle.

Case 132

16-month-old boy presenting with vomiting and impaired crawling/walking.
(sagittal, noncontrast scan; SE 600/15)

Case 133

8-year-old boy presenting with incoordination.
(axial, postcontrast scan; SE 800/17)

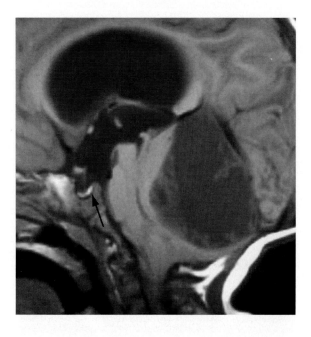

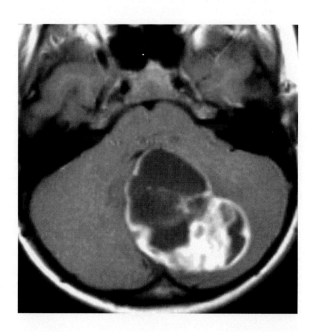

Although cerebellar astrocytomas are commonly cystic, solid masses may be seen in children and adults. The solid nature of some cerebellar astrocytomas is suggested by intermediate signal intensity, heterogeneity, and/or diffuse contrast enhancement (see Cases 151 and 164).

In other instances, homogeneous zones of long T1 and long T2 (as in Case 132) or well-defined nonenhancing areas (as in Case 133) may falsely suggest the presence of cysts. Both of the above tumors were solid at surgery, dem-

onstrating gelatinous tissue with microcystic histology that accounted for the pseudocystic MR appearance. As discussed in Case 126, the diagnosis of a cyst cannot be based on homogeneity of nonenhancing tissue.

The mass effect of these cerebellar tumors is impressive. Compare the diameter of the brainstem in Case 132 to Cases 120 and 121, and compare the brainstem morphology in Case 133 to Case 123.

DIFFERENTIAL DIAGNOSIS:
HETEROGENEOUSLY ENHANCING MASS EFFACING THE FOURTH VENTRICLE

Case 134

30-year-old man presenting with headaches
and ataxia.
(coronal, postcontrast scan; SE 650/15)

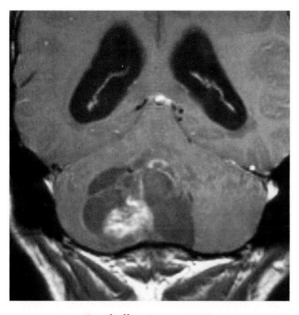

Cerebellar Astrocytoma

Case 135

15-year-old girl presenting with blurred vision and
found to have papilledema.
(coronal, postcontrast scan; SE 600/15)

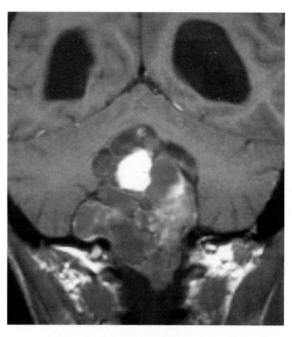

Ganglioglioma of the Brainstem

In both of these cases, a large mass near the midline of the posterior fossa has compressed the fourth ventricle, causing obstructive hydrocephalus. In each case the mass is lobulated and heterogeneous, with enhancing rims and nodules mixed with nonenhancing regions.

Although this appearance is well within the spectrum of cerebellar astrocytomas, it is not specific. The ganglioglioma in Case 135, extending dorsally from the brainstem to occupy and expand the vallecula, is an unusual tumor in the differential diagnosis. Other masses that could present a similar appearance in an adolescent or young adult would include hemangioblastomas of the cerebellum or brainstem and fourth ventricular masses such as ependymomas.

Note the caudal extension of the tumor in Case 135 through the foramen magnum to involve the cervical spinal canal. As illustrated here, the coronal and sagittal planes of MR are ideal for demonstrating lesions that span the craniocervical junction.

Case 136

48-year-old woman presenting with headaches
and ataxia.
(coronal, noncontrast scan; SE 700/16)

Case 137

40-year-old man complaining of neck pain
and arm numbness.
(axial, noncontrast scan; SE 2800/30)

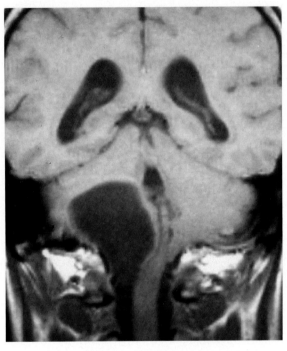

Cerebellar Hemangioblastoma

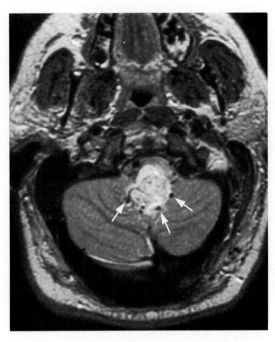

Hemangioblastoma of the Medulla

Hemangioblastomas are relatively uncommon tumors of the posterior fossa and spinal cord, usually seen in adults. These masses are often cystic and highly vascular. An intensely enhancing mural nodule is characteristic.

Clues to the diagnosis on noncontrast scans include the suspicion of a cystic tumor and the presence of prominent vessels within or surrounding the lesion. Case 136 demonstrates a rounded zone of homogeneously long T1 values involving the inferior right cerebellar hemisphere. An enhancing mural nodule was demonstrated on postcontrast scans, and the tumor proved to be grossly cystic at surgery. In Case 137, foci of low signal intensity at the margin of tumor tissue *(arrows)* suggest enlarged arteries or veins and favor a highly vascular neoplasm. (Compare to the discussion of glomus tumors in Cases 185 and 186.)

Another useful diagnostic feature is the usual superficial location of hemangioblastomas. These tumors characteristically arise at the pial surface of the cerebellum or brainstem. Multiplanar MR display is helpful in establishing this relationship.

Hemangioblastomas are among the tumors that may span the craniocervical junction, crowding the foramen magnum and causing occipital or cervical pain (as in Case 137). The foramen magnum should be carefully examined on all MR scans of the neck.

Case 138

46-year-old man presenting with neck pain
and headaches.
(sagittal, postcontrast scan; SE 500/15)

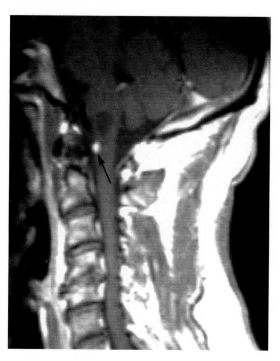

Hemangioblastoma of the Medulla

Case 139

16-year-old boy presenting with nausea
and vomiting.
(coronal, postcontrast scan; SE 600/15)

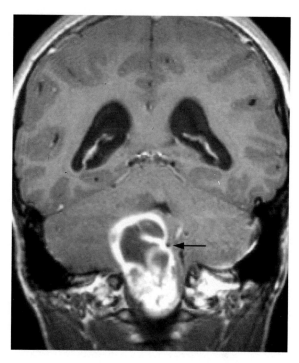

Cerebellar Hemangioblastoma

Intense contrast enhancement is characteristic of hemangioblastomas. The absence of this feature should suggest an alternative diagnosis. Enhancement may be seen throughout a solid hemangioblastoma or at the margin of cystic lesions. Marginal enhancement may occur only within a mural nodule or along the entire perimeter of a cyst.

The tiny nodule of enhancement in Case 138 *(arrow)* is located at one pole of the small, medullary cyst. The morphology of a mural nodule contacting the pial surface is highly suggestive of the diagnosis.

Case 139 presents a more complex hemangioblastoma, with solid tissue and rims of enhancement surrounding and separating several cystic loculations. "Flow voids" due to large vessels *(arrow)* can be identified at the perimeter of the tumor. The mass expands the cerebellar tonsil, which herniates caudally through the foramen magnum (compare to Case 303).

In 10% to 20% of cases, cerebellar hemangioblastomas are a manifestation of Von Hippel-Lindau disease. This neurocutaneous syndrome may also be associated with retinal angiomas, renal or pancreatic cysts, hypernephromas, pheochromocytomas, and hemangioblastomas of the spinal cord. Funduscopic examination and evaluation of the kidneys are warranted when a possible cerebellar hemangioblastoma is discovered.

Hemangioblastomas are often not encapsulated or well circumscribed at surgery or histologically. Postoperative recurrence has been reported in up to 20% of these tumors.

Occasionally, a partially cystic schwannoma within the cerebellopontine angle invaginates far into the adjacent brainstem and/or cerebellum to mimic the appearance of a superficial hemangioblastoma.

Case 140

44-year-old woman presenting with
mild incoordination.
(coronal, postcontrast scan; SE 600/15)

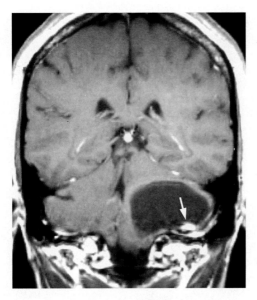

Hemangioblastoma

Case 141

14-year-old boy presenting with headaches
and blurred vision.
(coronal, postcontrast scan; SE 600/15)

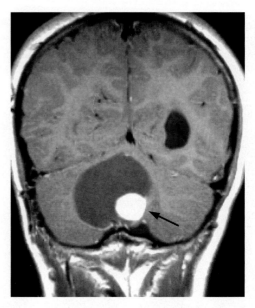

Cystic Cerebellar Astrocytoma
(same patient as Case 129)

The CT and MR appearance of hemangioblastomas and cystic cerebellar astrocytomas can be indistinguishable. In both cases, contrast enhancement may be confined to a mural nodule *(arrows),* while the remainder of the cyst wall is nonenhancing.

As mentioned in Cases 136 through 139, prominent vascular channels and contact with the pial surface are features regularly seen in hemangioblastomas and less commonly associated with astrocytomas. Cystic cerebellar astrocytomas typically demonstrate larger mural nodules, more irregular walls, and more septations than hemangioblasto-

mas. Angiography can be diagnostic in the evaluation of a cystic cerebellar tumor: the mural nodule of a hemangioblastoma is intensely vascular, while the mural nodule of a cystic astrocytoma is often hypovascular.

Angiography or contrast-enhanced MR scans in cases of hemangioblastoma may demonstrate additional small tumors of the cerebellum, brainstem, or cervical spinal cord that are inapparent on CT studies. Multiple hemangioblastomas, particularly involving the brain stem and spinal cord, usually imply Von Hippel-Lindau disease.

Case 142

28-year-old man presenting with ataxia.
(coronal, postcontrast scan; SE 600/15)

Case 143

79-year-old woman presenting with headaches
and dizziness.
(coronal, postcontrast scan; SE 700/15)

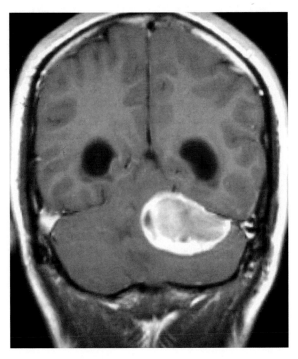

Cerebellar Hemangioblastoma

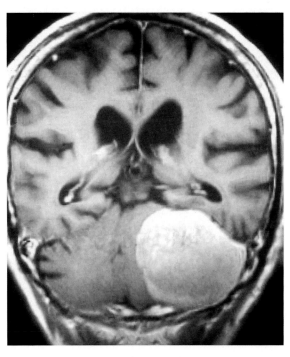

Tentorial Meningioma

The typical pial base of a hemangioblastoma may occasionally resemble the dural base of a meningioma. Since some meningiomas may demonstrate large vessels (see Cases 40 and 41) like hemangioblastomas, the two tumors can be confusingly similar in appearance. Contrast enhancement within meningiomas is usually more homogeneous than that of hemangioblastomas, as seen in the above cases. However, some hemangioblastomas are solidly enhancing, while some meningiomas are not (see Case 53).

The presence of relatively little mass effect for the size of the tumor, as in Case 143, favors a slowly growing mass such as a meningioma. By contrast, prominent edema and tonsillar herniation were demonstrated on other scans in association with the smaller but more rapidly enlarging hemangioblastoma in Case 142.

Angiography will usually distinguish between the above tumors, demonstrating pial supply to a hemangioblastoma and dural supply to a meningioma. A search for small additional lesions elsewhere in the cerebellum or brainstem is warranted to support the diagnosis of hemangioblastoma.

Medulloblastomas involving the cerebellar hemispheres of adults (so-called "cerebellar sarcomas") often reach the pial surface and should be included in this differential diagnosis (see Case 163). Metastases should also be considered whenever a cerebellar mass is encountered.

Case 144

9-year-old girl presenting with a two-week history
of headaches and new onset of diplopia.
(sagittal, noncontrast scan; SE 600/20)

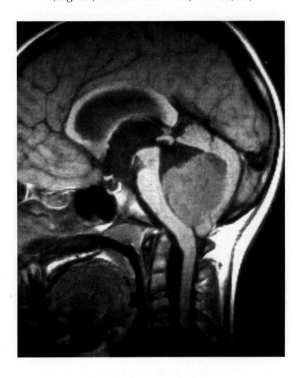

Case 145

10-year-old girl presenting with headaches.
(sagittal, noncontrast scan; SE 700/16)

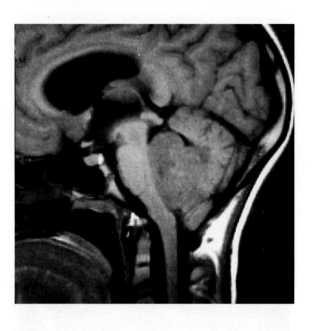

Medulloblastomas rank with cerebellar astrocytomas as the most common posterior fossa tumors in children. Medulloblastomas are highly cellular masses arising from primitive cells in the neuroepithelial roof of the fourth ventricle (external granular layer of the inferior medullary velum). Many pathologists classify these neoplasms as "primitive neuroectodermal tumors."

Medulloblastomas usually present as midline masses filling, expanding, and obstructing the fourth ventricle. The sagittal MR plane clearly demonstrates the fourth ventricular location of these tumors, as in the above examples.

In Case 144, both the brainstem and the cerebellum are displaced and compressed. Hydrocephalus has caused bowing of the corpus callosum and prominent inferior ballooning of the floor of the third ventricle. The ros-

tral fourth ventricle and aqueduct are distended due to the more caudal ventricular obstruction. The aqueduct has been shortened or "assimilated" into the superior expansion of the fourth ventricle.

Case 145 demonstrates the same features, which are slightly less severe. Note that in both cases the inferiorly displaced cerebellar tonsils enclose the caudal margin of the tumor, in contrast to Cases 152 and 153.

Medulloblastomas are often relatively homogeneous on MR scans, correlating with their usually uniform attenuation on CT studies. Calcification and cysts occur but are rarely prominent. Overall signal intensity on T1-weighted images is usually slightly less than that of the surrounding brainstem and cerebellum.

Case 146

8-year-old boy presenting with headaches.
(axial, noncontrast scan; SE 3000/75)

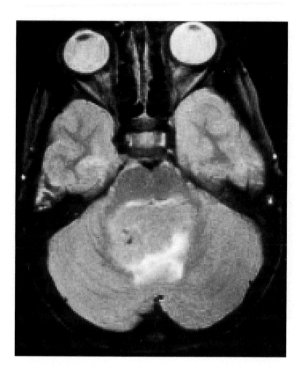

Case 147

9-year-old girl presenting with headaches
and diplopia.
(axial, noncontrast scan; SE 3000/90)

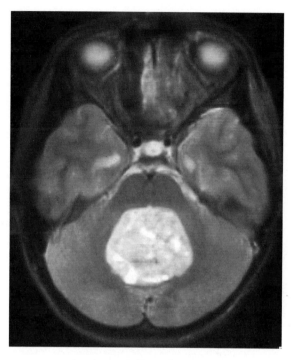

(same patient as Case 144)

Axial views demonstrate the midline location of most medulloblastomas in the pediatric age group. In the above cases the tumor has filled and enlarged the fourth ventricle, forming an expanded cast of this chamber.

Although mild heterogeneity can be seen within medulloblastomas (illustrated in Case 147), the overall impression is usually one of homogeneous tissue. Case 146 demonstrates that the signal intensity of medulloblastomas on T2-weighted images is often lower than other tumor types, reflecting dense cellularity and a high nuclear to cytoplasmic ratio. (Compare to germinomas, as in Case 272, and CNS lymphoma, as in Cases 313 and 314.) Occasional medulloblastomas present as homogeneous masses of high signal intensity on T2-weighted scans (see Case 670).

DIFFERENTIAL DIAGNOSIS:
UNIFORM MASS EXPANDING THE FOURTH VENTRICLE

Case 148

10-year-old girl presenting with ataxia.
(sagittal, noncontrast scan; SE 600/15)

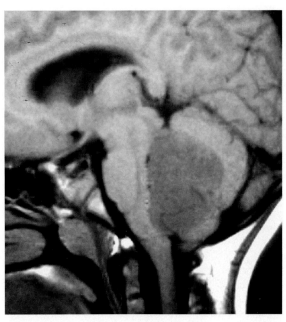

Medulloblastoma

Case 149

9-year-old girl presenting with headaches
and drowsiness.
(sagittal, noncontrast scan; SE 600/20)

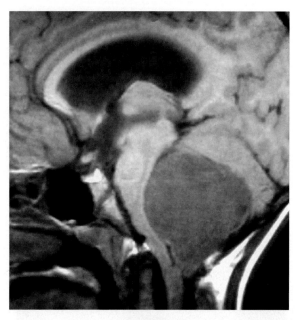

Astrocytoma
(solid)

The typical appearance of a medulloblastoma as in Case 148 can occasionally be mimicked by a midline astrocytoma arising near the margins of the fourth ventricle, illustrated by Case 149.

Medulloblastoma would be a reasonable diagnosis for the tumor in Case 149. The only unusual feature is the dorsal and caudal extension of the tumor into the vallecula and the foramen magnum. (This finding would be more sug-

gestive of ependymoma. but ependymomas are rarely as homogeneous as this tumor.)

Case 149 serves as a reminder that (1) many solid astrocytomas present as homogeneous masses on noncontrast scans (compare to Cases 126 and 132); (2) cystic or solid cerebellar astrocytomas may occupy the midline; and (3) very few CT or MR appearances are specific for a single pathology.

Case 150

9-year-old girl presenting with headaches
and diplopia.
(coronal, post-contrast scan; SE 800/20)

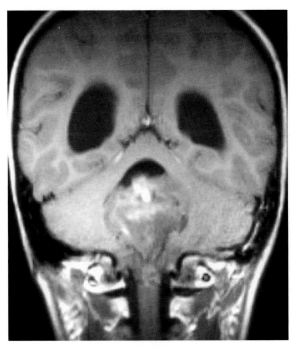

Medulloblastoma
(same patient as Cases 144 and 147)

Case 151

9-year-old girl presenting with headaches
and drowsiness.
(axial, postcontrast scan; SE 1000/20)

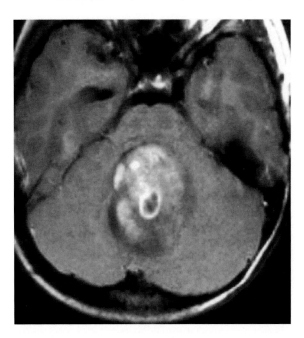

Astrocytoma
(same patient as Case 149)

These cases provide contrast-enhanced images for correlation with the previous noncontrast scans. In both instances, the pattern of enhancement is somewhat more heterogeneous than the precontrast appearance of the tumor.

Contrast enhancement in medulloblastomas is surprisingly variable in extent and morphology. The typical tumor enhances uniformly and intensely. However, heterogeneous patterns (as in Case 150) and relative lack of enhancement have been noted frequently on MR studies.

As mentioned in Cases 130 and 131, prominent contrast enhancement may be seen in cerebellar astrocytomas of low grade and relatively good prognosis.

Medulloblastomas are among the primary CNS neoplasms commonly associated with seeding of the cerebrospinal fluid. (Others include ependymoma, germinoma, pineal cell tumors, and malignant gliomas.) For this reason, a search for enhancing subarachnoid spaces is appropriate on initial and follow-up scans in these patients (see Case 160).

Compare Case 150 to Cases 134 and 135.

Case 152

23-year-old woman presenting with nausea,
dizziness, and headaches.
(sagittal, noncontrast scan; SE 800/17)

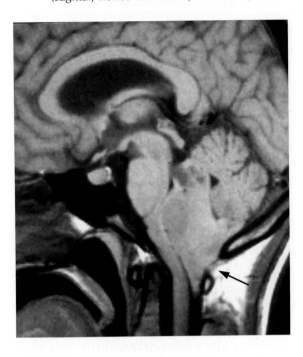

Case 153

22-month-old girl presenting with vomiting
and ataxia.
(sagittal, noncontrast scan; SE 600/20)

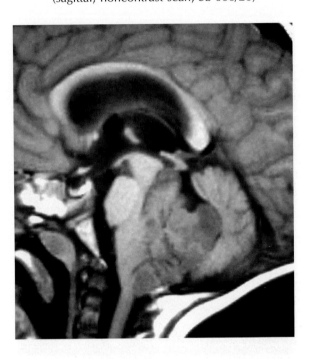

Ependymomas arising from the fourth ventricle may be encountered in children and adults. Their location mimics the more common medulloblastomas, but other MR features usually suggest the correct diagnosis. Ependymomas are frequently calcified, and they often contain cysts. Together with occasional hemorrhage, these components result in a more heterogeneous mixture of signal intensities than is usually seen in medulloblastomas. The areas of low signal intensity near the superior margin of the tumor in Case 152 correlated with large calcifications on the patient's CT scan.

Another important feature of ependymomas illustrated above is the common dorsal expansion through the foramen of Magendie into the vallecula. Further caudal extension through the foramen magnum is seen in both cases. This appearance of tumor flowing out of the fourth ventricle contrasts with the usually contained morphology of medulloblastomas, as seen in Cases 144 and 145. Ependy-

momas with extraventricular extension molding to the confines of the vallecula and subarachnoid space have been referred to as "plastic" ependymomas.

A third potential distinction between the typical MR appearances of ependymomas and medulloblastomas is their site of origin or attachment. Medulloblastomas are often more easily demarcated from the brainstem than from the vermis, where these tumors usually arise at the inferior medullary velum (see Case 144). By contrast, fourth ventricular ependymomas, as in Case 153, are often better separated from the vermis than from the dorsal brainstem, where they are frequently attached at surgery.

Like medulloblastomas, ependymomas typically fill and obstruct the fourth ventricle, causing hydrocephalus. Symptoms of nausea and vomiting may precede the development of overt hydrocephalus due to early tumor involvement of the dorsal medulla.

Case 154

15-year-old girl presenting with headaches.
(axial, noncontrast scan; SE 3000/80)

Case 155

13-year-old boy presenting with a stumbling gait.
(axial, noncontrast scan; SE 3000/75)

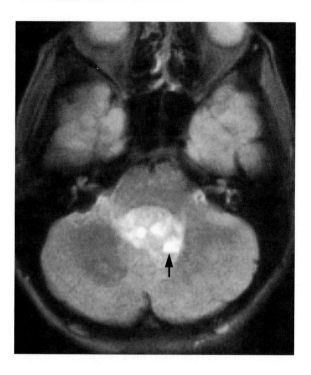

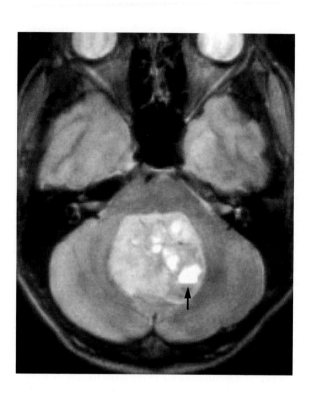

Both of these tumors contain small areas of long T2 that potentially represent cysts. A sedimentation level is present in at least one of the cystic areas in each case *(arrows)*, confirming a small fluid collection. While occasional medulloblastomas demonstrate comparable heterogeneity (see Case 147), this complex internal architecture is more characteristic of ependymomas. The background signal intensity of ependymomas on T2-weighted scans is usually intermediate, comparable to medulloblastomas (see Case 156 for another example).

Enhancement within ependymomas is often less homogeneous and intense than seen in medulloblastomas (see Cases 305 and 309). Tumor margins may be irregular and poorly defined, and lobulation is frequent.

Ependymomas of the fourth ventricle carry a poorer prognosis than medulloblastomas arising in the same location.

Case 156

22-month-old girl presenting with vomiting.
(axial, noncontrast scan; SE 3000/90)

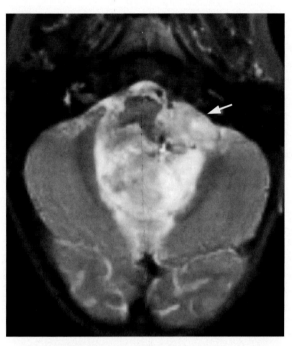

**Ependymoma Extending to the
Cerebellopontine Angle**
(same patient as Case 153)

Case 157

5-year-old boy presenting with headaches
and diplopia.
(coronal, noncontrast scan; SE 750/20)

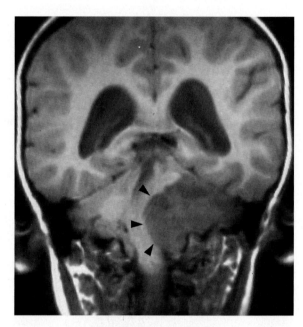

**Ependymoma Presenting in the
Cerebellopontine Angle**

In addition to the caudal extension illustrated in Cases 152 and 153, fourth ventricular ependymomas may grow laterally through the foramina of Luschka to accumulate in the cerebellopontine angle. In some cases the bulk of the tumor occupies this secondary location. In extreme cases the brainstem may be surrounded by cisternal neoplasm.

Case 156 illustrates a significant component of tumor within the left cerebellopontine angle *(arrow)*. This portion of the mass is causing displacement and rotation of the brainstem, with probable distortion of the ipsilateral cranial nerves.

Prominent asymmetrical extension of a fourth ventricular tumor into the cerebellopontine angle favors the diagnosis of ependymoma. Medulloblastomas may grow anteriorly into the anterolateral recesses of the fourth ventricle, but such extension is usually more symmetrical (see Case 670) and less bulky than that seen with ependymomas.

The large, lobulated extraaxial mass within the cerebellopontine angle cistern in Case 157 was found to be an ependymoma arising from the lateral recess of the fourth ventricle. A postcontrast scan showed heterogeneous enhancement throughout the lesion. The body of the fourth ventricle was deformed by mass effect but was surgically free of tumor.

DIFFERENTIAL DIAGNOSIS:
CEREBELLOPONTINE ANGLE MASS IN A CHILD

Case 158

7-year-old girl presenting with dysphagia.
(sagittal, noncontrast scan; SE 600/20)

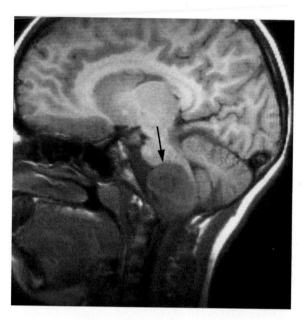

Exophytic Glioma of the Medulla

Case 159

5-year-old boy presenting with headaches
and diplopia.
(sagittal, noncontrast scan; SE 600/20)

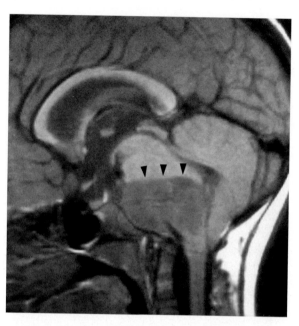

Ependymoma
(same patient as Case 157)

The differential diagnosis of a cerebellopontine angle mass in a child includes exophytic extension of intraaxial tumors as well as extraaxial neoplasms. In Case 158, the bulk of the exophytic brainstem glioma has accumulated anterolateral to the medulla. The cisternal component of the lesion is causing posterior displacement and compression of the uninvolved medulla and pons. Cerebellar astrocytomas can also extend exophytically to present as cerebellopontine angle masses in either children or adults.

Case 159 is a sagittal view of the tumor illustrated in Case 157. Ependymoma should be considered in the differential diagnosis of a cerebellopontine angle mass in a child. Choroid plexus papilloma, meningioma, schwannoma, histiocytosis, rhabdomyosarcoma, and metastasis (e.g., neuroblastoma or lymphoma) are other possibilities, although all are rare.

The relatively low signal intensity within the clivus in Case 159 probably represents residual hematopoietic marrow. There was no clival involvement by neoplasm. Fatty replacement of the clivus usually occurs by age 6.

Case 160A

8-year-old boy, six months after resection of a
fourth ventricular medulloblastoma.
(axial, noncontrast scan; SE 2500/45)

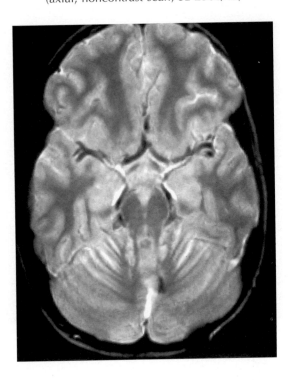

Case 160B

Same patient.
(coronal, postcontrast scan; SE 1000/20)

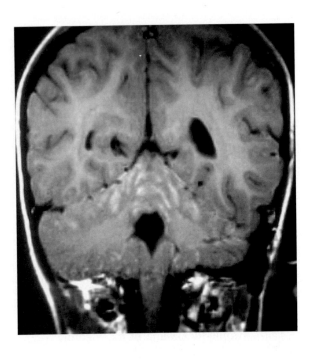

In addition to the caudal or lateral extension of fourth ventricular tumors discussed in Cases 152 through 157, ependymomas and medulloblastomas can spread by seeding of CSF spaces. Evidence of such fluid-borne leptomeningeal metastases may be present at the time of diagnosis or develop subsequently, as in this case. Involvement of the spinal canal is common.

In Case 160A, the presence of leptomeningeal tumor is suggested by superficial areas of high signal intensity following the cortical contour of the cerebellum. These linear or curvilinear zones of long T2 may represent tumor within sulci and/or reactive edema in adjacent cerebellar folia. The overall pattern of high water content with a cortical or gyriform morphology may resemble subacute infarction (see Cases 536 and 537).

In Case 160B, the multiple foci of contrast enhancement apparently within cerebellar parenchyma represent cross-sections of subarachnoid tumor filling the sulci between folia. Meningeal tumor frequently takes the form of a uniform coating or "frosting" on the surface of the brain or spinal cord (see also Cases 30, 905, and 906). Large nodular components may develop at any location within sulci or cisterns.

Meningeal involvement by medulloblastomas, ependymomas, and metastases from other primary CNS or systemic tumors is often most apparent over the superior surface of the cerebellum. Coronal postcontrast scans are especially useful in demonstrating such pathology.

Case 161

1-year-old boy presenting with hydrocephalus.
(axial, postcontrast scan; SE 700/15)

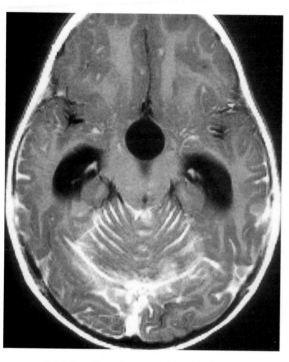

CSF Seeding from a Pineoblastoma

Case 162

58-year-old woman presenting with bilateral
hearing loss.
(axial, postcontrast scan; SE 600/15)

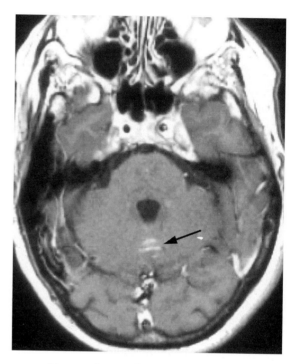

Metastatic Carcinoma of the Breast

Leptomeningeal involvement by tumor may represent CSF seeding from intracerebral neoplasms or metastatic spread of extracranial masses. Case 161 illustrates the former mechanism. Enhancing tumor fills sulci between cerebellar folia, comparable to the appearance in Case 160. Supratentorial subarachnoid spaces are also occupied by enhancing neoplasm. Primary brain tumors with a propensity for CSF spread include medulloblastomas, ependymomas, germinomas, pineal cell tumors, malignant gliomas, and choroid plexus tumors (see Cases 280 and 299).

The patient in Case 162 presented with hearing loss due to meningeal metastases involving the internal auditory canals (IAC) (see Case 177). The focal but definite enhance-

ment within superior vermian sulci *(arrow)* suggested that the IAC lesions might reflect meningeal disease. As a result, CSF cytology was obtained and metastatic adenocarcinoma was discovered. The systemic tumors that most commonly cause leptomeningeal metastases are melanoma, carcinoma of the breast, and carcinoma of the lung.

Abnormal meningeal enhancement may be seen in a number of nonneoplastic conditions. Among these are various forms of meningitis (see Case 386), the acute phase of cerebral infarction (see Cases 484 and 485), dural sinus thrombosis (see Case 386-2), and Sturge-Weber syndrome (see Case 770).

Case 163

40-year-old man presenting with ataxia.
(coronal, noncontrast scan; SE 700/16)

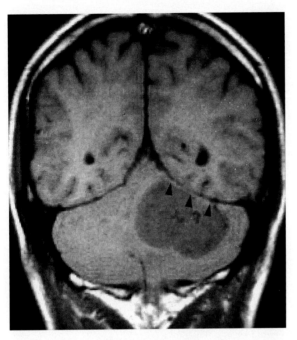

Medulloblastoma

Case 164

23-year-old woman presenting with ataxia.
(coronal, postcontrast scan; SE 600/15)

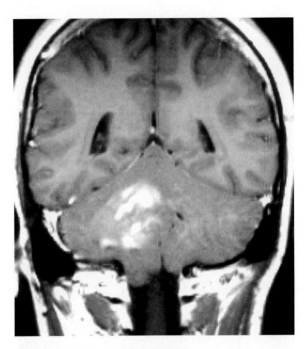

Astrocytoma

Metastases and hemangioblastomas are the most frequently encountered cerebellar masses in adults. However, the common cerebellar tumors of childhood may also occur in older patients, as illustrated in these cases.

Medulloblastomas in adults are often hemispheric. Such tumors are frequently associated with prominent fibrosis and have been called "desmoplastic medulloblastomas" or "cerebellar sarcomas." The mass in Case 163 was relatively isointense to cerebral cortex on a T2-weighted scan, reflecting dense cellularity and resembling most fourth ventricular medulloblastomas in children.

Adult, hemispheric medulloblastomas often reach the cerebellar surface, a feature shared by hemangioblastomas. Exophytic growth can mimic extraaxial masses in the cerebellopontine angle. Alternatively, an infiltrating pattern of growth may occur, resembling the appearance of Lhermitte-Duclos disease (see Case 165).

A CT scan in Case 163 had demonstrated a uniformly en-

hancing mass reaching the superior surface of the cerebellum, and a tentorial meningioma was suspected. The coronal MR plane demonstrates a thin rim of compressed cerebellar parenchyma *(arrowheads)* separating the tumor from the tentorium and establishing the diagnosis of an intraaxial neoplasm.

The astrocytoma in Case 164 demonstrates intense but patchy enhancement and is somewhat poorly defined. (Compare to the juvenile cerebellar astrocytomas in Cases 128-134.) The tumor has caused ipsilateral tonsillar herniation.

Cerebellar astrocytomas that are histologically categorized as "diffuse" are more commonly solid, occur in older patients, and carry a substantially worse prognosis than "pilocytic" tumors.

Primary or metastatic lymphoma should also be considered in the differential diagnosis of cerebellar masses in adults (see Cases 313 and 326.)

LHERMITTE-DUCLOS DISEASE (DYSPLASTIC GANGLIOCYTOMA OF THE CEREBELLUM)

Case 165A

36-year-old man presenting with ataxia.
(axial, noncontrast scan; SE 700/20)

Case 165B

Same patient.
(axial, noncontrast scan; SE 2300/80)

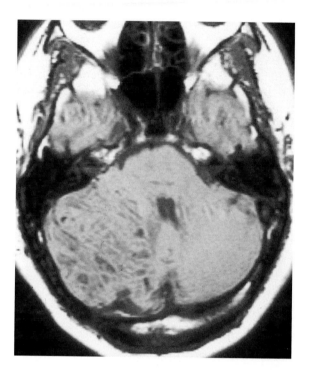 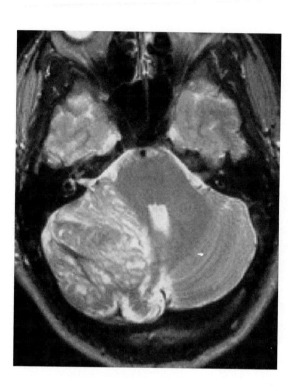

Lhermitte-Duclos disease is an unusual cause of a cerebellar mass in an adult. This lesion is viewed by some pathologists as a hypertrophic malformation or hamartoma. However, the associated masses have been demonstrated to enlarge over time and to recur after resection, acting much like low grade neoplasms.

The entity is now commonly referred to as "dysplastic gangliocytoma of the cerebellum." It most frequently affects young men. Gross pathology demonstrates localized thickening of cerebellar folia. Microscopic examination shows large, dysplastic neurons within the granular layer of cerebellar cortex and excessive myelination of axons in the molecular layer.

The unusual pattern of undulating, thickened folia seen in this case is characteristic of the disorder and correlates with the hypertrophic folia seen pathologically. Relatively isointense cerebellar cortex is surrounded by an overall background of prolonged T1 and T2 values in the above images. Other reported cases have demonstrated more extensive high intensity abnormality on T2-weighted scans.

This patient had undergone prior resection of a right cerebellar mass. Follow-up studies over a period of years documented recurrence of the lesion.

Case 166

43-year-old woman presenting with right-sided
hearing loss.
(coronal, noncontrast scan; SE 1000/16).

Case 167

60-year-old woman presenting with right facial
numbness and a ten-year history of right-sided
hearing loss.
(coronal, noncontrast scan; SE 600/16).

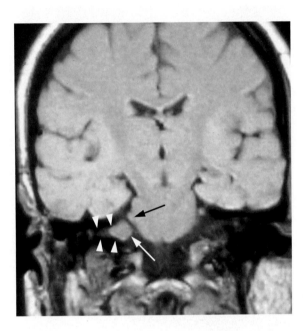

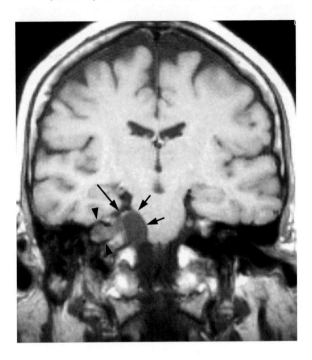

Acoustic schwannomas represent about 10% of primary intracranial tumors and account for the majority of masses in the cerebellopontine angle. They are typically well-defined lesions with smooth, rounded margins, centered at the internal auditory meatus.

In Case 166, the small schwannoma *(white arrow)* extends from the medial aspect of the internal auditory canal *(arrowheads)* into the cerebellopontine angle cistern, without contacting the adjacent fifth cranial nerve *(black arrow)*. The uniform, intermediate intensity of this mass is typical of small schwannomas.

Case 167 illustrates a larger, more complex schwannoma. The solid component of this tumor expands the IAC *(arrowheads;* compare to Case 166) and extends through the porus acusticus. A large cyst is present more medially, deforming the pons *(short arrows)* and elevating the fifth cranial nerve *(long arrow;* compare to the normal fifth nerve on the left side).

Cysts are commonly found in association with acoustic

schwannomas. Many such "cysts" represent loculations of CSF surrounded by thickened arachnoid membranes adjacent to a tumor. Cystic degeneration within schwannomas is also common. When a partially cystic schwannoma invaginates into adjacent parenchyma, the appearance may resemble a hemangioblastoma arising at the pial surface.

Almost all patients who present with acoustic schwannomas have hearing loss, the presence or absence of which can be of value in the differential diagnosis. Facial numbness due to distortion of the fifth nerve (as in Case 167) is a common secondary symptom of large eighth nerve tumors. The seventh cranial nerve is resistant to compressive dysfunction, and facial paresis rarely accompanies acoustic schwannomas.

Because most schwannomas arise from the vestibular portion of the eighth nerve, these tumors are most accurately termed "vestibular schwannomas." However, longstanding usage and the predominance of auditory symptoms explain the common "acoustic" nomenclature.

Case 168

20-year-old man presenting with right-sided hearing
loss and facial numbness.
(axial, noncontrast scan; SE 2800/80)

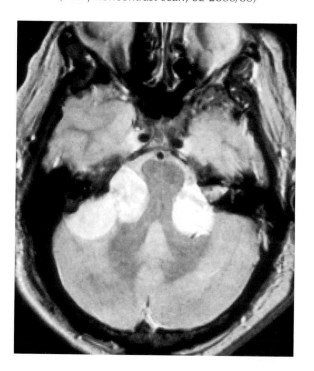

Case 169

67-year-old woman presenting with right-sided
hearing loss.
(axial, noncontrast scan; SE 3000/90)

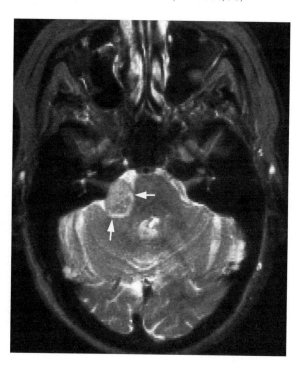

Schwannomas typically demonstrate high signal intensity on long TR spin echo images. Even large tumors may remain quite homogeneous, as in Case 168. However, a heterogeneous pattern of mixed tissue components is common in schwannomas exceeding two centimeters in diameter.

Occasional eighth nerve tumors are relatively isointense on T2-weighted scans. Case 169 illustrates this appearance. Note that the ipsilateral IAC is not appreciably expanded (compare to Case 170).

In Case 168, the cisternal components of the slowly growing schwannomas have gradually invaginated far into the adjacent parenchyma. Only a thin band of compressed tissue separates the tumors from the fourth ventricle. Proximity to the ventricular system is not a reliable criterion for distinguishing between intraaxial and extraaxial lesions.

The extraaxial origin of a cerebellopontine angle mass is usually indicated by contralateral brainstem displacement, causing widening of the ipsilateral cisterns at the margins

of the tumor. This cisternal widening is seen anteriorly on both sides in Cases 168 and 169 (also see Case 170).

Bilateral acoustic schwannomas as in Case 168 strongly suggest the diagnosis of neurofibromatosis, even if the disorder has not been previously recognized. "Bilateral acoustic neurofibromatosis" (BANF) has now been designated "type 2 neurofibromatosis" and is clinically and genetically distinct from the more common "type 1 neurofibromatosis" or Von Recklinghausen's disease (which is discussed in Cases 764-767). In addition to acoustic schwannomas at early ages, patients with type 2 neurofibromatosis may present with schwannomas of other cranial nerves and with multiple cranial meningiomas (see Cases 66 and 67).

The bilateral acoustic schwannomas in type 2 neurofibromatosis are often very asymmetrical in size. When an eighth nerve tumor is detected in a young adult, a careful search should be made for a smaller, contralateral lesion.

Case 170

38-year-old woman presenting with right-sided
hearing loss.
(axial, postcontrast scan; SE 600/20)

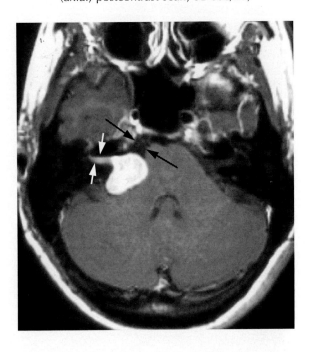

Case 171

73-year-old woman following transmastoid
resection of a left-sided acoustic schwannoma.
(axial, postcontrast scan; SE 600/15)

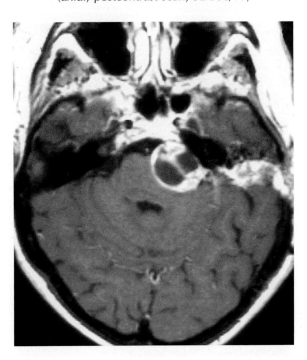

Contrast enhancement in schwannomas is usually intense. This characteristic allows detection of even very small eighth nerve lesions (see Case 175).

Uniformly enhancing schwannomas must often be considered in the differential diagnosis of meningiomas, particularly in the posterior fossa and parasellar regions. However, nonenhancing zones are common within large schwannomas, as illustrated by the recurrent tumor in Case 171.

Case 170 is a good example of ipsilateral cisternal widening *(black arrows)* in association with an extraaxial mass. This case also demonstrates the common appearance of a

bulbous cisternal schwannoma in continuity with a stem or pedicle of enhancement occupying the mildly expanded IAC *(white arrows)*. The degree of IAC erosion is not necessarily related to the overall size of an acoustic schwannoma, which may expand exophytically in the adjacent cistern.

High signal intensity within the left mastoid region in Case 171 is mainly due to a fat graft placed at the time of previous surgery. Contrast-enhanced scans performed with fat saturation techniques are useful to eliminate potential confusion between fat packing and enhancing tumor in cases with a history of transmastoid surgery.

DIFFERENTIAL DIAGNOSIS:
ENHANCING MASS WITHIN THE CEREBELLOPONTINE ANGLE

Case 172

38-year-old woman presenting with left facial pain.
(coronal, postcontrast scan; SE 700/20)

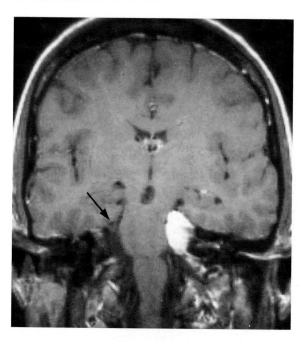

Meningioma

Case 173

38-year-old woman presenting with mild ataxia
and tinnitus.
(axial, postcontrast scan; SE 600/15)

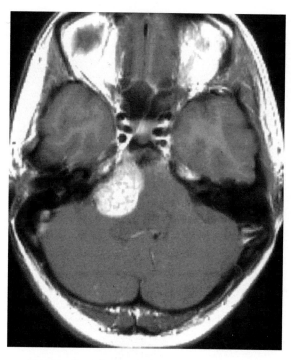

**Metastatic Adenocarcinoma (Intraaxial) of
Unknown Origin**

A number of pathologies may present as enhancing extraaxial masses within the cerebellopontine angle cistern. Meningioma is the most common benign tumor to mimic acoustic schwannoma in this location, as in Case 172.

The CT and MR appearance of meningiomas and acoustic schwannomas may be very similar. However, several potential discriminating features can be noted. Relatively low signal intensity on T2-weighted images is more common in meningiomas than schwannomas (but see Case 169). Most posterior fossa meningiomas are centered above or below the internal auditory canal, rather than at the internal auditory meatus. Cerebellopontine angle meningiomas can extend into the IAC, but few are associated with significant widening of the canal or with hearing loss. Finally, cerebellopontine angle meningiomas typically have a broader base against the petrous bone than acoustic schwannomas.

Other benign lesions in the CT differential diagnosis of an enhancing cerebellopontine angle mass often have characteristic MR appearances (e.g., aneurysms and glomus jugulare tumors).

Malignant neoplasms can also present in the cerebellopontine angle. Extraaxial, dural-based metastases in this location may occur with carcinomas of the prostate, breast, and lung. Lymphoma should also be considered in this differential diagnosis.

Case 173 demonstrates that superficial parenchymal lesions may grow exophytically to mimic an extraaxial mass. The apparent dural base, intense enhancement, and sharp definition of this mass closely resemble the expected characteristics of a meningioma. The only disconcerting feature is the unusual texture within the lesion. As discussed in Chapter 2, meningiomas are usually quite homogeneous or demonstrate radial or circular tissue patterns.

The meningioma in Case 172 distorts the left fifth cranial nerve near its entrance to the pons (compare to the normal trigeminal nerve on the right; *arrow*), causing the patient's facial pain.

Case 174

73-year-old woman presenting with reduced speech discrimination in the left ear.
(axial, noncontrast scan; RSE 4082/96)

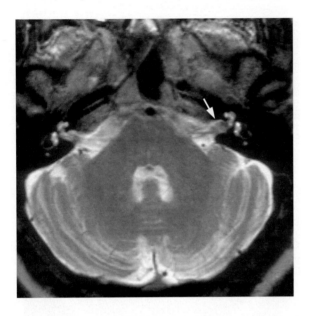

Case 175

46-year-old man presenting with right-sided hearing loss and vertigo.
(axial, postcontrast scan; SE 600/15)

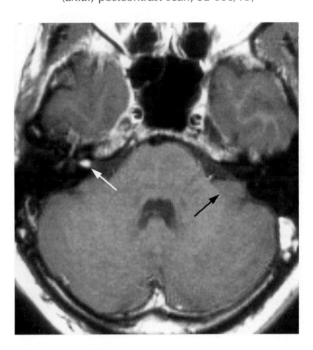

Symptoms of hearing loss or impaired discrimination can be caused by very small acoustic schwannomas compressing the cochlear nerve within the internal auditory canal. Tumors arising within the confines of the IAC typically cause symptoms at an earlier stage than masses that predominantly involve the cisternal portion of the nerve.

Intracanalicular acoustic schwannomas may be identified as soft tissue masses within the IAC on noncontrast MR images. Definition of small intracanicular lesions is favored by strongly T2-weighted scans with high spatial resolution (e.g., rapid spin echo sequences using a 512 matrix), such as Case 174.

Contrast-enhanced MR scans reliably demonstrate intracanalicular schwannomas measuring only a few millimeters in diameter. The tumor in Case 175 *(white arrow)* is a tiny mass, entirely within the confines of the IAC.

Both cases demonstrate soft tissue nodules near the posterior margin of the cerebellopontine angle cistern *(black arrow, Case 175)*, which represent the normal flocculus of the cerebellum. These rounded structures are occasionally misinterpreted as extraaxial masses, especially if head tilt causes asymmetrical visualization. However, the normal flocculus is located posterior to the internal auditory canal and does not enhance appreciably.

DIFFERENTIAL DIAGNOSIS:
FOCAL CONTRAST ENHANCEMENT IN THE REGION OF THE INTERNAL AUDITORY CANAL

Case 176

55-year-old man presenting with vertigo.
(coronal, postcontrast scan; SE 600/15)

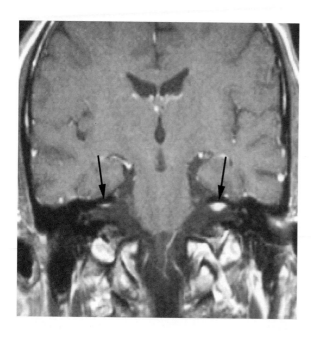

Normal Petrosal Veins

Case 177

58-year-old woman presenting with bilateral
hearing loss.
(axial, postcontrast scan; SE 600/15)

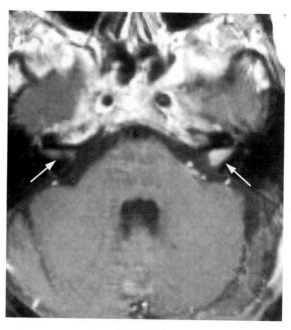

**Meningeal Metastases from Carcinoma
of the Breast**
(same patient as Case 162)

Normal vascular structures can cause contrast enhancement near or within the internal auditory canal, mimicking a small acoustic schwannoma. The petrosal venous system is typically located slightly superior and medial to the internal auditory meatus. Considerable right/left asymmetry in the size of these veins is common, as illustrated in Case 176 *(arrows)*. Attention to the margins of the IAC and comparison with the contralateral side will usually establish the nature of an enhancing vascular pseudotumor.

Areas of fatty marrow within the petrous apex are common and are frequently asymmetrical (see Case 189). These focal zones of high signal intensity can be mistaken for enhancing masses on T1-weighted postcontrast images. Attention to the precise location of the high signal region with respect to the IAC usually resolves confusion. A fat saturation scan can be performed in ambiguous cases. Precontrast T1-weighted images or fat saturation sequences will also distinguish rare lipomas of the internal auditory canal from enhancing schwannomas.

Abnormal contrast enhancement within the IAC on MR studies is not specific for acoustic schwannomas. Hemangiomas or inflammation of the facial nerve can present a similar appearance. Meningeal disease (e.g., carcinomatosis as in Case 177 or sarcoidosis) can extend into the IAC with associated abnormal enhancement. Finally, reactive meningeal changes following surgery to remove a schwannoma can lead to intracanalicular enhancement, so postoperative scans must be interpreted cautiously.

In Case 177, the patient's bilateral hearing loss was the presenting symptom of metastatic breast carcinoma. The presence of abnormal meningeal enhancement involving the superior vermis (see Case 162) as well as the internal auditory canals led to CSF cytology, which in turn established the diagnosis.

Enhancement of the membranous labyrinth may be noted on IAC studies performed to "rule out acoustic schwannomas." This evidence of labyrinthitis may correlate with the patient's symptoms and should be sought on otherwise negative scans of the petrous bones.

Case 178A

39-year-old woman presenting with right
facial pain.
(axial, noncontrast scan; SE 600/15)

Case 178B

Same patient.
(axial, postcontrast scan; SE 600/15)

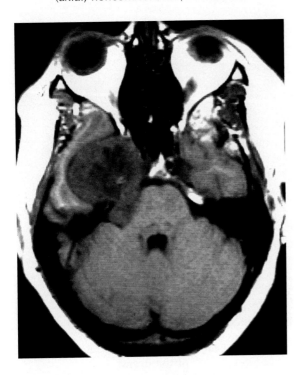

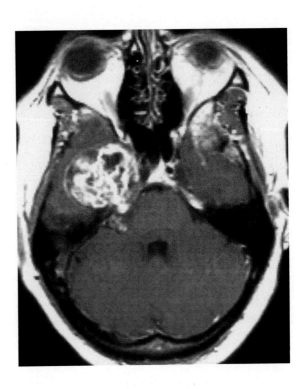

Trigeminal schwannomas commonly arise near the gasserian ganglion, which is located within Meckel's cave in the posterior portion of the cavernous sinus.

Small trigeminal schwannomas may cause local widening of the cavernous sinus and should be included in the differential diagnosis discussed in Cases 254 and 255. Care must be taken not to overread apparent asymmetry in the morphology of normal Meckel's caves caused by rotation or tilt of the head (see Case 373).

Larger tumors often acquire a dumbbell shape with parasellar and posterior fossa components. The middle fossa expansion of trigeminal schwannomas is characteristically extradural, while extension posteriorly along the cisternal course of the fifth nerve represents an intradural mass.

The precontrast appearance of the schwannoma in Case 178A is nonspecific and cannot be distinguished from a parasellar meningioma. (A T2-weighted scan demonstrated a granular texture and high signal intensity comparable to Case 179.) However, the irregular enhancement pattern in

Case 178B is characteristic of large trigeminal schwannomas and would be distinctly unusual for a meningioma (compare to Case 60).

Lymphoma and metastasis should be considered in the differential diagnosis of enhancing masses spanning the petrous apex. Parasagittal chordomas may also cross the petrous apex and can demonstrate speckled or "swiss cheese" enhancement patterns.

Trigeminal schwannomas are among the lesions to be sought in patients with tic douloureux. A more classic finding in such cases is looping of a vessel near the "entry zone" of the fifth cranial nerve as it joins the pons (see discussion of Cases 640 and 641). In most cases of trigeminal neuralgia, scans are unremarkable and symptoms are attributed to "microvascular compression" of the fifth nerve.

Neuritis (e.g., due to herpes) and meningeal neoplasm should be considered in the differential diagnosis of thickening and/or enhancement of the cisternal segment of the trigeminal nerve (see Cases 182 and 183).

Case 179

73-year-old woman with weakness and atrophy of
the right side of the tongue.
(axial, noncontrast scan; SE 2500/45)

Case 180

22-year-old woman presenting with diplopia due to
a right fourth nerve paresis.
(axial, noncontrast scan; SE 2800/70)

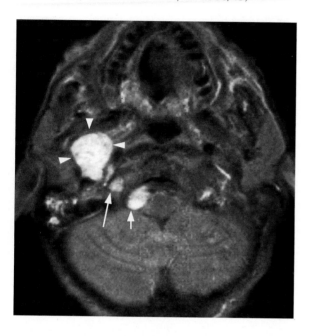

Hypoglossal Schwannoma

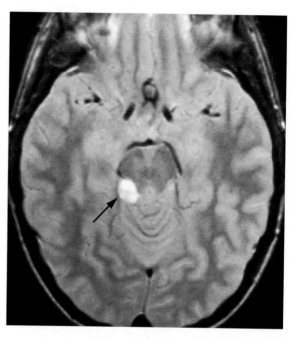

Presumed Fourth Nerve Schwannoma

Schwannomas of other cranial nerves usually have MR characteristics comparable to acoustic and trigeminal tumors. High signal intensity on T2-weighted images and intense contrast enhancement are typical.

Case 179 demonstrates a small nodule of tumor in the posterior fossa *(short arrow)* as well as a larger extracranial mass along the carotid sheath *(arrowheads)*. A bridging component occupies the expanded hypoglossal canal *(long arrow)*. This dumbbell morphology following the course of a cranial nerve through a foramen is highly suggestive of a schwannoma, in this case arising from the hypoglossal nerve. The well-defined, smoothly rounded margins of the lesion are characteristic, as is the high signal intensity on a long TR spin echo image. There is no evidence of prominent vascular channels, which would be expected in a glomus tumor of this size (compare to Case 185).

The small extraaxial mass within the right perimesencephalic cistern in Case 180 has not been resected. However, the location and signal characteristics are suggestive of a schwannoma involving the trochlear nerve. A meningioma arising near the tentorial hiatus would be an alternative possibility. Schwannomas of cranial nerves supplying the extraocular muscles are a rare cause of diplopia (see Case 181 for another example).

High signal intensity within the right mastoid process in Case 179 indicates mucosal thickening and opacification. This finding probably reflects obstruction or dysfunction of the eustachian tube due to the parapharyngeal component of the schwannoma.

Mononeuropathies unassociated with tumors may involve cranial nerves, especially the second (optic neuritis), seventh (Bell's palsy), and twelfth. Sarcoidosis is a potential etiology in such cases, along with viral syndromes, Lyme disease, and "idiopathic" inflammation.

Case 181

53-year-old man presenting with diplopia due to
left oculomotor palsy.
(coronal, postcontrast scan; SE 600/15)

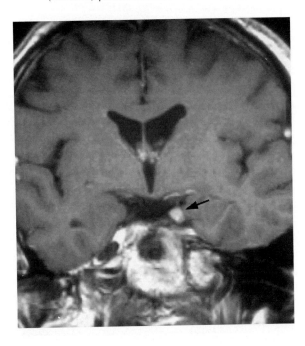

Third Nerve Schwannoma

Case 182

11-year-old girl, several months after resection of a
supratentorial primitive neuroectodermal tumor.
(coronal, postcontrast scan; SE 600/15)

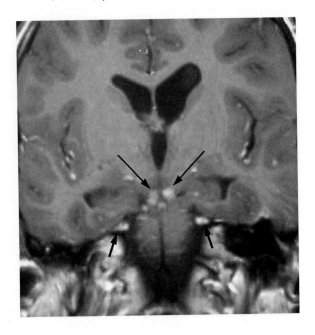

**Meningeal Tumor Coating the Third
and Fifth Cranial Nerves**

Abnormal enlargement and enhancement of a cranial nerve may reflect a mass arising from the nerve itself (e.g., schwannoma, hemangioma) or meningeal disease adherent to its surface. Case 181 illustrates the intense contrast enhancement typical of small schwannomas. The left third nerve *(arrow)* is involved between the interpeduncular fossa and the cavernous sinus.

Case 182 demonstrates abnormal enlargement and enhancement of both third nerves *(long arrows)* as they leave the midbrain within the interpeduncular fossa. Also apparent is abnormal enhancement of the cisternal segments of the fifth cranial nerves bilaterally *(short arrows;* compare

to the normal nonenhancing trigeminal nerves in Case 176). CSF seeding from primary intracranial tumors may result in tumor deposits affecting one or more cranial nerves, as seen here. Meningeal carcinomatosis from systemic neoplasms (e.g., melanoma and breast carcinoma; see Case 177) can cause a similar appearance.

Inflammatory meningeal disease (e.g., tuberculosis, sarcoidosis, and meningovascular syphilis) and neuritis (e.g., Lyme disease, herpes zoster oticus and ophthalmicus) should be included in the differential diagnosis of abnormally enhancing cranial nerves.

Case 183

17-year-old girl.
(axial, postcontrast scan; SE 500/25)

Case 184

31-year-old woman.
(coronal, postcontrast scan; SE 600/15)

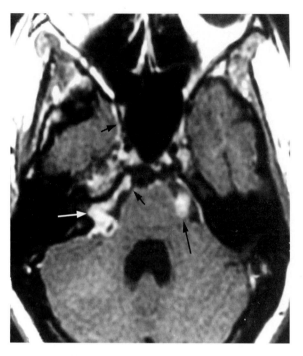

Meningeal Seeding from a Spinal Ependymoma

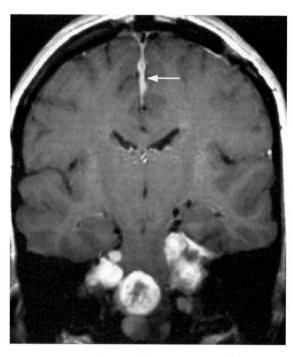

Multiple Schwannomas Associated with Type 2 Neurofibromatosis

As discussed on the previous page, cranial nerve masses may originate from the nerves themselves or from leptomeningeal pathology.

Case 183 illustrates intracranial seeding from an ependymoma of the spinal canal. Involvement of the left fifth cranial nerve *(long black arrow)* and the right internal auditory canal *(white arrow)* could be mistakenly assumed to represent multiple schwannomas in type 2 neurofibromatosis, as in Case 184. Abnormal thickening and enhancement of meninges elsewhere *(small black arrows)* is a clue to the presence of leptomeningeal disease, as is the associated communicating hydrocephalus.

Along with systemic metastases, the possibility of a spinal source should be considered when a cranial scan suggests meningeal tumor with no apparent primary lesion.

In Case 184, schwannomas involve many of the cranial nerves in the posterior fossa. One or more of the masses could alternatively represent a coexisting meningioma. Mild meningiomatosis of the falx is present *(arrow;* compare to Case 67).

Multiple enhancing cranial nerves with less mass-like morphology may represent inflammatory pathology (e.g., meningitis, Lyme disease, syphilis, sarcoidosis) as well as meningeal carcinomatosis.

Case 185A

70-year-old woman presenting with dysphagia.
(sagittal, noncontrast scan; SE 800/16)

Case 185B

Same patient.
(axial, noncontrast scan; SE 2500/100)

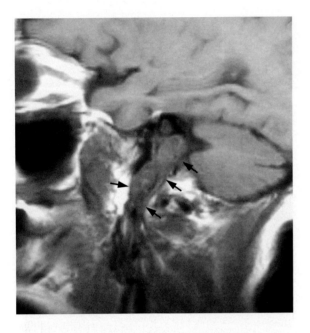

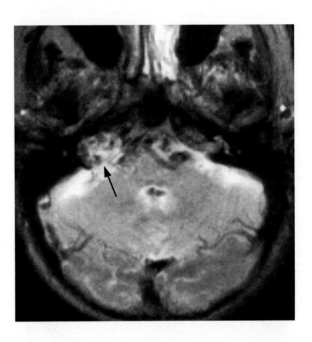

Glomus tumors ("chemodectomas," "paragangliomas") originate from paraganglionic cells in numerous locations, including the carotid sinus (carotid body tumor), jugular bulb (glomus jugulare), and middle ear (glomus tympanicum). Glomus tumors are multiple in about 3% of spontaneous cases and about 25% of familial cases. Although most of these neoplasms are histologically benign, they may be locally invasive. Associated bone erosion is often irregular and poorly defined, suggesting malignancy.

Glomus jugular tumors typically enlarge the jugular foramen and span the skull base, as seen in this case. The sagittal view (Case 185A) demonstrates that the region of the jugular foramen is expanded and filled with the intensity of soft tissue rather than the signal void of flowing blood (*arrows;* compare to Case 188B). The tumor is seen to ex-

tend below the skull base, involving the cervical portion of the internal jugular vein.

A useful feature in distinguishing glomus tumors from a normal jugular bulb (or from other mass lesions such as schwannomas) is the typical granular texture of glomus lesions due to "flow voids" within the highly vascular tissue. On spin echo images these small circular and tubular areas of low signal intensity cause a characteristic "salt and pepper" pattern. Compare this appearance in Case 185B to the more homogeneous texture of the jugular foramen in Case 188A.

The zones of low signal intensity within the left cerebellopontine angle cistern in Case 185B were due to tortuous looping of the distal left vertebral artery.

DIFFERENTIAL DIAGNOSIS:
INTENSELY ENHANCING MASS NEAR THE JUGULAR FORAMEN

Case 186

63-year-old man presenting with dysfunction of
cranial nerves IX-XII on the left.
(axial, postcontrast scan; SE 650/15)

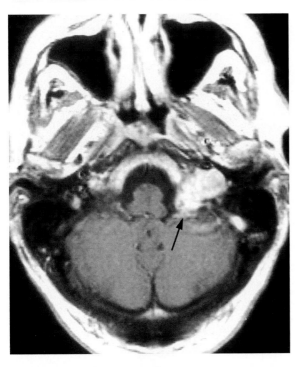

Glomus Jugulare Tumor

Case 187

86-year-old man presenting with dysfunction of
cranial nerves IX-XI on the left.
(coronal, postcontrast scan; SE 600/15).

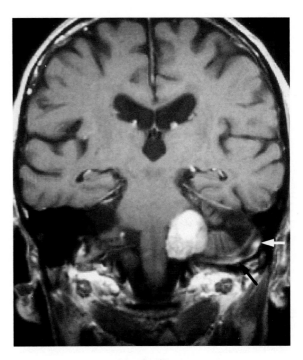

Meningioma

Intense contrast enhancement is a characteristic of glomus tumors. The mass in Case 186 has expanded the jugular foramen and extends medially into the cerebellopontine angle cistern. The cisternal component of the tumor continued superiorly to reach the level of the internal auditory canal, where it mimicked an acoustic schwannoma. Care must be taken to establish the rostral and caudal limits of cisternal masses; in this case, the lesion could be followed inferiorly into an enlarged jugular foramen.

The extraaxial tumor in Case 187 is located slightly posterior to the junction of the sigmoid sinus *(arrows)* and jugular vein. It was not associated with prominent vessels or erosion of the jugular foramen, making a glomus tumor very unlikely. However, a schwannoma of one of the lower cranial nerves could represent a very similar appearance.

Dural-based metastases and lymphoma should be included in the differential diagnosis of solidly enhancing masses near the jugular bulb.

Case 188A

66-year-old man presenting with bilateral
hearing loss.
(axial, noncontrast scan; SE 3600/22)

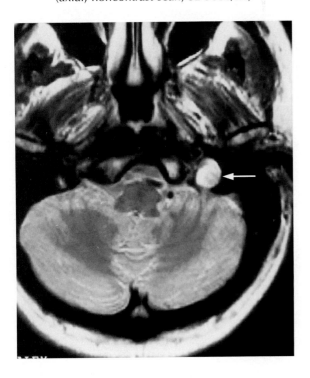

Case 188B

Same patient.
(sagittal, noncontrast scan; SE 760/17)

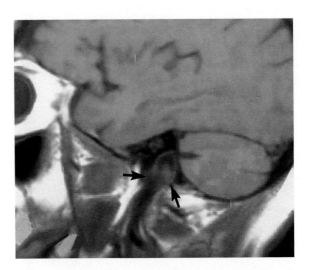

High signal intensity fills the large left jugular foramen in Case 188A *(arrow)*. This appearance could suggest a mass, such as a glomus jugulare tumor or a schwannoma. Instead, the finding represents normal slow flow within a large jugular vein.

MR scans performed with motion-refocusing pulse sequences, after contrast injection, and/or in circumstances of slow jugular flow, may normally demonstrate isointense or high signal within the jugular vein. The combination of a large jugular foramen and prominent intraluminal signal may falsely mimic a neoplasm.

Several clues help to differentiate a normal jugular bulb from a foraminal tumor on MR scans. First, the bony margins of normally large foramina are more smoothly rounded and better defined than the erosive appearance usually seen with glomus tumors. (This quality may be better appreciated on CT examinations.)

Second, as illustrated in Case 185B, glomus tumors of medium or large size usually contain multiple "flow voids," which give the lesion a characteristic coarse texture. This pattern is distinct from the more amorphous morphology of slow flow within a large vessel.

When axial scans through the jugular foramen are indeterminate, sagittal or coronal images may convincingly demonstrate a patent vein. A typical whorled pattern of variable flow is present within the jugular vein of Case 188B, unlike the clear visualization of a transcranial mass in Case 185A.

Finally, MR venography may be used to assess a questionable jugular foramen, as illustrated on the next page. Single slice gradient echo images in the axial plane may also establish flow-related enhancement within a patent jugular vein.

Case 188C

Same patient.
(axial source image from a two-dimensional,
time-of-flight angiographic series)

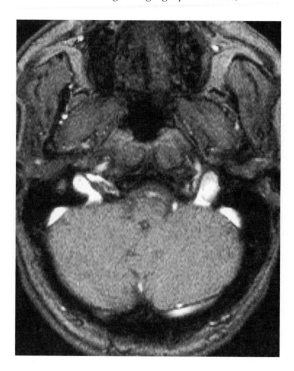

Case 188D

Same patient.
(submentovertex reformation of the entire
imaging volume)

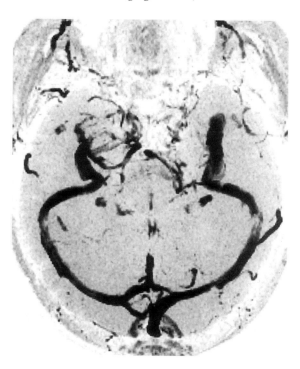

MR angiography can contribute to the assessment of many arterial pathologies (see Cases 547, 548, 600, and 601). The MR evaluation of venous flow is also helpful in several clinical settings. Documentation of dural sinus thrombosis and jugular foramen patency are two such applications. Phase-contrast techniques or two-dimensional time-of-flight studies are usually employed to image the slow flow encountered within major cerebral veins.

In Case 188C, flow-related enhancement produces high signal intensity within both jugular foramina. Although the intensity within the large left foramen is slightly heterogeneous (reflecting different flow velocities and phases), there is no "filling defect" displacing flow from any segment of the foramen.

Case 188D presents a composite view of the entire stack of two-dimensional images obtained. The transverse and sigmoid sinuses and jugular veins are well visualized bilaterally. In particular, the prominent signal intensity within the left jugular foramen in Case 188A is seen to correlate with a large, patent jugular bulb.

Localized areas of reduced signal intensity are present within the transverse sinuses bilaterally. This common normal variant may be caused by arachnoid granulations or by complex flow patterns near the entrance of major tributory veins (such as the vein of Labbé).

MR venography (looking for dural sinus stenosis or occlusion) may be useful in patients who evidence increased intracranial pressure with no apparent pathology on routine MR images.

111

Case 189A

47-year-old man presenting with a right sixth
nerve palsy.
(axial, postcontrast scan; SE 600/20)

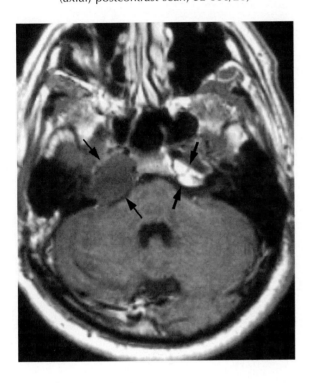

Case 189B

Same patient.
(axial, noncontrast scan; SE 3000/90)

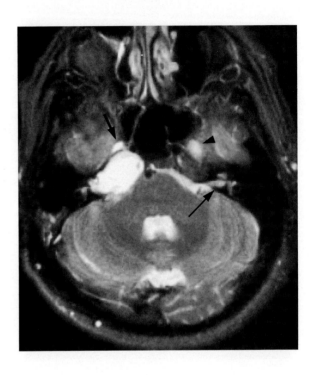

The petrous apex can be involved by a number of benign and malignant neoplasms. Among the former are primary epidermoid tumors. These gradually enlarging masses result from accumulation of squamous debris within a rest of keratinizing epithelium enclosed during formation of the skull. They are distinct from the secondary cholesteotomas that may develop as a complication of inflammatory disease in the middle ear and mastoid region.

Epidermoid tumors of the petrous apex are characteristically expansile lesions, with thinning rather than destruction of bony margins. Like intracranial epidermoid tumors, these masses usually demonstrate long T1 and long T2 values, as seen in this case. Minimal contrast enhancement may be present at the perimeter of the lesion, but the center is nonenhancing. This combination of features (long T1, expansion of bone, and lack of enhancement) is highly suggestive of the correct diagnosis.

An unusual mucocele or abscess within an apical petrous air cell could be considered in the differential diagnosis. An eccentric skull base chordoma (see Case 195) or a schwannoma might resemble the appearance of Case 189B but would be expected to enhance.

Case 189A demonstrates fatty marrow within the left petrous apex *(thick arrows)*, a common normal variant that is often asymmetrical. On non–fat-suppressed coronal postcontrast scans, similar areas can be mistaken for enhancement in a mass involving the cerebellopontine angle (e.g., acoustic schwannoma). Note that the signal intensity of this region is substantially decreased on the T2-weighted scan (Case 189B).

Conversely, CSF within the internal auditory canals is much more apparent on T2-weighted images *(long arrow,* Case 189B) than on T1-weighted scans. Comparing the right and left sides in this image, it is clear that the petrous apex tumor has extended posteriorly to involve the right IAC. The anterior margin of the mass displaces and compresses Meckel's cave *(short arrow;* compare to the normal left side indicated by the *arrowhead).*

CHOLESTEROL GRANULOMAS OF THE PETROUS APEX

Case 190A

42-year-old man with a history of chronic right
otitis media.
(sagittal, noncontrast scan; SE 600/15)

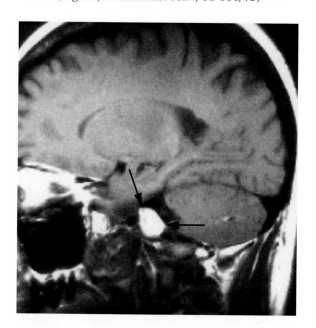

Case 190B

Same patient.
(axial, noncontrast scan; SE 3000/90)

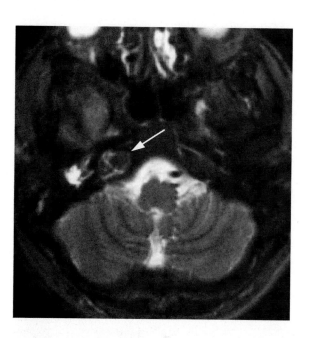

Cholesterol granulomas are among the benign pathologies that may involve the petrous apex. These lesions represent obstructed air cells that have become filled with old blood products from recurrent small hemorrhages.

Like primary epidermoid tumors, cholesterol granulomas are expansile, slowly growing masses. However, these two pathologies follow nearly opposite patterns of signal intensity. The presence of methemoglobin causes cholesterol granulomas to characteristically demonstrate high signal intensity on noncontrast T1-weighted images, as shown in Case 190A *(arrows)*. The presence of deoxyhemoglobin and/or hemosiderin usually results in low signal intensity on T2-weighted scans, as seen in Case 190B *(arrow)*. (The high signal intensity within the right middle ear in Case

190B represents inflammatory disease secondary to obstruction of the eustachian tube.)

The list of benign expansile bone tumors of the skull base also includes osteoblastomas and aneurysmal bone cysts. Like cholesterol granulomas, aneurysmal bone cysts contain blood products, usually evident as sedimentation levels within a multiloculated architecture.

Fatty marrow within the petrous apex is characterized by short T1 and short T2 values (see Case 189). The lack of bone expansion should distinguish this normal variation from a cholesterol granuloma. In equivocal cases, a scan using fat-suppression techniques can establish the nature of T1-shortening within the petrous apex.

Case 191

75-year-old woman presenting with
pharyngeal pain.
(axial, noncontrast scan; SE 3000/75)

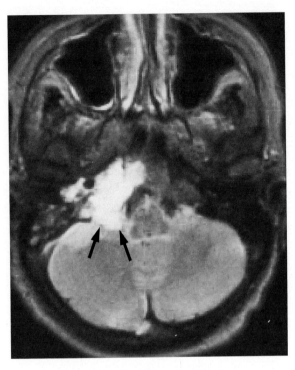

Metastatic Carcinoma of the Lung

Case 192

4-year-old girl presenting with left-sided hearing
loss and facial paresis.
(axial, postcontrast scan; SE 700/16)

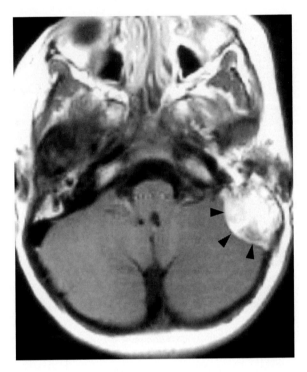

Rhabdomyosarcoma

Both systemic and local neoplasms can cause destruction of the petrous bone in children and adults. Metastases and myeloma should be considered in the differential diagnosis of Case 191, with the long T2 values making lymphoma less likely. Chordomas, chondromas, and chondrosarcomas can all arise near the petrooccipital synchondrosis; these may demonstrate lobulated contours and high signal intensity on T2-weighted images (see Case 194). Direct extension of a nasopharyngeal or parotid carcinoma into the skull base should also be considered, although such tumors are usually of lower signal intensity on T2-weighted scans than seen here (see Cases 197 and 199). Occasionally the

bone destruction of a glomus jugulare tumor mimics a malignant skull base lesion, but the anterior location and homogeneous texture of the mass in Case 191 argue against this possibility.

In Case 192, an intensely enhancing tumor destroys the posterior portion of the petrous bone. An epidural component of the lesion bulges medially into the posterior fossa. Lymphoma, neuroblastoma, and granulocytic sarcoma (leukemia) would be included with rhabdomyosarcoma in the differential diagnosis. Langerhans cell histiocytosis may also cause destructive petrous lesions in the pediatric age group.

Case 193A

38-year-old woman presenting with headaches.
(axial, noncontrast scan; SE 2500/45)

Case 193B

Same patient.
(axial, postcontrast scan; SE 550/20)

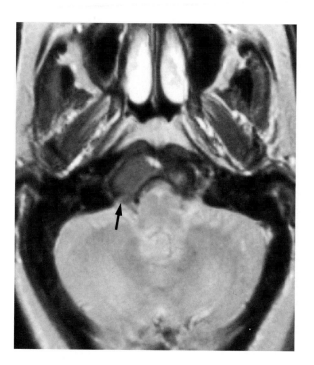

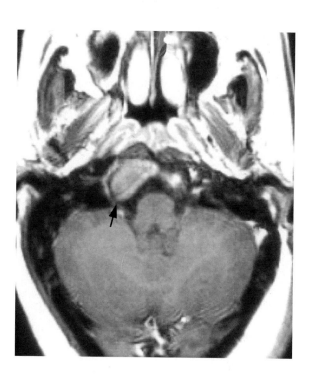

Fibrous dysplasia may involve the skull base in children or adults and should be considered in the different diagnosis of osseous pathology. Location within the basisphenoid or basiocciput is common. The lesions are frequently discovered incidentally, as in this case.

On noncontrast scans, fibrous dysplasia typically demonstrates homogeneous, finely granular low-to-intermediate signal intensity, corresponding to the characteristic "ground-glass" texture on radiographs and CT scans. Occasional cases have a cystic or bubbly appearance, particu-

larly centrally. The affected right side of the clivus in Case 193A is intermediate in intensity between the diploic bone on the left side of the clivus and the dense cortial bone in the petrous regions.

Fibrous dysplasia commonly causes expansion of bone, with notable preservation of cortical margins. Intense contrast enhancement is usual, as in Case 193B.

Metastatic carcinoma of the prostate can involve the skull base with low signal intensity on T2-weighted scans and a uniform, granular texture resembling fibrous dysplasia.

Case 194A

5-year-old girl presenting with right arm weakness.
(sagittal, noncontrast scan; SE 700/16)

Case 194B

Same patient.
(axial, noncontrast scan; SE 2500/90)

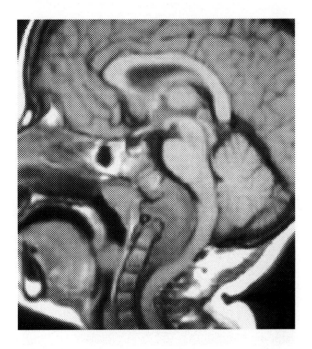

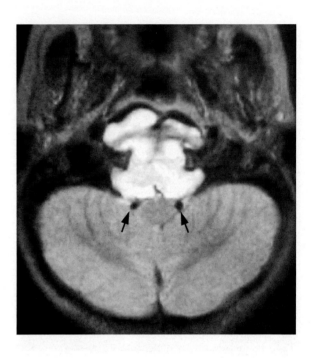

Chordomas arise from remnants of the primitive noto-chord, most frequently involving the clivus (35%) or sacrum (50%). Chordomas may also originate in the petrous or parasellar regions (see Case 195), mimicking other petrous tumors or parasellar meningiomas.

In Case 194A, a large soft tissue mass expands from the caudal aspect of the clivus. The tumor has grown inferiorly to occupy the ventral two thirds of the foramen magnum and cervical spinal canal. There is marked posterior displacement and distortion of the cervicomedullary junction. Prominent nasopharyngeal soft tissue is present, which can be a normal variant in children due to hypertrophy of lymphoid structures (i.e., adenoids).

The axial scan in Case 194B demonstrates that the clivus has been completely replaced by tumor, which is symmetrically centered in the midline. The very high signal intensity and lobulated character of the mass are characteristic features of chordomas, although other cases demonstrate greater heterogeneity. Components of T1- and T2-shortening may be present due to hemorrhage.

Calcification occurs within chordomas but is less well appreciated on MR scans than on CT images. Occasional chordomas demonstrate short T1 components (see Case 195), reflecting hemorrhage, mucinous content, or the effects of matrix calcification. Enhancement within chordomas may be minimal, mottled, or quite homogeneous (see Case 195B).

The posterior fossa component of the lesion in Case 194B causes posterior displacement of the distal vertebral arteries *(arrows)*. A shallower component of tumor extends anteriorly, causing ventral displacement of overlying nasopharyngeal tissue.

Occasional clivus chordomas project intracranially from an intact skull base, mimicking a clivus meningioma. Chordomas may also occur in the prepontine region with no bony attachment, arising from notochordal remnants in this location.

Case 195A

58-year-old man presenting with right-sided hearing loss and sixth nerve palsy.
(coronal, noncontrast scan; SE 600/11)

Case 195B

Same patient.
(axial, postcontrast scan; SE 750/11)

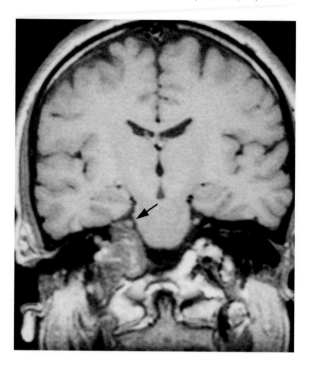

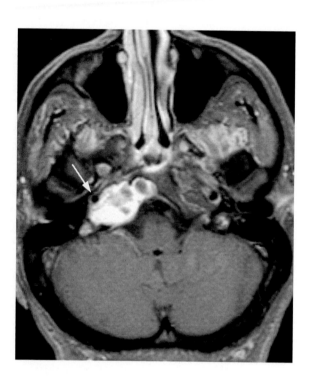

As mentioned on the previous page, chordomas of the skull base may arise several centimeters away from the midline to present as unilateral, parasagittal lesions.

The tumor in Case 195A erodes the petrous apex as it traverses the skull base on the right. The fifth cranial nerve can be identified at the superior margin of the mass *(arrow)*. The region of the internal auditory meatus is occupied and destroyed by neoplasm (compare to the normal left side). Small areas of T1-shortening within the mass may represent hemorrhage, mucinous material, or the effect of localized calcification within the tumor matrix.

Intense enhancement is present throughout most of the lesion in Case 195B. Other chordomas enhance less homogeneously and intensely. Although clearly destructive, the above chordoma is well defined, retaining a mildly lobulated contour.

Chondromas and chondrosarcomas may also occur in the area of the petrooccipital and sphenooccipital synchrondroses. These lesions should be considered along with chordoma in the differential diagnosis of midline or parasagittal skull base masses.

The petrous segment of the right internal carotid artery is identified by "flow void" at the lateral margin of the tumor in Case 195B *(arrow)*.

DIFFERENTIAL DIAGNOSIS:
CLIVAL MASS

Case 196

45-year-old woman presenting with bitemporal hemianopsia and diplopia.
(sagittal, noncontrast scan; SE 600/15)

Case 197

51-year-old woman presenting with bilateral sixth nerve palsies.
(sagittal, noncontrast scan; SE 600/15)

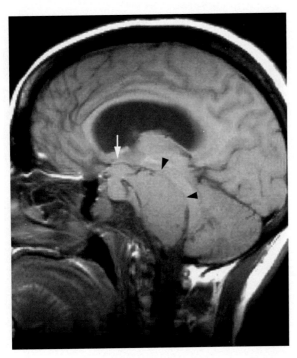

Meningioma

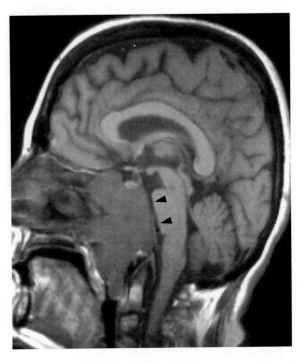

Nasopharyngeal Carcinoma

Chordomas are among several benign and malignant neoplasms that can involve the clivus.

In Case 196, a clival meningioma has permeated the basiocciput and basisphenoid. The low signal intensity within the involved bone represents reactive sclerosis. Tumor is present within the sphenoid sinus, sella turcica, and suprasellar cistern in addition to the large prepontine component. The optic chiasm is elevated and thinned *(arrow)*. The brainstem is posteriorly displaced and compressed.

Case 197 demonstrates direct extension of a nasopharyngeal carcinoma through the skull base. The clivus and the body of the sphenoid bone have been destroyed. The tumor crosses the prepontine cistern to flatten the anterior margin of the pons *(arrowheads)*.

A similar appearance could be caused by a skull base matastasis, myeloma, lymphoma, or a rare carcinoma of the sphenoid sinus. As demonstrated in Cases 207 and 208, large pituitary adenomas should also be considered in this differential diagnosis.

DIFFERENTIAL DIAGNOSIS:
REPLACEMENT OF THE BASISPHENOID

Case 198

67-year-old man presenting with headaches.
(sagittal, noncontrast scan; SE 550/20)

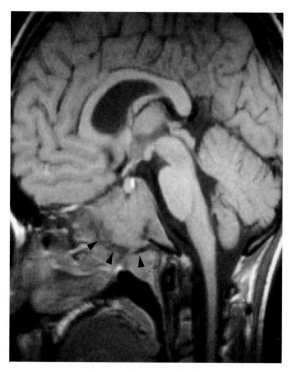

Metastatic Carcinoma of the Colon

Case 199

51-year-old woman presenting with bilateral sixth nerve palsies.
(axial, noncontrast scan; SE 2800/90)

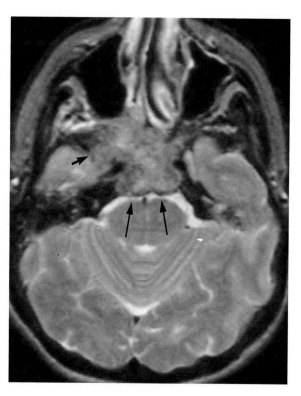

Nasopharyngeal Carcinoma
(same patient as Case 197)

Metastatic disease is a leading consideration when a destructive lesion of the skull base is discovered in an adult. The colon carcinoma in Case 198 replaces the sphenoid bone, with tumor tissue bulging into the pharynx and eroding the clivus. The sphenoid sinus has been obliterated, and the sella is surrounded by neoplasm. Myeloma (or solitary plasmocytoma) should also be considered in the differential diagnosis of this homogeneous, mildly lobulated mass.

Malignancies with dense cellularity and/or a fibrous stroma may be of relatively low intensity on T2-weighted images, as seen in Case 199 (compare to Case 194B). This unexciting signal pattern can belie a very aggressive tumor.

The carcinoma in Case 199 has destroyed the clivus, and tumor tissue interfaces with a flattened prepontine cistern *(long arrows)*. The tumor has invaded the cavernous sinuses and the pterygopalatine fossae bilaterally, with greater involvement on the right side *(short arrow)*.

A mucocele of the sphenoid sinus is a rare cause of a homogeneous mass replacing the skull base. Such lesions are characteristically well defined and expansile. Their signal intensity may be either high or low on either T1- or T2-weighted images, depending on the viscosity and inspissation of the contents. A similar appearance can be caused by a craniopharyngioma of the skull base, as illustrated in Case 235.

Compare Case 198 to the pituitary adenoma in Case 207, noting the difference in size of the sella turcica. Similarly, compare the malignant carcinoma in Case 199 to the benign adenoma in Case 208.

Postcontrast scans using fat-saturation techniques are often helpful in defining the extent of a lesion within the skull base.

REFERENCES

Albright AL, Packer RJ, Zimmerman R, Rorke LB, et al: Magnetic resonance scans should replace biopsies for the diagnosis of diffuse brain stem gliomas: a report from the children's cancer group. *Neurosurgery* 33:1026-1030, 1993.

Altman NR, Naidich TP, Braffman BH: Posterior fossa malformations. *AJNR* 13;691-724, 1992.

Anderson RE, Laskoff JM: Ramsay Hunt syndrome mimicking intracanalicular acoustic neuroma on contrast-enhanced MR. *AJNR* 11:409, 1990.

Asari S, Katayama S, Itoh T, Tsuchida S, et al: CT and MRI of haemorrhage into intracranial neuromas. *Neurosurgery* 35:247-250, 1993.

Ashley DG, Zee C-S, Chandrasoma PT, Segall HD: Lhermitte-Duclos disease: CT and MR findings. *J Comput Assist Tomgr* 14:984-987, 1990.

Baldwin D, King TT, Chevretton E, Morrison AW: Bilateral cerebellopontine angle tumors in neurofibromatosis type 2. *J Neurosurg* 74:910-915, 1991.

Beges C, Revel MP, Gaston A, et al: Trigeminal neuromas: assessment of MRI and CT. *Neuroradiology* 34:179-183, 1992.

Bilaniuk LT: Adult infratentorial tumors. *Semin Roentgenol* 25:155-173, 1990.

Bosley TM, Cohen DA, Schatz NJ, Zimmerman RA, et al: Comparison of metrizamide computed tomography and magnetic resonance imaging in evaluation of lesions at the cervicomedullary junction. *Neurology* 35:485-492, 1985.

Bourgouin PM, Tampieri D, Grahovac SZ, et al: CT and MR imaging findings in adults with cerebellar medulloblastoma: comparison with findings in children. *AJR* 159:609-612, 1992.

Brown RV, Sage MR, Brophy BP: CT and MR findings in patients with chordomas of the petrous apex. *AJNR* 11:121-124, 1990.

Byrne JV, Kendall Be, Kingsley DPE, et al: Lesions of the brain stem: assessment by magnetic resonance imaging. *Neuroradiology* 31:129, 1989.

Casselman JW, Dejonge I, Neyt L, et al: MRI in craniofacial fibrous dysplasia. *Neuroradiology* 35:234-237, 1993.

Casselman JW, Kuhweide R, Ampe W, Meeus L, et al: Pathology of the menbraneous labyrinth: comparison of T1-and T2-weighted and gadolinium-enhanced spin-echo and 3DFT-CISS imaging. *AJNR* 14:59-69, 1993.

Celli P, Ferrante L, Acqui M, et al: Neuromas of the third, fourth, and sixth cranial nerves: a survey and report of a new fourth nerve case. *Surg Neurol* 38:216-224, 1992.

Chaljub G, Van Fleet R, Guinto FC Jr, et al: MR imaging of clival and paraclival lesions. *AJR* 159:1069-1074, 1992.

Chang T, Teng MMH, Lirng JF: Posterior cranial fossa tumors in childhood. *Neuroradiology* 35:274-278, 1993.

Cohen TI, Powers SK, Williams DW III: MR appearance of intracanalicular eighth nerve lipoma. *AJNR* 13:1188-1190, 1992.

Curati WL, Graif M, Kingsley DPE, et al: Acoustic neuromas: Gd-DTPA enhancement in MR imaging. *Radiology* 158:447-451, 1986.

Curati WL, Graif M, Kingsley DPE, et al: MRI in acoustic neuroma: a review of 35 patients. *Neuroradiology* 28:208-214, 1986.

Daniels DL, Czervionke LF, Pojunas KW, et al: Facial nerve enhancement in MR imaging. *AJNR* 8:605-607, 1987.

Daniels DL, Czervionke LF, Millen SJ, Haberkamph TJ, et al: MR imaging of facial nerve enhancement in Bell palsy or after temporal bone surgery. *Radiology* June 171:807-809, 1989.

Daniels DL, Millen SJ, Meyer GA, et al: MR detection of tumor in the internal auditory canal. *AJNR* 8:249-252, 1987.

Daniels DL, Pech P, Pojunas KW, et al: Trigeminal nerve: anatomic correlation with MR imaging. *Radiology* 159:577-583, 1986.

Daniels DL, Schenck JF, Foster T, et al: Magnetic resonance imaging of the jugular foramen. *AJNR* 6:699-703, 1985.

David R, Lamki N, Fan S, et al: The many faces of neuroblastoma. *Radiographics* 9:859-882, 1989.

Dietz RR, Davis WL, Harnsberger HR, et al: MR imaging and MR angiography in the evaluation of pulsatile tinnitus. *AJNR* 15:879-889, 1994.

Domingues RC, Taveras JM, Reimer P, Rosen BR: Foramen magnum choroid plexus papilloma with drop metastases to the lumbar spine. *AJNR* 12:564-565, 1991.

Donna J, Halperin EC, Friedman HS, Boyko OB: Subfrontal recurrence of medulloblastoma. *AJNR* 13:1617-1618, 1992.

Elster AD, Arthur DW: Intracranial hemangioblastomas: CT and MR findings. *J Comput Assist Tomogr* 12:736-739, 1988.

Enzmann DR, O'Donohue J: Optimizing MR imaging for detecting small tumors in the cerebellopontine angle and internal auditory canal. *AJNR* 8:99-106, 1987.

Epstein FJ, Farmer J-P: Brain stem glioma growth patterns. *Neurosurgery* 78:408-412, 1993.

Filling-Katz MR, Choyke PL, Patronas NJ, et al: Radiologic screening for von Hippel-Lindau Disease: the role of Gd-DTPA enhanced MR imaging of the CNS. *J Comput Assist Tomogr* 13:743:755, 1989.

Gelbarski SS, Telian SA, Niparko JK: Enhancement along the normal facial nerve in the facial canal: MR imaging and anatomic correlation. *Radiology* 183:391-394, 1992.

Gelbarski SS, Tucci DL, Telian SA: The cochlear nuclear complex: MR location and abnormalities. *AJNR* 14:1311-1318, 1993.

Gentry LR, Jacoby CG, Turski PA, et al: Cerebellopontine angle-retromastoid mass lesions: comparative study of diagnosis with MR imaging and CT. *Radiology* 162:513-520, 1987.

Greenberg JJ, Oot RF, Wismer GL, et al: Cholesterol granulomas of the petrous apex: MR and CT evaluation. *AJNR* 9:1205-1214, 1988.

Griffin C, De La Paz R, Enzmann D: MR and CT correlation of cholesterol cysts of the petrous bone. *AJNR* 8:825-829, 1987.

Gusnard DA: Cerebellar neoplasms in children. *Semin Roentgenol* 25:263-278, 1990.

Han MH, Jabour BA, Andrews JC, et al: Noneoplastic enhancing lesions mimicking intracanalicular acoustic neuroma on gadolinium-enhanced MR images. *Radiology* 179:795-796, 1991.

Ho VB, Smirniotopoulos JG, Murphy FM, Rushing EJ: Radiologic-pathologic correlation: hemangioblastoma. *AJNR* 13:1343-1352, 1992.

Hudgins PA, Davis PC, Hoffman JC Jr: Gadopentetate Dimeglumine-enhanced MR imaging in children following surgery for brain tumor: spectrum of meningeal findings. *AJNR* 12:301-308, 1991.

Hueftle M, Han J, Kaufman B, et al: MR imaging of brainstem gliomas. *J Comput Assist Tomogr* 9:263, 1985.

Hutchins LG, Harnsberger HR, Hardin CW, et al: The radiological assessment of trigeminal neuropathy. *AJNR* 10:1031-1038, 1989.

Jan M, Dweik A, Destrieux C, Djebbari Y: Fronto-orbital sphenoidal fibrous dysplasia. *Neurosurgery* 34:544-547, 1994.

Kane AG, Robles HA, Smirniotopoulos JG, et al: Diffuse pontine astrocytoma. *AJNR* 14:941-945, 1993.

Kimura F, Kim KS, Friedman H, et al: MR imaging of the normal and abnormal clivus. *AJNR* 11:1015-1021, 1990.

Kingsley DPE, Brooks GB, Leung AW-L, Johnson MA: Acoustic neuromas: evaluation by magnetic resonance imaging. *AJNR* 6:1-5, 1985.

Kochi M, Mihara Y, Takada A, et al: MRI of subarachnoid dissemination of medulloblastoma. *Neuroradiology* 33:264-268 1991.

Koci TM, Chiang F, Mehringer CM, et al: Adult cerebellar medulloblastoma: imaging features with emphasis on MR. *AJNR* 14:929-939, 1993.

Laine FL, Nadel L, Brain IF: CT and MR imaging of the central skull base: 2. Pathologic spectrum. *Radiographics* 10:797, 1990.

Larson TL, Wong ML: Primary mucocele of the petrous apex: MR appearance. *AJNR* 13:203-204, 1992.

Lee BCP, Deck MDF, Kneeland JB, Cahill PT: MR imaging of the craniocervical junction. *AJNR* 6:209-213, 1985.

Lee BPC, Kneeland JB, Walker RW, et al: MR imaging of brain stem tumors. *AJNR* 6:159-164, 1985.

Lee SR, Sanches J, Mark As, et al: Posterior fossa hemangioblastomas: MR imaging. *Radiology* 171:463-468, 1989.

Lee Y-Y, Van Tassel P, Bruner JM, et al: Juvenile pilocytic astrocytomas: CT and MR characteristics. *AJNR* 10:363-370, 1989.

Leproux F, De Toffel B, Aesch, B, Cotty P: MRI of cranial chordomas: the value of gadolinium. *Neuroradiology* 35:543-545, 1993.

Lhuillier FM, Doyon DL, Halimi PhM, et al: Magnetic resonance imaging of acoustic neuromas: pitfalls and differential diagnosis. *Neuroradiology* 34:144-149, 1992.

Lizak PF, Woodruff WW: Posterior fossa neoplasms: multiplanar imaging. *Semin US CT MR* 13:182-206, 1992.

Lyons MK, Kelly PJ: Posterior fossa ependymoma: report of 30 cases and review of the literature. *Neurosurgery* 28:659-672, 1991.

Maleci A, Cervoni L, Delfini R: Medulloblastoma in children and in adults: a comparative study. *Acta Neurochir (Wien)* 19:62-67, 1992.

Mark AS, Blake P, Atlas SW, et al: Gd-DTPA enhancement of the cisternal portion of the oculomotor nerve on MR imaging. *AJNR* 13:1463-1470, 1992.

Mark AS, Fitzgerald D: Segmental enhancement of the cochlea on contrast-enhanced MR: correlation with the frequency of hearing loss and possible sign of perilymphatic fistula and autoimmune labyrinthitis. *AJNR* 14:991-996, 1993.

Mark AS, Seltzer S, Harnsberger HR: Sensorineural hearing loss: more than meets the eye? *AJNR* 14:37-46, 1993.

Martin N, Sterkers O, Mompoint D, Nahum H: Facial nerve neuromas: MR imaging. *Neuroradiology* 34:62-67, 1992.

Mathews VP, Broome DR, Smith RR, et al: Neuroimaging of disseminated germ cell neoplasms. *AJNR* 11-319-324, 1990.

McCormick PC, Bello JA, Post KD: Trigeminal schwannoma. *J Neurosurg* 69:850-860, 1988.

Meyers SP, Hirsch WL Jr, Curtin HD, et al: Chordomas of the skull base: MR features. *AJNR* 13:1627-1636, 1992.

Meyers SP, Hirsch WL, Curtin HD, Barnes L, et al: Chondrosarcomas of the skull base: MR imaging features. *Radiology* 184:103-108, 1992.

Meyers SP, Kemp SS, Tarr RW: MR imaging features of medulloblastomas. *AJR* 158:865-895, 1992.

Mikhael MA, Ciric IS, Wolff AP: Differentiation of cerebellopontine angle neuromas and meningiomas with MR imaging. *J Comput Assist Tomogr* 9:852-856, 1985.

Mikhael MA, Cirie IS, Wolff AP: MR diagnosis of acoustic neuromas. *J Comput Assist Tomogr* 11:232-235, 1987.

Mueller DP, Moore SA, Sato RY, Yuh WTC: MR spectrum of medulloblastoma. *Clin Imaging* 16:250-255, 1992.

Mulkens TH, Parizel PM, Martin JJ, et al: Acoustic schwannoma: MR findings in 84 tumors. *AJR* 160:395-398, 1993.

Neuman HPH, Eggert HR, Scheremet R, et al: Central nervous system lesions in von Hippel-Lindau syndrome. *J Neurol Neurosurg Psychiatr* 55:898-901, 1992.

Okada Y, Aoki S, Barkovich AJ, et al: Cranial bone marrow in children: assessment of normal development with MR imaging. *Radiology* 171:161-164, 1989.

Olsen WL, Dillon WP, Kelly WM, et al: MR imaging of paragangliomas. *AJNR* 7:1039-1042, 1986.

Oot RF, Melville GE, New PFJ, et al: The role of MR and CT in evaluating clival chondroma and chondrosarcomas. *AJNR* 9:715-723, 1988.

Peterman SB, Steiner RE, Bydder GM, et al: Nuclear magnetic resonance imaging (NMR) of brain stem tumors. *Neuroradiology* 27:202-207, 1985.

Pollack IF, Sekhar LN, Jannetta PJ, Janecka JP: Neurilemmomas of the trigeminal nerve. *J Neurosurg* 70:737-745, 1989.

Press GA, Hesselink JR: MR imaging of cerebellopontine angle and internal auditory canal lesions at 1.5 T. *AJNR* 9:241-252, 1988.

Remley KB, Coit WE, Harnsberger HR, et al: Pulsatile tinnitus and the vascular tympanic membrane: CT, MR, and angiographic findings. *Radiology* 174:383-390, 1990.

Rippe DJ, Boyko OB, Friedman HS, et al: Gd-DTPA-enhanced MR imaging of leptomeningeal spread of primary intracranial CNS tumors in children. *AJNR* 11:329-332, 1990.

Rollins N, Mendelsohn D, Mulne A, et al: Recurrent medulloblastoma: frequency of tumor enhancement on Gd-DTPA MR imaging. *AJNR* 11:583-587, 1990.

Sartoretti-Schefer S, Wichmann W, Valavanis A: Idiopathic, herpetic, and HIV-associated facial nerve palsies: abnormal MR enhancement patterns. *AJNR* 15:479-486, 1994.

Sato Y, Wazir M, Smith W, et al: Hippel-Lindau disease: MR imaging. *Radiology* 166:241, 1988.

Seltzer S, Mark AS: Contrast enhancement of the labyringh on MR scans in patients with sudden hearing loss and vertigo: evidence of labyrinthine disease. *AJNR* 12:13-16, 1991.

Sen CN, Sekhar LN, Schramm VL, et al: Chordoma and chondrosarcoma of the cranial base: an 8-year experience. *Neurosurgery* 25:921-941, 1989.

Sevick RJ, Dillon WP, Engstrom J, et al: Trigeminal neuropathy: Gd-DTPA enhanced MR imaging. *J Comput Assist Tomogr* 15:605-611, 1991.

Shanley DJ, Vassallo CJ: Atypical presentation of Lhermitte-Duclos disease: preoperative diagnosis with MRI. *Neuroradiology* 34:102-103, 1992.

Sherman J, Citrin C, Barkovich A, et al: MR imaging of the tectum. *AJNR* 8:59, 1987.

Shigeki A, Dillon WP, Barkovich AJ, Normal D: Marrow conversion before pneumatization of the sphenoid sinus: assessment with MR imaging. *Radiology* 172:373-375, 1989.

Smirniotopoulos JG, Uye NC, Rushing EJ: Cerebellopontine angle masses: radiologic-pathologic correlation. *Radiographics* 13:1131-1146, 1993.

Smith RR, Grossman RI, Goldberg HI, et al: MR imaging of Lhermitte-Duclos disease: a case report. *AJNR* 10:187, 1989.

Som PM, Dillon WP, Sze G, et al: Benign and malignant sinonasal lesions with intracranial extension: differentiatio with MR imaging. *Radiology* 172:763-766, 1989.

Spoto GP, Press GA, Hesselink JR, Solomon M: Intracranial ependymoma and subependymoma: MR manifestations. *AJNR* 11:83-91, 1990.

Stroink AR, Hoffman HJ, Hendrick EB, Humphreys RP: Diagnosis and management of pediatric brain stem gliomas. *J Neurosurg* 65:745-750, 1986.

Strong JA, Hatten HP Jr, Brown MT, et al: Pilocytic astrocytoma: correlation between the initial imaging features and clinical aggressiveness. *AJR* 161:369-372, 1993.

Sze G, Vichanco LS, Brant-Zawadzki M, et al: Chordomas: MR imaging. *Radiology* 166:187-191, 1988.

Tali ET, Yuh WTC, Nguyen HD, et al: Cystic acoustic schwannoma: MR characteristics. *AJNR* 14:1241-1247, 1993.

Tach RR, Sze G, Leslie DR: Trigeminal neuralgia: MR imaging features. *Radiology* 172:767-770, 1989.

Tien RD, Dillon WP: Herpes trigeminal neuritis and rhombencephalitis on Gd-DTPA-enhanced MR imaging. *AJNR* 11:413, 1990.

Tien RD, Dillon WP, Jackler RK: Contrast-enhanced MR imaging of the facial nerve in 11 patients with Bell's palsy. *AJNR* 11:735-741, 1990.

Valvassori GE, Morales FJ, Palacios E, Dobben GE: MR of the normal and abnormall internal auditory canal. *AJNR* 9:115-120, 1988.

Vandertop WP, Hoffman HJ, Drake JM, et al: Focal midbrain tumors in children. *Neurosurgery* 31:186-194, 1992.

Vieco PT, Del Carpio-O'Donovan R, Melanson D, et al: Dysplastic gangliocytoma (Lhermitte-Duclos disease): CT and MR imaging. *Pediatr Radiol* 22:366-369, 1992.

Vogl T, Bruning R, Schedel H, et al: Paraganglioma of the jugular bulb and carotid body: MR imaging with short sequences and Gd-DTPA enhancement. *AJNR* 10:823-827, 1989.

Von Gils APG, Van Den Berg R, Falke THM, et al: MR diagnosis of paraganglioma of the head and neck: value of contrast enhancement. *AJR* 162:147-153, 1994.

West MS, Russell EJ, Breit R, et al: Calvarial and skull base metastases: comparison of nonenhanced and Gd-DTPA-enhanced MR images. *Radiology* 174:85-92, 1990.

Williams DW, Elster AD, Ginsberg LE, Stanton C: Recurrent Lhermitte-Duclos disease: report of two cases and association with Cowden's disease. *AJNR* 13:287-290, 1992.

Yano M, Tajima S, Tanaka Y, et al: Magnetic resonance imaging of craniofacial fibrous dysplasia. *Ann Plast Surg* 30:371-374, 1993.

Yuh WT, Wright DC, Barloon TJ, et al: MR imaging of primary tumors of the trigeminal nerve and Meckel's cave. *AJNR* 9:665-670, 1988.

CHAPTER 5

Pituitary, Suprasellar, and Parasellar Masses

Case 200

77-year-old man complaining that "the side vision in both eyes has gone."
(sagittal, noncontrast scan; SE 700/17)

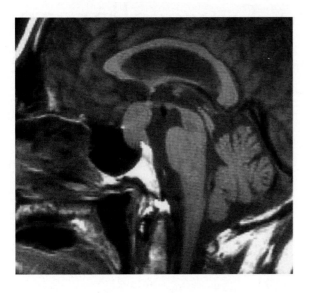

Case 201

53-year-old man presenting with bitemporal hemianopsia.
(sagittal, noncontrast scan; SE 600/20)

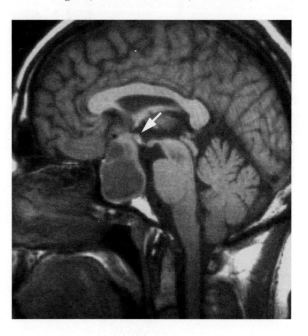

The most reliable CT or MR feature of pituitary adenomas is their origin within the sella turcica. Large adenomas may have confusing suprasellar or parasellar components, heterogeneous signal intensity, and variable enhancement patterns. When a complex lesion is encountered at the skull base, expansion of the sella turcica near the geographic center of the mass is a key clue to pituitary etiology.

On T1-weighted images, the signal intensity of uncomplicated pituitary adenomas is comparable to that of brain parenchyma, as seen in Case 200. Large adenomas often contain cystic or necrotic areas that demonstrate longer T1 values than the surrounding tumor tissue, as illustrated by Case 201. A third pattern of signal intensity is seen when subacute hemorrhage causes areas of T1-shortening within an adenoma (see Cases 211 and 212).

In Case 200, the sella is moderately enlarged. A suprasellar component of the tumor elevates the optic chiasm *(arrow)*, causing bitemporal hemianopsia.

Case 201 demonstrates gross expansion of the sella. The adenoma bulges into the sphenoid sinus and erodes the clivus. Suprasellar extension of the tumor has elevated and flattened the anterior recesses of the third ventricle and the optic chiasm *(arrow)*.

Pathologies other than pituitary adenomas may cause cystic-appearing masses within the sella turcica. Intrasellar craniopharyngiomas, Rathke's pouch cysts, and rare pituitary abscesses can present in this manner.

The relative severity of optic nerve compression or bitemporal hemianopsia (from pressure on the optic chiasm) depends on the congenitally variable proximity of the optic chiasm to the optic canals as well as on the size and location of a suprasellar mass.

Case 202

55-year-old man presenting with blurred vision.
(axial, noncontrast scan; SE 2500/30)

Case 203

50-year-old woman presenting with diplopia.
(axial, noncontrast scan; SE 3000/90)

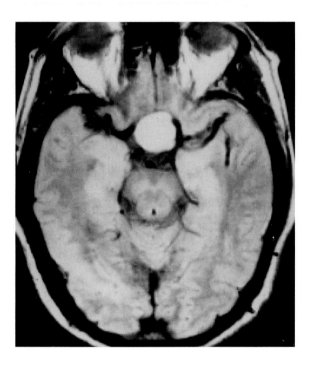

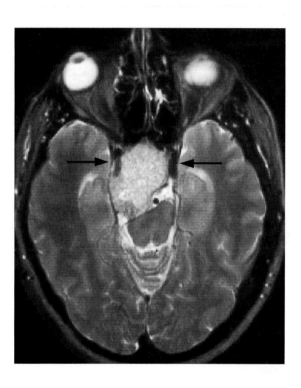

Nonhemorrhagic pituitary adenomas usually demonstrate intermediate or high signal intensity on T2-weighted images. Low intensity may be noted in the presence of hemorrhage or dense calcification.

High signal intensity on T2-weighted scans may reflect cystic degeneration within an adenoma (as in Case 202) and/or high water content of viable tumor tissue. Adenomas of relatively low intensity on long TR spin echo sequences are often more fibrous and more

difficult to resect than adenomas with high intensity on such sequences.

The adenoma in Case 203 is a large mass that has caused lateral displacement of the internal carotid arteries *(arrows)*. In addition, a retrosellar component deforms the right cerebral peduncle. Such lateral and posterior expansion of pituitary tumors may distort cranial nerves III through VI, leading to ophthalmoplegia and diplopia as in this case.

Case 204

41-year-old man presenting with bitemporal
hemianopsia.
(sagittal, postcontrast scan; SE 600/15)

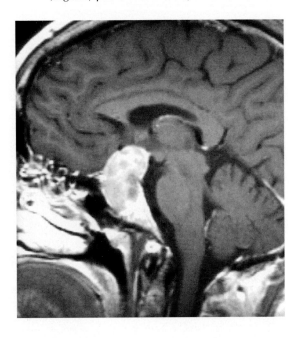

Case 205

53-year-old man presenting with bitemporal
hemianopsia.
(coronal, postcontrast scan; SE 700/20)

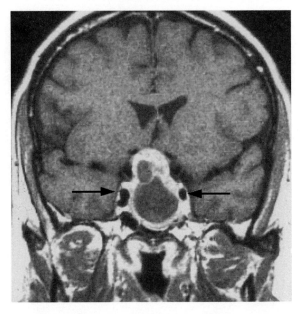

(same patient as Case 201)

Many pituitary adenomas demonstrate uniform, intense contrast enhancement, as in Case 204. The suprasellar extension of such tumors may resemble other suprasellar masses (e.g., meningioma, germinoma, or hypothalamic glioma). However, the lesion in Case 204 arises from an expanded sella turcica, establishing the correct diagnosis. (It is rarer for a suprasellar meningioma to grow inferiorly and enlarge the sella turcica; see Case 210.)

Case 205 presents a postcontrast scan of the cystic/necrotic adenoma shown in Case 201. Large adenomas often contain nonenhancing regions due to cysts, hemorrhage, or necrosis. Sometimes the entire tumor has this appearance, with only a rim of contrast enhancement. The suprasellar extension of such a rim-enhancing adenoma can mimic a craniopharyngioma (see Case 234).

Pituitary abscesses may closely resemble a cystic or necrotic intrasellar neoplasm. Abscesses may be relatively in-

dolent, causing few symptoms and no systemic signs of infection. However, they are usually smaller than the lesion in Case 205, typically demonstrating a very round shape with a uniformly thin rim of enhancement.

Coronal MR scans demonstrate the position and caliber of the parasellar internal carotid arteries, seen as "flow voids" within the cavernous sinus in Case 205 (*arrows;* see also Cases 215 and 216). Since the medial margin of the enhancing cavernous sinus is usually difficult to distinguish from enhancing adenoma, encasement of the internal carotid artery can be important evidence of cavernous sinus invasion.

In both of these cases, the suprasellar portion of the tumor has elevated the floor of the third ventricle. The optic chiasm, which resides in a notch between the ventricle's optic and infundibular recesses, can be presumed to be displaced and stretched.

Case 206A

38-year-old man presenting with blurred
vision and headaches.
(sagittal, noncontrast scan; SE 600/15)

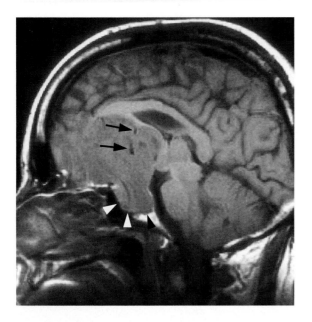

Case 206B

Same patient.
(coronal, postcontrast scan; SE 600/15)

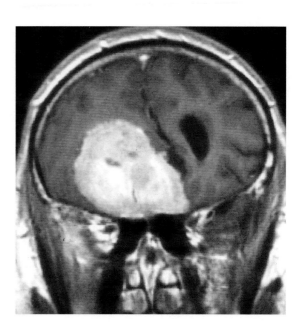

Nonsecreting pituitary adenomas may become very large before compression of the optic chiasm causes symptoms. Here a huge subfrontal mass is continuous with an expanded sella turcica (*arrowheads,* Case 206A), establishing the origin of the tumor.

"Flow voids" of low signal intensity near the superior margin of the mass *(arrows)* represent encased branches of the anterior cerebral arteries. Encasement of basal arteries is characteristic of parasellar meningiomas (see Case 42) but can also be associated with pituitary adenomas, more commonly involving the cavernous segments of the internal carotid arteries (see Cases 215 and 216).

Suprasellar extension of a pituitary adenoma may be grossly asymmetrical, as seen in Case 206B. The appearance of the tumor on this image is indistinguishable from a subfrontal meningioma.

Esthesioneuroblastoma or "olfactory neuroblastoma" is a rare tumor that can also present as an enhancing subfrontal mass in young patients (see Case 307). The characteristic origin of this neoplasm from the region of the cribriform plate and ethmoid roof usually differentiates such tumors from meningiomas or pituitary adenomas.

Case 207

66-year-old man presenting with headaches.
(sagittal, noncontrast scan; SE 600/20)

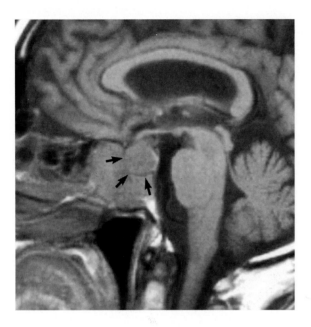

Case 208

59-year-old woman.
(axial, noncontrast scan; SE 2500/90)

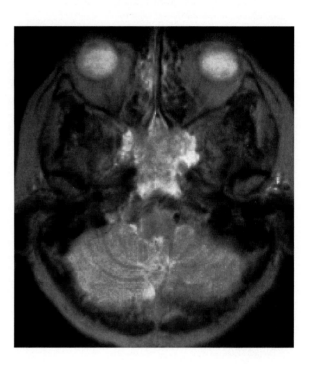

Some pituitary adenomas grow predominantly inferiorly, filling the sphenoid sinus and eroding the skull base. The above cases demonstrate large defects in the middle of the sphenoid bone and clivus due to inferior extension of pituitary tumors. Such bone destruction may mimic the skull invasion of a nasopharyngeal neoplasm (compare to Case 197). Metastasis and myeloma are also prime considerations when lesions of the skull base are encountered in adults (see Case 198).

Compare the relatively homogeneous tissue texture and intermediate signal intensity of the tumor in Case 208 to the squamous cell carcinoma in Case 199. Benign and malignant neoplasms of the skull base may present surprisingly similar MR features, requiring careful attention to associated findings. Note the ghost of an expanded sella within the lesion in Case 207 *(arrows)* and compare to Case 198.

Sagittal and coronal MR scans are valuable for simultaneously defining the pharyngeal and intracranial components of masses involving the skull base (see Case 194 for an additional example).

Case 209

50-year-old woman presenting with impaired
vision in the left eye.
(coronal, postcontrast scan; SE 600/15)

Case 210

41-year-old man presenting with
bitemporal hemianopsia.
(coronal, postcontrast scan; SE 550/20)

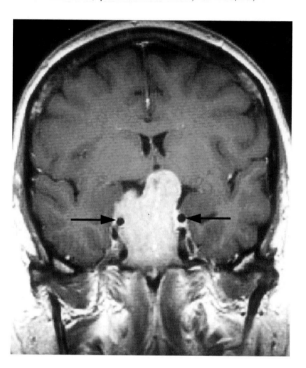

Pituitary Adenoma

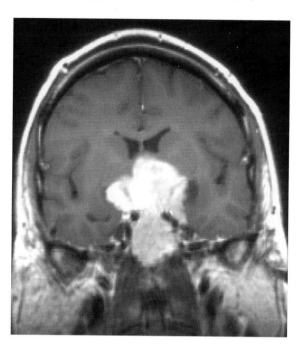

Meningioma

The distinction between a pituitary tumor with suprasellar extension and a suprasellar mass growing into the sella may be difficult. Both of the above tumors have expanded the sella turcica, eroded the sphenoid bone, and accumulated in the suprasellar cistern. They are transsphenoidal masses that present substantial surgical risks for cranial nerve injury and postoperative CSF leak.

The enhancement patterns of the two lesions are indistinguishable. The wide separation of the cavernous segments of the internal carotid arteries in Case 209 *(arrows)*

is typical of an originally intrasellar tumor, providing a clue to the diagnosis. The marked enlargement of the sella and the broad continuity between the intrasellar and suprasellar components also favor a pituitary adenoma in this case.

The meningioma in Case 210 represents the opposite extreme from the small lesion in Case 224. The size of a tumor at the time of clinical presentation depends on the location of the lesion with respect to adjacent neural structures.

Case 211

21-year-old man presenting with headaches.
(sagittal, noncontrast scan; SE 700/17)

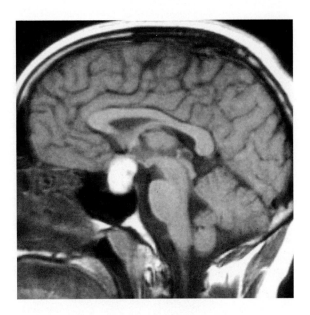

Case 212

15-year-old girl presenting with amenorrhea.
(sagittal, noncontrast scan; SE 600/20)

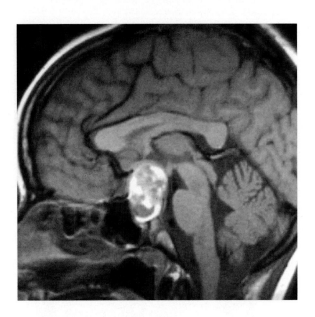

Hemorrhage is commonly noted within pituitary adenomas at the time of diagnosis or during treatment. Some observers suggest an increased incidence of pituitary hemorrhages in patients receiving bromocriptine therapy.

Acute bleeding into an adenoma may cause sudden enlargement of the tumor, with compression of the optic apparatus and adenohypophysis. The associated rapid development of visual impairment and endocrine dysfunction (usually accompanied by headache) has been called "pituitary apoplexy."

Much more commonly, the hemorrhages within an adenoma are small and subclinical. That is, the presence of blood products in a pituitary adenoma is usually *not* correlated with a catastrophic or even recognizable clinical event.

The pattern of hemorrhage within pituitary adenomas is variable. Both of the above cases demonstrate diffuse T1-shortening due to methemoglobin, with a homogeneous distribution in Case 211 and more heterogeneity in Case 212. Both tumors extend into the suprasellar region, with elevation of the third ventricle and optic chiasm.

Homogeneous T1-shortening normally occurs within the moderately enlarged pituitary glands of pregnant women. This physiological change should not be mistaken for hemorrhage when such patients present with headache or other nonspecific symptoms. (The pituitary glands of newborn infants demonstrate similar T1-shortening, probably reflecting the intrauterine hormonal environment.)

Craniopharyngiomas and Rathke's cleft cysts can also present as intrasellar and suprasellar masses of high signal intensity on T1-weighted images (see Cases 228 and 240).

Case 213

35-year-old woman presenting with
bitemporal hemianopsia.
(coronal, noncontrast scan; SE 600/17)

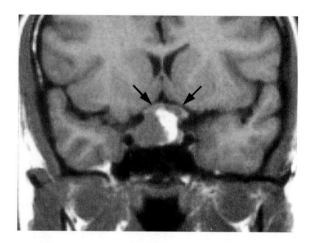

Case 214

17-year-old woman presenting with amenorrhea
and bitemporal hemianopsia.
(axial, noncontrast scan; SE 2500/120)

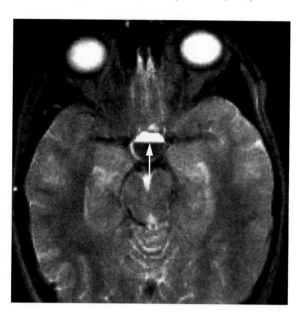

In Case 213, T1-shortening due to methemoglobin is seen within the left side of the pituitary adenoma. This evidence of subacute hemorrhage was not correlated with any acute event in the patient's history. A postcontrast scan demonstrated a nonenhancing zone corresponding exactly to the area of precontrast T1-shortening.

The optic chiasm is stretched over the superior pole of the adenoma in Case 213, accounting for the patient's presentation with bitemporal visual field cuts *(arrows)*. However, the cavernous sinuses do not appear to be invaded by tumor (compare to Cases 215 and 216).

Case 214 demonstrates a sedimentation level of blood products within the cystic, suprasellar component of a pituitary adenoma. The marked T2-shortening of the dependent component is characteristic of liquid collections containing blood products (compare to the sedimentation level within the subdural hematoma in Case 576). The presence of a sedimentation level is the most reliable MR or CT indication that a lesion is truly cystic (see also Cases 86 and 129).

Case 215

30-year-old woman presenting with sudden onset of a painful left third nerve palsy.
(coronal, noncontrast scan; SE 700/22)

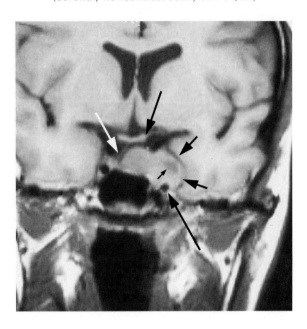

Case 216

36-year-old woman presenting with diplopia.
(coronal, postcontrast scan; SE 650/20)

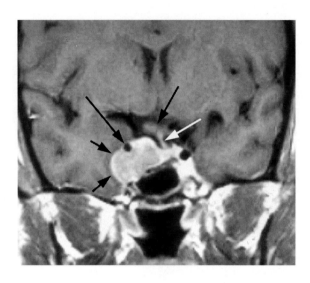

Pituitary adenomas may grow laterally to involve the cavernous sinus, sometimes with little expansion of the sella itself. Such tumors may mimic other parasellar masses such as meningioma, trigeminal schwannoma, lymphoma, or metastasis (see Cases 253-255).

Even with the perspective of coronal MR imaging, it may be difficult to distinguish displacement and compression of the cavernous sinus from actual tumor invasion. Invasion is suspected when the signal intensity of the adenoma extends to the lateral wall of the cavernous sinus, when the sinus is widened with convex margins *(short black arrows),* and when the cavernous segment of the internal carotid artery is clearly encased.

In Case 215, the internal carotid artery *(longest black arrow)* is depressed, while in Case 216 it is elevated. In both cases, the vessel is mildly narrowed. Like parasellar meningiomas, pituitary adenomas may be associated with encasement of adjacent arteries.

Coronal MR scans provide excellent definition of the optic chiasm *(medium length black arrows)* and pituitary infundibulum *(white arrows),* which are key suprasellar landmarks. In both of the above cases, eccentric origin of the adenoma causes contralateral displacement of the infundibulum. The optic chiasm is not deformed in either case.

The acute onset of the third nerve palsy in Case 215 could represent an episode of infarction within the cavernous extension of the tumor (in turn possibly corresponding with the small area of low intensity seen laterally; *tiny arrow).* As noted on the previous pages, hemorrhage is common in pituitary adenomas. Acute infarction can also cause rapid swelling of an adenoma, leading to sudden visual or endocrine compromise ("pituitary apoplexy").

Case 217A

22-year-old woman presenting with amenorrhea
and high serum prolactin levels.
(sagittal, noncontrast scan; SE 600/15)

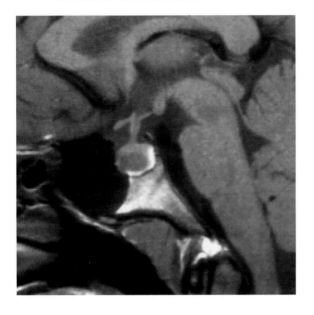

Case 217B

Same patient.
(coronal, noncontrast scan; RSE 4000/96)

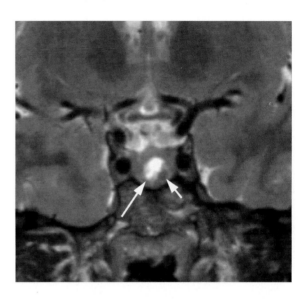

Secreting adenomas of the pituitary may cause significant endocrine symptoms even when small. (Compare the size of the above tumor to the non-secreting adenomas in Cases 206 and 207.) Tumors less than ten millimeters in diameter have been termed "microadenomas." Prolactinomas are the most frequent microadenomas to produce symptoms, usually amenorrhea and/or galactorrhea in a young woman.

Axial CT and MR scans are often normal in the presence of microadenomas. Sagittal and coronal MR scans without contrast material may demonstrate the tumors as focal zones of altered T1 and/or T2 values.

In Case 217A, a mass of uniformly low signal intensity occupies the inferior portion of the sella turcica. The T2-weighted coronal scan in Case 217B confirms that the lesion is within the pituitary gland. The majority of the mass is sharply defined by high signal intensity *(long arrow)*. A nodule of low intensity is present inferiorly on the left *(short arrow)*.

Microadenomas may have either higher or lower signal intensity than surrounding pituitary tissue on T2-weighted scans, with the former pattern being more common. Low intensity within adenomas on T2-weighted images may reflect blood products (see Cases 213 and 214), calcification, or densely fibrous texture.

See Case 218-2 for postcontrast images of this lesion.

Case 218

18-year-old woman presenting with galactorrhea.
(coronal, postcontrast scan; SE 600/20)

Case 218-1

21-year-old man with acromegaly.
(coronal, postcontrast scan; SE 600/15)

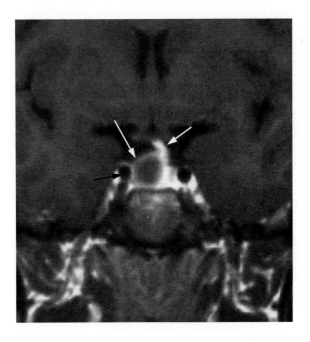

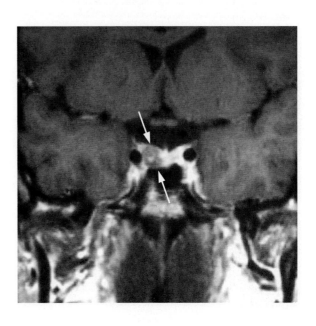

In many cases, microadenomas are best defined by coronal scans performed immediately after the injection of contrast material. The tumors are usually outlined on such images as "filling defects" within otherwise enhancing pituitary tissue. This appearance must be correlated with secondary findings and the clinical presentation, since other nonenhancing regions (e.g., small cysts) are common within the gland.

Secondary findings of a pituitary microadenoma on coronal scans include increased height of the gland, eccentric superior convexity, deviation of the pituitary infundibulum, and focal erosion of the sellar floor. Each of these features can be an isolated normal finding, but their association suggests a responsible mass.

Case 218 illustrates a microadenoma within the right side of the sella (*long arrow*). The mass is large enough to cause superior convexity of the pituitary gland and contralateral displacement of the infundibulum (*short arrow*). The lumen of the right internal carotid artery is not surrounded or displaced, suggesting that the tumor does not involve the cavernous sinus.

The small growth hormone–secreting microadenoma in Case 218-1 does not affect the overall contour of the gland or the position of the infundibulum. Even smaller microadenomas may be clinically manifest as Cushing's disease, acromegaly, or amenorrhea/galactorrhea.

A small area of artifact is often encountered at the junction of the sphenoid sinus septum and the sellar floor. This localized abnormality can mimic or obscure a microadenoma. The pseudolesion is best identified by recognizing its relationship to the sphenoid septum.

Case 218-2A

22-year-old woman presenting with amenorrhea.
(coronal scan performed sixty seconds after
injection of contrast; GRE 125/6/80°)

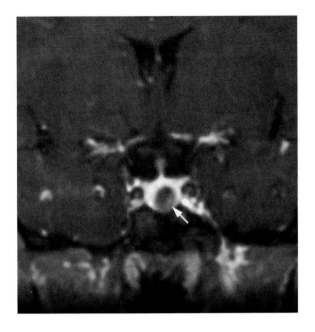

Case 218-2B

Same patient.
(coronal scan performed eight minutes after
injection of contrast; SE 550/20)

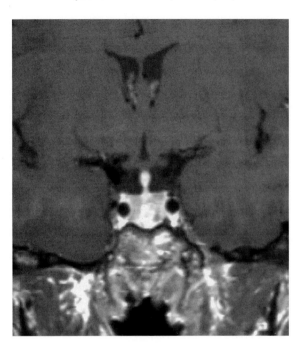

Scans performed during the early phases of pituitary enhancement may demonstrate microadenomas more clearly than images obtained several minutes after the injection of contrast material. The signal intensity of many microadenomas increases steadily on delayed postcontrast scans, with the tumor becoming progressively less distinct from surrounding pituitary tissue.

Case 218-2 illustrates this pattern. The majority of the adenoma is nonenhancing on the early scan (Case 218-2A), with a tiny nodule of active enhancement at the left inferior margin of the lesion *(arrow)*. However, within a few minutes the adenoma accumulates contrast to a level slightly exceeding the enhancement of surrounding pituitary tissue (Case 218-2B; note that the small nodule of early enhancement is now seen as a relative filling defect).

Occasional microadenomas demonstrate the reverse pattern, with more rapid and more intense enhancement than normal pituitary tissue. This differential may be appreciable for only a brief period (about a minute) during the arrival of contrast material, so that dynamic scans are necessary to convincingly document the finding.

Case 219

36-year-old woman with a history of
transsphenoidal hypophysectomy.
(sagittal, noncontrast scan; SE 700/17).

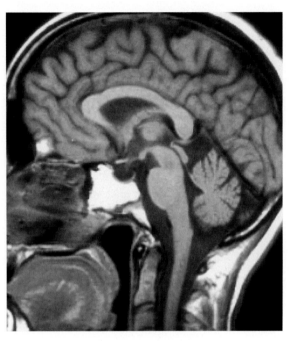

Secondary "Empty Sella"

Case 220

20-year-old woman complaining of headaches.
(coronal, noncontrast scan; SE 600/20)

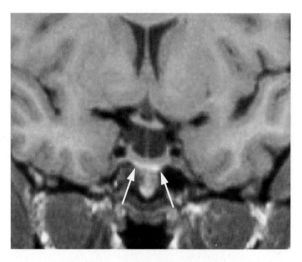

Primary "Empty Sella" Syndrome

Following removal of a pituitary macroadenoma, residual normal pituitary tissue may occupy only a small portion of the large sella turcica. The remainder of the sella is then filled with CSF, resulting in an "empty" appearance. Case 219 demonstrates this situation. The high signal intensity of fat packing within the sphenoid sinus identifies this "empty" sella as postsurgical.

Case 220 illustrates a primary "empty" sella. This "syndrome" is often discovered in otherwise healthy, middle-aged, overweight patients (especially women) with vague complaints (especially headache). Associated pituitary dysfunction is rare. Occasional visual symptoms may be caused by prolapse of the optic chiasm, more commonly seen with secondary "empty" sellas following necrosis or removal of pituitary tumors.

Primary "empty sella" syndrome is caused by an unusually large aperture in the diaphragm sella, allowing spinal fluid from the suprasellar cistern to extend into the sella. The intrasellar cistern participates in normal CSF pulsations and can cause gradual expansion of the sella, closely resembling the enlargement seen with pituitary adenomas.

A number of cystic-appearing lesions can occur within the sella turcica, including some pituitary adenomas, abscesses, cysts, craniopharyngiomas, and dermoid cysts. A primary "empty sella" can be distinguished from these potential intrasellar masses if the thin pituitary infundibulum is seen to traverse the intrasellar fluid space, reaching the pituitary gland at the floor of the sella (*arrows,* Case 220).

A transsphenoidal meningocele or encephalocele could superficially resemble an "empty" sella, with CSF values filling the midsphenoid region. Distorted optic nerves may traverse the cephalocele, mimicking a thick pituitary infundibulum. Associated traction deformity of the hypothalamic region should establish the correct diagnosis in such cases.

Occasionally a small pituitary adenoma may be found within an otherwise "empty" sella. The latter does not exclude the former, and symptomatic cases of "empty sella" need to be carefully analyzed.

Case 221

10-year-old girl presenting with small stature.
(sagittal, noncontrast scan; SE 600/20)

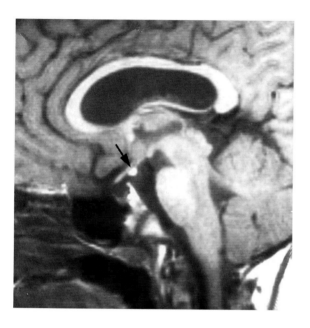

Case 222

6-year-old boy with panhypopituitarism.
(coronal, noncontrast scan; SE 600/20)

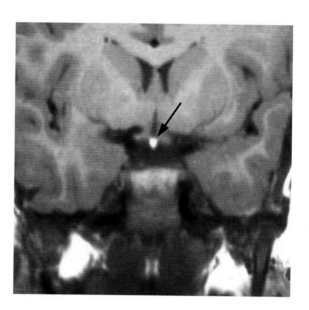

The pituitary glands in Cases 219 and 220 appear small because of chronic compression. They are functionally intact. By contrast, the pituitary gland in Case 221 above is small because of developmental hypoplasia and is functionally insufficient. The sella turcica in Case 221 is also small, supporting the diagnosis of congenital pituitary abnormality.

Failure of development of the pituitary infundibulum and hypoplasia of the adenohypophysis may be isolated abnormalities or part of a midline dysgenesis syndrome (see Cases 728 and 729). In Case 221, the optic chiasm is small and the septum pellucidum was absent, suggesting the diagnosis of septooptic dysplasia (de Morsier's syndrome). Associated pituitary insufficiency is often the most clinically significant component of this syndrome.

The normal neurohypophysis demonstrates high signal intensity on T1-weighted images. The cause of this T1-shortening has been extensively debated. The finding seems to reflect enhanced relaxation of water protons in the vicinity of neurosecretory vesicles, which function in the storage and secretion of oxytocin and vasopressin. On sagittal MR images, the neurohypophyseal focus of T1-shortening lies immediately anterior to the dorsum sella and has been referred to as the "posterior pituitary bright spot." (See Cases 115, 126, 132, and 198 for normal examples.)

In both of the above cases, an ectopic zone of T1-shortening representing the functional neurohypophysis is seen along the floor of the third ventricle at the base of the infundibulum *(arrows)*. This "bright spot" has failed to develop in the normal intrasellar location due to impaired formation of or damage to the pituitary infundibulum, which normally transmits carrier-bound neuropeptide hormones from the hypothalamus to the neurohypophysis. Similar development of an "ectopic posterior pituitary gland" along the floor of the third ventricle may occur in cases of post-traumatic transsection of the infundibulum.

Case 223

8-year-old boy being evaluated for small stature.
(coronal, postcontrast scan; SE 600/17)

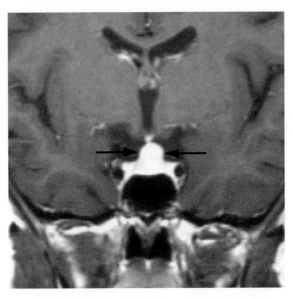

Pituitary Hyperplasia Due to Hypothyroidism

Case 224

54-year-old woman complaining of diminished
visual acuity in the right eye.
(coronal, postcontrast scan; SE 600/15)

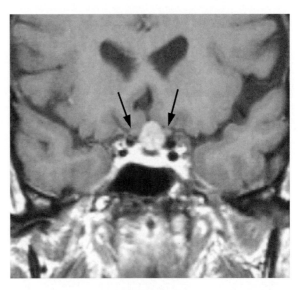

Meningioma

Adenomas of the pituitary gland are one of several uniformly enhancing masses that may be encountered in the suprasellar region. Case 223 demonstrates that pituitary hyperplasia may also present with suprasellar extension and a mass-like contour *(arrows)*. This possibility should be considered when a symmetrical pituitary "mass" is found in appropriate clinical settings (e.g., hypothyroidism or pregnancy). The snowman contour of hypertrophic pituitary tissue in Case 223 resolved within months of treatment with thyroid hormone.

Lymphocytic adenohypophysitis, an idiopathic inflammatory process usually occurring in women during the peripartum period, may cause an appearance very similar to Case 223. Masses arising from the pituitary infundibulum should also be considered in the differential diagnosis, as illustrated on the next page.

Meningiomas are among the extrapituitary masses to present as midline, suprasellar lesions. The tumor in Case 224 lies between the optic nerves *(arrows)*. In contrast to Case 223, the meningioma is separated from the pituitary gland.

In children, chiasmatic/hypothalamic gliomas, unusual craniopharyngiomas, and histiocytosis should be considered when a uniformly enhancing suprasellar mass is encountered. In adolescents or young adults, germinomas may present in this manner. Optic neuritis occasionally causes a similar appearance (see Case 795).

DIFFERENTIAL DIAGNOSIS:
THICKENING AND ENHANCEMENT OF THE PITUITARY INFUNDIBULUM

Case 225

15-year-old boy presenting with diabetes insipidus.
(coronal, postcontrast scan; SE 700/15)

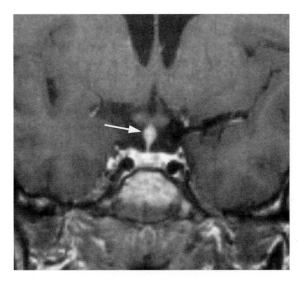

Langerhans Cell Histiocytosis

Case 226

40-year-old woman presenting with nausea,
dizziness, and decreased vision.
(coronal, postcontrast scan; GRE sequence)

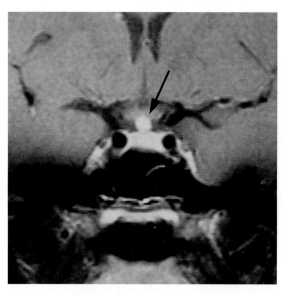

Metastatic Carcinoma of the Breast

A number of pathologies can involve the pituitary infundibulum in children and adults. Histiocytosis may occur at this site in young patients (as in Case 225) and should be included in the differential diagnosis of other pediatric suprasellar masses (such as germinoma and optic/hypothalamic glioma).

Langerhans cell histiocytosis is among the suprasellar pathologies commonly presenting with diabetes insipidus. (Others are sarcoidosis and suprasellar germinomas.) Diabetes insipidus in histiocytosis may precede the appearance of a hypothalamic or infundibular mass and/or persist after a mass has resolved.

Histiocytosis may also involve the cerebral hemispheres, with single or multiple lesions and a tendency to affect the temporal lobes. Some of the parenchymal lesions in histiocytosis may represent a secondary autoimmune or cross-reacting pathophysiology.

Lymphocytic adenohypophysitis (see discussion of Case 223) may cause infundibular thickening in young adults. Granulomatous inflammatory disorders such as sarcoidosis and tuberculosis can also present as infundibular masses.

Metastatic disease may lead to intrasellar or suprasellar masses, as demonstrated in Case 226. Carcinomas of the breast are the most common systemic tumors to involve the pituitary stalk or gland.

Case 227

46-year-old woman, one year after
surgery for craniopharyngioma.
(sagittal, noncontrast scan; SE 600/20)

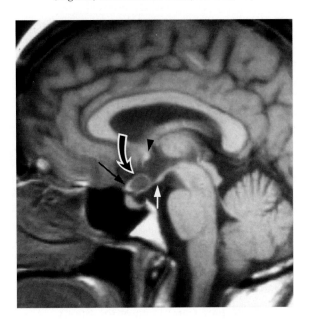

Case 228

8-year-old girl presenting with headaches
and weight gain.
(sagittal, noncontrast scan; SE 600/15)

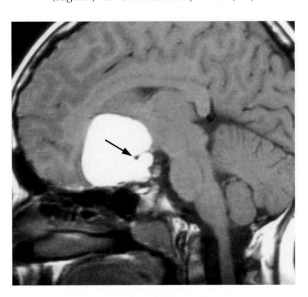

Craniopharyngiomas can present a variety of signal intensities, sizes, and morphologies on MR scans. These masses most commonly involve the suprasellar region, alone or in combination with intrasellar components. Although midline location is typical, laterally eccentric tumors do occur (see Case 249).

The signal intensity of craniopharyngiomas on T1-weighted scans may be low, intermediate, or high. Low intensity often reflects a cystic lesion, as was true of the recurrent craniopharyngioma in Case 227. Solid tumors may be relatively isointense to brain tissue.

Short T1 components within craniopharyngiomas most often represent high protein content within cystic regions of the tumor. Experimental studies and analysis of fluid from tumor cysts have suggested that protein concentrations up to 10% (10,000 mg/dl) have little effect on T1 re-

laxation. Appreciable T1-shortening is usually correlated with protein concentrations in the range of 10% to 30%. The mass in Case 228 contained viscous material with no evidence of hemorrhage or cholesterol.

The small lesion in Case 227 *(large, curved arrow)* occupies the anterior recesses of the third ventricle, immediately posterior to the optic chiasm *(black arrow)*. Other anatomical details on this mid-sagittal MR image include the anterior commissure *(arrowhead)* and the mamillary bodies *(white arrow)*.

The tumor in Case 228 encases the elevated A1 segment of the anterior cerebral artery *(arrow)*.

Postsurgical recurrence is a recognized tendency of craniopharyngiomas, and postoperative radiation therapy may be advocated for these "benign" lesions.

Case 229

4-year-old boy presenting with headaches.
(axial, noncontrast scan; SE 3000/90)

Case 230

17-year-old girl evaluated for worsening
school performance.
(axial, noncontrast scan; SE 2500/90)

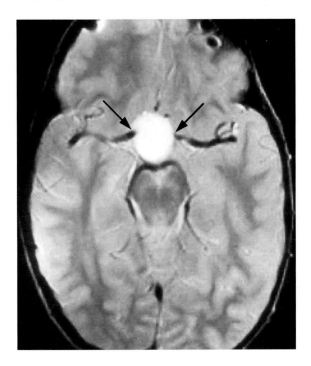

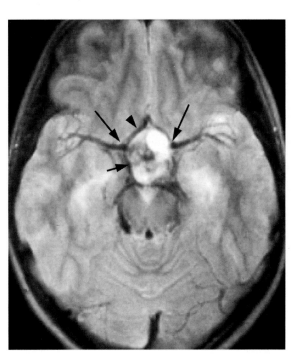

Craniopharyngiomas are included in the differential diagnosis of suprasellar masses in all age groups. The child and adolescent illustrated above join the adult on the previous page and the elderly patient in Case 234 to illustrate the age range of these tumors.

On T2-weighted images, the signal intensity of craniopharyngiomas may be homogeneously high or complex and heterogeneous. Homogeneity may reflect a uniformly solid tumor or a cystic lesion, as was found in Case 229. Low signal intensity components within craniopharyngiomas like Case 230 may be due to calcification or blood products causing T2-shortening.

Calcification, a hallmark of craniopharyngiomas on CT scans, is more difficult to appreciate on MR studies. A correlative CT examination can help to narrow the differential diagnosis when a nonspecific suprasellar mass is encountered on MR images.

Both of the above tumors fill the suprasellar region, spanning the distance between the supraclinoid internal carotid arteries *(long arrows)*. The anterior cerebral and posterior communicating arteries are stretched along the margins of such masses (*arrowhead* and *short arrow,* Case 230). Tumor adherence to these vessels (and to the optic chiasm) makes complete resection difficult.

Case 231

40-year-old man presenting with headaches
and bitemporal hemianopsia.
(sagittal, noncontrast scan; SE 600/15)

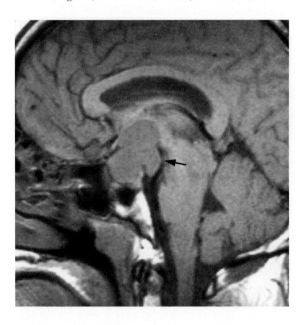

Case 232

4-year-old boy presenting with headaches.
(sagittal, noncontrast scan; SE 600/15)

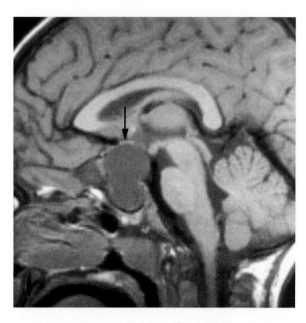

(same patient as Case 229)

The stereotype of craniopharyngiomas as heterogeneous suprasellar lesions is applicable to a minority of these tumors. Many craniopharyngiomas are surprisingly homogeneous, and up to 70% demonstrate an intrasellar component.

In both of the above cases, the continuity between the suprasellar tumor and an expanded sella turcica would raise the question of pituitary adenoma (although this would be a rare diagnosis in a child). Craniopharyngiomas may closely resemble pituitary adenomas as combined intrasellar and suprasellar masses.

One clue to the diagnosis of craniopharyngioma is prominent retrosellar extension. A lobulation growing posteriorly into the interpeduncular cistern is a common feature of these tumors (*arrow,* Case 231).

Although the above lesions are comparably homogeneous, the tumor in Case 231 proved to be solid at surgery, while the mass in Case 232 was grossly cystic. Homogeneity is not a reliable indication of fluid content, as discussed in Chapter 4.

Cases 231 and 232 demonstrate marked elevation of the floor of the third ventricle and optic chiasm (*arrow,* Case 232). Superior enlargement of craniopharyngiomas may obstruct the foramina of Monro to cause hydrocephalus, which is beginning to develop in Case 231. Such cases may mimic the presentation of a colloid cyst of the third ventricle. However, colloid cysts rarely exceed one centimeter in diameter before causing symptoms and are not associated with intrasellar components.

Occasional craniopharyngiomas are completely intrasellar in location. This possibility should be considered in the differential diagnosis of an intrasellar adenoma.

Case 233

40-year-old man presenting with headaches
and visual field deficits.
(sagittal, postcontrast scan; SE 600/15)

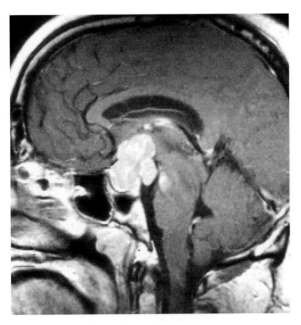

(same patient as Case 231)

Case 234

82-year-old woman presenting with decreased
visual acuity.
(sagittal, postcontrast scan; SE 600/15)

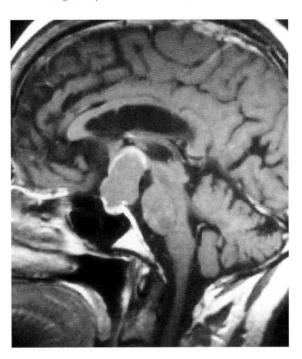

Contrast enhancement in craniopharyngiomas may be minimal or intense. Patterns include homogeneous enhancement of solid tumors and rim enhancement surrounding cystic components.

Case 233 illustrates uniform contrast enhancement throughout the intrasellar, suprasellar, and retrosellar portions of the tumor presented in Case 231.

Enhancement in Case 234 is limited to a thin rim at the perimeter of the large mass. In a younger patient with a smaller tumor, this appearance of a homogeneous, minimally enhancing suprasellar mass may resemble a low grade glioma of the hypothalamus or optic chiasm (see Case 243) or a hypothalamic hamartoma (see Cases 250 and 251).

Case 235A

10-year-old girl presenting with headaches.
(sagittal, noncontrast scan; SE 600/15)

Case 235B

Same patient.
(axial, noncontrast scan; SE 3000/80)

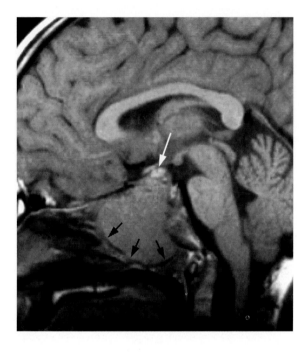

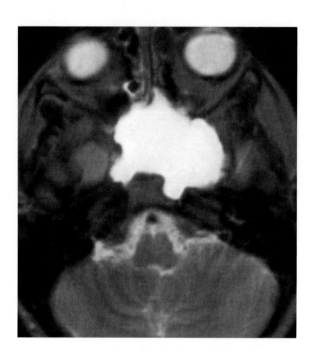

Although the majority of craniopharyngiomas are suprasellar and/or intrasellar in location, infrasellar lesions may occur along the course of Rathke's pouch. Such masses can fill and expand the basisphenoid and/or sphenoid sinus, as seen in this case.

The sagittal scan in Case 235A demonstrates that the sella turcica and pituitary gland have been displaced superiorly (*white arrow*) to nearly reach the optic chiasm and floor of the third ventricle. The inferior margin of the tumor bulges below the skull base into the nasopharynx (*black arrows*).

Uniformly high signal intensity is seen throughout the lesion in Case 235B, suggesting homogeneous fluid content.

This appearance combines with lobulated lateral and posterior extensions of the mass to resemble a chordoma such as Case 194B. However, contrast enhancement was limited to the margin of the lesion, favoring the diagnosis of a cystic craniopharyngioma. The center of the mass within the sphenoid bone is also more anterior than the usual clival origin of midline chordomas (compare to Case 194A).

A mucocele of the sphenoid sinus should be considered in the differential diagnosis when a lesion like Case 235 is encountered in an adult. The sphenoid sinus is rarely pneumatized in children, and mucoceles of any sinus are uncommon in the pediatric population.

CHORISTOMAS (GRANULAR CELL TUMORS)

Case 237A

49-year-old woman presenting with memory loss.
(axial, noncontrast scan; SE 2200/80)

Case 237B

Same patient.
(coronal, postcontrast scan; SE 500/15)

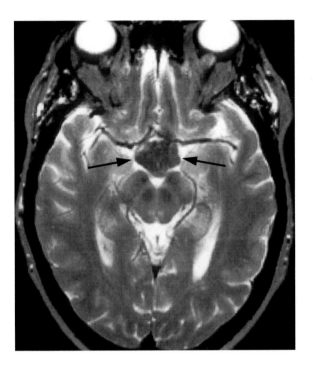

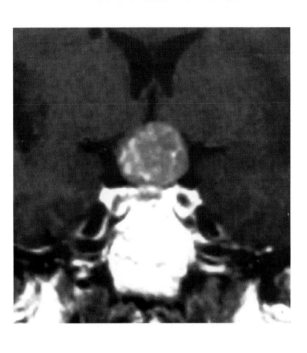

Choristomas are unusual tumors of the suprasellar and/or posterior pituitary region. These masses have been described under many different names, including "granular cell tumor," "myoblastoma," and "pituicytoma." Choristomas probably arise from astrocytic cells of the neurohypophyseal axis, although this identification is controversial.

The tumors may be intrasellar and/or suprasellar in location. They are slowly growing lesions, causing symptoms by compression of the adenohypophysis or optic chiasm.

The few reported MR scans of choristomas have had vari-able appearances. The tumor in Case 237 demonstrates impressively low signal intensity on the T2-weighted image. Enhancement is somewhat nodular and subdued. This pattern differs from the pituitary adenomas and craniopharyngiomas illustrated previously, but overlaps the spectrum of optic/hypothalamic gliomas.

Choristomas can be highly vascular tumors. If this diagnosis is suggested preoperatively, the surgeon may consider a craniotomy rather than a transsphenoidal approach to the mass.

Case 238

14-year-old girl presenting with decreased
vision and diabetes insipidus.
(sagittal, noncontrast scan; SE 600/20)

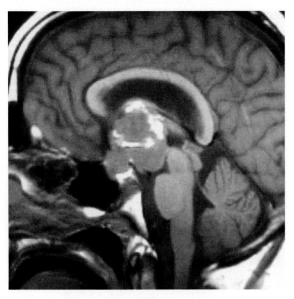

Germinoma

Case 239

59-year-old woman presenting with a third
nerve palsy.
(sagittal, noncontrast scan; SE 600/17)

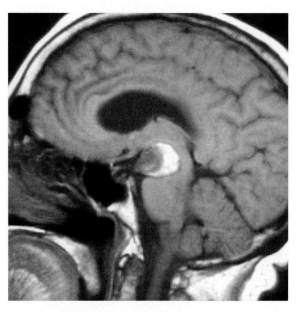

Thrombosed Aneurysm of the Basilar Tip

The differential diagnosis of a suprasellar mass containing high signal intensity on T1-weighted scans includes many lesions in addition to craniopharyngiomas, as illustrated above and on the next page.

The appearance of Case 238 resembles a craniopharyngioma, with patchy T1-shortening and prominent retrosellar extension. The center of the mass is suprasellar, arguing against pituitary adenoma (although the lesion does have an intrasellar extension). At surgery, the tumor was found to be a suprasellar germinoma containing hemorrhage. (Compare to the hemorrhagic pituitary adenoma in Case 213 and to an axial scan of this patient presented as Case 285.)

Suprasellar germinomas are most common in adolescent girls. A clinical clue to the diagnosis is the common presentation with diabetes insipidus (which is rarely an initial symptom of craniopharyngiomas or hypothalamic gliomas). A general discussion of this pathology is presented in Case 272.

Patent aneurysms are easily distinguished from other suprasellar masses on MR scans by their characteristic absence of signal or "flow void." (This differential diagnosis is much more difficult on CT studies.) However, thrombosed aneurysms can present a pattern of mixed signal intensity that may resemble heterogeneous suprasellar tumors such as craniopharyngiomas.

In Case 239, a thrombosed aneurysm arising from the tip of the basilar artery occupies the interpeduncular fossa. Layers of varying signal intensity within the mass are due to thrombus of differing age. This laminated internal architecture is a hallmark of thrombosed aneurysms and is usually most apparent on T2-weighted scans (see Case 604).

Cavernous angiomas occasionally involve the suprasellar region and optic chiasm. Evidence of T2-shortening usually accompanies T1-shortening within these lesions, assisting differential diagnosis (see Cases 627-630).

Case 240

36-year-old woman presenting with
decreased vision.
(sagittal, noncontrast scan; SE 600/30)

Case 241

40-year-old woman presenting with headaches.
(sagittal, noncontrast scan; SE 500/17)

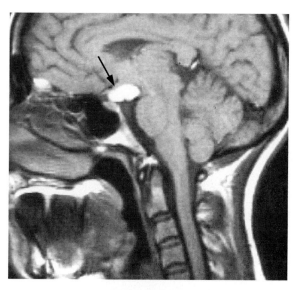

Rathke's Cleft Cyst

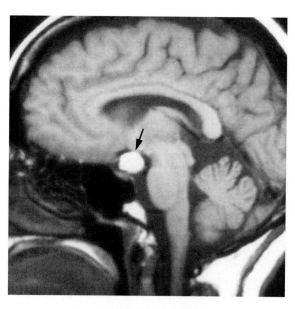

Suprasellar Dermoid Cyst

Rathke's cleft cysts are related to craniopharyngiomas, since they are derived from remnants of the epithelium embryologically lining Rathke's cleft. Like craniopharyngiomas, these masses can be intrasellar and/or suprasellar in location. The cysts are usually simple, lined by a single epithelial layer. They may contain thickly mucinous material, serous fluid, or cellular debris. Their signal intensity on T1-weighted images can be correspondingly high, low, or intermediate. Contrast enhancement is usually absent or minimal, which may aid in differential diagnosis.

Case 240 demonstrates T1-shortening within a Rathke's cleft cyst of the suprasellar and retrosellar regions. The optic chiasm is mildly displaced at the anterosuperior margin of the mass *(arrow).*

The normal neurohypophysis demonstrates T1-shortening and is quite round on coronal scans. This appearance may falsely suggest an intrasellar mass such as a Rathke's cleft cyst. The usually midline position of the neurohypophysis in the posterior portion of the sella turcica helps to correctly identify this structure.

The suprasellar region is a common location for intracranial dermoid cysts (see Case 286). The signal intensity of these masses depends on the proportion of lipid and proteinaceous components within the lesion. When sebaceous material predominates, T1-shortening is apparent as in Case 241. Fat saturation scans would suppress the high signal intensity in this case, unlike Case 240.

Lipomas may also arise along the floor of the third ventricle and could present an appearance comparable to Case 241 (see Case 252).

Case 242

4-year-old girl complaining of headaches.
(sagittal, noncontrast scan; SE 600/15)

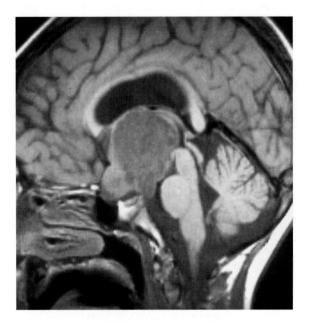

Case 243

48-year-old woman presenting with visual
field deficits.
(coronal, noncontrast scan; SE 800/17)

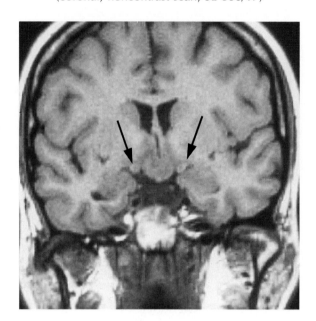

Hypothalamic gliomas rank with optic gliomas and cra-niopharyngiomas as the most common suprasellar masses in children. They are rarer in adults.

Case 242 illustrates that some hypothalamic gliomas are bulky, complex lesions. A mixture of solid and cystic components is common, with the latter demonstrating longer T1 values than the former. The lobulation and heterogeneity of hypothalamic gliomas like Case 242 may resemble the appearance of a craniopharyngioma. These two pathologies should both be considered in the differential diagnosis of a complex suprasellar mass in a child. (See also Case 284.)

Other hypothalamic gliomas are low grade, homogeneous lesions with minimally abnormal signal intensity and little contrast enhancement, as illustrated in Case 243. The CT attenuation values of such tumors may be low, making them difficult to distinguish from the adjacent third ventricle. Evidence of mass effect may be subtle, best demonstrated on coronal and sagittal MR scans.

In Case 243, the floor of the third ventricle is abnormally bulbous, with obliteration of the normal "slit" of CSF in the anterior recesses. The optic tracks (arrows) are well seen on either side of the tumor.

The mass in Case 243 demonstrated high signal intensity on a T2-weighted scan as well as increased size and enhancement on a follow-up study. These features help to distinguish a low grade hypothalamic glioma from hypothalamic hamartomas (see Cases 250 and 251). Clinical correlation (i.e., presence or absence of hypothalamic and chiasmal symptoms) may assist in this differential diagnosis.

Case 244

52-year-old man presenting with reduced
visual fields and acuity.
(axial, noncontrast scan; RSE 6000/104)

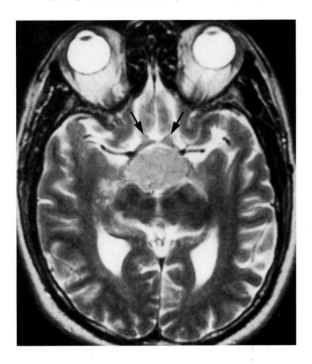

Case 245

4-year-old boy presenting with increasing
irritability and clumsiness.
(axial, noncontrast scan; SE 3000/90)

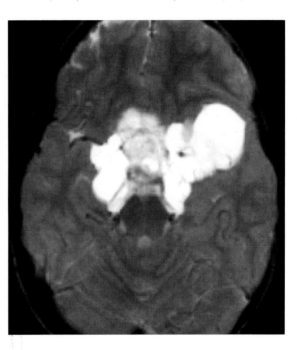

As discussed in Chapter 3, low grade gliomas are usually better defined on MR scans than on CT studies. Such tumors differ more from surrounding normal brain in magnetic relaxation behavior than they do in x-ray absorption. T2-weighted images are particularly helpful in defining these lesions.

The signal intensity of hypothalamic gliomas may be intermediate to high on long TR spin echo images. In Case 244, the homogeneous suprasellar component of the tumor is only slightly higher in signal intensity than adjacent brain. The mass spans the distance between the supraclinoid internal carotid arteries. The optic chiasm is draped across the anterior margin of the tumor *(arrows)*. A postcontrast scan of this glioma closely resembled Case 237B.

Case 245 demonstrates multiple, bilateral, high intensity cysts, extending into the parasellar and retrosellar regions. Some of the cysts enhanced peripherally after contrast injection while others did not, suggesting reactive loculations of the subarachnoid space. (Compare to the cysts seen adjacent to acoustic schwannomas, as discussed in Cases 166 and 167.) The solid midline component of the mass demonstrates less marked hyperintensity.

Although hypothalamic gliomas are intraaxial tumors, they frequently extend exophytically into basal cisterns as seen above. This behavior may combine with lobulated morphology to closely mimic the appearance of craniopharyngiomas.

Case 246

10-year-old boy presenting with headaches
and papilledema.
(sagittal, postcontrast scan; SE 600/15)

Case 247

2-year-old girl, one year after biopsy
of a suprasellar glioma.
(axial, postcontrast scan; SE 600/15)

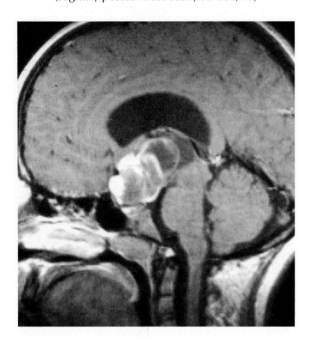

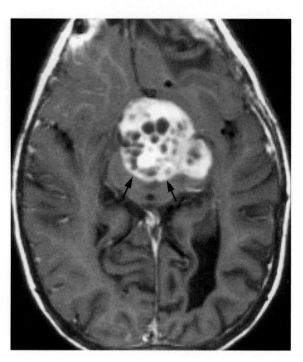

Contrast enhancement within hypothalamic gliomas is variable in extent and morphology. Low grade lesions may demonstrate minimal enhancement. Larger and more aggressive tumors may enhance relatively homogeneously (see Case 248) or in complex patterns, as shown above.

The multiple rims of enhancement in Case 246 could also be seen in a craniopharyngioma. In this case the tumor fills both the suprasellar cistern and the majority of the third ventricle, causing obstructive hydrocephalus.

Case 247 illustrates a more solid pattern of enhancement containing multiple small cysts or zones of necrosis. Posterior extension of this lobulated tumor has caused substan-

tial compression and deformity of the midbrain *(arrows)*. (An area of long T1 values in the inferior left frontal lobe reflects previous surgery.)

It may be difficult or impossible to distinguish between hypothalamic and chiasmatic origin of a large, lobulated, suprasellar glioma. Eccentric location suggests a tumor arising along the wall of the third ventricle (i.e., hypothalamus), while erosion of the chiasmatic sulcus favors a mass originating in the chiasm. Such distinctions are often not meaningful, since bulky tumors arising from either the chiasm or the hypothalamus usually invade the adjacent structures.

Case 248

14-year-old boy presenting with deteriorating vision.
(coronal, postcontrast scan; SE 600/15)

Case 249

40-year-old man presenting with bitemporal hemianopsia.
(coronal, postcontrast scan; SE 600/15)

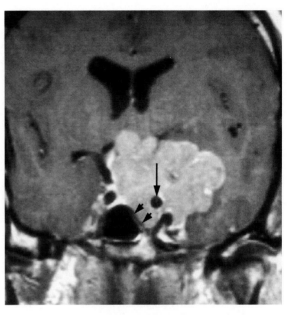

Hypothalamic Glioma

Craniopharyngioma
(same patient as Cases 231 and 233)

These cases demonstrate that both hypothalamic gliomas and craniopharyngiomas may grow laterally to involve the parasellar region and extend along the proximal middle cerebral artery.

The glioma in Case 248 enhances with a relatively solid and homogenous pattern. A smaller mass of this type would be included in the differential diagnosis of Cases 223 and 224. Note that the margins of this intraaxial mass are more infiltrating and less well defined than the cystic and nodular tumors in Cases 245-247 or than the extraaxial lesion in Case 249.

Case 249 is another example of intrasellar involvement by a craniopharyngioma. The floor of the sella is depressed on the left *(small arrows)*. Enhancing tumor surrounds the left internal carotid artery within the cavernous sinus (*large arrow;* compare to Cases 215 and 216). A substantial portion of this lobulated lesion occupies the middle cranial fossa.

Compare the above cases to the tumors in Cases 209 and 210.

Case 250

40-year-old woman complaining of headaches.
(sagittal, noncontrast scan; SE 600/17)

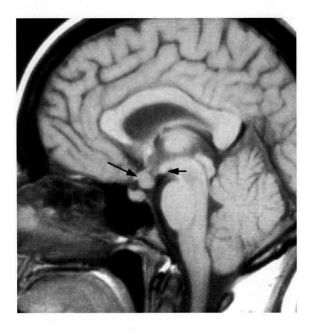

Case 251

27-year-old man presenting with dizziness.
(coronal, postcontrast scan; SE 1000/20)

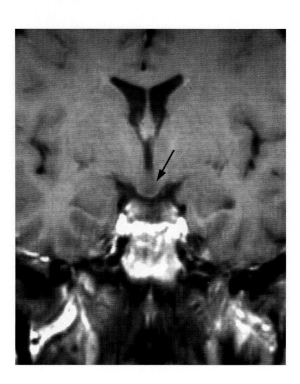

Hypothalamic hamartomas are typically midline masses that arise along the floor of the third ventricle and project inferiorly into the suprasellar and retrosellar cisterns. These low grade lesions have traditionally been referred to as "hamartomas of the tuber cinereum." They may be asymptomatic, although in children (especially boys), they are often associated with precocious puberty. "Gelastic" seizures (laughing spells) are another typical clinical manifestation of hypothalamic hamartomas, seeming to be associated with broadly based tumors deforming the mamillary bodies.

Hamartomas of the hypothalamus are usually about one centimeter in diameter when discovered. They are typically quite round and are located anterior to the mamillary bod-

ies (*short arrow,* Case 250; the *long arrow* indicates the optic chiasm). These masses consist predominantly of mature ganglion cells and are nearly isointense to gray matter on all pulse sequences. They do not demonstate abnormal contrast enhancement.

Case 251 illustrates a midline mass at the inferior margin of the hypothalamus. Signal intensity in the center of the lesion *(arrow)* is comparable to cortical gray matter. These features, combined with the absence of abnormal contrast enhancement, make hamartoma the most likely diagnosis. A low grade hypothalamic glioma could not be excluded (compare to Case 243), and a follow-up scan would be warranted.

Case 252A

36-year-old woman presenting with headaches.
(sagittal, noncontrast scan; SE 600/20)

Case 252B

Same patient.
(axial, noncontrast scan; SE 2500/45)

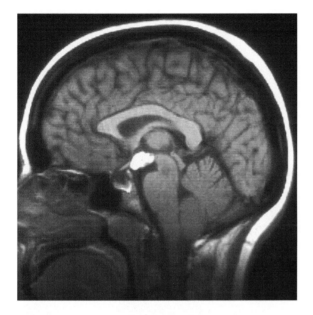

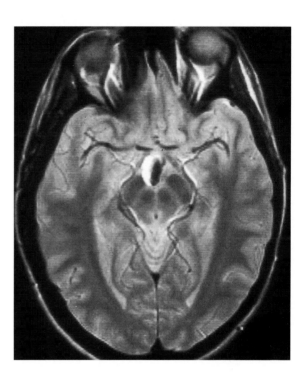

Like hamartomas, lipomas may occur along the floor of the third ventricle, as illustrated in this case. They are usually midline masses that are slightly retrosellar. Short T1 values reflecting lipid protons characterize the lesion on short TR spin echo sequences; this high signal intensity would be suppressed on a fat saturation study. As demonstrated in Case 241, suprasellar dermoid cysts can present an appearance similar to a lipoma in this location.

Most fat-containing masses demonstrate a relative loss of signal intensity on T2-weighted MR images, as seen in Case 252B. The lipoma occupying the interpeduncular cistern is now lower in intensity than CSF, a reversal of the relationship in Case 252A.

Masses with T1-shortening due to proteinaceous contents (e.g., Rathke's pouch cysts) usually demonstrate higher signal intensity than seen here on T2-weighted scans. Blood products may cause shortening of both T1 and T2 similar

to this case, but the morphology of such signal changes is usually characteristic (see Cases 238 and 239).

The MR distinction between lipid material and other causes of T1-shortening within a cerebral lesion can be based on (1) the use of pulse sequences that selectively suppress the signal from water or lipid protons or (2) the presence of chemical shift artifact.

Chemical shift artifact is encountered when a fatty mass is "shifted" or misregistered in space with respect to its aqueous surroundings. Because lipid protons resonate at a slightly lower frequency than water protons, the computer has erroneously placed the lipoma in Case 252B a little closer to the low end of the frequency axis than its true location. As a result, the right side of the lipoma appears to overlap the aqueous tissue along its right margin, while a false gap is created between the left side of the lipoma and the adjacent parenchyma.

Case 253A

17-year-old boy presenting with right-sided
orbital pain and ophthalmoplegia.
(coronal, noncontrast scan; SE 800/10)

Case 253B

Same patient.
(coronal, postcontrast scan; SE 800/19)

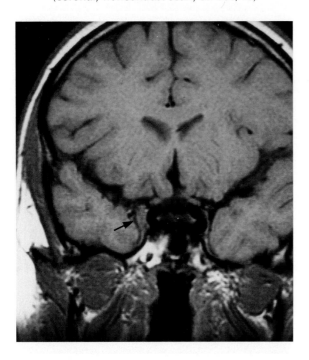

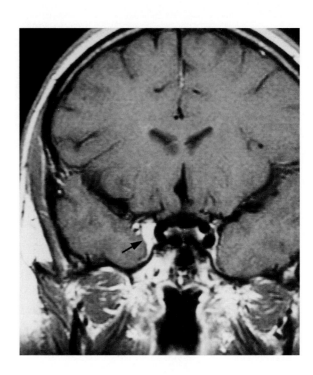

Idiopathic inflammation of the cavernous sinus causing painful ophthalmoplegia is a condition known as "Tolosa-Hunt" syndrome. The disorder is probably related to orbital pseudotumor (see Case 807). (In some cases, orbital and parasellar inflammation communicates through the superior orbital fissure.) Like orbital pseudotumor, Tolosa-Hunt syndrome usually responds to treatment with steroids.

MR scans of patients with Tolosa-Hunt syndrome usually demonstrate mild but definite widening of the ipsilateral cavernous sinus, as seen in Case 253A *(arrow)*. The homogeneous tissue within the sinus is relatively isointense to gray matter on T1-weighted scans and characteristically hypointense on T2-weighted images. The latter appearance is nonspecific and can be noted in parasellar meningiomas, metastases, and lymphoma. Conversely, such a mass within the cavernous sinus should not be presumed to represent neoplasm without a trial of steroid therapy.

Intense contrast enhancement within the thickened parasellar tissue is usual, as illustrated in Case 253B. Again this appearance does not distinguish Tolosa-Hunt syndrome from intracavernous tumors. Encasement of the internal carotid artery may be present, comparable to parasellar meningiomas or lateral extension of pituitary adenomas.

Other inflammatory processes that can involve the cavernous sinus and produce similar MR findings include sarcoidosis and Wegener's granulomatosis.

DIFFERENTIAL DIAGNOSIS:
MASS EXPANDING THE CAVERNOUS SINUS

Case 254

68-year-old woman presenting with right
facial numbness.
(coronal, noncontrast scan; SE 700/15)

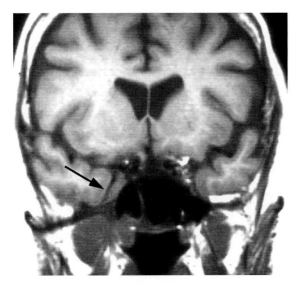

Adenoid Cystic Carcinoma of the Pharynx

Case 255

61-year-old woman presenting with diplopia.
(axial, noncontrast scan; SE 2500/90)

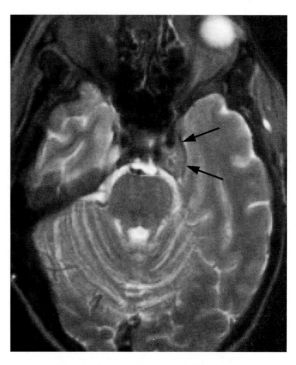

Metastatic Carcinoma of the Breast

Extracranial tumors of the head and neck may extend intracranially by direct invasion and/or perineural spread. Case 254 illustrates the latter mechanism: a pharyngeal carcinoma has tracked back along branches of the fifth cranial nerve to involve the cavernous sinus *(arrow)*, which demonstrates abnormal thickness and signal intensity.

The foramen ovale and the cavernous sinus should be closely examined in all cases of pharyngeal tumor for evidence of perineural spread. Adenoid cystic carcinoma is particularly prone to perineural extension, but the more common squamous cell carcinomas of the pharynx may exhibit similar behavior. Melanomas of the head and neck can also traverse the skull base in this manner.

Tumor can cross the floor of the middle cranial fossa in the opposite direction as well. Parasellar masses such as trigeminal schwannomas and meningiomas may pass through and expand the foramen ovale, giving rise to large parapharyngeal components.

In Case 255, the left cavernous sinus is abnormally thickened by a homogeneous mass. The relatively low signal intensity of the lesion on this T2-weighted scan falls within the spectrum of meningiomas, lymphoma, and hematogenous metastases.

Both of the above lesions demonstrated intense contrast enhancement. The MR diagnosis in such cases cannot be specific, and clinical correlation is required.

In addition to meningioma, metastasis, and lymphoma, lesions to be considered in the differential diagnosis of a homogeneous parasellar mass include lateral extension of a pituitary adenoma, cranial nerve schwannoma, Tolosa-Hunt syndrome (see Case 253), sarcoidosis, Wegener's granulomatosis, and lateral extension of sphenoid sinusitis or mucocele. Chordomas, chondromas, and cavernous angiomas occur in the parasellar region but typically demonstrate signal characteristics distinct from the above cases. Similarly, distention of the cavernous sinus by an aneurysm or a carotid/cavernous fistula is usually accompanied by characteristic patterns of signal change (see Chapter 10).

REFERENCES

Abrahams JJ, Trefelner E, Boulware SD: Idiopathic growth hormone deficiency: MR findings in 35 patients. *AJNR* 12:155-160, 1991.

Ahmadi J, Destian S, Apuzzo MLJ, et al: Cystic fluid in craniopharyngiomas: MR imaging and quantitative analysis. *Radiology* 182:783-785, 1992.

Ahmadi J, North CM, Segall HD, et al: Cavernous sinus invasion by pituitary adenomas. *Am J Neuroradiol* 6:893-898, 1985.

Albright AL, Lee PA: Neurosurgical treatment of hypothalamic harmartomas causing precocious puberty. *J Neurosurg* 78:77-82, 1993.

Appignani B, Landy H, Barnes P: MR in idiopathic central diabetes insipidus of childhood. *AJNR* 14:1407-1410, 1993.

Barkovich AJ, Fram EK, Norman D: Septo-optic dysplasia: MR imaging. *Radiology* 171:189-192, 1989.

Barral V, Brunelle F, Brauner R, et al: MRI of hypothalamic hamartomas in children. *Pediatr Radiol* 18:449, 1988.

Beningfield SJ, Bonnici F, Cremin BJ: Magnetic resonance imaging of hypothalamic hamartomas. *Br J Radiol* 61:1177, 1988.

Benshoff ER, Katz BH: Ectopia of the posterior pituitary gland as a normal variant: assessment with MR imaging. *AJNR* 11:709, 1990.

Boecher-Schwartz HG, Fries G, Bornemann A, et al: Suprasellar granular cell tumor. *Neurosurgery* 31:751-754, 1992.

Boyko OB, Curnes JT, Oakes WJ, Burger PC: Hamartomas of the tuber cinereum: CT, MR, and pathologic findings. *AJNR* 12:309-314, 1991.

Brooks BS, Gammal TE, Allison JD, et al: Frequency and variation of the posterior pituitary bright signal on MR images. *AJNR* 10:943-948, 1989.

Buchfelder M, Nistor R, Fahlbusch R, Huk WJ: The accuracy of CT and MR evaluation of the sella turcica for detection of adrenocorticotropic hormone-secreting adenomas in Cushing disease. *AJNR* 14:1183-1190, 1993.

Burton EM, Ball WS Jr, Crone K, Dolan LM: Hamartoma of the tuber cinereum: a comparison of MR and CT findings in four cases. *AJNR* 10:497-502, 1989.

Chakares DW, Curtin A, Ford G: Magnetic resonance imaging of pituitary and parasellar abnormalities. *Radiol Clin North Am* 27:265-282, 1989.

Chong BW, Kucharczyk W, Singer W, George S: Pituitary gland MR: a comparative study of healthy volunteers and patients with microadenomas. *AJNR* 15:675-679, 1994.

Chong BW, Newton TH: Hypothalamic and pituitary pathology. *Radiol Clin North Am* 31:1147-1184, 1993.

Colombo N, Berry I, Kucharczyk J, et al: Posterior pituitary gland: appearance on MR imaging in normal and pathological states. *Radiology* 165:481-485, 1987.

Cone L, Srinivasan M, Romanul FCA: Granular cell tumor (choristoma) of the neurohypophysis: two cases and a review of the literature. *AJNR* 11:403-406, 1990.

Cox TD, Elster AD: Normal pituitary gland: changes in shape, size, and signal intensity during the 1st year of life at MR imaging. *Radiology* 179:721-724, 1991.

Crenshaw WB, Chew FS: Rathke's cleft cyst. *AJR* 158:1312, 1993.

Daniels EL, Czervonike LF, Bonneville JF, et al: MRI of the cavernous sinus value of spin-echo and gradient recalled echo images. *AJR* 1009-1014, 1988.

Daniels DL, Pech P, Mark L, et al: Magnetic resonance imaging of the cavernous sinus. *AJNR* 6:187-192, 1985.

Daniels PL, Pojunas KW, Kilgore DP, et al: MR of the diaphragm sellae. *AJNR* 7:765-769, 1986.

Davis P, Hoffman J, Malko J, et al: Gd-DTPA and MR imaging of pituitary adenoma. *AJNR* 8:817, 1987.

Davis PC, Hoffman JC, Spencer T, et al: MR imaging of pituitary ad-

enoma. CT, clinical, and surgical consideration. *AJNR* 8:107-112, 1987.

Dina TS, Feaster SH, Laws ER Jr, Davis DO: MR of the pituitary gland postsurgery: serial MR studies following transsphenoidal resection. *AJNR* 14:763-769, 1993.

Doppman JL, Frank JA, Dwyer AJ, et al: Gadolinium-DTPA-enhanced MR imaging of ACTH-secreting microadenomas of the pituitary gland. *J Comput Assist Tomogr* 12:728-736, 1988.

Doraiswamy PM, Potts JM, Axelson DA, et al: MR assessment of pituitary gland morphology in healthy volunteers: age- and gender-related differences. *AJNR* 13:1295-1300, 1992.

Dwyer AJ, Frank JA, Doppman JL, et al: Pituitary adenomas in patients with Cushing disease: initial experience with Gd-DTPA-enhanced MR imaging. *Radiology* 163:421-426, 1987.

El Gammal T, Brooks BS, Hoffman WH: MR imaging of the ectopic bright signal of posterior pituitary regeneration. *AJNR* 10:323-328, 1989.

El-Kalliny M, Van Loveren H, Keller JT, Tew Jr J: Tumors of the lateral wall of the cavernous sinus. *Neurosurgery* 77:508-514, 1992.

Elster AD: Imaging of the sella: anatomy and pathology. *Semin US CT MR* 14:182-194, 1993.

Elster AD: Modern imaging of the pituitary. *Radiology* 187:1-14, 1993.

Elster AD: Sellar susceptibility artifacts: theory and implications. *AJNR* 14:129-136, 1993.

Elster AD, Chen MV, Williams D III, Key LL: Pituitary gland: MR imaging of physiologic hypertrophy in adolescents. *Radiology* 174:681-686, 1990.

Finelli DA, Kaufman B: Varied microcirculation of pituitary adenomas at rapid, dynamic, contrast-enhanced MR imaging. *Radiology* 189:205-210, 1993.

Freeman MP, Kessler RM, Allen JH, Price AC: Craniopharyngioma: CT and MR imaging in nine cases. *J Comput Assist Tomogr* 11:810-814, 1987.

Fujisawa I, Asato R, Okumura R, et al: Magnetic resonance imaging of neurohypophyseal germinomas. *Cancer* 68:1009-1014, 1991.

Fujisawa I, Kikuchi K, Nishimura K, et al: Transection of the pituitary stalk. Development of an ectopic posterior lobe assessed with MR imaging. *Radiology* 165:487-489, 1987.

Fujisawa I, Nishimura K, Asato R, et al: Posterior lobe of the pituitary in diabetes insipidus: MR findings. *J Comput Assist Tomogr* 11:221-225, 1987.

Giacometti AR, Joseph GJ, Peterson JE, Davis PC: Comparison of full- and half-dose Gadolinium-DTPA: MR imaging of the normal sella. *AJNR* 14:123-128, 1993.

Gudinchet F, Brunelle F, Barth MO, et al: MR imaging of the posterior hypophysis in children. *AJNR* 10-511-514, 1989.

Hahn FJ, Leibrock LG, Huseman CA, et al: The MR appearance of hypothalamic hamartoma. *Neuroradiology* 30:65-68, 1988.

Halimi P, Sigal R, Doyon D, et al: Post-traumatic diabetes insipidus: MR demonstration of pituitary stalk rupture. *J Comput Assist Tomogr* 12:135-140, 1988.

Harrison MJ, Morgello S, Post KD: Epithelial cystic lesions of the sella and parasellar region: a continuum of ectodermal derivatives? *J Neurosurg* 80:1018-1025, 1994.

Hashimoto M, Yanaki T, Nakahara N, Masuzawa T: Lymphocytic adenohypophysitis: an immunohistochemical study. *Surg Neurol* 36:137-144, 1991.

Hershey BL: Suprasellar masses: diagnosis and differential diagnosis. *Semin US CT MR* 14:215-231, 1993.

Hirsch WL, Hryshko FG, Sekhar LN, et al: Comparison of MR imaging. CT and angiography in the evaluation of the enlarged cavernous sinus. *AJNR* 9:907-915, 1988.

Hoyt WF, Kaplan S, Grumbach MM, et al: Septo-optic dysplasia and pituitary dwarfism. *Lancet* 1:893-894, 1970.

Hua F, Asato R, Miki Y, et al: Differentiation of suprasellar non-neoplastic cysts from cystic neoplasms by Gd-DTPA MRI. *J Comput Assist Tomogr* 16:747-749, 1992.

Hutchins WW, Crues JV III, Miya P, Pojunas KW: MR demonstration of pituitary hyperplasia and regression after therapy for hypothyroidism. *AJNR* 11:410, 1990.

Johnsen DE, Woodruff WW, Allen IS, et al: MR imaging of the sellar and juxtasellar regions. *Radiographics* 11:727-758, 1991.

Kaard HP, Khangure MS, Waring P: Extraaxial parasellar cavernous hemangioma. *AJNR* 11:1259-1261, 1990.

Karnaze MG, Sartor K, Winthorp JD, et al: Suprasellar lesions: evaluation with MR imaging. *Radiology* 161:77-82, 1986.

Kaufman B, Kaufman BA, Arafah B, et al: Large pituitary gland adenomas evaluated with magnetic resonance imaging. *Neurosurgery* 21:540-546, 1987.

Kaufman B, Tomsak RL, Kaufman BA, et al: Herniation of the suprasellar visual system and third ventricle into empty sellae: Morphologic and clinical considerations. *AJNR* 10:65-76, 1989.

Kelly WM, Kucharczyk J, et al: Posterior pituitary ectopia: an MR feature of pituitary dwarfism. *AJNR* 9:453-460, 1988.

Knosp E, Steiner E, Kitz K, Matula C: *Neurosurgery* 33:610-618, 1993.

Komiyama M, Hakuba A, Yasui T, et al: Magnetic resonance imaging of intracavernous pathology. *Neurol Med Chir (Tokyo)* 29:573-578, 1989.

Kucharczyk W, Davis DO, Kelly WM, et al: Pituitary adenoma: high-resolution MRI at 1.5 T. *Radiology* 161:761-765, 1986.

Kucharczyk W, Peck WW, Kelly WM, et al: Rathke cleft cysts: CT, MR imaging, and pathologic features. *Radiology* 165:491-495, 1987.

Kucharczyk W, Lenkinski RE, Kucharczyk J, Henkelman RM: The effect of phospholipid vesicles on the NMR relaxation of water: an explanation for the MR appearance of the neurohypophysis? *AJNR* 11:693-700, 1990.

Kulkarni MV, Lee KF, McArdle CB, et al: 1.5 T MR imaging of pituitary microadenomas: technical considerations and CT correlation. *AJNR* 9:5-12, 1988.

Kuroiwa T, Okabe Y, Hasuo K, et al: MR imaging of pituitary dwarfism. *AJNR* 12:161-164, 1991.

Kuroiwa T, Okabe Y, Hasuo K, et al: MR imaging of pituitary hypertrophy due to juvenile primary hypothyroidism: a case report. *Clin Imaging* 15:202-205, 1991.

Kyle CA, Laster RA, Burton EM, Sanford RA: Subacute pituitary apoplexy: MR and CT appearance. *J Comput Assist Tomogr* 14:40-44, 1990.

Laine FJ, Braun IF, Jensen ME, et al: Perineural tumor extension through the foramen ovale: evaluation with MR imaging. *Radiology* 174:65-71, 1990.

Lee BCP, Deck MDF: Sellar and juxtasellar lesion detection with MR. *Radiology* 157:143-148, 1985.

Levine SN, Benzel EC, Fowler MR, et al: Lymphocytic adenohypophysitis: clinical, radiological, and magnetic resonance imaging characterization. *Neurosurgery* 22:937-941, 1988.

Lundin P, Bergstrom K, Nyman R, et al: Macroprolatinomas: serial MR imaging in long-term bromocriptine therapy. *AJNR* 13:1279-1291, 1992.

Lundin P, Nyman R, Burmas P, et al: MRI of pituitary microadenomas with reference to hormonal activity. *Neuroradiology* 34:43-51, 1992.

Maggio WW, Cail WS, Brookeman JR, et al: Rathke's cleft cyst: computed tomographic and magnetic resonance imaging appearances. *Neurosurgery* 21:60-62, 1987.

Maghnie M, Arico M, Villa A, et al: MR of the hypothalamic-pituitary axis in Langerhans cell histiocytosis. *AJNR* 13:1365-1371, 1992.

Mark AS, Phister SH, Jackson DE Jr, Kolsky MP: Traumatic lesions of the suprasellar region: MR imaging. *Radiology* 182:49-52, 1992.

Meyer JR, Quint DJ, McKeever PE, et al: Giant Rathke cleft cyst. *AJNR* 15:533-536, 1994.

Michael AS, Paige ML: MR imaging of intrasellar meningiomas simulating pituitary adenomas: *J Comput Assist Tomogr* 12:944, 1988.

Mikhael MA, Ciric IS: MR imaging of pituitary tumors before and after surgical and/or medical treatment. *J Comput Assist Tomogr* 12:441-445, 1988.

Miki Y, Asato R, Okumura R, et al: Anterior pituitary gland in pregnancy: hyperintensity at MR. *Radiology* 187:229-231, 1993.

Moses AM, Clayton B, Hochhauser L: Use of T1-weighted MR imaging to differentiate between primary polydipsia and central diabetes insipidus. *AJNR* 13:1273-1278, 1992.

Mucelli RSP, Frezza F, Magnaldi S, Proto G: Magnetic resonance imaging in patients with panhypopituitarism. *Eur J Radiol* 2:42-46, 1992.

Naheedy MH, Haag JR, Azar-Kia B, et al: MRI and CT of sellar and parasellar disorders. *Radiol Clin North Am* 25:819-848, 1987.

Nakumura T, Schorner W, Bittner RC, et al: Value of paramagnetic contrast agent gadolinium-DTPA in the diagnosis of pituitary adenomas: *Neuroradiology* 30:481, 1988.

Nemoto Y, Inoue Y, Fukuda T, et al: MR appearance of Rathke's cleft cysts. *Neuroradiology* 30:155-159, 1988.

Newton DR, Dillon WP, Norman D, et al: Gd-DTPA-enhanced MR imaging of pituitary adenomas. *AJNR* 10:949-954, 1989.

Nichols DA, Laws ER Jr, Houser OW, Abboud CP: Comparison of magnetic resonance imaging and computed tomography in the preoperative evaluation of pituitary adenomas. *Neurosurgery* 22:380-385, 1988.

Ostrov SG, Quencer RM, Hoffman JC Jr, et al: Hemorrhage within pituitary adenomas: how often associated with pituitary apoplexy syndrome? *AJNR* 10:503-510, 1989.

Paakko E, Talvensaari K, Pyhtinen J, Lanning M: Decreased pituitary gland height after radiation treatment to the hypothalamic-pituitary axis evaluated by MR. *AJNR* 15:537-542, 1994.

Peck WW, Dillon WP, Norman D, et al: High resolution MR imaging of microadenomas at 1.5 T: experience with Cushing's disease. *AJNR* 9:1085-1991, 1988.

Pigeau I, Sigal R, Halimi P, et al: MRI features of craniopharyngiomas at 1.5 Tesla: a series of 13 cases. *J Neuroradiol* 15:276, 1988.

Pojunas KW, Daniels DL, Williams AL, Haughton VM: MR imaging of prolactin-secreting microadenoma. *AJNR* 7:209-213, 1986.

Pusey E, Kortman KE, Flannigan BD, et al: MR of craniopharyngiomas: tumor delineation and characterization. *AJNR* 8:439-444, 1987.

Rodriguez LA, Edwards MSB, Levin VA: Management of hypothalamic gliomas in children: an analysis of 33 cases. *Neurosurgery* 26:242-247, 1990.

Ross DA, Norman D, Wilson CB: Radiologic characteristics and results of surgical management of Rathke's cysts in 43 patients. *Neurosurgery* 30:173-179, 1992.

Rubinstein D, Symonds D: Gas in the cavernous sinus. *AJNR* 15:561-566, 1994.

Sakamoto Y, Takahashi M, Korogi Y, et al: Normal and abnormal pituitary glands: gallopentetate dimeglumine-enhanced MR imaging. *Radiology* 178:441-445, 1991.

Sakurai K, Fujita N, Harada K, et al: Magnetic susceptibility artifact in spin-echo MR imaging of the pituitary gland. *AJNR* 13:1301-1308, 1992.

Sartor K, Karnaze MG, Winthrop JD, et al: MR imaging in infra-, para- and retrosellar mass lesions. *Neuroradiology* 29:19-29, 1987.

Savino PJ, Grossman RI, Schatz NJ, et al: High-field magnetic resonance imaging in the diagnosis of cavernous sinus thrombosis. *Arch Neurol* 43:1081-1082, 1986.

Schubiger O, Haller D: Metastases to the pituitary hypothalamic axis. *Neuroradiology* 34:131-134, 1992.

Schwartzberg DG: Imaging of pituitary gland tumors. *Semin US CT MR* 13:207-223, 1992.

Scotti G, Yu CY, Dillon WP, et al: MR imaging of cavernous sinus involvement by pituitary adenomas. *AJNR* 9:657-664, 1988.

Sigal R, Monnet O, De Baere T, et al: Adenoid cystic carcinoma of the head and neck: evaluation with MR imaging and clinical-pathologic correlation in 27 patients. *Radiology* 184:95-102, 1992.

Simmons GE, Suchnicki JE, Rak KM, Damiano TR: MR imaging of the pituitary stalk: size, shape, and enhancement pattern. *AJNR* 159:375-377, 1992.

Stadnik T, Stevenaert A, Beckers A, et al: Pituitary microadenomas: diagnosis with two and three dimensional MR imaging at 1.5 T before and after injection of gadolinium. *Radiology* 176:419-428, 1990.

Steiner E, Imhof H, Knosp E: Gd-DTPA-enhanced high resolution MR imaging of pituitary adenomas. *Radiographics* 9:587-598, 1989.

Steiner E, Knosp E, Herold CJ, et al: Pituitary adenomas: findings of postoperative MR imaging. *Radiology* 185:521-527, 1992.

Sumida M, Uozumi T, Mukada K, et al: Rathke cleft cysts: correlation of enhanced MR and surgical findings. *AJNR* 15:525-532, 1994.

Tien R, Dillon WP: MR imaging of cavernous hemangioma of the optic chiasm. *J Comput Assist Tomogr* 13:1087, 1989.

Tien R, Kucharczyk J, Kucharczyk W: MR imaging of the brain in patients with diabetes insipidus. *AJNR* 12:533-542, 1991.

Tien RD, Newton TH, McDermott MW, et al: Thickened pituitary stalk on MR images in patients with diabetes insipidus and Langerhans cell histiocytosis. *AJNR* 11:703-708, 1990.

Voelker JL, Campbell RL, Muller J: Clinical radiographic and pathological features of Rathke's cleft cysts. *J Neurosurg* 74:535-544, 1991.

Vogl TJ, Stemmler J, Scriba PC, et al: Sarcoidosis of the hypothalamus and pituitary stalk. *Eur J Radiol* 2:76-78, 1992.

Weissbuch SS: Explanation and implications of MR signal changes within pituitary adenomas after bromocriptine therapy. *AJNR* 7:214-216, 1986.

Whyte AM, Sage MR, Brophy BP: Imaging of large Rathke's cleft cysts by CT and MRI: report of two cases. *Neuroradiology* 35:258-260, 1993.

Wolpert SM, Osborne M, Anderson M, et al: The bright pituitary gland—a normal MR appearance in infancy. *AJNR* 9:1-3, 1988.

Young SC, Grossman RI, Goldberg HI, et al: MR of vascular encasement in parasellar masses: comparison with angiography and CT. *AJNR* 9:35-38, 1988.

Yousem DM, Atlas SW, Grossman RI, et al: MR imaging of Tolosa-Hunt syndrome. *AJNR* 10:1181-1184, 1989.

Yuh WTC, Fisher DJ, Nguyen HD, et al: Sequential MR enhancement pattern in normal pituitary gland and in pituitary adenoma. *AJNR* 15:101-108, 1994.

Zimmerman RA: Imaging of intrasellar, suprasellar and parasellar tumors. *Semin Roentgenol* 25:174-197, 1990.

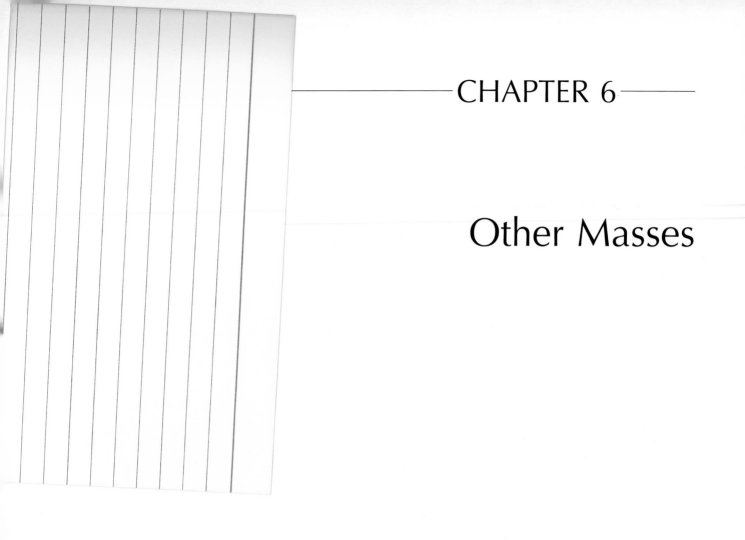

CHAPTER 6

Other Masses

Case 256

27-year-old man with a history
of sudden collapse.
(coronal, noncontrast scan; SE 800/16)

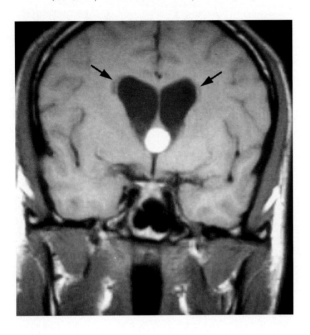

Case 257

44-year-old man presenting with headaches.
(coronal, noncontrast scan; SE 700/17)

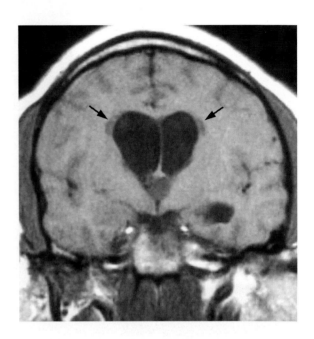

Colloid cysts of the third ventricle characteristically present as round, midline masses at the foramina of Monro. These lesions arise from the anterior roof of the third ventricle. They are typically about one centimeter in diameter at the time of diagnosis, although larger cysts are occasionally encountered (see Case 263).

The signal intensity of colloid cysts may be high, low, or intermediate on either T1-weighted or T2-weighted scans. Short T1 values as in Case 256 may reflect thickly proteinaceous material and/or the presence of paramagnetic metals. Low intensity on T1-weighted images, seen in Case 257, usually correlates with a more watery content.

Coronal and sagittal MR scans add anatomical detail and new tissue contrast to the CT evaluation of lesions near the foramina of Monro. The coronal examinations in the above cases precisely localize the lesions to the junction of the lateral and third ventricles, differentiating the cysts from other potential suprasellar or hypothalamic masses. (Compare to Cases 243 and 251.)

The strategic position of colloid cysts leads to hydrocephalus as the masses enlarge. The lateral ventricles are distended in both of the above cases, and periventricular edema is present *(arrows)*.

Colloid cysts of the third ventricle are occasionally associated with single or recurrent episodes of explosive headache or collapse, as in Case 256. Such sudden events are probably due to a rapid increase in intracranial pressure, caused by acute ventricular obstruction by a somewhat mobile cyst.

Case 258

59-year-old man complaining of severe,
intermittent headaches.
(axial, noncontrast scan; SE 2800/90)

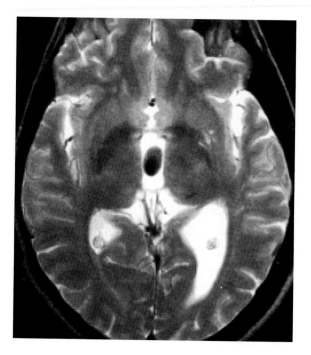

Case 259

19-year-old woman presenting with headaches.
(axial, noncontrast scan; SE 2500/45)

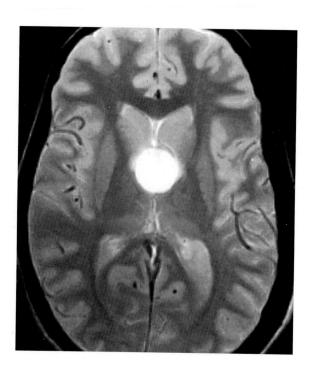

The content of colloid cysts varies from liquid to gelatinous to caseous in consistency. Together with variable amounts of paramagnetic materials, this range of hydration and inspissation can cause a variety of signal intensities on long TR spin echo images.

The cyst in Case 258 is well-defined as a low intensity filling defect within the superior portion of the third ventricle. By contrast, the larger cyst of Case 259 demonstrates uniformly high intensity.

Occasional colloid cysts are nearly isointense to surrounding tissues on both T1-weighted and T2-weighted MR scans. Such lesions may be more easily diagnosed as high attenuation masses on CT studies.

In a young patient with a relatively large midline mass as in Case 259, the possibility of craniopharyngioma, hypotha-lamic glioma, suprasellar germinoma, or suprasellar extension of a pituitary adenoma could be considered. Coronal and sagittal views assist in the differential diagnosis by demonstrating that a colloid cyst arises from the superior margin of the third ventricle, above other potential suprasellar masses.

The size of a colloid cyst does not correlate precisely with the presence or severity of hydrocephalus. The large cyst in Case 259 is not associated with ventricular enlargement or periventricular edema.

The origin of colloid cysts is controversial. Recent studies have suggested that these lesions are more closely related to endodermally derived cysts (e.g., Rathke's cleft cysts) than to neuroepithelium.

Case 260

34-year-old man presenting with hydrocephalus.
(sagittal, postcontrast scan; SE 600/15)

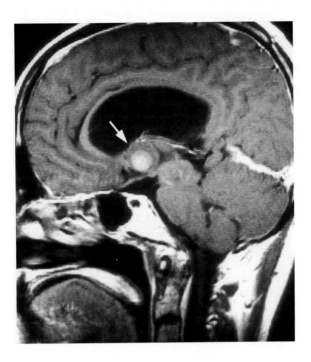

Case 261

41-year-old man presenting with loss
of consciousness.
(axial, noncontrast scan; SE 2500/45)

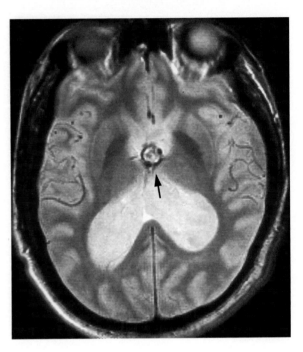

Most colloid cysts are simple, round masses of uniform signal intensity. Occasional lesions have a more complex character, as illustrated above.

Concentric layering of different signal intensities may cause a target-like appearance within some colloid cysts, as seen in Case 260. The central zone of short T1 values was apparent on precontrast scans. (Contrast enhancement within colloid cysts is unusual; see Case 263.)

Case 261 demonstrates a colloid cyst with mixed signal intensity and irregular margins. At surgery, the cyst was found to have ruptured, with partial evacuation of its contents and presumed collapse of previously bulging contours.

Prominent enhancement of the dura and deep venous system in Case 260 had no clinical correlation apart from hydrocephalus and increased intracranial pressure.

Case 262

5-year-old boy presenting with headaches.
(coronal, noncontrast scan; SE 800/16)

Case 263

19-year-old woman presenting with headaches.
(coronal, postcontrast scan; SE 550/20)

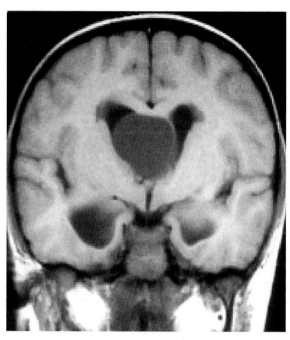

Cystic Astrocytoma of the Septum Pellucidum

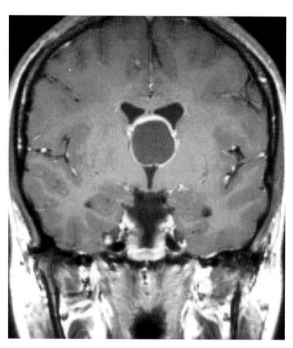

Colloid Cyst of the Third Ventricle
(same patient as Case 259)

Not all cystic masses at the foramen of Monro are colloid cysts. Suprasellar or third ventricular cysts (e.g., craniopharyngioma or cysticercosis) can enlarge superiorly to occupy a similar location (see Cases 234 and 265).

Deep frontal lesions may also involve the midline. Gliomas commonly arise near the frontal horns and frequently extend into the septum pellucidum. In Case 262, the midline cystic tumor resembles Case 263 but is located superior to the foramina of Monro.

Conversely, large colloid cysts can mimic other midline masses. The rim of peripheral contrast enhancement in Case 263 combines with the size of the cyst to suggest a neoplasm (compare to Case 234). Peripheral contrast enhancement is occasionally associated with colloid cysts on CT or MR scans, usually reflecting surrounding reactive inflammatory tissue rather than enhancement of the cyst's epithelium. Central contrast enhancement is rare.

Despite its somewhat unusual size and enhancement, the lesion in Case 263 is clearly centered at the level of the foramina of Monro. Recognition of this characteristic location helps to clarify the diagnosis.

Case 264

55-year-old man presenting with headaches.
(coronal, postcontrast scan; SE 500/15)

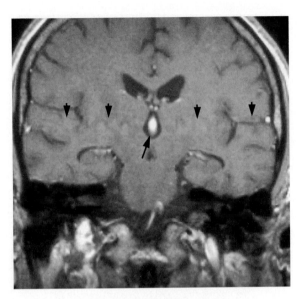

Normal CSF Pulsation

Case 265

17-year-old girl presenting with decreased vision.
(axial, noncontrast scan; SE 2500/28)

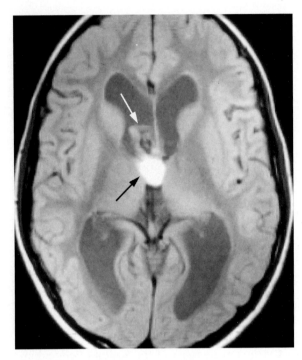

Craniopharyngioma

A number of artifacts and pathologies can resemble the appearance of a colloid cyst within the third ventricle.

The scan in Case 264 was the most posterior section of a series that centered on the sella turcica. High signal intensity within the third ventricle *(long arrow)* represents the entry of unsaturated CSF protons into the imaging volume from normal bidirectional flow through the aqueduct (see Cases 657 and 658). Identification of this finding as a flow phenomenon is supported by the band of phase artifact passing through the "lesion" *(short arrows)*.

Case 265 demonstrates that suprasellar pathologies may grow superiorly to obstruct the foramina of Monro and mimic a colloid cyst. This craniopharyngioma demonstrates both homogeneous *(black arrow)* and heterogeneous *(white arrow)* components. Coronal and sagittal scans usually establish the origin and nature of such lesions.

DIFFERENTIAL DIAGNOSIS:
MASS NEAR THE FORAMINA OF MONRO

Case 266

16-year-old boy presenting with a seizure.
(coronal, postcontrast scan; SE 1000/17)

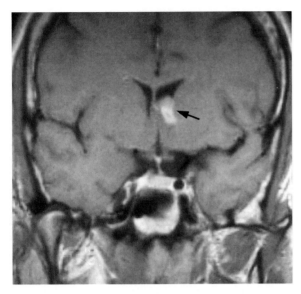

Subependymal Giant Cell Astrocytoma
(in tuberous sclerosis)

Case 267

43-year-old woman presenting with headaches.
(coronal, postcontrast scan; SE 600/15)

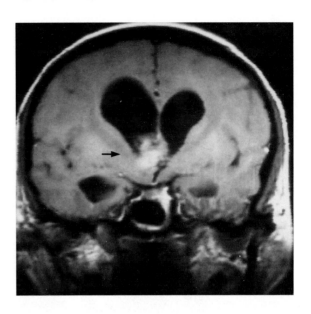

Meningioma

A number of tumors can arise near the foramina of Monro and should be considered in the differential diagnosis of colloid cysts.

Tuberous sclerosis is discussed in Cases 750-762. Subependymal tubers often occur along the margins of the lateral ventricles. Lesions near the foramina of Monro are particularly prone to develop into giant cell astrocytomas, characterized by an enlarging and enhancing mass as in Case 266. These tumors may cause unilateral or bilateral hydrocephalus, but they behave otherwise as low grade neoplasms. Subependymal tubers and giant cell astrocytomas typically occur along the lateral margin of the foramina of Monro, in contrast to the medial location of colloid cysts.

The intraventricular meningioma occupying the right foramen of Monro in Case 267 is an unusual mass in this lo-

cation. (Compare to the more typical trigone meningiomas in Cases 64 and 65.) The enhancing tumor is sufficiently bulky to compress the left foramen of Monro while it occludes the right, causing bilateral hydrocephalus like a colloid cyst. The overall appearance is similar to a glial neoplasm arising from the septum pellucidum. The "fleshy" texture and lobulated margins of the meningioma also resemble a choroid plexus papilloma (see Case 302).

Ependymomas, subependymomas, oligodendrogliomas, and astrocytomas can all arise at the ventricular margin and project into the frontal horn. (Compare the above scans to Cases 115 and 118.)

A small mass along the superior margin of the pituitary gland in Case 266 is incidentally noted on the right side, associated with deviation of the infundibulum.

PINEAL CYSTS

Case 268

47-year-old woman complaining of dizziness.
(sagittal, postcontrast scan; SE 650/20)

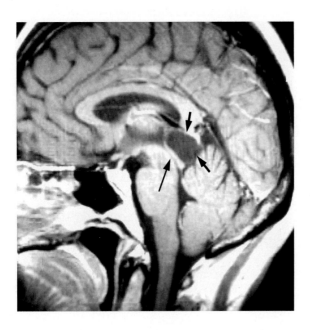

Case 269

31-year-old woman being evaluated
for multiple sclerosis.
(coronal, postcontrast scan; SE 600/15)

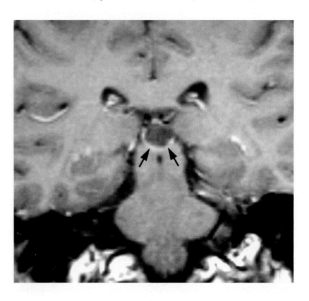

Pineal cysts are commonly encountered as incidental findings on MR studies. Small cysts within the substance of the pineal gland rarely cause diagnostic concern. Larger cysts may replace and expand the gland, causing localized mass effect and raising the question of a pineal neoplasm.

The signal intensity of pineal cysts is typically somewhat higher than that of ventricular CSF, as in the above cases. Hemorrhage into a pineal cyst occasionally causes more marked signal abnormality (T1-shortening and T2-shortening). Contrast enhancement is often seen at the perimeter of the cyst (*arrows,* Case 269), due to displaced residual parenchyma and/or adjacent vessels. Contrast material may accumulate within the center of a pineal cyst on delayed scans and may remain for a day or more.

Benign pineal cysts are typically simple, round lesions with uniform peripheral enhancement. However, heterogeneous cysts with eccentric, nodular contrast enhancement (presumably representing displaced pineal tissue) have been reported. Such features raise the possibility of a cystic pineal neoplasm (e.g., pineocytoma) and warrant follow-up observation.

Large pineal cysts commonly cause moderate compression of the underlying midbrain tectum, as illustrated by the above cases (note the aqueductal narrowing in Case 268; *long arrow).* The majority of patients with this finding have no related symptoms. Rarely, clinical evidence of dorsal midbrain dysfunction (Parinaud's syndrome) or radiographic signs of aqueductal compromise are encountered.

Compare the above scans to the arachnoid cysts of the quadrigeminal cistern in Cases 683 and 684.

DIFFERENTIAL DIAGNOSIS:
FOCAL LESION INVOLVING THE MIDBRAIN TECTUM

Case 270

10-year-old boy originally presenting with
hydrocephalus.
(axial, noncontrast scan; SE 3000/30)

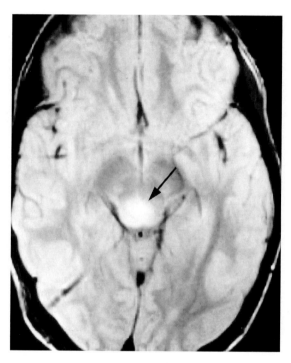

Brainstem Glioma
(same patient as Case 124)

Case 271

31-year-old woman presenting with vague arm
and leg numbness.
(axial, noncontrast scan; SE 2800/45)

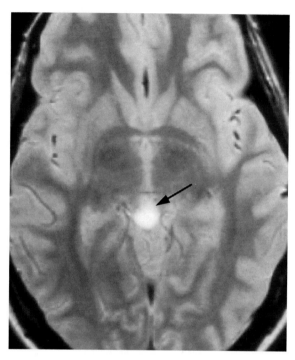

Pineal Cyst
(same patient as Case 269)

As discussed in Chapter 4, focal gliomas may be encountered in the midbrain tectum, usually in children (see Cases 124 and 125). Such lesions cause aqueductal compression and obstructive hydrocephalus. (A ventricular shunt has been placed in Case 270.)

The signal intensity of a pineal cyst is often higher than that of CSF, probably due to the combined effects of higher protein concentration and less pulsation. This difference is typically most apparent on spin echo scans with intermediate weighting (long TR, short TE values), as in Case 271. Such prominent signal abnormality of a pineal cyst may mimic intraaxial pathology arising from the quadrigeminal plate. Careful attention to sagittal scans will establish the extrinsic nature of a pineal lesion.

Case 272A

19-year-old man presenting with blurred vision
and headaches.
(sagittal, noncontrast scan; SE 600/20)

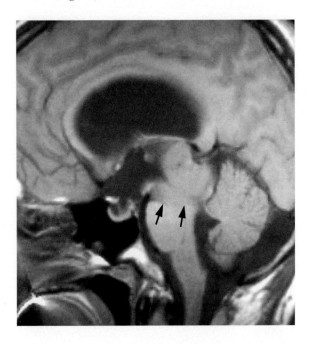

Case 272B

Same patient.
(axial, noncontrast scan; SE 3000/90)

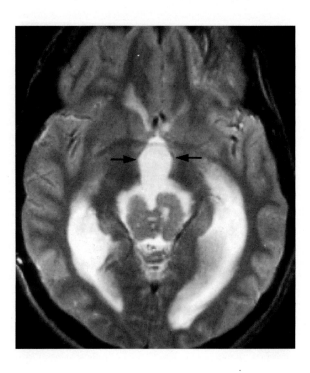

Germ cell tumors are the most common pineal masses. Within this category, germinomas are the most frequent pathology. (Other pineal germ cell tumors include teratoma, choriocarcinoma, embryonal cell carcinoma, and endodermal sinus tumor.) Pineal germinomas occur with a 9 to 1 male predominance. (Girls more often have suprasellar versions of this tumor; see Cases 238 and 285.) Germinomas may also present in the basal ganglia, particularly in boys and young men.

Pineal germinomas are often quite homogeneous in signal intensity, as seen above. The T2-weighted scan in Case 272B demonstrates the tumor to be nearly isointense to gray matter. This finding is associated with highly cellular neoplasms and has been noted in germinomas, medulloblastomas, primary CNS lymphomas, and densely cellular gliomas. Hemorrhage may occur within germinomas, as in other germ cell tumors of the pineal gland.

Pineal neoplasms often grow anteriorly along the walls of the third ventricle. Bilobed anterior extensions of the germinoma in Case 272B are well outlined by a halo of intense edema. This pattern of ventral growth may mimic an intraaxial lesion of the diencephalon or hypothalamus.

The clinical presentation of pineal tumors usually reflects hydrocephalus from obstruction of the posterior third ventricle and aqueduct, as in this case. The sagittal view of Case 272A demonstrates inferior bulging of the floor of the third ventricle and stretching of the corpus callosum. The axial plane in Case 272B documents widening of the third ventricle *(arrows)* and dilatation of the temporal and occipital horns of the lateral ventricles. Occasional germinomas are associated with precocious puberty, predominantly in males.

Germinomas are usually radiosensitive. Even bulky masses may disappear completely without recurrence after a course of radiation therapy.

DIFFERENTIAL DIAGNOSIS:
HOMOGENEOUS MASS IN THE PINEAL REGION

Case 273

25-year-old woman presenting with headaches
and weight loss.
(sagittal, noncontrast scan; SE 600/20)

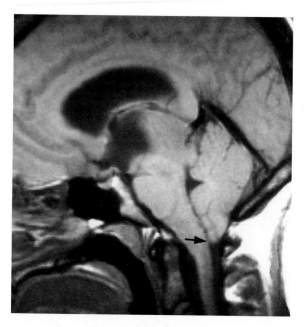

Diencephalic Glioma

Case 274

43-year-old woman presenting with headaches
following an automobile accident.
(sagittal, noncontrast scan; SE 600/15)

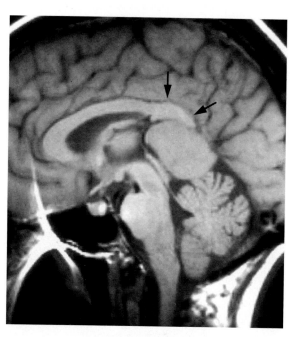

Subsplenial Meningioma

The differential diagnosis of pineal region masses includes a number of intraaxial and extraaxial pathologies. Gliomas of the brainstem or thalamus may extend into the pineal region to mimic a primary pineal tumor. For example, Case 273 is quite similar in appearance to Case 272A. The potential resemblance of pineal tumors and gliomas is increased by the tendency of the former to invaginate ventrally into adjacent parenchyma (see Case 272B).

A number of clues can contribute to distinguishing gliomas from pineal tumors: (1) eccentricity is more typical of gliomas arising in the pineal region than of true pineal neoplasms; (2) gliomas often demonstrate higher signal intensity than pineal tumors on T2-weighted images (compare Cases 270 and 272B); and (3) contrast enhancement of pineal tumors is usually intense, while that of deep gliomas may be much less impressive. None of these considerations is individually reliable, but their combination can be helpful.

Meningiomas are among the extrapineal lesions that may occur in the quadrigeminal region. The tumor in Case 274 is clearly extraaxial, with elevation of the splenium *(arrows)* and flattening of the quadrigeminal plate. Homogeneous contrast enhancement within a meningioma may resemble that of a germinoma.

On CT scans, a patent vein of Galen "aneurysm" would also be included in this differential diagnosis. The characteristic appearance of flow in such lesions is diagnostic on MR studies (see Cases 610 and 611). However, the MR appearance of a thrombosed vein of Galen aneurysm may resemble a hemorrhagic pineal neoplasm.

The cerebellar tonsils in Case 273 extend below the plane of the foramen magnum with peg-like morphology *(arrow)* suggesting a Chiari I hindbrain malformation as well as caudal displacement. (Compare to Case 272A, where the posterior fossa is not "tight" despite comparable hydrocephalus and mesencephalic mass effect.)

Case 275

12-year-old boy presenting with headaches, papilledema, and markedly elevated serum levels of human chorionic gonadotropin.
(axial, noncontrast scan; SE 2500/90)

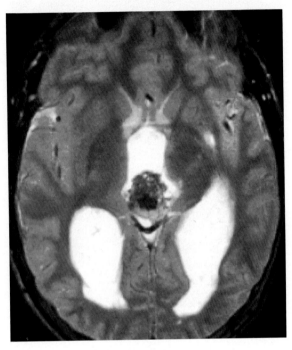

Choriocarcinoma

Case 276

4-year-old girl presenting with increased intracranial pressure.
(axial, noncontrast scan; SE 2800/90)

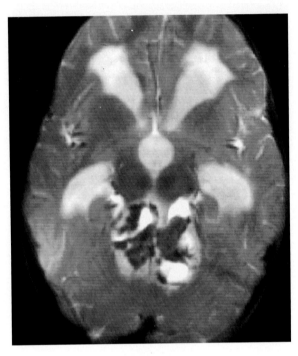

Teratoma

Germ cell tumors of the pineal gland other than germinomas are uncommon masses of variable appearance. They are often more heterogeneous than germinomas, with frequent cysts, calcification, and hemorrhage. Lipid components may be present in pineal teratomas.

The choriocarcinoma in Case 275 occupies the typical position of a pineal neoplasm in the midline at the posterior margin of the third ventricle. Obstruction of the aqueduct has caused hydrocephalus. Areas of T2-shortening within the mass suggest hemorrhage or calcification. (T1-shortening indicating subacute blood products was present on T1-weighted scans.)

The teratoma in Case 276 is even more complex. Multiple cysts with high signal intensity are intermixed with solid tissue and low intensity foci suggesting hemorrhage and/or calcification. This coarse, heterogeneous texture is typical of intracranial teratomas (see Case 283). Similar complexity can occur within pineoblastomas.

It is not possible to reliably distinguish among the several types of pineal germ cell tumors on the basis of MR characteristics. Even pathological determinations are difficult, since mixed cell types are frequent in these masses. Serum levels of human chorionic gonadotropin (HCG) and alpha fetoprotein (AFP) can assist in the differential diagnosis: choriocarcinomas are often associated with high HCG levels (as in Case 275), while teratomas may cause elevation of serum AFP.

Case 277

19-year-old man presenting with headaches.
(coronal, postcontrast scan; SE 600/17)

Case 278

12-year-old boy presenting with headaches.
(coronal, postcontrast scan; SE 700/20)

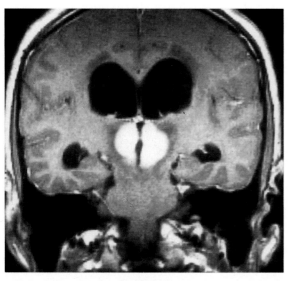

Germinoma
(same patient as Case 272)

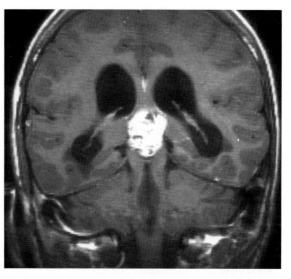

Choriocarcinoma
(same patient as Case 275)

Germinomas usually demonstrate intense, homogeneous contrast enhancement, as in Case 277. Parenchymal invasion along the margins of the third ventricle in this case is well demonstrated by the coronal plane.

The enhancement pattern of nongerminomatous germ cell tumors of the pineal gland is typically more heterogeneous. In Case 278, the overall appearance remains one of solid enhancement. In other cases, particularly of teratoma, enhancement may be less prominent. Large, nonenhancing regions in such tumors may reflect cysts, lipid material, coarse calcification, and/or necrosis.

Germinomas are among the primary CNS neoplasms associated with distant meningial or ventricular implants due to CSF seeding. A search for isointense or enhancing cisterns and sulci is therefore appropriate in these patients. Contrast-enhanced MR scans are more sensitive than CT studies for the detection of meningeal dissemination of tumor (see Cases 160-162).

Hydrocephalic enlargement of the lateral ventricles is present in both of the above cases, with prominent periventricular edema in Case 277.

Case 279

9-year-old boy presenting with headaches
and diplopia.
(sagittal, noncontrast scan; SE 600/15)

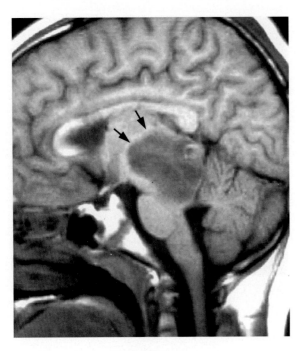

Pineoblastoma

Case 280

1-year-old boy presenting with hydrocephalus.
(axial, postcontrast scan; SE 600/15)

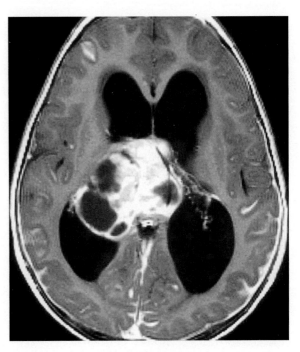

Pineoblastoma

Tumors of true pineal cell origin are much less common than germ cell tumors. Pineocytomas are relatively well-differentiated pineal cell neoplasms. They may be homogeneously solid or grossly cystic masses. Intense contrast enhancement is usual and comparable to germinomas, although pineocytomas are more likely to have lobulated margins.

Pineoblastomas are less well-differentiated and more malignant. Many neuropathologists classify these lesions in the category of "primitive neuroectodermal tumors." They often present as bulky and heterogeneous masses.

Case 279 demonstrates mixed signal intensity, with areas of subacute hemorrhage interspersed among long T1 components. On T2-weighted scans, pineoblastomas may be relatively isointense, reflecting dense cellularity and analogous to germinomas, or high in intensity (see Case 281). A mixed appearance comparable to Case 276 may be encountered. Contrast enhancement is usually prominent and heterogeneous, as in Case 280.

Like germinomas, pineocytomas and pineoblastomas frequently demonstrate CSF spread. Ventricular and meningeal metastases may be present at the time of diagnosis or on follow-up studies. Many sulci in Case 280 are filled with enhancing tumor (compare to Case 299B).

DIFFERENTIAL DIAGNOSIS:
PINEAL REGION MASS WITH AN ECCENTRIC, INTRAAXIAL COMPONENT

Case 281

8-year-old girl with a long history of headaches and a two-week history of nausea, vomiting, and ataxia.
(axial, noncontrast scan; SE 2500/28)

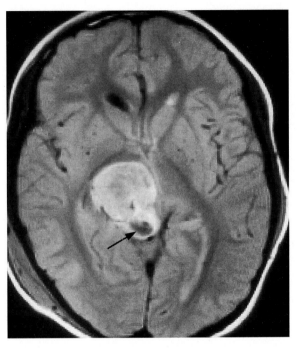

Pineoblastoma

Case 282

25-year-old woman presenting with headaches and weight loss.
(axial, noncontrast scan; SE 3000/45)

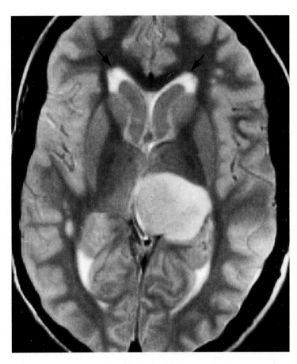

Thalamic Glioma
(same patient as Case 273)

Occasionally a pineal tumor invaginates or invades far into adjacent parenchyma. When such ventral extension is eccentric or unilateral, as in Case 281, the appearance may resemble an intraaxial tumor such as Case 282. (Compare Case 281 to the more symmetrical parenchymal invasion of the germinoma in Case 272B.)

Both of the above lesions demonstrate high signal intensity on long TR spin echo scans. Many pineal tumors show less prolongation of T2 due to dense cellularity and a high nuclear to cytoplasmic ratio. The area of focal low intensity at the posterior margin of the tumor in Case 281 *(arrow)* correlated with calcification on a CT scan.

Hydrocephalus has been shunted in Case 281. Periventricular edema is apparent in Case 282.

Case 283A

16-year-old girl presenting with worsening
headaches.
(sagittal, noncontrast scan; SE 600/15)

Case 283B

Same patient.
(axial, postcontrast scan; SE 600/15)

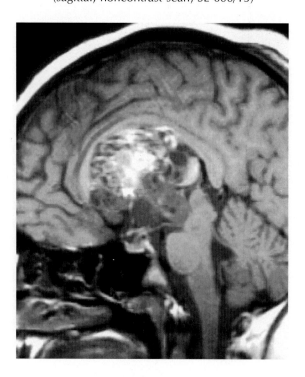

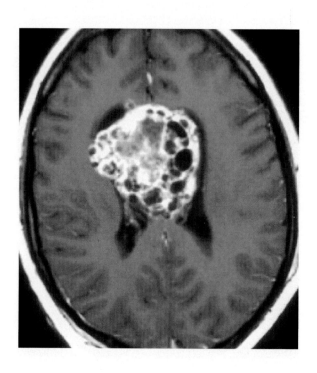

Teratomas are among the germ cell tumors that may originate in the pineal region. Teratomas may also occur in hemispheric locations, sometimes presenting as congenital tumors in neonates.

The mass in Case 283 does involve the posterior portion of the third ventricle, but the bulk of the midline lesion is centered at the level of the lateral ventricles. The extensive areas of T1-shortening on the noncontrast scan (Case 283A) may represent lipid components and/or subacute hemor-

rhage, both of which are common in teratomas. A fat saturation MR sequence or correlation with a CT scan would distinguish between these possibilities.

Contrast enhancement within the lesion is intense (Case 283B), outlining multiple cysts or necrotic areas. Cysts are frequently found within teratomas, combining with hemorrhage, fat, and calcification to cause the strikingly heterogeneity characteristic of these tumors.

DIFFERENTIAL DIAGNOSIS:
HETEROGENEOUS, SUPRASELLAR MASS IN A CHILD

Case 284

2-year-old girl presenting with irritability.
(axial, postcontrast scan; SE 600/15)

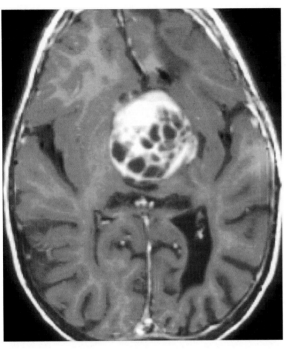

Hypothalamic Glioma

Case 285

14-year-old girl presenting with decreased vision
and diabetes insipidus.
(axial, noncontrast scan; SE 2500/90)

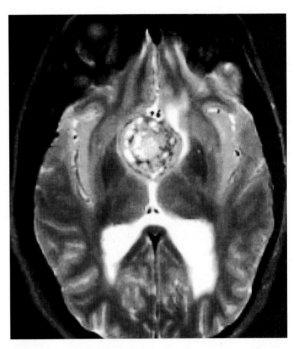

Suprasellar Germinoma
(same patient as Case 238)

As discussed in Cases 242-248, hypothalamic gliomas may demonstrate complex morphology with multiple cystic components. The heterogeneous architecture of the tumor in Case 284 closely resembles the appearance of the teratoma in Case 283 (as well as mimicking more common craniopharyngiomas).

Case 285 presents a T2-weighted scan of the hemorrhagic suprasellar germinoma seen in Case 238. The relatively low signal intensity of the tumor is due to dense cellularity and T2-shortening associated with blood products within the mass. The margin of the lesion is defined by a zone of surrounding edema. Central cystic areas are seen as high intensity foci, with an overall pattern resembling Cases 283 and 284.

As noted earlier, germinomas are the most common tumors of the pineal region. In a suprasellar location these lesions have been called "ectopic pineolomas" or "atypical teratomas." Most patients with suprasellar germinomas are teenagers or young adults presenting with diabetes insipidus or visual impairment. The sex incidence for germinomas in this location is nearly equal, in contrast to the 9:1 male predominance in the pineal region.

Case 286

40-year-old woman presenting with headaches.
(axial, noncontrast scan; SE 600/17)

Case 287

45-year-old woman presenting with headaches.
(axial, noncontrast scan; SE 600/11)

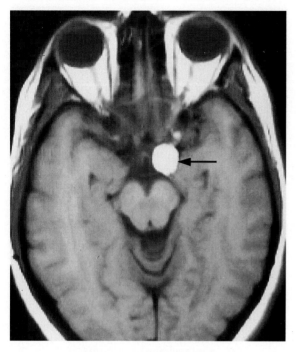

(same patient as Case 241)

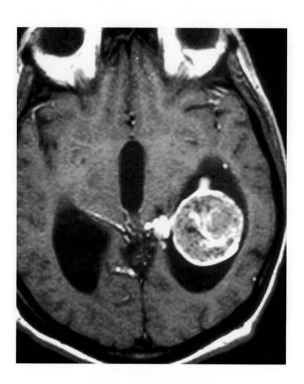

Dermoid tumors or "cysts" are benign masses arising from ectodermal cells enclosed intracranially during embryogenesis. In addition to squamous epithelium, dermoid cysts may contain skin appendages such as hair follicles, sweat glands, and sebaceous glands. Slow proliferation of these tissues leads to gradual accumulation of a pilosebaceous mass, with the congenital lesions often presenting in adulthood.

The lipid content of dermoid cysts causes high signal intensity on T1-weighted scans. This T1-shortening may entirely fill the lesion, as in Case 286, or be mixed with lower intensity proteinaceous material, as illustrated in Case 287. The internal architecture of a dermoid cyst may be correspondingly simple or complex.

Many dermoid cysts are found in the parasellar region, as illustrated by Case 286 *(arrow)*. Other common locations include the posterior fossa, near the fourth ventricle or between the cerebellar hemispheres. Intraventricular lesions such as Case 287 are rare.

The occurrence of T1-shortening within a parasellar lesion is not specific for dermoid cysts. Craniopharyngiomas, Rathke's pouch cysts, hemorrhage into pituitary adenomas, cavernous hemangiomas, or an "ectopic" neurohypophysis can present a similar appearance (see Cases 238-241). Lipomas may also be located along the floor of the third ventricle in the retrosellar region, with prominent T1-shortening (see Case 252).

A fat saturation pulse sequence was performed in Case 287 and demonstrated markedly reduced signal intensity throughout the mass.

Case 288A

67-year-old man presenting with a seizure.
(coronal, noncontrast scan; SE 600/15)

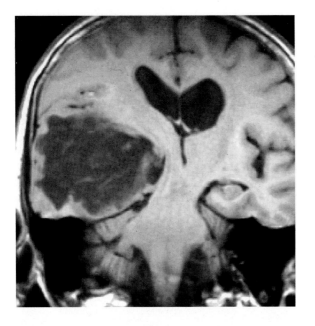

Case 288B

Same patient.
(axial, noncontrast scan; SE 3000/90)

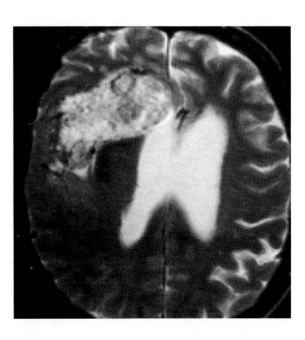

While many dermoid cysts are small lesions, others may become very large masses. The dermoid cyst in Case 288 originated in the right parasellar region and invaginated far into the adjacent temporal and frontal lobes.

Not all cranial (or spinal) dermoid cysts demonstrate T1-shortening. Mixed or low intensity on T1-weighted images may be noted, depending on the amount of contained hair and proteinaceous material and on the proportion of liquid and solid components. Small areas of T1-shortening were present on scans anterior to Case 288A, but the majority of the lesion was of low signal intensity on T1-weighted images. Dermoid cysts combining low signal intensity and lobulated margins may resemble the typical MR appearance of an epidermoid cyst (see Cases 292 and 293).

Case 288B provides a T2-weighted scan of the same lesion, better demonstrating the complex internal architecture. The relatively isointense components within the mass would be unusual in an epidermoid cyst (compare to Cases 295 and 296).

CT scans often demonstrate peripheral calcification surrounding a dermoid cyst. This characteristic feature is rarely appreciated on MR studies. Teratomas can also demonstrate both lipid material and calcification, but the latter is usually more dense and central. Lipomas are a third type of lesion in which lipid material may be seen with adjacent calcification apparent on CT scans but poorly demonstrated on MR studies.

Case 289A

45-year-old woman presenting with headaches.
(sagittal, noncontrast scan; SE 500/16)

Case 289B

Same patient.
(axial, noncontrast scan; SE 600/11)

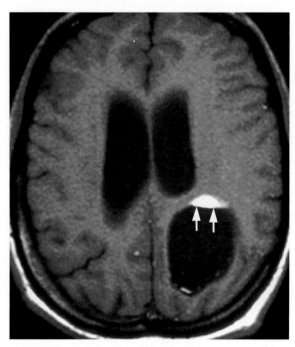

(same patient as Case 287)

Dermoid cysts may leak or rupture, releasing their content into the subarachnoid space and/or ventricular system. The resultant appearance of scattered lipid droplets within sulci and cisterns is demonstrated in Case 289A. A similar pattern can be caused by intracranial droplets of Pantopaque, an oily contrast material previously used for myelography and posterior fossa cisternography.

Cisternal fat droplets demonstrate low attenuation on CT scans and may be mistaken for pneumocephalus. An MR study such as Case 289A clearly distinguishes between air bubbles and fat droplets within the subarachnoid space when the clinical context is ambiguous (e.g., following head trauma).

In Case 289B, a layer of lipid material floats at the non-dependent margin of the dilated trigone of the left lateral ventricle *(arrows)*. Similar fat/fluid levels may rarely be seen within ventricles or cisterns in association with leaking teratomas.

Intraventricular rupture or leakage of fatty material is often clinically silent. Some patients experience a severe chemical meningitis, particularly when the contents of a ruptured cyst extend beyond the ventricles to involve the subarachnoid spaces.

Case 290

18-year-old woman presenting with dizziness.
(coronal, noncontrast scan; SE 600/20)

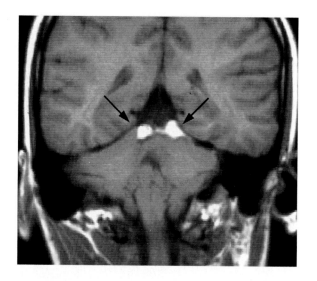

Case 291

82-year-old woman presenting with left body
seizures following head trauma.
(coronal, noncontrast scan; SE 600/15)

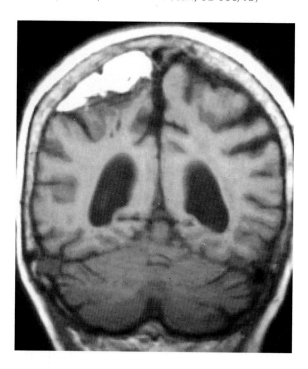

Lipomas present as high intensity lesions on T1-weighted images, potentially resembling dermoid cysts or other pathologies associated with T1-shortening. Several characteristic locations of intracranial lipomas may assist in differential diagnosis.

Interhemispheric lipomas are common, often associated with hypoplasia or agenesis of the corpus callosum (see Cases 724-727). Lipomas bordering the floor of the third ventricle have been illustrated in Case 252.

A third common location for intracranial lipomas is the quadrigeminal cistern, demonstrated in Case 290. Lipomas at this site may be unilateral or bilateral, usually measuring only a few millimeters in diameter. The absence of lipid material in other CSF spaces helps to distinguish small cisternal lipomas from free fat due to rupture of a dermoid cyst.

The convexity location of the lipoma in Case 291 is unusual. Such a lesion could be mistaken for a subacute subdural hematoma in the setting of recent head trauma and relevant symptoms. Although the overall morphology of the lipoma is plaque-like, the mild lobulation of the margins suggests the diagnosis (and would be atypical for subdural hemorrhage). The nature of the lesion was confirmed by homogeneously decreased signal intensity on a T2-weighted scan and on a fat saturation sequence.

Case 292

51-year-old man presenting with facial numbness
and incoordination of the right arm.
(sagittal, noncontrast scan; SE 550/20)

Case 293

47-year-old man presenting with temporal
lobe seizures.
(axial, postcontrast scan; SE 600/15)

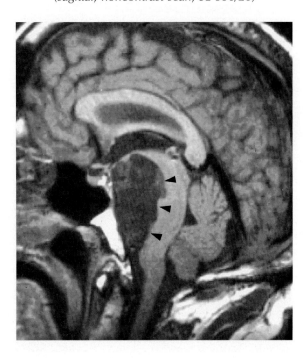

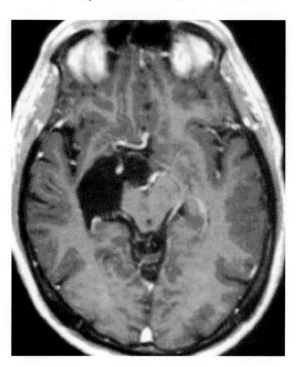

The signal intensity of most epidermoid cysts remains close to that of CSF on a variety of pulse sequences. However, subtle differences are usually apparent. In Case 292, the large prepontine lesion is slightly but definitely higher and less homogeneous in intensity than the CSF within the third ventricle.

Rare epidermoid cysts demonstrate short T1 values (and associated T2-shortening) resembling dermoid cysts. Such masses usually contain viscous liquid components rather than lipid material, with high signal intensity on T1-weighted scans due to enhanced relaxation of *water* protons.

MR is helpful in defining the characteristically lobulated surface of epidermoid cysts. In Case 292 the interface be-

tween the lesion and the brainstem is notably irregular, a feature that would be unusual for an arachnoid cyst (see Cases 693-695). The slow growth of this benign mass has led to impressive displacement and deformity of the brainstem (see Case 295) as well as marked superior bowing of the floor of the third ventricle.

The prepontine and cerebellopontine angle cisterns are common sites for epidermoid cysts. Another frequent location is the suprasellar and parasellar area, demonstrated in Case 293. Masses in this region may be midline or eccentric. Associated compression of the medial temporal lobes may present clinically as seizures or impairment of memory.

Note the lack of contrast enhancement in Case 293, which is characteristic of epidermoid cysts (see also Case 294A).

Case 294A

44-year-old man presenting with
intractable hiccups.
(axial, postcontrast scan; SE 600/15).

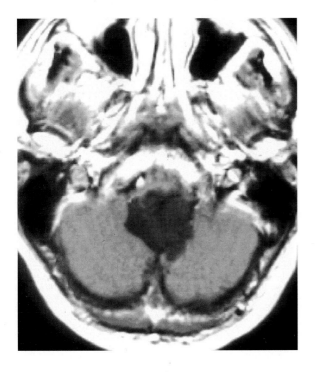

Case 294B

Same patient.
(axial, noncontrast scan; SE 3000/90).

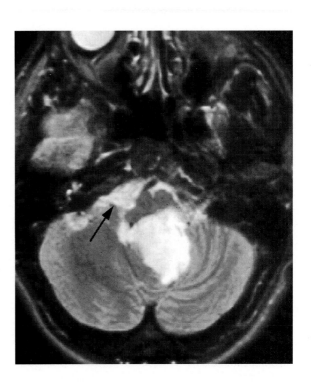

Epidermoid cysts are occasionally found within the fourth ventricle. Although rarely associated with hydrocephalus, such masses can grow to distort the brainstem. In this case the dorsal medulla is deformed, correlating with the patient's presenting symptoms. His hiccups resolved following resection of the lesion.

The MR features in this case match the characteristics of epidermoid cysts described on the preceding and following pages: homogeneous long T1 and long T2 values, lobulated margins, and lack of contrast enhancement. A small component of the tumor has extended through the right fo-

ramen of Luschka into the cerebellopontine angle (*arrow*; compare to the ependymoma in Case 156).

The differential diagnosis of an intraventricular mass with signal intensity similar to CSF would include tumors such as pilocytic astrocytoma (see Case 149) and cysts such as cysticercosis. Most glial and neuroectodermal neoplasms occupying the fourth ventricle would demonstrate areas of contrast enhancement, unlike epidermoid (or dermoid) masses. The margins of cysticercosis cysts are usually smoothly rounded rather than finely lobulated, and the cysts are rarely as large as the lesion in this case.

Case 295

51-year-old man presenting with facial numbness
and incoordination of the right arm.
(axial, noncontrast scan; SE 3000/45)

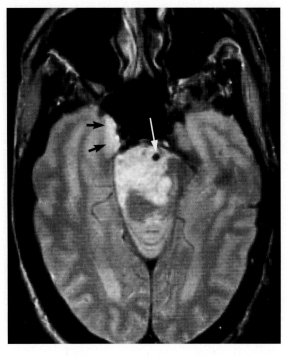

(same patient as Case 292)

Case 296

23-year-old woman presenting with right-sided
facial pain and nystagmus.
(axial, noncontrast scan; SE 3000/90)

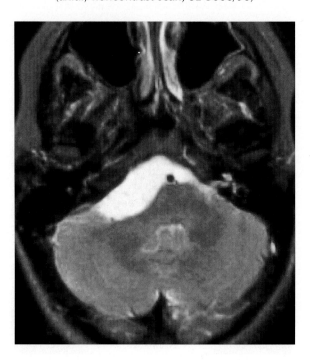

The signal intensity of epidermoid cysts is typically high on T2-weighted scans. The combination of long T1 and long T2 values within these lesions matches the appearance of CSF. As a result, epidermoid cysts may resemble CSF-containing masses and/or be difficult to distinguish from adjacent cisterns.

The greatest difference in signal intensity between epidermoid cysts and CSF is often noted on "intermediate" spin echo images obtained with long TR and short TE values. In Case 295, the intensity of the prepontine epidermoid cyst is slightly greater than that of CSF in the occipital horns. The lobulated contour of the mass is apparent, as is the marked deformity of the brainstem. Both of these features are hallmarks of a prepontine epidermoid cyst. Even more characteristic is the manner in which the mass has surrounded the vessels and cranial nerves in the region, insinuating itself between the basilar artery *(white arrow)* and the displaced midbrain.

The posterior fossa mass in Case 295 has grown into Meckel's cave on the right *(black arrows)*. Epidermoid cysts are among the lesions with a tendency to span the petrous apex (compare to Cases 60 and 178) and among the masses that may be responsible for trigeminal neuralgia or facial numbness.

Case 296 demonstrates a more smoothly marginated epidermoid cyst with prepontine and cerebellopontine angle components. This lesion more closely resembles an arachnoid cyst (compare to Case 297). Careful inspection of all pulse sequences for subtle heterogeneity within the lesion, mild divergence of signal intensity from that of spinal fluid, subtle lobulation of lesion margins, and/or encasement rather than displacement of cranial nerves and vessels may suggest the nonfluid nature of the lesion. Diffusion imaging may be useful in ambiguous cases.

DIFFERENTIAL DIAGNOSIS:
EXTRAAXIAL POSTERIOR FOSSA MASS WITH CSF-LIKE SIGNAL INTENSITY

Case 297

31-year-old man presenting with a left
sixth nerve palsy.
(axial, noncontrast scan; SE 3000/90)

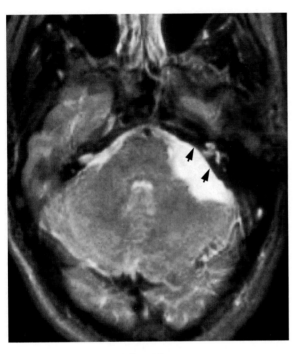

Arachnoid Cyst

Case 298

68-year-old man presenting with diplopia.
(axial, noncontrast scan; SE 2500/90)

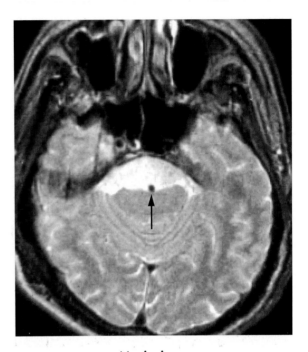

Meningioma

A number of extraaxial lesions can present as posterior fossa masses with homogeneously long T1 and T2 values.

Arachnoid cysts are described in Chapter 11. They are common in the cerebellopontine angle and may closely resemble an epidermoid cyst in this location. A clue to the correct diagnosis in Case 297 is the mild erosion of the adjacent petrous bone *(arrows)*. Overlying bone erosion is commonly associated with arachnoid cysts but is rarely seen at the margins of epidermoid tumors.

The prepontine mass in Case 298 is a reminder that meningiomas can demonstrate homogeneous low intensity on T1-weighted scans and high intensity on long TR sequences (compare to Case 38). Note the anterior extension to involve the right cavernous sinus, comparable to Case 295.

This tumor could be confused with a prepontine epidermoid cyst on noncontrast scans. However, a postcontrast study would show intense enhancement throughout the meningioma, distinguishing it from a nonenhancing epidermoid tumor.

Occasional acoustic schwannomas are homogeneous masses with high signal intensity on T2-weighted scans and could be included in this differential diagnosis. Like meningiomas, acoustic schwannomas are characterized by abnormal contrast enhancement.

There is marked posterior displacement of the basilar artery *(arrow)* and flattening of the pons in Case 298. Compare this prepontine mass effect to Cases 194A and 196.

Case 299A

2-year-old girl presenting with hemiparesis.
(coronal, noncontrast scan; RSE 3400/102)

Case 299B

Same patient.
(coronal, postcontrast scan; SE 900/11)

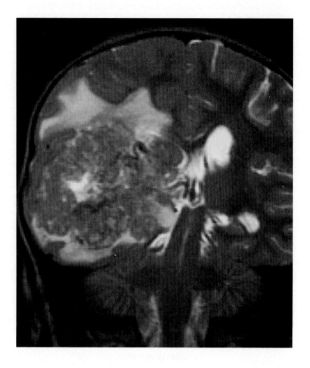

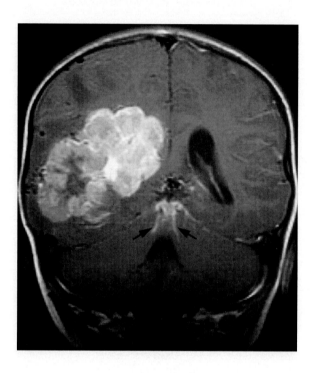

Choroid plexus papillomas in children are most common in the lateral ventricles, particularly on the left. They usually arise from the trigone and are often massive when discovered. Even "benign" papillomas may demonstrate bulky involvement of the adjacent hemisphere, frequently associated with large cysts.

The lobulated, heterogeneous mass in Case 299A is centered in the region of the right lateral ventricular trigone. The tumor fills the ventricle and extends into adjacent cerebral parenchyma, with surrounding edema. Relatively low signal intensity within the lesion on this T2-weighted scan reflects both dense cellularity (compare to germinomas as in Case 272B and lymphoma as in Cases 313 and 314) and diffuse calcification, which was apparent on a CT scan. Large vascular channels are present in the mass, which also contains small cysts or necrotic foci.

Intense contrast enhancement, as demonstrated in Case 299B, is typical of choroid plexus tumors. These neoplasms are highly vascular, with prominent angiographic stains fed by the anterior and posterior choroidal arteries.

Aggressive-appearing choroid plexus papillomas in children can be indistinguishable on CT or MR studies from choroid plexus carcinomas or from malignant ependymomas (see Case 300). The tumor in this case proved to be a carcinoma arising from the choroid plexus. A clue to malignant histology is the presence of meningeal seeding, which is demonstrated over the surface of the superior vermis in Case 299B (*arrow*; compare to Cases 160-162). CSF-borne dissemination of choroid plexus papillomas occurs but is not common.

Choroid plexus papillomas and carcinomas are among the intracranial tumors that may be present at birth. They are often associated with hydrocephalus, sometimes due to excessive production of spinal fluid. More commonly, secondary communicating hydrocephalus develops after repeated tumor hemorrhages with high CSF loads of protein and cells.

DIFFERENTIAL DIAGNOSIS:
MASS WITHIN THE LATERAL VENTRICULAR TRIGONE

Case 300

2-year-old girl presenting with increased
intracranial pressure.
(axial, noncontrast scan; SE 2500/25)

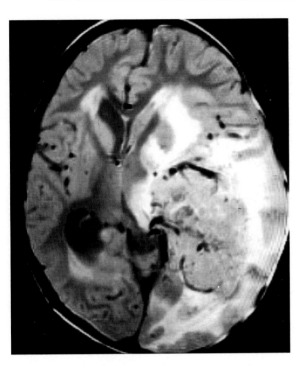

Malignant Ependymoma

Case 301

76-year-old woman.
(axial, postcontrast scan; SE 600/15)

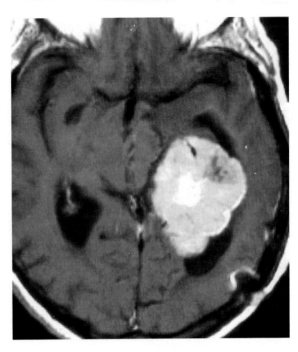

Meningioma

The tumor in Case 300 presents an aggressive appearance. Multiple, large circular and tubular "flow voids" suggest high vascularity, while extensive surrounding edema indicates hemispheric invasion. These features resemble the choroid plexus carcinoma in Case 299. Surgery instead disclosed a malignant ependymoma. A primitive neuroectodermal tumor could also be considered in the differential diagnosis (see Case 306).

Case 301 demonstrates a mass that is completely intraventricular, characterized by predominantly homogeneous contrast enhancement. This appearance and the location of the lesion within the trigone of the lateral ventricle are typical for intraventricular meningiomas in adults.

The uniform enhancement of the lobulated mass in Case 301 resembles Case 299B. However, a lateral ventricular tumor in an adult is unlikely to represent a choroid plexus papilloma or carcinoma. Diagnostic possibilities other than meningioma include metastasis, astrocytoma (see Case 113), oligodendroglioma (see Case 114), ependymoma, central neurocytoma (see Case 308), arteriovenous malformation, or an inflammatory lesion (e.g., granuloma, parasitic or fungal mass).

Case 302

2-month-old boy with hydrocephalus.
(sagittal, noncontrast scan; SE 800/16)

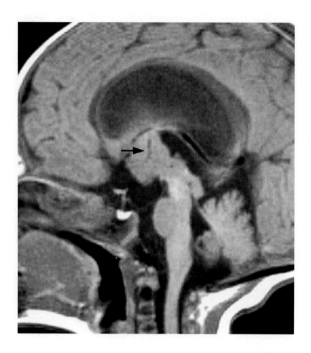

Case 303

46-year-old woman presenting with neck
pain and nausea.
(coronal, noncontrast scan; SE 700/16)

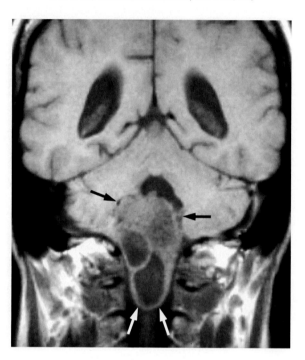

Choroid plexus papillomas are occasionally encountered in the third ventricle, as illustrated in Case 302. The fleshy or papillary character of the homogeneous mass and the presence of prominent "flow voids" *(arrow)* implying high vascularity are clues to the diagnosis, even in this unusual location. The associated hydrocephalus is probably due to obstruction of the third ventricle.

In adults, choroid plexus papillomas occur most commonly in the fourth ventricle, particularly caudally. This location and the frequent presence of calcification can suggest the correct diagnosis.

The scan in Case 303 shows a lesion with two components. The superior half of the tumor *(black arrows)* deforms the fourth ventricle. Dense calcification was seen in this tissue on a CT scan but causes only mild reduction in signal intensity on MR. The caudal half of the tumor *(white arrows)* is a bilocular cyst extending into the cervical spinal canal. This component was inapparent on the patient's CT scan, again demonstrating the superiority of MR for evaluation of lesions involving or traversing the skull base.

DIFFERENTIAL DIAGNOSIS:
FOURTH VENTRICULAR MASS IN AN ADULT

Case 304

72-year-old woman presenting with hydrocephalus.
(sagittal, noncontrast scan; SE 600/17)

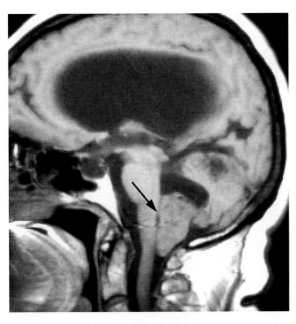

Choroid Plexus Papilloma

Case 305

47-year-old woman presenting with dysmetria,
nausea and dizziness.
(coronal, postcontrast scan; SE 800/15)

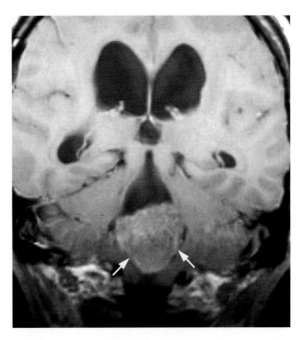

Ependymoma

A variety of pathologies can cause masses occupying or bordering the fourth ventricle in adults. As mentioned on the previous pages, the fourth ventricle is the most common site for choroid plexus papillomas outside the pediatric age group. Such tumors frequently contain calcification and are often found at the caudal end of the ventricle, as in Case 304.

Ependymomas of the fourth ventricle, such as Case 305, are occasionally encountered in young or middle-aged adults. As discussed in Case 163, medulloblastomas in adults tend to be hemispheric rather than midline.

Metastases within the brainstem or cerebellar vermis may mimic other fourth ventricular tumors. The differential diagnosis of a fourth ventricular mass in an adult also includes unusual glioma, subependymoma, hemangioblastoma, arteriovenous malformation, rare epidermoid or dermoid tumors (see Case 294), and an inflammatory mass or cyst.

Case 306A

9-year-old boy presenting with behavioral
changes and headaches.
(sagittal, noncontrast scan; SE 600/15)

Case 306B

Same patient.
(axial, noncontrast scan; SE 3000/45)

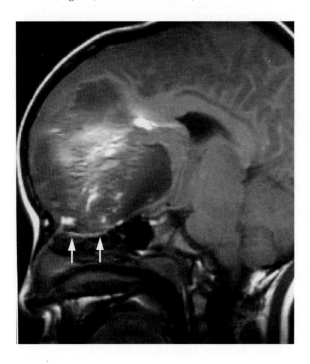

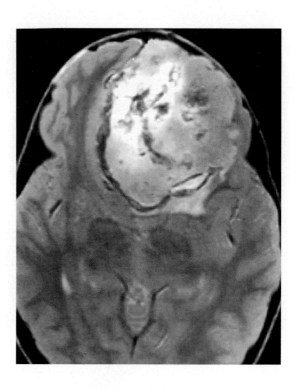

Primitive neuroectodermal tumors (PNET) arise from un-differentiated neuroepithelial cells with the capacity for glial and/or neuronal maturation. Pathologists group a number of malignancies under this heading, including medulloblastomas (see Cases 144-148) and pineoblastomas (see Cases 279-281).

Primitive neuroectodermal tumors of the cerebral hemispheres are rare. These lesions, which have also been called "cerebral neuroblastomas," are usually seen in children. Bulky, heterogeneous masses like Case 306 are typical. Intratumoral hemorrhage, indicated by the patchy zones of T1-shortening in Case 306A, is common. Cysts and calcification are also frequent, with the latter feature better appreciated on CT scans. The mixture of cystic and solidly enhancing components of a PNET may closely resemble the lobulations of a teratoma like Case 283 or a malignant glioma like Case 98.

Although the heterogeneous character of the mass in Case 306 suggests an aggressive malignancy, the large size of the lesion with little surrounding edema indicates that the tumor may have been enlarging slowly for some time. Supporting this possibility is bony remodelling with depression of the cribriform plate (arrows, Case 306A).

Like medulloblastomas and pineoblastomas, cerebral PNETs may be associated with CSF dissemination. Multiple intradural, extramedullary spinal masses developed within months in this case.

ESTHESIONEUROBLASTOMAS ("OLFACTORY NEUROBLASTOMAS")

Case 307A

3-year-old boy presenting with headaches
and papilledema.
(sagittal, noncontrast scan; SE 700/20)

Case 307B

Same patient.
(axial, noncontrast scan; SE 2500/90)

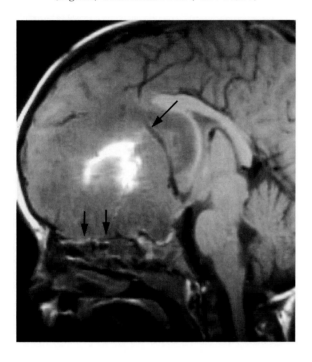

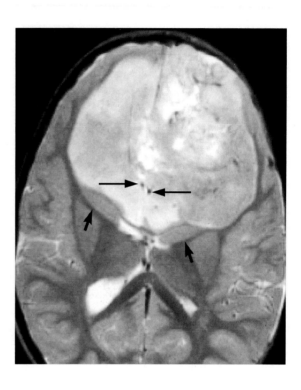

Esthesioneuroblastomas or "olfactory neuroblastomas" are uncommon tumors originating from neuroepithelial sensory cells of the olfactory system. These masses arise near the cribriform plate and may present in the ethmoid-nasal region and/or intracranially. In either case, the tumors can be centered in the midline or predominantly unilateral. Esthesioneuroblastomas are seen in both children and adults.

The MR appearance of esthesioneuroblastomas is variable. The tumors may be homogeneous or heterogenous, with short or long T2 values and mild or intense contrast enhancement. Characteristic location is the most helpful diagnostic clue.

In Case 307A, a very large subfrontal mass is based in the region of the cribriform plate *(short arrows)*. The corpus callosum is markedly displaced, and the anterior cerebral artery *(long arrow)* is encased by tumor. Hemorrhage is present at the center of the lesion.

Marked invagination of the mass into the frontal lobes is apparent in Case 307B. There is posterior displacement and splaying of the caudate nuclei *(short arrows)* and extreme thinning of surrounding frontal lobe white and gray matter. The anterior cerebral arteries are seen in cross-section, surrounded by tumor *(long arrows)*. The impressive lack of reactive edema and the marked cerebral deformity argue for a slowly growing lesion of extraaxial origin.

The differential diagnosis for a subfrontal mass in a child is quite limited. Meningiomas would be unusual in this location at this age. Subfrontal extension of pituitary adenomas occurs in adults (see Case 206) but would be rare in a child. Craniopharyngiomas tend to expand laterally or posteriorly rather than anteriorly (see Cases 233 and 249), although this diagnosis would be considered here since the mass does involve the suprasellar region. An exophytic glioma of the hypothalamus/optic chiasm could be included in the differential diagnosis for the same reason.

Note that the extraaxial tumor in Case 307, like the intraaxial glioma in Case 82, adjoins the anterior falx. This proximity does not necessarily imply dural origin of the lesion (i.e., a diagnosis of meningioma).

Case 308A

31-year-old man presenting with headaches,
most severe on awakening.
(sagittal, noncontrast scan; SE 600/15)

Case 308B

Same patient.
(axial, noncontrast scan; SE 3000/90)

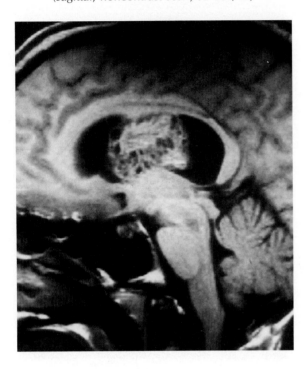

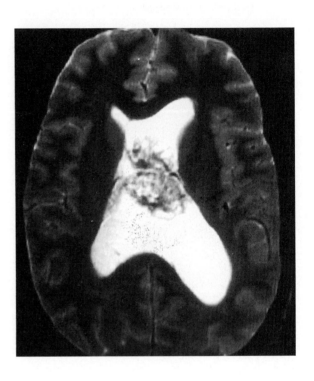

A group of intraventricular tumors with characteristic imaging features and favorable clinical prognosis has been recognized over the past decade. These masses, called "central neurocytomas," resemble oligodendrogliomas at traditional light microscopy. However, when examined by electron microscopy, the lesions demonstrate neuronal differentiation. The tumors are comprised of small, uniform, well-differentiated cells and may be considered to be a mature intraventricular form of neuroblastoma.

Central neurocytomas are typically heterogeneous masses containing multiple cysts and calcifications and occasional hemorrhage. The tumors are most often located within the body of a lateral ventricle, usually attached to the septum pellucidum. Case 308 illustrates these characteristic features.

Contrast enhancement in central neurocytomas is variable but often less uniform or extensive than might be expected in a glioma of corresponding size.

Unlike intraventricular gliomas, neurocytomas rarely recur after resection. Adjunctive radiation therapy may therefore not be required. For this reason, it is important to recognize the imaging clues to the diagnosis, alerting the pathologist to perform electron microscopy and/or specific immunohistochemical stains for accurate classification.

DIFFERENTIAL DIAGNOSIS:
MASS INVOLVING THE SEPTUM PELLUCIDUM

Case 309

22-year-old woman presenting with headaches
and nausea.
(coronal, postcontrast scan; SE 600/20)

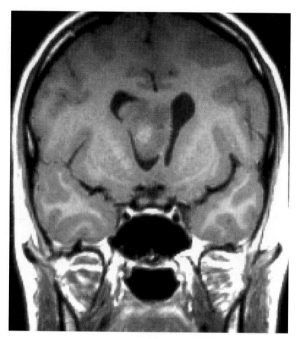

Ependymoma
(same patient as Case 115)

Case 310

66-year-old man presenting with headaches
and confusion.
(axial, noncontrast scan; SE 2500/90)

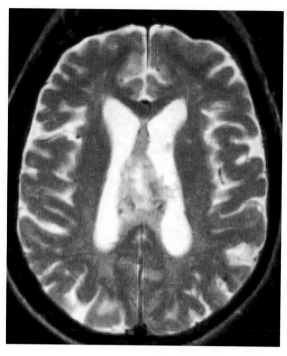

Grade III Astrocytoma

Central neurocytomas are among several tumors that can originate from or invade the septum pellucidum. Ependymomas and subependymomas can arise from the lateral ventricular margins laterally or medially. The mass in Case 309 demonstrates a broad base along the septum pellucidum. The relative homogeneity of this tumor argues against the diagnosis of central neurocytoma (compare to Case 308A). The lack of more prominent contrast enhancement is somewhat unusual for an ependymoma.

Case 310 illustrates invasion of the septum pellucidum by a malignant glioma of the corpus callosum. Although the lesion demonstrates heterogeneous signal intensity, the diffuse septal infiltration and thickening in this case are distinct from the more focal and mass-like morphology of most central neurocytomas (compare to Case 308B).

Gliomas commonly occur near the lateral ventricles and frequently invade the septum pellucidum. Thickening of the septum suggests intraaxial origin of an otherwise ambiguous deep frontal lobe lesion. This finding is most commonly associated with gliomas but can also be seen with other pathologies (e.g., primary CNS lymphoma).

Case 311

38-year-old man with AIDS, presenting
with confusion.
(sagittal, noncontrast scan; SE 600/15)

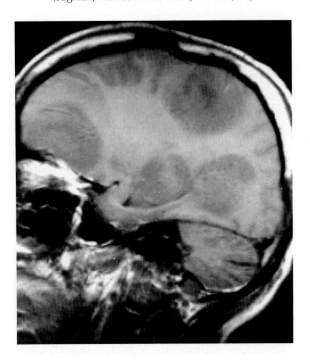

Case 312

74-year-old woman presenting with blurred
vision and impaired memory.
(coronal, noncontrast scan; SE 550/20)

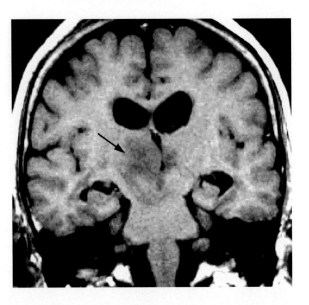

Primary CNS lymphoma ("reticulum cell sarcoma," "microglioma," "immunoblastic lymphoma") is an increasingly common cause of single or multiple intracranial masses. Primary CNS lymphomas are infrequent in otherwise healthy individuals. They are much more common in patients who are immunosuppressed due to disease (e.g., AIDS) or medication (e.g., transplant regimens). Primary lymphoma of the CNS is more common than parenchymal involvement by systemic lymphoma, which more typically infiltrates the meninges or the ventricular surface (see Cases 386-1 and 390).

Primary CNS lymphomas can assume a variety of appearances and may mimic other pathologies. Both lobar and deep hemisphere lesions may occur. Frequent areas of involvement include the basal ganglia, corpus callosum, cerebellum, and periventricular white matter.

On T1-weighted scans, the signal intensity of CNS lymphomas is usually low to intermediate, as illustrated above. The multiple lesions in Case 311 are predominantly lobar and demonstrate well-defined T1-prolongation. The deep hemisphere mass in Case 312 is less well demarcated from surrounding parenchyma. (Compare the involvement along the margins of the third ventricle in Case 312 to the ventral extension of a pineal germinoma in Case 277.)

The lesions of primary CNS lymphoma often regress in response to steroid therapy and may wax and wane spontaneously. Clues to the diagnosis include involvement of deep hemisphere structures, multicentricity, steroid response, and a clinical association with immunosuppression.

Case 313

31-year-old woman presenting with ataxia.
(axial, noncontrast scan; SE 3000/90)

Case 314

73-year-old man presenting with a seizure.
(axial, noncontrast scan; SE 3000/90)

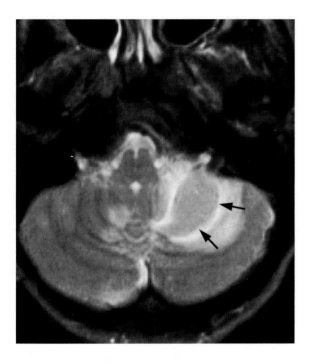

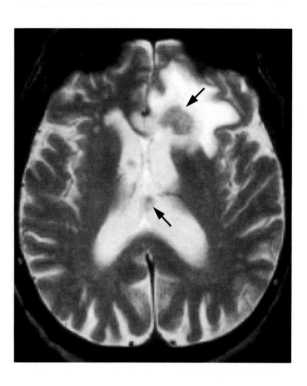

In both of these cases, a rim of high intensity edema surrounds a tumor *(arrows)* that is nearly isointense to gray matter. This lack of T2-prolongation is characteristic of primary CNS lymphoma, reflecting the dense cellularity and high nuclear to cytoplasmic ratio of these tumors. (Compare to medulloblastomas and germinomas, such as Cases 146 and 272B).

As seen above and on the previous page, primary CNS lymphomas are usually homogeneous lesions. An exception to this rule occurs in AIDS patients, when central necrosis is commonly observed (see Cases 323 and 324).

Lymphoma should be one of the diagnoses considered when a cerebellar mass is encountered in a young adult, such as Case 313. Other possibilities include lateral medulloblastoma, hemangioblastoma, and astrocytoma (see Cases 163 and 164).

The periventricular location of the frontal lesion in Case 314 is typical for CNS lymphoma. Additional nodules along the septum pellucidum are more easily seen on a postcontrast scan of this patient, presented in Case 321.

Case 315

74-year-old woman presenting with loss of
short-term memory.
(axial, noncontrast scan; SE 3000/90)

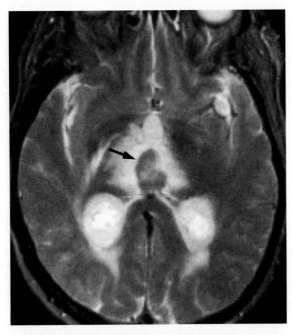

Primary CNS Lymphoma
(same patient as Case 312)

Case 316

19-year-old man presenting with blurred
vision and headaches.
(axial, noncontrast scan; SE 3000/90)

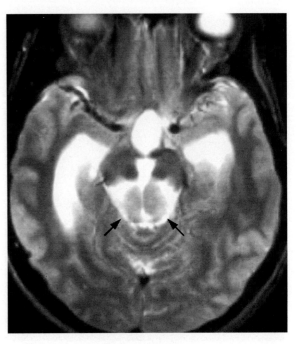

Pineal Germinoma
(same patient as Case 272)

The character of these two lesions is very similar. The central tumor in each scan demonstrates relatively low signal intensity, comparable to gray matter. This lack of T2-prolongation is attributable to the close packing of small cells that characterizes these pathologies. In both cases, the tumor involves the walls of the third ventricle. Both masses are outlined by a halo of edema, and both have caused obstructive hydrocephalus.

The scan features of Case 315 closely match the tumors on the previous page. Deep hemisphere, periventricular location is a common finding in primary CNS lymphoma, seen also in Cases 319-321.

Case 317

69-year-old man presenting with confusion.
(axial, postcontrast scan; SE 600/15)

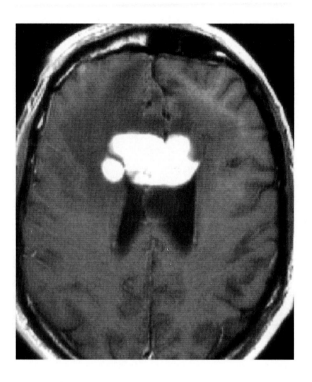

Case 318

76-year-old man presenting with right hemiparesis.
(coronal, postcontrast scan; SE 600/15)

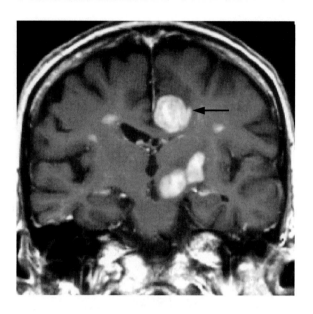

Contrast enhancement within CNS lymphomas may be solid or peripheral. Intense, uniform enhancement is common, as seen in these cases.

CNS lymphoma is among the pathologies that may involve and cross the corpus callosum. (Other tumors in this category are gliomas and occasional metastases.) The large mass occupying the genu and anterior body of the corpus callosum in Case 317 is surrounded by bifrontal edema. A malignant glioma could cause an identical appearance, although central necrosis with irregular rim enhancement would be more common (see Case 97).

The multiple enhancing nodules in Case 318 predominantly involve the basal ganglia and periventricular regions. This deep distribution is typical for CNS lymphoma and would be less common for metastatic disease (compare to Case 14).

The faintly laminated or target-like morphology within the largest mass in Case 318 *(arrow)* is a frequent feature of primary CNS lymphoma, seen also in Cases 325 and 326.

In rare instances, cerebral masses due to primary CNS lymphoma do not enhance. Pathological examination of such lesions may demonstrate intraluminal tumor obstructing arteries within the neoplasm. In any event, the absence of contrast enhancement does not exclude the diagnosis of CNS lymphoma.

Nonenhancing lymphoma occasionally mimics progressive multifocal leukoencephalopathy in an immunocompromised patient. Fungal disease (e.g., aspergillosis) may also present as multiple nonenhancing masses in this context.

Case 319

31-year-old man with AIDS, presenting
with headaches.
(coronal, postcontrast scan; SE 600/15)

Case 320

80-year-old woman presenting with dizziness.
(axial, postcontrast scan; SE 600/15)

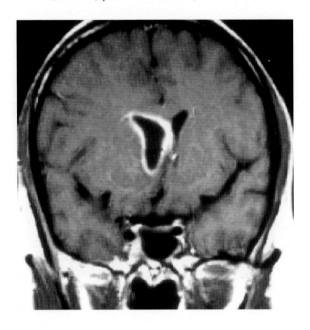

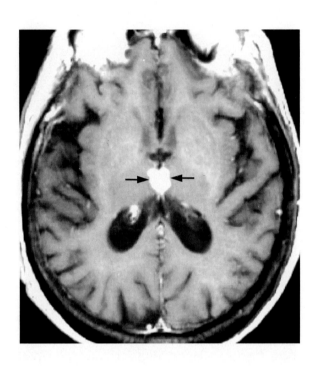

Periventricular involvement by primary CNS lymphoma is common. It may take the form of localized masses (see Cases 312 and 314) or more diffuse infiltration along ventricular margins. The latter pattern is demonstrated in the scans above.

In Case 319, an enhancing layer of subependymal tumor follows the contour of the right frontal horn. Relatively uniform thickening of this enhancing rind mimics the appearance of inflammatory ventriculitis (compare to Case 389). Slight thickening of the tumor layer is present medially within the septum pellucidum (see discussion of Cases 309 and 310).

The solid appearance of the third ventricular lesion in Case 320 represents the meeting in the midline of bilateral tumor layers involving the walls of the third ventricle. Reactive edema is present in the thalamus bilaterally.

Case 321

73-year-old man presenting with a seizure.
(axial, postcontrast scan; SE 800/17)

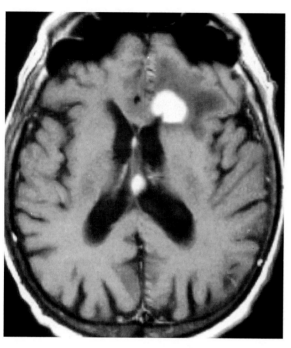

Primary CNS Lymphoma
(same patient as Case 314)

Case 322

8-year-old boy complaining of headaches.
(axial, postcontrast scan; SE 720/17)

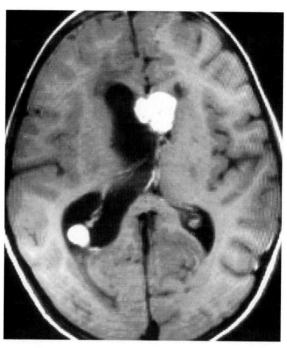

**Recurrent Astrocytoma, Originally of the
Septum Pellucidum**
(same patient as Case 262, three years later)

As discussed previously and illustrated by Case 321, primary CNS lymphoma may cause multiple tumor nodules along ventricular margins.

A similar appearance may represent implants due to CSF seeding by a glial neoplasm, medulloblastoma, germinoma, pineal cell tumor, primitive neuroectodermal tumor, or systemic metastasis. The original septal glioma in Case 322 was a cystic lesion without aggressive features (see Case 262). However, the eventual development of recurrent tumor along ventricular margins is a poor prognostic sign.

Unilateral hydrocephalus on the right in Case 322 was due to an obstructing tumor nodule at the right foramen of Monro.

Case 323

28-year-old man.
(axial, noncontrast scan; SE 2500/90)

Case 324

38-year-old man.
(axial, postcontrast scan; SE 600/15)

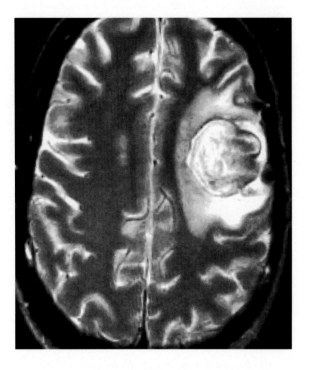

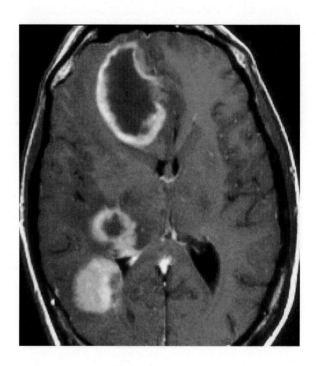

Patients with AIDS have a high incidence of primary CNS lymphoma. This diagnosis should be considered (along with toxoplasmosis; see Cases 418-422) whenever a cerebral mass is discovered in an HIV-positive individual. Deep hemisphere involvement and multiple masses are common, as in the simultaneous presence of inflammatory lesions.

CNS lymphomas in AIDS patients are often inhomogenous, with large areas of central necrosis. The masses may contain zones of high signal intensity on T2-weighted scans, as seen in Case 323. This heterogeneity and T2-prolongation differ from the appearance of typical primary CNS lymphomas, as illustrated in Cases 313 to 315.

Masses due to CNS lymphoma in AIDS patients frequently demonstrate peripheral contrast enhancement, as in Case 324. Similar lesions are occasionally seen as solitary tumors in nonimmunocompromised adults, closely resembling a malignant glioma. (Compare the frontal mass in Case 324 to Cases 99 and 100.)

The combination of solid and rim-enhancing lesions in Case 324 could represent either variation in the appearance of CNS lymphoma or the coexistence of inflammatory lesions and tumor. The clinical course usually makes this distinction. None of the masses in Case 324 responded to therapy for toxoplasmosis, while all subsequently "melted" with steroids. Prominent (but temporary) response to steroids and radiation therapy is characteristic of primary CNS lymphoma.

DIFFERENTIAL DIAGNOSIS:
ENHANCING MASS WITH LAYERED INTERNAL STRUCTURE

Case 325

76-year-old woman presenting with
word-finding difficulty.
(axial, postcontrast scan; SE 600/15)

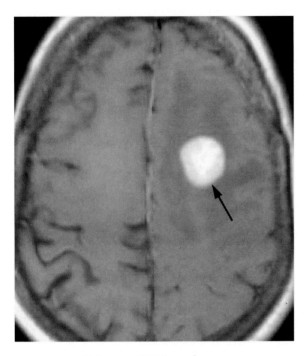

Primary CNS Lymphoma

Case 326

24-year-old man presenting with ataxia
and severe headaches.
(coronal, postcontrast scan; SE 600/15)

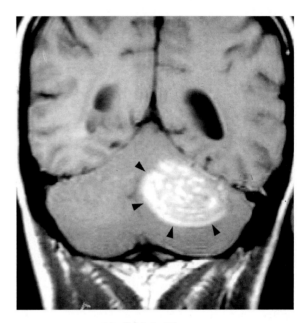

Hodgkin's Disease

Lymphomas of both CNS and systemic origin may demonstrate complex internal organization on MR studies. As mentioned in Case 318, the nodules of primary CNS lymphoma may contain layers of varying signal intensity on precontrast or postcontrast scans. Case 325 faintly illustrates this pattern.

A target-like morphology is by no means specific for CNS lymphoma. Toxoplasmosis abscesses can present a similar appearance in AIDS patients. Thin rings may also be observed within the demyelinating plaques of multiple sclerosis (see Cases 339 and 340).

The mass in Case 325 is a little unusual by virtue of its midhemisphere location. However, this lesion makes the point that CNS lymphoma should be considered whenever one or more solidly enhancing cerebral or cerebellar masses are discovered in an adult. Specifically, CNS lym-

phoma should be included in the differential diagnosis of metastatic disease.

Like some metastases, the mass in Case 325 has incited extensive surrounding edema. The reactive edema is more responsible for mass effect and associated symptoms than the underlying tumor.

Systemic lymphoma uncommonly involves brain parenchyma. Lymphomatous meningial infiltration or subependymal spread is more frequent (see Cases 386-1 and 390). Occasional intraaxial masses such as Case 326 are encountered. The laminated, granular texture within this cerebellar lesion would be unusual for more common tumors (compare to Cases 138-141, 163, and 164). Like Case 313, Case 326 indicates that lymphoma (primary or systemic) should be included in the differential diagnosis of a cerebellar mass in a young adult.

REFERENCES

Ahmadi J, Savabi F, Apuzzo MLJ, et al: Magnetic resonance imaging and quantitative analysis of intracranial cystic lesions: surgical implication. *Neurosurgery* 35:199-207, 1994.

Bolen JW, Lipper MH, Caccamo D: Juxtaventricular central neurocytoma: CT and MR findings. *J Comput Assist Tomogr* 13:495-497, 1989.

Buetow PC, Smirniotopoulos JG, Done S: Congenital brain tumors: a review of 45 cases. *AJNR* 11:793-799, 1990.

Casadei GP, Komori T, Scheithauer BW, et al: Intracranial parenchymal schwannoma. *J Neurosurg* 79:217-222, 1993.

Coates TL, Hinshaw DBJ Jr, Peckman N, et al: Pediatric choroid plexus neoplasms: MR, CT, and pathologic correlation. *Radiology* 173:81-88, 1989.

Cordoliani Y-S, Derosier C, Pharaboz C, et al: Primary cerebral lymphoma in patients with AIDS: MR findings: 17 cases. *AJNR* 159:841-847, 1992.

Davis PC, Wichman RD, Takei Y, Hoffman JCJ: Primary cerebral neuroblastoma: CT and MR findings in 12 cases. *AJNR* 11:115-120, 1990.

DeAngelis LM: Cerebral lymphomas presenting as a nonenhancing lesion on computed tomographic/magnetic resonance scan. *Ann Neurol* 33:308-311, 1993.

Dina TS: Primary central nervous system lymphoma versus toxoplasmosis in AIDS. *Radiology* 179:823-838, 1991.

Donati F, Vasella F, Kaiser G, Blumberg A: Intracranial lipomas. *Neuropediatrics* 23:32-38, 1992.

Eghwrudjakpor PO, Kurisaka M, Fukuoka M, Mori K: Intracranial lipomas. *Acta Neurochir (Wien)* 110:124-128, 1991.

Fain JS, Tomlinson FH, Bernd W, et al: Symptomatic glial cysts of the pineal gland. *J Neurosurg* 80:454-460, 1994.

Figueroa RE, El Gammal T, Brooks BS, et al: MR findings on primitive neuroectodermal tumors. *J Comput Assist Tomogr* 13:773-778, 1989.

Fleege MA, Miller GM, Fletcher GP, et al: Imaging characteristics with histologic correlation. *AJNR* 15:161-166, 1994.

Friedman DP: Extrapineal abnormalities of the tectal region: MR imaging findings. *AJR* 159:859-866, 1992.

Gao P, Osborn AG, Smirniotopoulos JG, Harris CP: Epidermoid tumor of the cerebellopontine angle. *AJNR* 13:863-872, 1992.

Goergen SK, Gonzales MF, McLean CA: Intraventricular neurocytoma: radiologic features and review of the literature. *Radiology* 182:787-792, 1992.

Golzarian J, Baleriaux D, Bank WO, et al: Pineal cyst: normal or pathological? *Neurosurgery* 35:251-253, 1993.

Gualdi GF, Di Biasi C, Trasimeni G, et al: Unusual MR and CT appearance of an epidermoid tumor. *AJNR* 12:771-772, 1991.

Hahn FJ, Ong E, McComb RD, et al: MR imaging of ruptured intracranial dermoid. *J Comput Assist Tomogr* 10:888-889, 1986.

Hashimoto M, Fujimoto K, Shinoda S, Masuzawa T: Magnetic resonance imaging of ganglion cell tumors. *Neuroradiology* 35:181-184, 1993.

Hassoun J, Söylemezoglu F, Gambarelli D, et al: Central neurocytoma: a synopsis of clinical and histological features. *Brain Pathol* 3:297-306, 1993.

Hoffman HJ, Otsubo H, Hendrick EB, et al: Intracranial germ cell tumors in children. *J Neurosurg* 74:545-551, 1991.

Horowitz BL, Chari MV, James R: MR of intracranial epidermoid tumors: correlation of in vivo imaging with in vitro C-13 spectroscopy. *AJNR* 11:299-302, 1990.

Hunt SJ, Johnsen PC, Coons SW, Pittman HW: Neonatal intracranial teratomas. *Surg Neurol* 34:336-342, 1990.

Jelinek J, Smirniotopoulos JG, Parisi JE, Kanzer M: Lateral ventricular neoplasms of the brain: differential diagnosis based on clinical, CT, and MR findings. *AJNR* 11:567-574, 1990.

Ken JG, Sobel DF, Copeland B, et al: Choroid plexus papillomas of the foramen of Luschka: MR appearance. *AJNR* 12:1201-1203, 1991.

Kilgore DP, Strother CM, Starshak RJ, Haughton VM: Pineal germinoma: MR imaging. *Radiology* 158:435-438, 1986.

Klein P, Rubinstein LJ: Benign symptomatic glial cysts of the pineal gland: a report of seven cases and review of the literature. *J Neurol Neurosurg Psychiatr* 52:991-995, 1989.

Koeller KK, Dillon WP: Dysembryoplastic neuroepithelial tumors: MR appearance. *AJNR* 13:1319-1325, 1992.

Komatsu Y, Narushima K, Kobayashi E, et al: CT and MR of germinoma in the basal ganglia. *AJNR* 10:59, 1989.

Latack JT, Kartush JM, Kemink JL, et al: Epidermoidomas of the cerebellopontine angle and temporal bone: CT and MR aspects. *Radiology* 157:361-366, 1985.

Lee DH, Norman D, Newton TH: MR imaging of pineal cysts. *J Comput Assist Tomogr* 11:586-690, 1987.

Li C, Yousem DM, Hayden RE, Doty RL: Olfactory neuroblastoma: MR evaluation. *AJNR* 14:1167-1171, 1993.

Lunardi P, Missori P: Supratentorial dermoid cysts. *J Neurosurg* 75:262-266, 1991.

Maeder PP, Holtas SL, Basibuyuk LN, et al: Colloid cysts of the third ventricle: correlation of MR and CT findings with histology and chemical analysis. *AJNR* 11:575-581, 1990.

Mamourian AC, Towfight J: Pineal cysts: MR imaging. *AJNR* 7:1081-1086, 1986.

Mamourian AC, Yarnell T: Enhancement of pineal cyst on MR images. *AJNR* 12:773-774, 1991.

Markus H, Kendall BE: MRI of a dermoid cyst containing hair. *Neuroradiology* 35:256-257, 1993.

Matthews VP, Broome DR, Smith RR, et al: Neuroimaging of disseminated germ cell neoplasms. *AJNR* 11:319, 1990.

Miyazawa N, Yamazaki H, Wakao T, Nukui H: Epidermoid tumors of Meckel's cave: case report and review of the literature. *Neurosurgery* 25:951-954, 1989.

Morita A, Ebersold MJ, Olsen KD, et al: Esthesioneuroblastoma: prognosis and management. *Neurosurgery* 32:706-715, 1993.

Muller-Forell W, Schroth G, Egan PJ: MR imaging in tumors of the pineal region. *Neuroradiology* 30:224-231, 1988.

Musolino A, Cambria S, Rizzo G, Cambria M: Symptomatic cysts of the pineal gland: stereotactic diagnosis and treatment of two cases and review of the literature. *Neurosurgery* 32:315-321, 1993.

Nakagawa H, Iwasaki S, Kichikawa K, et al: MR imaging of pineocytoma: report of two cases. *AJNR* 11:185, 1990.

Nakagawa H, Iwasaki S, Kichikawa K, et al: MR imaging of pineocytoma: report of two cases. *AJNR* 11:195-198, 1990.

Newton DR, Larson TC III, Dillon WP, Newton TH: Magnetic resonance characteristics of cranial epidermoid and teratomatous tumors. *AJNR* 8:945, 1987.

Olson JJ, Beck DW, Crawford SC, Menezes AH: Comparative evaluation of epidermoid tumors with computed tomography and magnetic resonance imaging. *Neurosurgery* 21:357-360, 1987.

Packer RJ, Perilongo G, Johnson D, et al: Choroid plexus carcinoma of childhood. *Cancer* 69:580-585, 1992.

Robles HA, Smirniotopoulos JG, Figueroa RE: Understanding the radiology of intracranial primitive neuroectodermal tumors from a pathological perspective: a review. *Semin US CT MR* 13:170-181, 1992.

Roman-Goldstein SM, Goldman DL, Howieson J, et al: MR in primary CNS lymphoma in immunologically normal patients. *AJNR* 13:1207-1213, 1992.

Roosen N, Gahlen D, Stork W, et al: Magnetic resonance imaging of colloid cysts of the third ventricle. *Neuroradiology* 29:10-14, 1987.

Savader SJ, Murtagh FR, Savader BL, et al: Magnetic resonance imaging of intracranial epidermoid tumors. *Clin Radiol* 40:282, 1989.

Schwaighofer BW, Hesselink JR, Press GA, et al: Primary intracranial CNS lymphoma: MR manifestations. *AJNR* 10:725-730, 1989.

Scotti G, Scialfa G, Colombo N, et al: MR in the diagnosis of colloid cysts of the third ventricle. *AJNR* 8:370-372, 1987.

Shen WC, Yang CF: Epidermoid cyst with variable contents shown on CT and MRI. *Neuroradiology* 33(suppl):317-318, 1991.

Shoemaker EI, Romano AS, Gado M: Neuroradiology case of the day: choroid plexus papilloma, third ventricle. *AJR* 152:1333-1338, 1989.

Smirniotopoulos JG, Rushing EJ, Mena H: Pineal region mass: differential diagnosis. *Radiographics* 12:577-595, 1992.

Smith AS, Benson JE, Blaser SI, et al: Diagnosis of ruptured intracranial dermoid cyst: value of MR over CT. *AJNR* 12:175-180, 1991.

Smoker WRK, Townsend JJ, Reichman MV: Neurocytoma accompanied by intraventricular hemorrhage: case report and literature review. *AJNR* 12:765-770, 1991.

Som PM, Lidov M, Brandwein M, et al: Sinonasal esthesioneuroblastomas with intracranial extension: marginal tumor cysts as a diagnostic MR finding. *AJNR* 15:1259-1262, 1994.

Steffev DJ, De Filipp GJ, Spera T, Gabrielsen TO: MR imaging of primary epidermoid tumors. *J Comput Assist Tomogr* 12:438-440, 1988.

Stephenson TF, Spitzer RM: MR and CT appearance of ruptured intracranial dermoid tumors. *Comput Radiol* 11:249, 1987.

Tampieri D, Melanson D, Ethier R: MR imaging of epidermoid cysts. *AJNR* 10:351-356, 1989.

Tatler GLV, Kendall BE: The radiological diagnosis of epidermoid tumors. *Neuroradiology* 33(suppl):324-325, 1991.

Tien RD: Intraventricular mass lesions of the brain: CT and MR findings. *AJR* 157:1283-1290, 1991.

Tien RD, Barkovich AJ, Edwards MSB: MR imaging of pineal tumors. *AJNR* 11:557-565, 1990.

Todo T, Kondo T, Shinoura N, Yamada R: Large cysts of the pineal gland: report of two cases. *Neurosurgery* 29:101-106, 1992.

Truwit CL, Barkovich AJ: Pathogenesis of intracranial lipoma: an MR study in 42 patients. *AJNR* 11:665-674, 1990.

Vion-Dury J, Vincentilli F, Jiddane M, et al: MR imaging of epidermoid cysts. *Neuroradiology* 29:333-338, 1987.

Waggenspack GA, Guinto FC Jr: MR and CT of masses of the anterosuperior third ventricle. *AJNR* 10:105-110, 1989.

Wagle WA, Jaufmann B, Mincy JE: Magnetic resonance imaging of fourth ventricular epidermoid tumors. *Arch Neurol* 48:438-440, 1991.

Wichmann W, Schubiger O, Von Demling A, et al: Neuroradiology of central neurocytoma. *Neuroradiology* 33:143-148, 1991.

Wilms G, Casselman J, Demaerel Ph, et al: CT and MRI of ruptured intracranial dermoids. *Neuroradiology* 33:149-151, 1991.

Wilms G, Marchal G, Van Hecke P, et al: Colloid cysts of the third ventricle: MR findings. *J Comput Assist Tomogr* 14:527-531, 1990.

Yasargil MG, Von Ammon K, Von Deimling A, et al: Central neurocytoma: histopathological variants and therapeutic approaches. *J Neurosurg* 76:32-37, 1992.

Yuh WTC, Barloon TJ, Jacoby CG, et al: MR of fourth ventricular epidermoid tumors. *AJNR* 9:794-798, 1988.

Zee C-S, Segall H, Apuzzo M, et al: MR imaging of pineal region neoplasms. *J Comput Assist Tomogr* 15:56-63, 1991.

Zimmerman RA: Central nervous system lymphoma. *Radiol Clin North Am* 28:697-722, 1990.

Zimmerman RA: Pediatric supratentorial tumors. *Semin Roentgenol* 25:225-248, 1990.

CHAPTER 7

White Matter Disorders

Case 327

37-year-old woman presenting with a two-day
history of worsening hemiparesis.
(sagittal, noncontrast scan; SE 600/20)

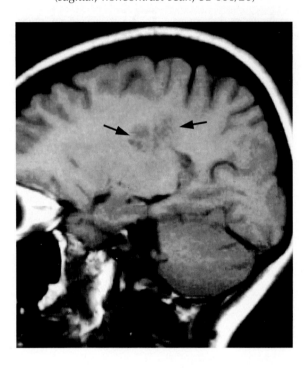

Case 328

51-year-old woman with a ten-year history
of multiple sclerosis.
(sagittal, noncontrast scan; SE 600/17)

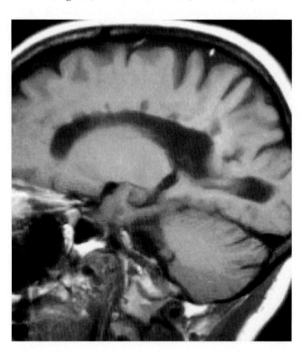

The MR appearance of multiple sclerosis is widely variable, depending on acuity and extent of disease. Active demyelination usually presents as a zone of moderate T1-prolongation, as in Case 327 *(arrows)*. Such lesions are typically 1 to 2 cm in diameter, with mildly indistinct margins due to associated edema. (Compare to the hazy borders of similar plaques in the left hemisphere of Case 330.) Relatively rapid onset of related symptoms may mimic cerebral ischemia.

Older multiple sclerosis plaques are typically smaller, more sharply defined, and somewhat lower in signal intensity on T1-weighted scans. Periventricular lesions in Case 328 illustrate this appearance. The characteristically prominent T1-prolongation of established demyelinating foci can

be a useful feature in differential diagnosis (on either T1-weighted spin echo or inversion recovery pulse sequences). If multiple small lesions seen on a T2-weighted scan are not well-defined on a T1-weighted image, they are unlikely to represent multiple sclerosis.

Both of the above cases demonstrate the typical involvement of periventricular white matter by demyelinating disease. Sagittal scans (T1- or T2-weighted) are particularly useful for assessing lesions within the corpus callosum (see Cases 331, 332, and 359).

Cases 339, 347, and 348 illustrate additional variations in the appearance of multiple sclerosis on T1-weighted images.

Case 329

44-year-old woman presenting with numbness
of the legs and feet.
(axial, noncontrast scan; SE 2500/45)

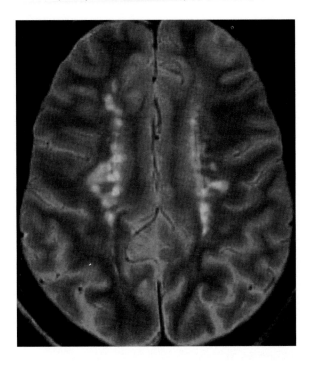

Case 330

56-year-old woman presenting with right
body numbness.
(axial, noncontrast scan; SE 2500/90)

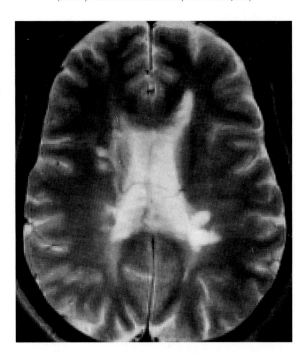

The detection of plaques in multiple sclerosis was one of the first and most dramatic demonstrations of the contrast sensitivity of magnetic resonance imaging. Although CT scans may disclose many abnormalities in patients with demyelinating disease, MR is the procedure of choice for evaluating these cases. Negative MR scans are rare in a setting of clinically documented multiple sclerosis. (Spinal cord involvement should be considered in such instances.)

Areas of demyelinatination are well defined as foci of high signal intensity on long TR spin echo scans. Periventricular involvement is characteristic. However, lesions due to multiple sclerosis may be found in any area of white matter, including myelinated tracts within gray matter nuclei such as the basal ganglia.

Deep hemisphere lesions often demonstrate a relatively elliptical shape, with the long axis directed toward the ventricular margin. This characteristic morphology ("Dawson's finger"), which can be helpful in differential diagnosis, has been attributed to the perivenular pathophysiology of demyelination. (See Case 496 for an additional example of this appearance.)

The above cases illustrate two commonly encountered types of lesions. The small, uniform, sharply defined foci of high signal intensity in Case 329 and predominating in the right corona radiata of Case 330 are typical of old plaques demonstrated during quiescent clinical periods. The larger lesions with less distinct margins found in the left corona radiata of Case 330 suggest active demyelination with associated edema. Such lesions often demonstrate contrast enhancement (see Cases 349 and 350) and may correlate with new symptoms.

As can be surmised from these cases, the MR pattern of multiple sclerosis can vary from strikingly symmetrical to markedly asymmetrical, depending on the number and activity of individual lesions.

Case 331

46-year-old man presenting with facial numbness.
(sagittal, noncontrast scan; SE 600/15)

Case 332

39-year-old woman presenting with leg weakness.
(sagittal, noncontrast scan; SE 600/16)

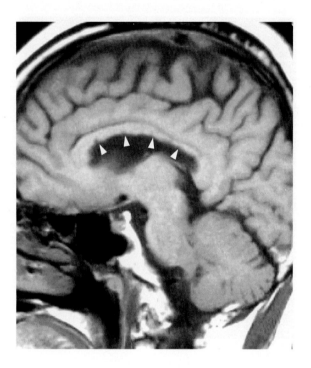

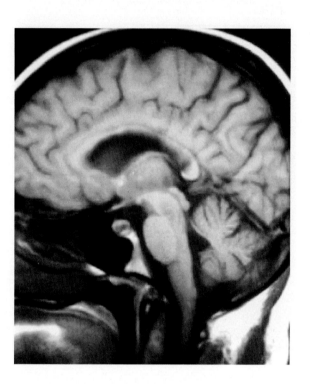

The corpus callosum is routinely involved by multiple sclerosis. Demyelinating foci within the transversely oriented commisure are often better demonstrated on sagittal or coronal views than on axial images.

A particularly common location for plaques is the inferior surface of the corpus callosum or "callosal-septal interface," as seen in Case 331 *(arrowheads)*. Lesions within the substance of the corpus callosum or spanning its diameter are also encountered, as in Case 332.

Long-standing multiple sclerosis is typically associated with callosal atrophy, reflecting both direct involvement and secondary loss of volume due to hemispheric disease (see Case 359).

Like the findings illustrated in Cases 343 to 346, the presence of callosal lesions can be a helpful clue to the diagnosis of multiple sclerosis when hemispheric abnormalities are nonspecific. Foci of ischemic change may mimic multiple sclerosis in the centrum semiovale or periventricular regions but rarely involve the corpus callosum.

DIFFERENTIAL DIAGNOSIS:
FOCAL SIGNAL ABNORMALITIES IN DEEP HEMISPHERE WHITE MATTER

Case 333

41-year-old woman presenting with numbness
of the left arm and face.
(axial, noncontrast scan; SE 2500/15)

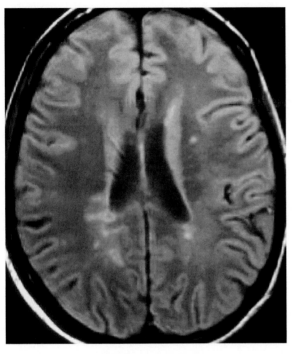

Multiple Sclerosis

Case 334

18-year-old woman presenting with dizziness.
(axial, noncontrast scan; SE 2500/90)

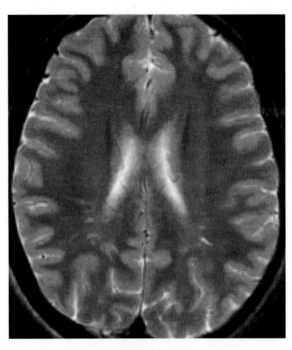

Prominent Perivascular Spaces
(normal variant)

Plaques of multiple sclerosis are well demonstrated as high signal foci on spin echo sequences with long TR and short TE values, as in Case 333. Subependymal lesions are better defined by such "intermediate" or "balanced" sequences than by more heavily T2-weighted scans. On the latter images, shallow demyelinating foci may be difficult to distinguish from adjacent CSF of high signal intensity (compare Cases 330 and 333).

"Fluid-attenuated" inversion recovery pulse sequences ("FLAIR") are also useful for defining plaques of demyelination in the brain or spinal cord. The low signal intensity of CSF on such images contrasts with the high intensity of parenchymal lesions.

Case 334 illustrates a normal developmental variant. Unusually wide sleeves of CSF often accompany small arteries from the cerebral surface into the hemisphere, representing "giant" Virchow-Robin spaces. Such perivascular spaces have a linear, radial pattern on scans paralleling the direction of penetrating arteries, as is usually true on axial images in the deep parietal region.

Scans perpendicular to penetrating arteries (e.g., axial images at the vertex) demonstrate prominent perivascular spaces as a field of tiny dots that are smaller, more uniform, and more peripheral than typical plaques of multiple sclerosis. Prominent perivascular spaces are usually inconspicuous on long TR short TE spin echo images, in contrast to the clear definition of demyelinating foci on such scans.

See Case 382 for a more subtle presentation of prominent perivascular spaces in deep parietal white matter.

Case 335

40-year-old man presenting with a six-week
history of left hemiparesis.
(axial, noncontrast scan; SE 3000/90)

Case 336

30-year-old woman complaining of patchy
bilateral arm and leg numbness.
(axial, noncontrast scan; SE 2500/45).

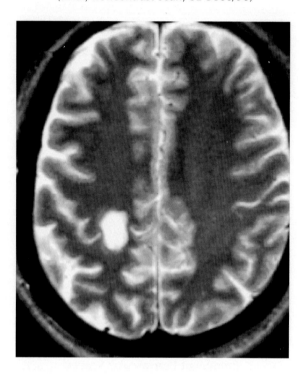

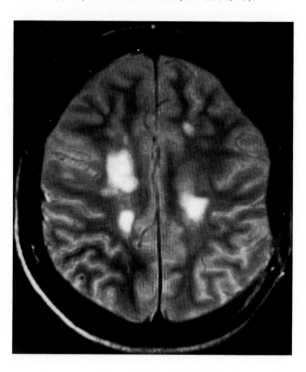

Although small lesions within periventricular white matter are characteristic of multiple sclerosis, larger and more peripheral plaques are commonly encountered. When such foci are solitary, as in Case 335, the appearance is nonspecific. Correlation with clinical findings and/or other suggestive MR features of multiple sclerosis (see Cases 343-346) is necessary for diagnosis.

Multiple sclerosis is one of several pathologies to be considered in the presence of multiple subcortical lesions, as demonstrated in Case 336. A similar pattern may be seen in acute disseminated encephalomyelitis (see Cases 363-365), progressive multifocal leukoencephalopathy (see Cases 369-371), systemic lupus erythematosus (see Cases 431-433), and metastatic disease (see Cases 6 and 372).

Case 337

18-year-old woman presenting with worsening
left hemiparesis.
(axial, noncontrast scan; SE 3000/28)

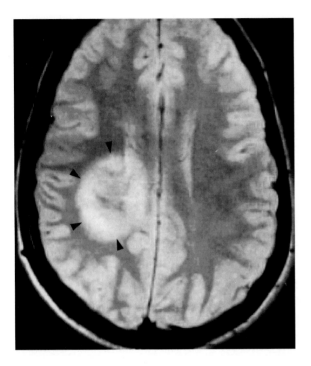

Case 338

29-year-old woman presenting with numbness
and clumsiness of the right arm.
(axial, noncontrast scan; SE 3000/28)

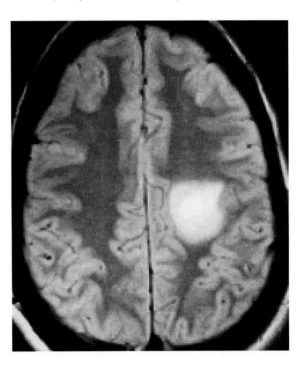

Regions of active demyelination in multiple sclerosis may measure several centimeters in diameter, mimicking cerebral neoplasms on CT and MR scans. Such lesions are usually located in the centrum semiovale, as in the above cases. They may also occur within the corpus callosum. Associated contrast enhancement is typically present and may be solid or peripheral. Marginal enhancement is often asymmetrical.

A giant focus of demyelinating disease should be considered whenever a deep hemisphere "tumor" is encountered in a young adult. A round shape and relative lack of mass effect (see Cases 343 and 344) can be clues to the correct diagnosis.

Case 339

21-year-old woman presenting with optic neuritis.
(sagittal, noncontrast scan; SE 600/20)

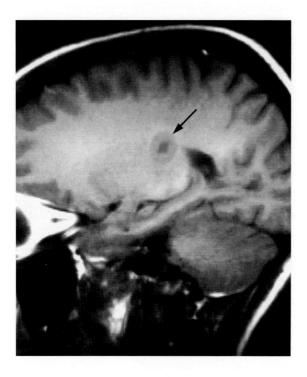

Case 340

29-year-old woman presenting with "trouble
controlling my right side."
(axial, noncontrast scan; SE 2500/90)

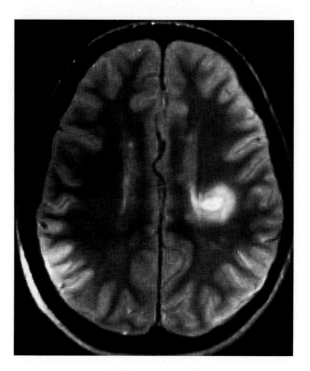

Active plaques sometimes demonstrate a relatively thin and uniform ring of altered signal intensity within a larger lesion. This feature is most commonly appreciated as a rim of relatively low intensity within an edematous zone on T2-weighted scans, as in Case 340. (A similar ring is faintly seen within the giant plaque in Case 338.) Less commonly, a peripheral ring of low intensity marginates the remainder of a lesion on T1-weighted scans, as illustrated in Case 339 (see also Case 347). In some cases, these findings correlate with a well-defined rim of enhancement on postcontrast scans.

The ring structure likely represents a zone of inflamma-
tion and reaction that corresponds to an intermediate stage of demyelination. The finding can suggest the diagnosis of multiple sclerosis in ambiguous cases. However, a similar thin rim can be seen on MR studies of cerebral abscesses (see Cases 405-408). "Target" morphologies have also been noted within masses due to toxoplasmosis and primary CNS lymphoma, especially in AIDS patients.

Cases 339 and 340 again illustrate that multiple sclerosis may present as a single focus of acute demyelination. The large size and indistinct margins of these lesions suggest active inflammation.

DIFFERENTIAL DIAGNOSIS:
MULTIPLE ROUND MASSES IN PERIVENTRICULAR AND SUBCORTICAL WHITE MATTER

Case 341

23-year-old woman presenting with vague
paresthesias.
(axial, noncontrast scan; SE 3000/28)

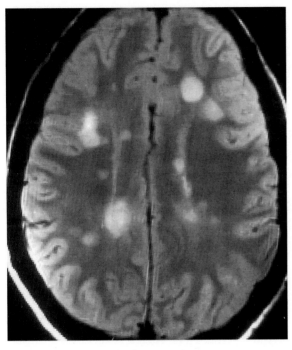

Multiple Sclerosis

Case 342

39-year-old man complaining of headaches.
(axial, noncontrast scan; SE 3000/25)

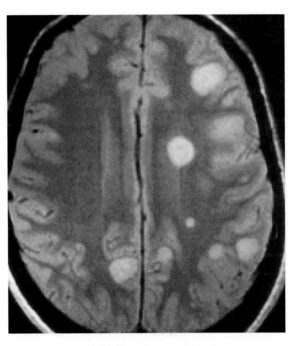

Metastatic Adenocarcinoma
(unknown primary)

Demyelinating foci may be sufficiently numerous and nodular to mimic metastatic lesions, as in Case 341. Clues to the correct diagnosis include the prominent involvement of periventricular regions and the clinical context.

Metastatic disease should be included in the differential diagnosis of multiple white matter lesions, even in young adults. The majority of the metastases in Case 342 are subcortical, with less involvement of periventricular areas.

Both multiple sclerosis and cerebral metastases may also present with a "miliary" pattern of smaller, more numerous foci of signal abnormality throughout cerebral white matter. Such lesions may demonstrate contrast enhancement and mimic infectious etiologies (see Cases 353 and 354).

Case 343

28-year-old woman.
(axial, noncontrast scan; SE 3000/28)

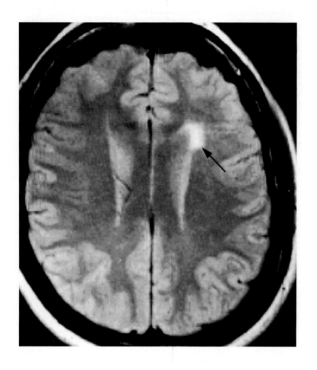

Case 344

37-year-old woman.
(axial, noncontrast scan; SE 3000/25)

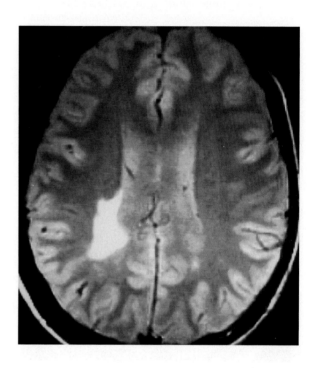

These patients illustrate another characteristic morphology occasionally demonstrated by lesions of multiple sclerosis. In both cases, a plaque is based along a corner of the ventricular margin. Despite the otherwise convex borders of the lesion, there is little effacement or compression of the ventricle. This lack of ventricular deformity is distinct from the appearance of a true subependymal mass (compare to Case 352) and can suggest the diagnosis of multiple sclerosis.

Case 345

34-year-old woman.
(axial, noncontrast scan; SE 2500/28)

Case 346

38-year-old woman.
(axial, noncontrast scan; SE 2500/28)

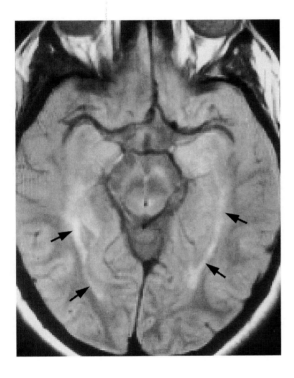

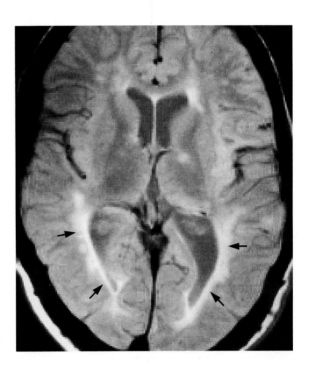

A relatively thin and uniform layer of high signal intensity is often seen along the margins of the lateral ventricles on long TR images in patients with multiple sclerosis. The etiology of this finding is unclear, since periventricular demyelination is typically more nodular and less confluent than the observed zone of signal abnormality.

Regardless of the cause, this finding can be a clue to the diagnosis of multiple sclerosis when hemispheric lesions are ambiguous. The margins of the temporal and occipital horns are commonly affected. A search for abnormal subependymal signal in these regions is warranted when demyelinating disease is suspected.

A uniform layer of periventricular signal abnormality may alternatively be due to ventriculitis (see Case 389) or subependymal tumor spread (see Cases 390 and 391).

Case 347

49-year-old woman presenting with
left hemiparesis.
(axial, postcontrast scan; SE 500/11)

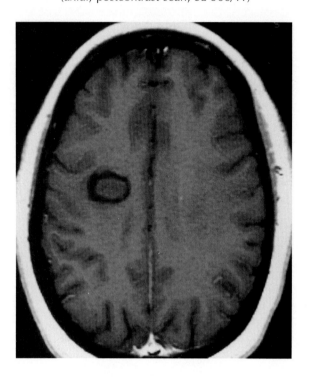

Case 348

54-year-old man with an eight-year history
of multiple sclerosis.
(axial, noncontrast scan; SE 500/16)

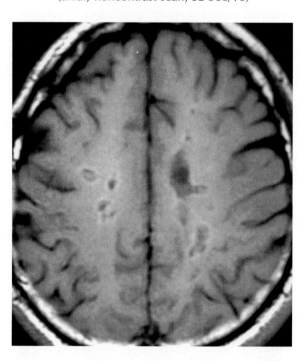

The margins of most subacute and chronic demyelinating plaques are well defined on T1-weighted scans because of uniform T1-prolongation within the lesions (see Case 328). Occasionally an additional rim of altered signal intensity is seen at the edge of a plaque, as illustrated above.

In Case 347 a margin of very low signal intensity surrounds an otherwise unremarkable solitary plaque. As discussed in Cases 339 and 340, such morphology presumably reflects a specific zone or stage of myelin breakdown and/or reactive inflammation. The biological or chemical

correlate of the finding has not been established. Notice the absence of associated contrast enhancement in this case.

Demyelinated areas in Case 348 are outlined by a thin rim of high signal intensity. The basis of such peripheral T1-shortening is undetermined but may relate to accumulation of myelin degradation products. The finding is normally noted in the context of long-standing disease. (Compare to the T1-shortening that often characterizes the capsule of cerebral abscesses; see Cases 405 and 406).

Case 349

49-year-old woman presenting with optic neuritis.
(axial, postcontrast scan; SE 600/15)

Case 350

54-year-old woman presenting with
incoordination and imbalance.
(axial, postcontrast scan; SE 600/15)

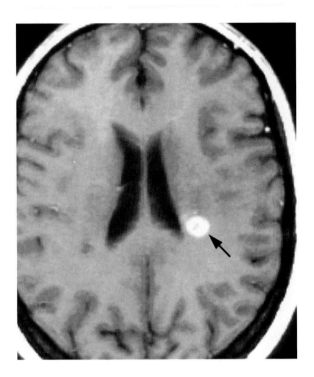

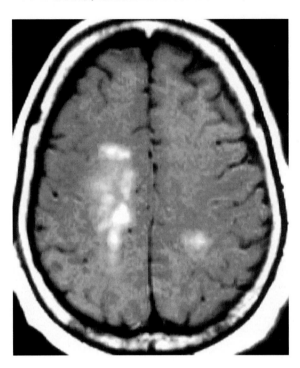

Active demyelinating plaques may demonstrate solid or peripheral patterns of contrast enhancement. In Case 349, the abnormal enhancement is discrete, nodular, and rim-like. Case 350 illustrates a more confluent and multifocal appearance.

Most enhancing plaques are small, but occasional lesions are large enough to resemble neoplasms (see Cases 337 and 338). Serial scans may demonstrate evolution of a plaque from an active enhancing phase to a quiescent, nonenhancing lesion over a period of several weeks. Although the presence of contrast enhancement within a plaque presumably indicates active inflammation, the majority of enhancing lesions are clinically silent.

Solitary lesions (as in Case 349) are occasionally seen on MR scans of patients with multiple sclerosis. While this appearance is nonspecific, it does fall within the spectrum of demyelinating disease. Multiple sclerosis should be considered when such lesions are encountered, so that patients are not unnecessarily subjected to work-ups or therapies based on other diagnoses (e.g., angiography or anticoagulation for presumed subacute lacunar infarction).

Optic neuritis is a common manifestation of multiple sclerosis. Its occurrence together with or prior to cerebral symptoms may help to establish the diagnosis in ambiguous cases.

Case 351

30-year-old woman with a history of optic neuritis
and recent scattered paresthesias.
(axial, postcontrast scan; SE 600/15)

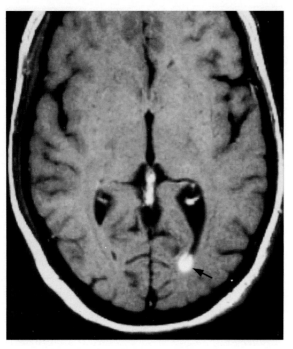

Multiple Sclerosis

Case 352

73-year-old man presenting with a seizure.
(axial, postcontrast scan; SE 800/17)

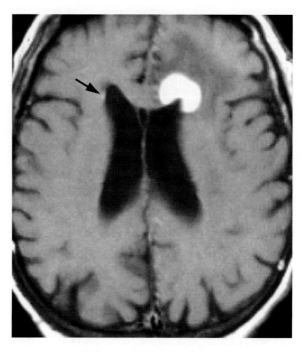

Primary CNS Lymphoma

A number of pathologies can cause localized periventricular enhancement. (Compare to the differential diagnosis of diffuse ependymal/subependymal enhancement in Cases 390 and 391.) Multiple sclerosis should be considered in the appropriate clinical context, as illustrated by Case 351.

Occasional systemic metastases present as subependymal nodules (see Case 19). Ependymal implants from CSF dissemination of primary CNS tumors (e.g., glioma or medulloblastoma; see Case 322) may also have this appearance.

Primary CNS lymphoma often involves the ventricular surface and subependymal region (see Cases 311-320). Note that the tumor in Case 352 causes more ventricular deformity than the usual "perched" plaques of multiple sclerosis (compare to Cases 343 and 344).

Extensive edema surrounds the enhancing nodule in Case 352. A tiny second focus of ependymal-based enhancement is seen along the lateral margin of the right frontal horn *(arrow)*.

Case 353

21-year-old woman presenting with blurred vision.
(axial, postcontrast scan; SE 600/15)

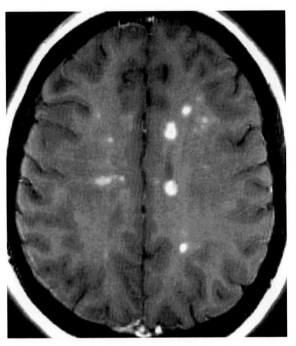

Multiple Sclerosis

Case 354

40-year-old woman presenting with nausea
and dizziness.
(axial, postcontrast scan; SE 817/11)

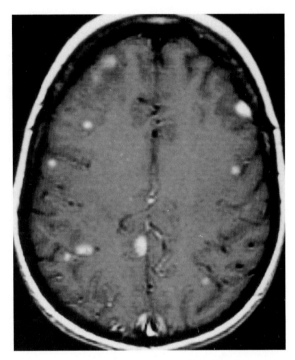

Metastatic Carcinoma of the Breast

The enhancing plaques of multiple sclerosis may be numerous and relatively uniform in size, as in Case 353. The pattern of such lesions can resemble the appearance of multiple metastases, illustrated by Case 354.

Plaques usually occupy a midhemisphere location. This distribution is more central than the peripheral position of most metastases near the gray-white matter junction. The clinical setting often distinguishes these two processes when overlapping MR patterns are encountered.

Additional pathologies in the differential diagnosis of multiple enhancing nodules include disseminated infection (e.g., cysticercosis, tuberculosis, histoplasmosis, toxoplasmosis), sarcoidosis, primary CNS lymphoma (see Case 318), subacute multifocal infarction (arterial or venous; see Case 490), vasculitis, and multiple cavernous angiomas.

Case 355

41-year-old man presenting with ataxia.
(axial, noncontrast scan; SE 2500/90)

Case 356

39-year-old man presenting with diplopia.
(axial, noncontrast scan; SE 3000/80)

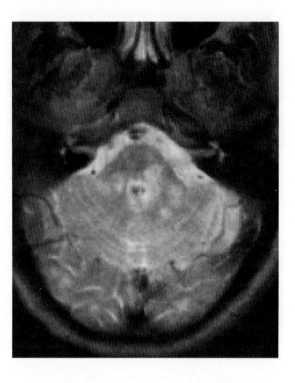

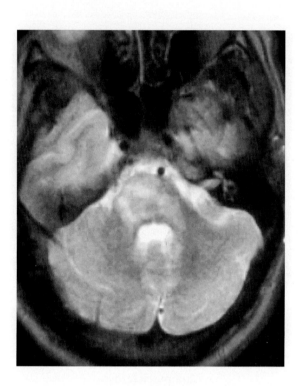

Multiple sclerosis frequently involves the brainstem and cerebellar peduncles. The pattern of demyelinating foci in these locations may be multinodular, as in Case 355, or confluent, as in Case 356.

The middle cerebellar peduncle is a particularly common site for demyelinating plaques. One or more small lesions within the brachium pontis in a young patient should suggest the possibility of multiple sclerosis (see Case 373 for another example).

Large areas of confluent brainstem demyelination and edema as in Case 356 may mimic a neoplasm. This appearance can be especially confusing in adolescents or younger children, who suffer brainstem gliomas more commonly than demyelinating disease. Also compare Case 356 to the appearance of central pontine myelinolysis in Case 375.

Case 357

58-year-old man presenting with headaches.
(axial, noncontrast scan; SE 3000/45)

Case 358

44-year-old woman presenting with diplopia.
(axial, noncontrast scan; SE 2800/90)

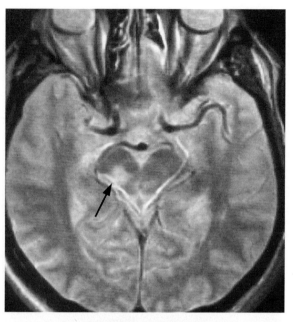

Metastatic Melanoma

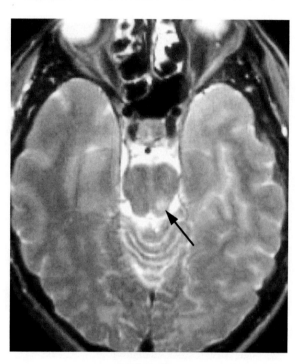

Multiple Sclerosis

Metastatic disease should be considered whenever focal brainstem lesions are encountered in adults. MRI has demonstrated that the incidence of metastasis to the brainstem (and spinal cord) is higher than appreciated by prior imaging techniques (see also Cases 20 and 21). The appearance of the small metastasis in Case 357 is nonspecific. The diagnosis was made by biopsy of a larger cerebral mass.

Case 358 illustrates a demyelinating plaque within the midbrain tectum. This lesion is also nonspecific. Characteristic accompanying foci of multiple sclerosis were present in the middle cerebellar peduncles and cerebral hemispheres.

Compare these cases to the differential diagnosis in Cases 520 and 521.

Mucosal thickening is present within the ethmoid sinuses in Case 358.

Case 359

39-year-old woman.
(sagittal, noncontrast scan; SE 600/16)

Case 360

41-year-old man.
(axial, noncontrast scan; SE 2500/28)

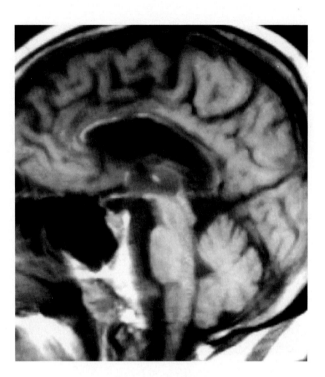

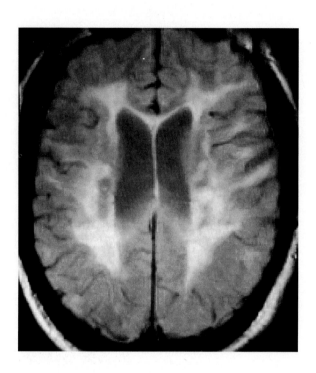

Long-standing multiple sclerosis is often associated with ventricular and sulcal enlargement, as seen in the above cases. This diagnosis is among the potential causes of prominent CSF spaces in a young patient (see discussion of Cases 457 and 458).

In Case 359, the sagittal plane documents extensive atrophy, both of the hemispheres and of the corpus callosum. The sulci on the medial surface of the frontal lobe are much too large for the patient's age. The corpus callosum is markedly thinned, with abnormal signal intensity and irregular margins indicating direct involvement by severe demyelinating disease.

Case 360 demonstrates large areas of abnormal intensity throughout the white matter, reflecting long-standing multiple sclerosis. Ventricular enlargement indicates associated volume loss. The pattern is bilateral and extensive, resembling a diffuse leukoencephalopathy (see Case 377), severe vascular insufficiency (as in Cases 514 and 515), or radiation change (see Case 517).

Another MR finding in some cases of long-standing multiple sclerosis is abnormally prominent or extensive low signal intensity within the basal ganglia and thalamus on T2-weighted images. This appearance has been suggested to reflect the accumulation of iron due to impaired peripheral axonal transport.

Case 361

11-year-old boy who developed somnolence and hemiparesis over a four-day period, two weeks after a viral illness.
(coronal, postcontrast scan; SE 1000/20)

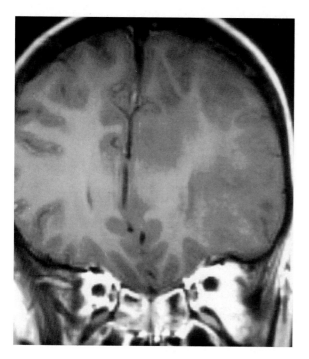

Case 362

23-year-old woman presenting with rapidly worsening hemiparesis three weeks after "the flu."
(axial, noncontrast scan; SE 600/17)

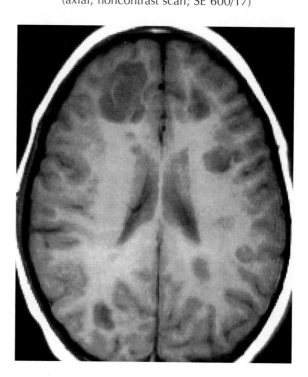

Acute disseminated encephalomyelitis (ADEM) is alternatively called "immune-mediated encephalitis," because the pathophysiology is believed to involve autoimmune demyelination. Patients typically give a history of antigenic challenge (e.g., virus or vaccination) days or weeks prior to the onset of symptoms.

ADEM primarily affects white matter, but deep gray matter is often involved. The pattern is highly variable. Large, geographical regions of edema and mass effect may develop, as seen in the left frontal lobe in Case 361. (See Case 363 for a T2-weighted axial scan of this patient.) Both symmetrical and asymmetrical presentations may be encountered.

In other cases of ADEM, smaller and more nodular lesions are scattered throughout the hemispheres, illustrated by Case 362 (see also Cases 364 and 365). Such lesions are typically a little larger than quiescent plaques of multiple sclerosis and have a more random distribution.

The demyelinating lesions of ADEM usually present as variably defined foci of low signal intensity on T1-weighted scans. Some cases of immune-mediated encephalitis are associated with hemorrhage, which can cause T1-shortening due to the presence of methemoglobin. This entity, previously called "acute hemorrhagic leukoencephalitis," progresses rapidly and carries a poor prognosis.

Contrast enhancement in ADEM is variable. Many lesions demonstrate little or no enhancement, as seen in Case 361. Other lesions enhance prominently, resembling the active plaques of multiple sclerosis (see Cases 349-353).

Case 363

11-year-old boy presenting with somnolence
and hemiparesis.
(axial, noncontrast scan; SE 3000/90)

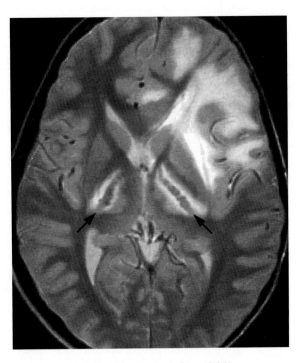

(same patient as Case 361)

Case 364

14-year-old boy with rapidly decreasing mental
status two weeks after chickenpox.
(axial, noncontrast scan; SE 2800/90)

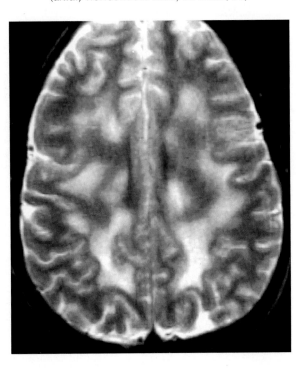

Zones of demyelination and edema in acute disseminated encephalomyelitis are well demonstrated as regions of high signal intensity on long TR images. The size and symmetry of hemispheric lesions are variable.

Case 363 demonstrates symmetrical involvement of the internal capsules (arrows), with grossly asymmetrical demyelination in the left frontal lobe. In Case 364, a patchy pattern of demyelination is diffuse and symmetrical, resembling a leukodystrophy (compare to Cases 377 and 380). Case 365 presents a third morphology in ADEM, with a mul-

tinodular appearance, and Case 379 illustrates confluent hemispheric edema.

Nonhemorrhagic cases of ADEM usually respond well to steroids. Clinical improvement often precedes resolution of the MR abnormalities, which may continue to evolve while symptoms are regressing. Both of the above boys were clinically normal within a month after presentation.

Like multiple sclerosis, ADEM frequently involves the brainstem, cerebellar peduncles, and cerebellum.

Case 365

23-year-old woman presenting with
progressive hemiparesis.
(axial, noncontrast scan; SE 2500/90)

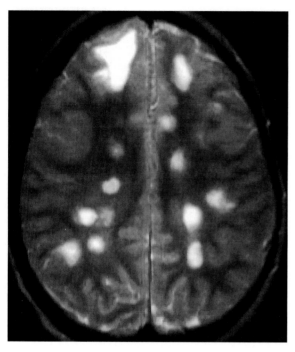

Acute Disseminated Encephalomyelitis
(same patient as Case 362)

Case 366

39-year-old man presenting with headaches.
(axial, noncontrast scan; SE 3000/90)

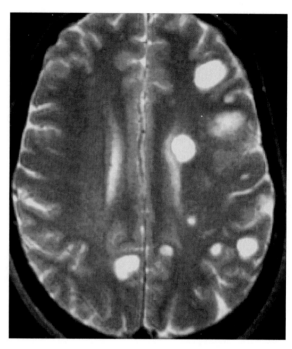

Metastatic Adenocarcinoma
(primary unknown)

ADEM may present as multiple nodular lesions scattered throughout the cerebral hemispheres, as in Case 365. The corpus callosum is commonly involved.

Such an appearance can resemble the pattern of cerebral metastases within subcortical and periventricular white matter, illustrated in Case 366. As discussed in Chapter 1, metastases are characteristically sharply defined and occasionally incite little edema. In such instances, metastatic disease in a young patient may resemble a demyelinating disorder.

The lesions of ADEM are typically larger and more scattered than the plaques of multiple sclerosis. However, the appearance of these two disorders can clearly overlap (compare Case 365 to Case 341). Characteristic associated findings in multiple sclerosis, as demonstrated in Cases 343 to 346, may assist in differential diagnosis. In other cases, clinical correlation and follow-up studies are necessary to distinguish between the two pathologies.

Unlike the typical relapsing course of multiple sclerosis, ADEM is usually monophasic. However, an episode of ADEM may extend over a period of four to six weeks.

Case 367

60-year-old man presenting with hemiparesis.
(sagittal, noncontrast scan; SE 600/17)

Case 368

57-year-old man presenting with confusion.
(coronal, noncontrast scan; SE 700/17)

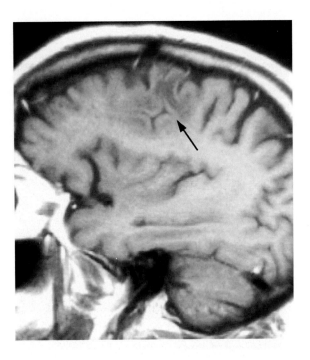

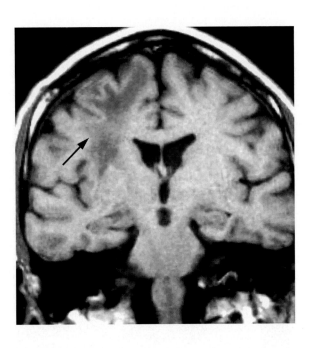

Progressive multifocal leukoencephalopathy (PML) is a demyelinating disorder representing infection by a papovavirus. The disease is usually seen in immunocompromised hosts. Lymphoma and leukemia have been common predisposing conditions, but a rapidly increasing proportion of PML cases now occurs in AIDS patients. Iatrogenic immunosuppression may also be implicated. (Compare with the epidemiology of primary CNS lymphoma, discussed in Cases 311 and 312).

The multifocal demyelination of PML often involves subcortical white matter, as seen in the above cases. Mass effect and contrast enhancement are rare, and hemorrhage is very uncommon.

Notice the relative sparing of the cortical ribbon in involved areas. This "heart of the gyrus" pattern with discretely subcortical edema is even more striking on T2-weighted images (see Case 370).

Case 369

28-year-old woman with systemic lymphoma.
(axial, noncontrast scan; SE 3000/45)

Case 370

57-year-old man presenting with confusion.
(axial, noncontrast scan; SE 2500/90)

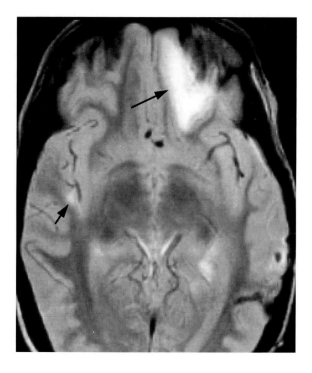

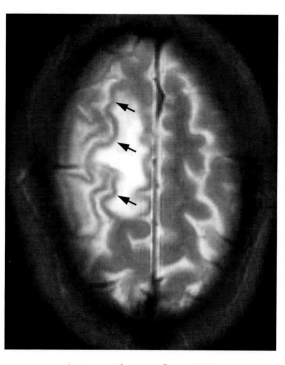

(same patient as Case 368)

PML may cause signal abnormality in subcortical or deep hemispheric white matter. Case 369 illustrates the variable size of such lesions. A large focus is present in the left frontal lobe *(long arrow)*, with much smaller lesions in the right superior temporal gyrus *(short arrow)* and near the apex of the left sylvian cistern.

Although cerebral involvement in PML is often bilateral and multifocal, symmetry is rare. Contrast enhancement is notably absent in most cases.

A prominent finding on many CT and MR scans in PML is the "heart of the gyrus" involvement demonstrated in Case 370. Individual gyri are thickened by edema of central white matter, with conspicuous sparing and margination of the overlying cortical ribbon *(arrows)*.

DIFFERENTIAL DIAGNOSIS:
MULTIFOCAL SUBCORTICAL EDEMA

Case 371

60-year-old man presenting with left hemiparesis.
(axial, noncontrast scan; SE 3000/75)

Case 372

50-year-old woman presenting with a seizure.
(axial, noncontrast scan; SE 2500/90)

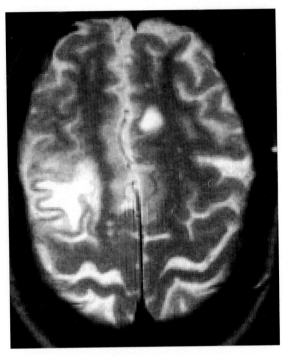

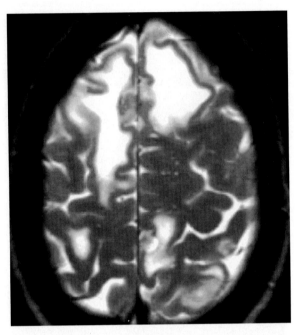

Metastatic Carcinoma of the Breast

Progressive Multifocal Leukoencephalopathy
(same patient as Case 367)

Although subcortical edema is characteristic of progressive multifocal leukoencephalopathy (PML), the finding is not specific. Case 372 demonstrates that edema associated with metastases near the gray/white junction may produce a similar appearance on noncontrast scans. The injection of contrast material should help to narrow the diagnosis: metastases inciting edema would be expected to enhance, while the lesions of PML usually do not.

The asymmetrical and multifocal appearance of PML may also resemble early cerebritis or venous infarction (usually secondary to dural sinus thrombosis). Correct diagnosis in such cases is aided by the concentration of findings in PML within white matter and the usual lack of contrast enhancement.

Another potential cause of multifocal subcortical signal abnormality in the clinical setting of immunosuppression is cyclosporin A toxicity in transplant patients (see Case 465). Cerebral vasculitis (e.g., granulomatous angiitis) is an additional pathology that may present with scattered areas of subcortical edema.

DIFFERENTIAL DIAGNOSIS:
LESION WITHIN THE BRACHIUM PONTIS

Case 373

37-year-old man presenting with left facial pain.
(axial, noncontrast scan; SE 3000/90)

Case 374

29-year-old man with AIDS.
(axial, noncontrast scan; SE 2500/90)

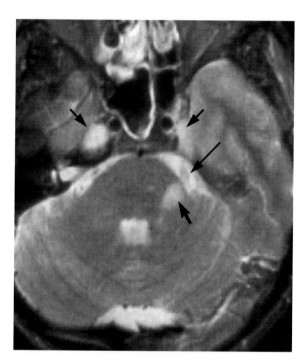

Multiple Sclerosis

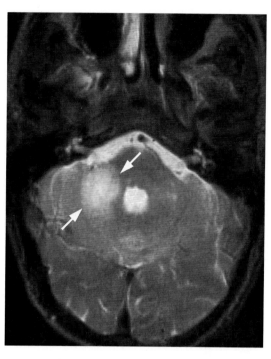

Progressive Multifocal Leukoencephalopathy

As discussed in Cases 355 and 356, the middle cerebellar peduncle is a common site of demyelination in multiple sclerosis. The lesion in Case 373 *(wide arrow)* is located at the junction of the pons and brachium pontis. The patient's facial pain probably indicates dysfunction of axons entering the pons from the trigeminal nerve *(long arrow)*. Multiple sclerosis is among the recognized etiologies of trigeminal neuralgia.

PML may also involve the brainstem and cerebellum. The morphology of such infratentorial lesions is usually less characteristic than the subcortical edema of cerebral foci.

The size and hazy definition of the lesion in Case 374 are compatible with active demyelination (compare to Case 340). Acute disseminated encephalomyelitis would be included in the differential diagnosis. PML should be considered as the etiology of focal demyelination in immunocompromised patients.

A rare cause of focal edema within the lateral pons is trigeminal neuritis (e.g., herpes), extending from the nerve into the brainstem.

CSF within Meckel's caves is well seen as areas of high signal intensity occupying the posterior portion of the cavernous sinuses in Case 373 *(small arrows)*. Head tilt can cause asymmetrical prominence of Meckel's cave on one side, falsely suggesting a posterior parasellar lesion on the side with better visualization (compare to Cases 295 and 298).

Case 375A

46-year-old man presenting with decreased level of consciousness and a history of alcohol abuse.
(sagittal, noncontrast scan; SE 600/20)

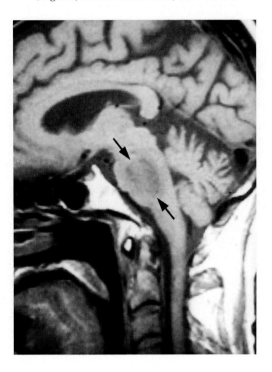

Case 375B

Same patient.
(axial, noncontrast scan; SE 2500/70)

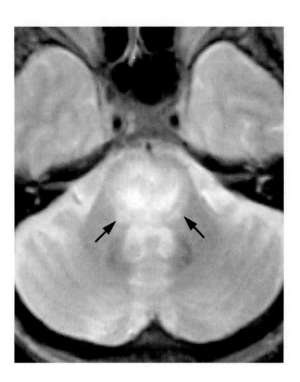

Central pontine myelinolysis (CPM) is an acute demyelinating process affecting the brainstem. It is incompletely understood but seems to correlate with the rapid correction (or overcorrection) of severe electrolyte abnormalities. The condition has also been called "osmotic demyelination syndrome" or "osmotic myelinolysis." Other factors (e.g., nutritional) may contribute.

CT scans may be abnormal in cases of CPM, but definition of the lesion is often vague. MR offers unequivocal documentation of this pathology, as seen above. The pons is expanded by a central zone of long T1 and T2 values suggesting edema. Pontine involvement is symmetrical, with relative sparing of peripheral tissue and tracts. The morphology of the involved region on axial images may be round, triangular, or butterfly-shaped. Contrast enhancement in CPM is unusual.

A similar demyelinating pathology ("extrapontine myelinolysis") can occur within the basal ganglia and cerebral hemispheres, together with or independent of pontine involvement (see Case 430). Conversely, other white matter disorders (e.g., PML) may involve the pons.

The characteristic MR findings of CPM may not develop until several days after the onset of symptoms. Symptoms usually begin a few days after the correction of hyponatremia.

Case 376A

48-year-old woman, four months after admission
for central pontine myelinolysis.
(sagittal, noncontrast scan; SE 600/28)

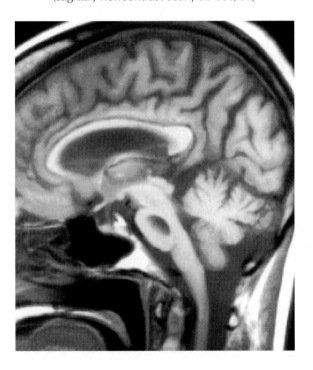

Case 376B

Same patient.
(axial, noncontrast scan; SE 2500/90)

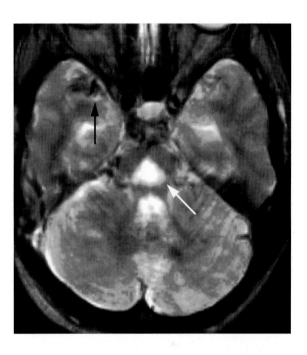

Some cases of CPM progress inexorably to death. Other patients recover completely, with resolution of scan abnormalities. A third group of patients demonstrates partial or complete clinical recovery with residual abnormality of the pons on follow-up MR studies.

In this case the pontine lesion is smaller and better defined than in Case 375, reflecting demarcation of old encephalomalacia. Involvement of the central pons with spar-

ing of peripheral tracts may result in a distinctive triangular shape of myelinolysis on axial images in early or late stages, as seen here *(white arrow,* Case 376B).

A prominent tangle of vessels in the anterior portion of the right middle cranial fossa *(black arrow,* Case 376B) represents proximal branches of the middle cerebral artery. This normal finding should not be mistaken for an arteriovenous malformation (compare to Cases 606-609).

Case 377A

10-year-old boy presenting with a one-year history of deteriorating school performance, behavior problems, and diminished reflexes.
(sagittal, noncontrast scan; SE 600/15)

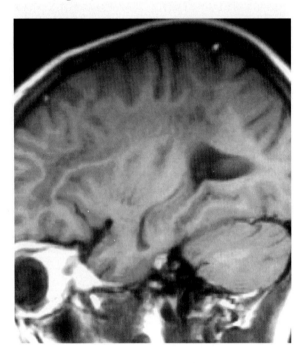

Case 377B

Same patient.
(axial, noncontrast scan; SE 2800/45)

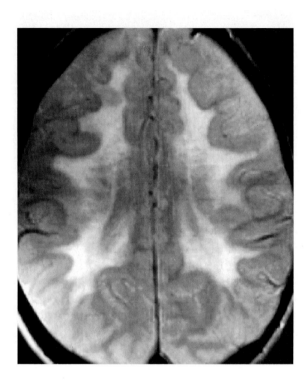

The demyelinating disorders described in the previous portion of this chapter are characterized by destruction of normally formed myelin. A number of other pathologies can be classified as "dysmyelinating," in that they cause abnormal or incomplete development of myelin.

Metachromatic leukodystrophy, one of the relatively common dysmyelinating disorders, is caused by insufficient activity of the enzyme arylsulfatase A. Most cases of metachromatic leukodystrophy present in infancy. The patient above represents the less frequent "juvenile" variant of the disease.

Unlike adrenoleukodystrophy (see Case 380), metachromatic leukodystrophy involves white matter throughout the cerebral hemispheres. Extensive, scalloped zones with long T1 and long T2 values typically fill the centrum semiovale.

Subcortical "U" fibers (see *arrows,* Case 378) are usually spared. A spotted appearance caused by islands of relatively normal white matter within involved regions has been noted in some cases, as seen above. Contrast enhancement is rare.

The prognosis in metachromatic leukodystrophy is poor. Bone marrow transplantation is considered for early cases to restore adequate enzyme levels.

When white matter abnormality is patchy or multifocal rather than diffuse, congenital and metabolic disorders should be included in the differential diagnosis along with leukodystrophy. (See the discussions of mitochondrial encephalomyopathy in Case 447 and tuberous sclerosis in Cases 760-762.)

DIFFERENTIAL DIAGNOSIS:
DIFFUSELY ABNORMAL WHITE MATTER IN A CHILD

Case 378

10-year-old boy presenting with behavior problems.
(axial, noncontrast scan; SE 2800/90)

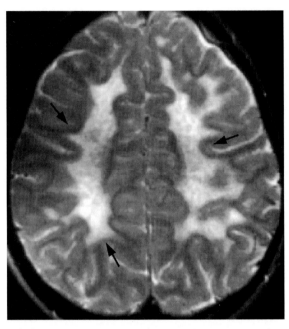

Metachromatic Leukodystrophy
(same patient as Case 377)

Case 379

4-year-old girl presenting with a three-day
history of increasing obtundation.
(axial, noncontrast scan; SE 2500/45)

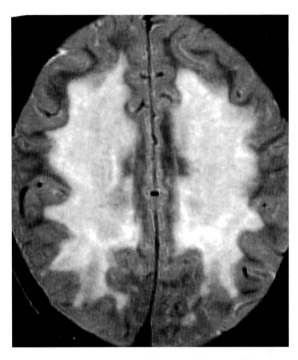

Acute Disseminated Encephalomyelitis

Widespread abnormality of cerebral white matter may be the result of either demyelinating or dysmyelinating disease. Case 379 represents the former etiology as an unusually severe and symmetrical example of ADEM (compare to Cases 361-365).

Case 378 demonstrates the widespread dysmyelination typically seen in metachromatic leukodystrophy. Note that subarcuate "U" fibers are spared *(arrows)*, as is typical of this disorder.

The time course of neurological deterioration is a useful clue to the categorization of white matter diseases. Demyelinating disorders are typically more rapidly progressive than dysmyelinating disease.

Extensive white matter damage has been noted pathologically and on imaging studies in children following chemotherapy administered alone or in combination with cerebral radiation. The phrase "disseminated necrotizing leukoencephalopathy" has been used for methotrexate-associated disease but may apply to other combinations of chemotherapy and/or radiation. Histological analysis of such cases suggests that the primary damage is astrocytic rather than neuronal.

Compare the diffuse white matter damage in the above cases to comparable adult scans in Cases 514 to 517.

Case 380A

8-year-old boy presenting with bilateral
hearing loss.
(axial, noncontrast scan; SE 2900/80).

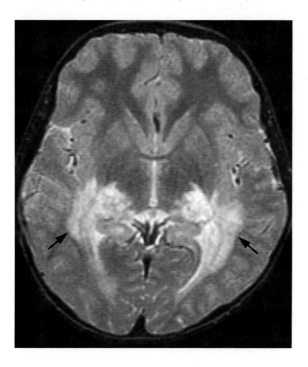

Case 380B

Same patient.
(axial, postcontrast scan; SE 600/27)

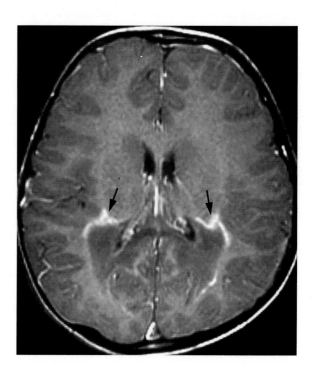

Adrenoleukodystrophy is an X-linked recessive dysmy-elinating disease caused by inadequate metabolism of very long chain fatty acids. Affected boys typically present between 5 and 10 years of age with progressive school problems and gait abnormality. Involvement of visual pathways in the temporal and occipital lobes or of auditory pathways within the brainstem (see Case 442) may lead to visual or hearing loss, as in this case. Associated adrenal hypofunction varies widely in severity.

Most cases of adrenoleukodystrophy demonstrate symmetrical abnormality of white matter beginning within the parietooccipital regions and spreading anteriorly. In Case 380, large, scalloped zones with long T1 and long T2 values are confined to the posterior portion of the cerebral hemispheres. (Compare this appearance to the more dif-fuse involvement of metachromatic leukodystrophy in Case 377 and to the similarly localized but morphologically distinct appearance of periventricular leukomalacia in Case 498.) Occasionally the margins or center of the white matter lesions demonstrate high signal intensity on precontrast T1-weighted scans, possibly reflecting lipid products of myelin metabolism.

The pattern of contrast enhancement in adrenoleukodystrophy is usually characteristic, as demonstrated in Case 380B. A "flame-shaped" zone of enhancement is present at the advancing edge of involvement (arrows).

Many atypical appearances of adrenoleukodystrophy have been reported, including frontal lobe predominance and unilateral, holohemispheric patterns.

DIFFERENTIAL DIAGNOSIS:
SYMMETRICAL SIGNAL ABNORMALITY IN DEEP PARIETAL WHITE MATTER

Case 381

21-month-old girl presenting with
developmental delay.
(axial, noncontrast scan; SE 2500/90)

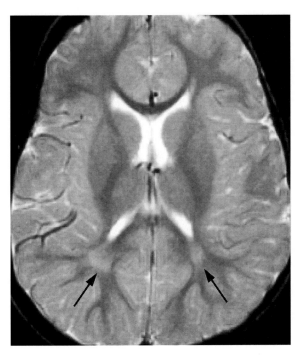

Normal Slow Myelination

Case 382

60-year-old woman presenting with confusion.
(axial, noncontrast scan; SE 2500/90)

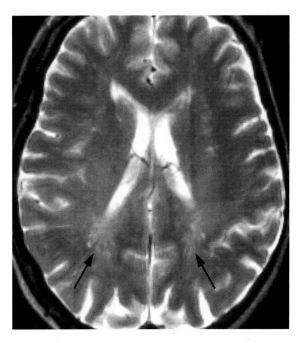

Prominent Perivascular Spaces

Two normal variants can cause symmetrical high signal intensity in deep parietal white matter on T2-weighted scans. These developmental variants should not be confused with demyelinating or dysmyelinating disorders.

The periventricular parietal region is the last zone of the cerebral hemispheres to become fully myelinated during normal maturation. At ages 2 or 3, this residual unmyelinated tissue (containing more water and demonstrating longer T2 values than myelinated areas) contrasts with the uniform background of surrounding white matter. Case 381 is a typical example *(arrows)*.

In adults, a hazy appearance of increased signal within the deep parietal regions can be seen normally due to prominent perivascular spaces. These sleeves of CSF surrounding penetrating vessels are often most prominent in the parietal lobes. If the individual perivascular spaces are large, they may be resolved as fine, radial, or linear structures (see Case 334). When the perivascular spaces are smaller (or spatial resolution of the scan is lower), the fluid within the spaces is averaged with adjacent tissue to cause a zone of high signal on T2-weighted scans. Case 382 illustrates this appearance *(arrows)*.

Case 383A

10-month-old girl presenting with
developmental delay.
(sagittal, noncontrast scan; SE 600/15)

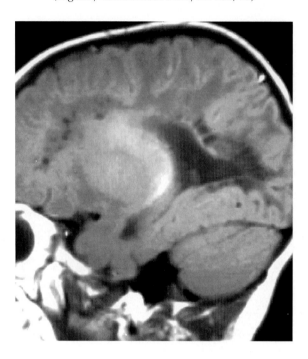

Case 383B

Same patient.
(coronal, noncontrast scan; SE 600/15)

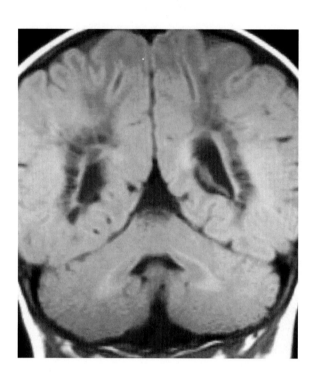

Canavan's disease is an autosomal recessive disorder caused by deficiency of the enzyme *N*-acetyl aspartase. The condition is also known as "spongiform leukoencephalopathy," because normal white matter is replaced by a mesh-like network of small cysts. This vacuolization is often very fine, causing homogeneously prolonged T1 and T2 values throughout cerebral white matter.

In some cases the cysts are large enough to be individually resolved, as seen above. This finding can be a clue to the diagnosis in an infant with otherwise nonspecific, "watery" white matter. The concentration of cysts in the periventricular white matter of Case 383 resembles several other pathologies (compare to Cases 384 and 704).

The typically diffuse and symmetrical involvement of Canavan's disease often causes T2-weighted images that re-

semble Cases 378 and 379. Subarcuate "U" fibers are characteristically involved, unlike metachromatic leukodystrophy (see Case 378). The internal capsule may be relatively spared.

Canavan's disease usually presents within the first year of life. Hypotonia and seizures typically accompany developmental delay. Prognosis is poor, with death occurring by age 2 or 3.

Head size can be a useful clinical discriminator in children with leukodystrophy. Patients with metachromatic leukodystrophy and adrenoleukodystrophy are usually normocephalic. If the affected child presents with a large head, Alexander's disease (characterized by frontal lobe predominance) or Canavan's disease (with more diffuse abnormality) should be considered.

MUCOPOLYSACCHARIDOSES: HURLER'S DISEASE (MPS TYPE 1H)

Case 384A

14-month-old girl presenting with
developmental delay.
(sagittal, noncontrast scan; SE 850/20)

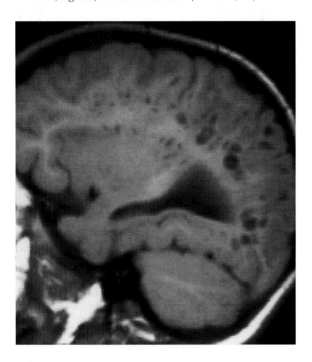

Case 384B

Same patient.
(coronal, noncontrast scan; SE 850/20)

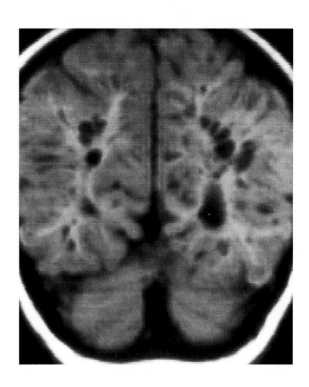

The mucopolysaccharidoses are systemic metabolic disorders with major neurological components. Although these syndromes are characterized by neuronal damage, they also involve white matter and may resemble traditional leukodystrophies (compare Cases 383 and 384).

Deficiencies of various lysosomal enzymes in these diseases impair degradation of mucopolysaccharides, leading to toxic intracellular accumulation or "storage" of these materials. Several of the mucopolysaccharidoses present with prominent visceral and skeletal abnormalities, including spinal involvement with potential compression of the spinal cord (e.g., Morquio's disease, or mucopolysaccharidosis type IV).

Hurler's syndrome results from deficiency of the enzyme alpha-L-iduronidase. Untreated patients usually die before age 10 due to cardiac or pulmonary failure. Bone marrow transplantation is currently considered in newly diagnosed cases.

Cerebral involvement in the mucopolysaccharidoses may be manifested as atrophy, patchy areas of long T1 and long T2 within white matter resembling a leukodystrophy, and/or focal cysts or cavities within the corpus callosum and periventricular tissue. Case 384 demonstrates the latter finding. Such "cribriform changes" are characteristic of the mucopolysaccharidoses, reflecting perivascular deposition of glycosaminoglycans.

Similar cystic areas within deep hemisphere white matter can also be seen among the leukodystrophies (e.g., Canavan's disease; see Case 383) and in the group of aminoacidopathies (e.g., maple syrup urine disease). There is considerable potential overlap in the MR appearance of disorders from different categories of metabolic disease.

REFERENCES

Atlas SW, Grossman RI, Goldberg HI, et al: MR diagnosis of acute disseminated encephalomyelitis. *J Comput Assist Tomogr* 10:798-801, 1986.

Baram TZ, Goldman AM, Percy AK: Krabbe's disease: specific MR and CT findings. *Neuroradiology* 36:111, 1986.

Barkhof F, Scheltens P, Frequin STFM, et al: Relapsing-remitting multiple sclerosis: sequential enhanced MR imaging vs clinical findings in determining disease activity. *AJR* 159:1041-1047, 1992.

Barkhof F, Thompson AJ, Kappos L, et al: Database for serial magnetic resonance imaging in multiple sclerosis. *Neuroradiology* 35:362-366, 1993.

Barkhof F, Valk J, Hommes OR, Scheltens P: Meningeal Gd-DTPA enhancement in multiple sclerosis. *AJNR* 13:397-400, 1992.

Barkhof F, Valk J, Hommes OR, et al: Gadopentetate Dimeglumine enhancement of multiple sclerosis lesions on long TR spin-echo images at 0.6 T. *AJNR* 13:1257-1260, 1992.

Barkovich AJ, Lyon G, Evrard P: Formation, maturation and disorders of white matter. *AJNR* 13:447-461, 1992.

Baum PA, Barkovich AJ, Koch TK, Berg BD: Deep gray matter involvement in acute disseminated encephalomyelitis. *AJNR* 15:1275-1283, 1994.

Bewermeyer H, Bamborschke S, Ebhardt G, et al: MR imaging in adrenoleukomyeloneuropathy. *J Comput Assist Tomogr* 9:793-796, 1985.

Brismar J, Brismar G, Gascon G, Oznan P: Caravan disease: CT and MR imaging of the brain. *AJNR* 11:805-810, 1990.

Caldemeyer KS, Edwards MK, Smith RR, Moran CC: Viral and post-viral demyelination central nervous system infection, neuroimaging. *Radiol Clin North Am* 3:305-317, 1993.

Caldemeyer KS, Harris TM, Smith RR, Edwards MK: Gadolinium enhancement in acute disseminated encephalomyelitis. *J Comput Assist Tomogr* 15:673-675, 1991.

Capra R, Marciano N, Vignolo LA, et al: Gadolinium-pentetic acid magnetic resonance imaging in patients with relapsing remitting multiple sclerosis. *Arch Neurol* 49:687-689, 1992.

Choi S, Enzmann DR: Infantile Krabbe disease: complementary CT and MR findings. *AJNR* 14:1164-1166, 1993.

Curé JK, Cromwell LD, Case JL, et al: Auditory dysfunction caused by multiple sclerosis: detection with MR imaging. *AJNR* 11:817-820, 1990.

Cutler JR, Aminoff MJ, Brant-Zawadzki M: Evaluation of patients with multiple sclerosis by evoked potentials and magnetic resonance imaging: a comparative study. *Ann Neurol* 20:645-648, 1986.

Demaerel P, Faubert C, Wilms G, et al: MR findings in leukodystrophy. *Neuroradiology* 33:368-371, 1991.

Dietrich R, Bradley WG, Zaragoza EG, et al: MR evaluation of early myelination patterns in normal and developmentally delayed infants. *AJNR* 9:69-76, 1988.

Drayer BP, Burger P, Hurwitz B, Dawson D, et al: Reduced signal intensity on MR images of thalamus and putamen in multiple sclerosis: increased iron content? *AJNR* 8:413-419, 1987.

Dunn V, Bale JF Jr, Zimmerman RA, et al: MRI in children with post-infectious disseminated encephalomyelitis. *Magn Reson Imaging* 4:25-32, 1986.

Ebner F, Millner MM, Justich E: Multiple sclerosis in children: value of serial MR studies to monitor patients. *AJNR* 11:1023-1027, 1990.

Edwards MK, Farlow MR, Stevens JC: Multiple sclerosis: MRI and clinical correlation. *AJNR* 7:595-598, 1986.

Farley TJ, Ketonen LM, Bodensteiner JB, Wang DD: Serial MRI and CT findings in infantile Krabbe disease. *Pediatr Neurol* 8:455-458, 1992.

Farlow MR, Markand ON, Edwards MK, et al: Multiple sclerosis: magnetic resonance imaging, evoked responses, and spinal fluid electrophoresis. *Neurology* 36:828-831, 1986.

Fazekas F, Offenbacher H, Fuchs S, et al: Criteria for an increased specificity of MRI interpretation in elderly subjects with suspected multiple sclerosis. *Neurology* 38:1822-1825, 1988.

Finelli DA, Tarr RW, Sawyer RN, Horwitz SJ: Deceptively normal MR in early infantile Krabbe disease. *AJNR* 15:167-171, 1994.

Gean-Marton AD, Vezina LG, Martin KL, et al: Abnormal corpus callosum: a sensitive and specific indicator of multiple sclerosis. *Radiology* 180:215-221, 1991.

Gebarski SS, Gabrielsen TO, Gilman S, et al: The initial diagnosis of multiple sclerosis: clinical impact of magnetic resonance imaging. *Ann Neurol* 17:469-474, 1985.

Gerard D, Healy ME, Hesselink JR: MR demonstration of mesencephalic lesions in osmotic demyelination syndrome (central pontine myelinolysis). *Neuroradiology* 29:582-584, 1987.

Giang DW, Poduri KR, Eskin TA, et al: Multiple sclerosis masquerading as a mass lesion. *Neuroradiology* 34:150-154, 1992.

Grossman RI, Braffman BH, Bronson JR, et al: Multiple sclerosis: serial studies of gadolinium-enhanced MR imaging. *Radiology* 169:117-122, 1988.

Grossman RI, Gonzalez-Scarano F, Atlas SW, et al: Multiple sclerosis: Gadolinium enhancement in MR imaging. *Radiology* 161:721-725, 1986.

Guilleux MH, Steiner RE, Young IR: MR imaging of progressive multifocal leukoencephalopathy. *AJNR* 7:1033-1035, 1986.

Haas G, Schroth G, Krageloh-Mann I, et al: Magnetic resonance imaging of the brain of children with multiple sclerosis. *Dev Med Child Neurol* 29:586, 1985.

Heier LA, Bauer CJ, Schwarts L, et al: Large Virchow-Robin spaces: MR-clinical correlation. *AJNR* 10:929-936, 1989.

Hirabuki N, Fujita N, Fujii K, et al: MR appearance of Virchow-Robin spaces along lenticulostriate arteries: spin-echo and two-dimensional fast low-angle shot imaging. *AJNR* 15:277-282, 1994.

Ho VB, Fitz CR, Yoder CC, Geyer CA: Resolving MR features in osmotic myelinolysis (central pontine and extrapontine myelinolysis). *AJNR* 14:163-167, 1993.

Holland BA, Haas DK, Norman D: MRI of normal brain maturation. *AJNR* 7:201, 1986.

Horowitz AL, Kaplan RD, Grewe G, et al: The ovoid lesions: a new MR observation in patients with multiple sclerosis. *AJNR* 10:303-305, 1989.

Huckman MS, Wong PWK, Sullivan T, et al: Magnetic resonance imaging compared with computed tomography in adrenoleukodystrophy. *Am J Dis Child* 150:1001-1003, 1986.

Inoue Y, Matsumura Y, Fukuda T, et al: MR imaging of the Wallerian degeneration in the brainstem: temporal relationships. *AJNR* 11:897-902, 1990.

Jackson A, Fitzgerald JB, Gillespie JE: The callosal-septal interface lesion in multiple sclerosis: effect of sequence and imaging plane. *Neuroradiology* 35:573-577, 1993.

Jackson JA, Leake DR, Schneiders NJ, et al: Magnetic resonance imaging in multiple sclerosis: results in 32 cases. *AJNR* 6:171-176, 1985.

Jacobs L, Kinkel WR, Polachini I, et al: Correlations of nuclear magnetic resonance imaging, computerized tomography, and clinical profiles in multiple sclerosis. *Neuroradiology* 36:27-34, 1986.

Jensen ME, Sawyer RW, Braun IF, Rizzo WB: MR imaging appearance in childhood adrenoleukodystrophy with auditory, visual, and motor pathway involvement. *Radiographics* 10:53-66, 1990.

Johnson MA, Desai S, Hugh-Jones K, Starer F: Magnetic resonance imaging of the brain in Hurler syndrome. *AJNR* 5:816-819, 1984.

Kepes JJ: Large focal tumor-like demyelinating lesions of the brain:

intermediate entity between multiple sclerosis and acute disseminated encephalomyelitis. A study of 31 patients. *Ann Neurol* 33:18-27, 1993.

Kermode AG, Thompson AJ, Tofts P, et al: Breakdown of the blood-brain barrier precedes symptoms and other MRI signs of new lesions in multiple sclerosis: pathogenetic and clinical implications. *Brain* 113:1477-1489, 1990.

Kesselring J, Miller DH, Robb SA, et al: Acute disseminated encephalomyelitis. MRI findings and the distinction from multiple sclerosis. *Brain* 113:291, 1990.

Kimura S, Unayama T, Mori T: The natural history of acute disseminated leukoencephalitis: a serial magnetic resonance imaging study. *Neuropediatrics* 23:192-195, 1992.

Koci TM, Chiang F, Chow P, et al: Thalamic extrapontine lesions in central pontine myelinolysis. *AJNR* 11:1229-1233, 1990.

Korogi Y, Takahashi M, Shinzato J, et al: MR findings in two presumed cases of mild central pontine myelinolysis. *AJNR* 14:651-654, 1993.

Krupp LB, Lipton RB, Swerdlow ML, et al: Progressive multifocal encephalopathy: clinical and radiographic features. *Ann Neurol* 17:344-349, 1985.

Kuhn MJ, Johnson KA, Davis KK: Wallerian degeneration: evaluation with MR imaging. *Radiology* 168:199-202, 1988.

Kuhn MJ, Mikulis DJ, Ayoub DM, et al: Wallerian degeneration after cerebral infarction: evaluation with sequential imaging. *Radiology* 172:179-182, 1989.

Kumar AH, Rosenbaum AE, Naidu S, et al: Adrenoleukodystrophy: correlating MR imaging with CT. *Radiology* 165:497-504, 1987.

Lee C, Dineen TE, Brack M, et al: The mucopolysaccharidoses: characterization by cranial MR imaging. *AJNR* 14:1285-1292, 1993.

Lee KH, Hashimoto SA, Hooge JP, et al: Magnetic resonance imaging of the head in the diagnosis of multiple sclerosis: a prospective 2-year follow-up with comparison of clinical evaluation, evoked potentials, oligoclonal banding, and CT. *Neurology* 41:657-660, 1991.

Levy JD, Cottingham KL, Campbell RJ, et al: Progressive multifocal leukomalacia and magnetic resonance imaging. *Ann Neurol* 19:399-401, 1986.

Lukes SA, Norman D, Mills C: Acute disseminated encephalomyelitis: CT and NMR findings. *J Comput Assist Tomogr* 7:182, 1983.

Mark AS, Atlas SW: Progressive multifocal leukoencephalopathy in patients with AIDS: appearance of MR images. *Radiology* 173:517-520, 1989.

McAdams HP, Geyer CA, Done SL, et al: CT and MR imaging of Canavan disease. *AJNR* 11:397, 1990.

McArdle CB, Richardson CJ, Nicholas DA, et al: Developmental features of the neonatal brain: MR imaging. *Radiology* 162:223-229, 1987.

Miller GM, Baker HL Jr, Okazaki H, Whisnant JP: Central pontine myelinolysis and its imitators: MR findings. *Radiology* 168:795-802, 1988.

Miromitz S, Sartor K, Gado M, Torack R: Focal signal intensity variations in the posterior internal capsule: normal MR findings and distinction from pathologic findings. *Radiology* 172:535-540, 1989.

Mirsen TR: Clinical correlates of white-matter changes on magnetic resonance imaging scans of the brain. *Arch Neurol* 48:1015, 1991.

Moriwaka F, Tashiro K, Maruo Y, et al: MR imaging of pontine and extrapontine myelinolysis. *J Comput Assist Tomogr* 12:446-449, 1988.

Murata R, Nakajima S, Tanaka A, et al: MR imaging of the brain in patients with mucopolysaccharidosis. *AJNR* 10:1165-1170, 1989.

Nesbit GM, Forbes GS, Scheithauer BW, et al: Multiple sclerosis: histopathologic and MR and/or CT correlation in 37 cases at biopsy and three cases at autopsy. *Radiology* 180:467-474, 1991.

Niebler G, Harris T, Davis T, Ross K: Fulminant multiple sclerosis. *AJNR* 13:1547-1551, 1992.

Nowell MA, Grossman RI, Hackney DB, et al: MR imaging of white matter diseases in children. *AJNR* 9:503, 1988.

Oba H, Araki T, Ohtomo K, et al: Amyotrophic lateral sclerosis: T2-shortening in motor cortex at MR imaging. *Radiology* 189:843-846, 1993.

Orita T, Tsurutani T, Izumihara A, Matsunaga T: Coronal MR imaging for visualization of Wallerian degeneration of the pyramidal tract. *J Comput Assist Tomogr* 15:802-804, 1991.

Osborn AG, Harnsberger HR, Smoker WRK, et al: Multiple sclerosis in adolescents: CT and MR Findings. *AJNR* 11:489-494, 1990.

Paty DW, Oger JJF, Kastrukoff LF, et al: MRI in the diagnosis of multiple sclerosis: a prospective study with comparison of clinical evaluation. Evoked potentials, oligoclonal banding, and CT. *Neurology* 38:180, 1988.

Powell T, Sussman JG, Davies-Jones GAB: MR imaging in acute multiple sclerosis: ring-like appearance in plaques suggesting the presence of paramagnetic free radicals. *AJNR* 13:1544-1546, 1992.

Quint DJ: Multiple sclerosis and imaging of the corpus callosum. *Radiology* 180:15-17, 1991.

Ragland RL, Duffis AW, Gendelman S, et al: Central pontine myelinolysis with clinical recovery: MR documentation. *J Comput Assist Tomogr* 13:316-318, 1989.

Rippe DJ, Edwards MK, D'Amour PG, et al: MR imaging of central pontine myelinolysis. *J Comput Assist Tomogr* 11:724-726, 1987.

Runge VM, Price AC, Kirshner HS, et al: The evaluation of multiple sclerosis by magnetic resonance imaging. *Radiographics* 6:203-212, 1986.

Runge VM, Price AC, Kishner HS, et al: Magnetic resonance imaging of multiple sclerosis: a study of pulse-technique efficacy. *AJNR* 5:691-702, 1984.

Sasaki M, Sakuragawa N, Takashima S, et al: MRI and CT findings in Krabbe disease. *Pediatr Neurol* 7:283-288, 1991.

Scotti G, Scialfa G, Biondi A, et al: Magnetic resonance in multiple sclerosis. *Neuroradiology* 28:319-323, 1986.

Sheldon JJ, Siddharthan R, Tobias J, et al: MR imaging of multiple sclerosis: comparison with clinical and CT examination in 74 patients. *AJNR* 6:683-690, 1985.

Sherman JL, Clawson LL, Citrin CH, et al: MR evaluation of amyotrophic lateral sclerosis (ALS). *AJNR* 8:941, 1987.

Simon JH, Holtas SL, Schiffer RB, et al: Corpus callosum and subcallosal-periventricular lesions in multiple sclerosis: detection with MR. *Radiology* 160:363-368, 1986.

Simon JH, Schiffer RB, Rudick RA, Herndon RM: Quantitative determination of MS-induced corpus callosum atrophy in vivo using MR imaging. *AJNR* 8:599-604, 1987.

Takeda K, Sakuta M, Saeki F: Central pontine myelinolysis diagnosed by magnetic resonance imaging. *Ann Neurol* 17:310, 1985.

Thompson AJ, Brown MM, Swash MM, et al: Autopsy validation of MRI in central pontine myelinolysis. *Neuroradiology* 30:175, 1988.

Uchiyama M, Hata Y, Tada S: MR imaging of adrenoleukodystrophy. *Neuroradiology* 33:25-29, 1991.

Udaka F, Sawada H, Seriv N, et al: MRI and SPECT findings in amyotrophic lateral sclerosis. *Neuroradiology* 34:389-393, 1992.

Uhlenbrook D, Seidel D, Genlen W, et al: MR imaging in multiple sclerosis: comparison with clinical, CSF, and visual evoked potential findings. *AJNR* 9:59-68, 1988.

Uhlenbrook D, Sehlen S: The value of T1-weighted images in the differentiation between MS, white matter lesions, and subcortical arteriosclerotic encephalopathy (SAE). *Neuroradiology* 31:203-212, 1989.

Van der Knaap MS, Valk J: MR of adrenoleukodystrophy: histopathologic correlations. *AJNR* 10:512-514, 1989.

Van der Knaap MS, Valk J, DeNeeling N, Nauta JJP: Pattern recognition in magnetic resonance imaging of white matter disorders in children and young infants. *Neuroradiology* 33:478-493, 1991.

Wallace CJ, Seland TP, Fong TC: Multiple sclerosis: the impact of MR imaging. *AJR* 158:849-857, 1992.

Wheeler AL, Truwit CL, Kleinschmidt-DeMasters BK, et al: Progressive multifocal leukoencephalopathy: contrast enhancement on CT scans and MR images. *AJR* 161:1049-1051, 1993.

Whiteman MLH, Post MJD, Berger JR, et al: Progressive multifocal leukoencephalopathy in 47 HIV-seropositive patients: neuroimaging with clinical and pathologic correlation. *Radiology* 187:233-240, 1993.

Wilms G, Marchal G, Kersschot E, et al: Axial vs sagittal T2-weighted brain MR images in the evaluation of multiple sclerosis. *J Comput Assist Tomogr* 15:359-364, 1991.

Yagishita A, Nakano I, Oda M, Hirano A: Location of the corticospinal tract in the internal capsule at MR imaging. *Radiology* 191:455-460, 1994.

Yetkin FZ, Houghton VM, et al: Multiple sclerosis: specificity of MR for diagnosis. *Radiology* 178:447-451, 1991.

CHAPTER 8

Inflammatory, Metabolic, and Degenerative Disorders

Case 385

1-year-old girl presenting with a two-day history of
fever and increasing irritability.
(axial, noncontrast scan; SE 3000/30)

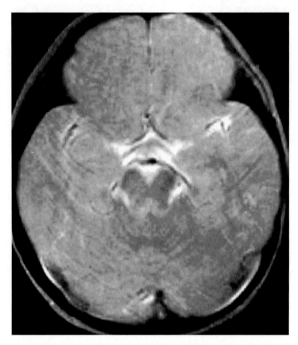

Bacterial Meningitis
(due to *Haemophilus influenzae)*

Case 386

3-year-old boy adopted from Eastern Europe,
presenting with a seizure.
(axial, postcontrast scan; SE 600/15)

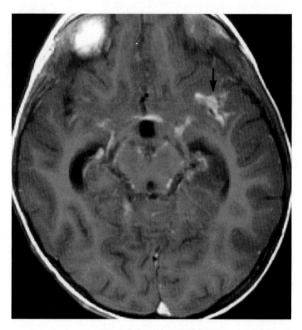

Tuberculous Meningitis

MR scans may be negative in the clinical setting of meningitis. In some cases communicating hydrocephalus is the only clue to meningeal pathology.

In other cases, cells, protein, and reactive tissue may alter the signal intensity within sulci and cisterns. This finding may be obvious or subtle on noncontrast scans.

In Case 385, basal cisterns are too "bright" for normal CSF given the intermediate weighting (long TR, short TE) of the pulse sequence. (Such "balanced" sequences often demonstrate the distinction between complex fluid and simple CSF more clearly than T1-weighted or T2-weighted scans.) Isointense or high intensity cisterns due to meningitis are most often associated with bacterial, fungal, or granulomatous pathogens and are most commonly found near the base of the brain.

Superficial contrast enhancement may confirm the suspicion of meningitis raised clinically or on noncontrast studies. Involvement may be generalized or localized. The pattern may be predominantly dural (linear, paralleling the cal-

varium) or pia-arachnoidal (with invaginations into cerebral sulci and cisterns).

Case 386 demonstrates a finely nodular layer of abnormal pial enhancement on the surface of the midbrain and along the medial margin of the uncus bilaterally. The left sylvian cistern is filled with enhancing material near the genu of the middle cerebral artery (*arrow;* compare to Case 402). Moderate communicating hydrocephalus is present, due to impaired cisternal circulation of CSF.

Contrast-enhanced MR scans (particularly using magnetization transfer suppression techniques) are more sensitive than CT studies in detecting inflammatory meningeal pathology. However, the degree of abnormal enhancement varies among the multiple potential etiologies of meningitis. For example, coccidiomycosis typically provokes an intense inflammatory response, while cryptococcus often incites minimal meningeal enhancement.

Sarcoidosis or syphilis in an adult could cause an appearance very similar to Case 386.

DIFFERENTIAL DIAGNOSIS:
LEPTOMENINGEAL ENHANCEMENT

Case 386-1

50-year-old woman presenting with headaches.
(axial, postcontrast scan; SE 600/15)

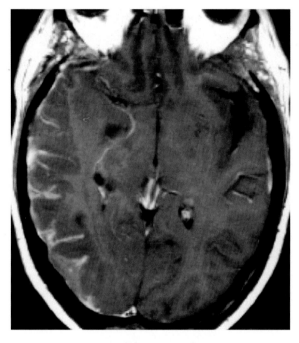

Non-Hodgkins Lymphoma

Case 386-2

51-year-old man with a three day history
of severe headaches.
(axial, postcontrast scan; SE 600/15)

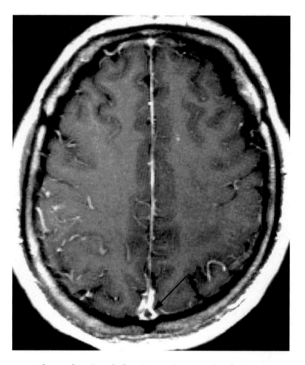

Thrombosis of the Superior Sagittal Sinus

Several noninflammatory pathologies can cause abnormal enhancement of the leptomeninges resembling menigitis.

Meningeal infiltration by tumor may be seen in association with systemic leukemia or lymphoma (as in Case 386-1), metastatic solid tumors (see Cases 30 and 31), or seeding from primary intracranial malignancies (see Cases 160-162).

Intracranial involvement by leukemia or lymphoma may also present as dural-based masses resembling meningiomas or metastatses from solid tumors (such as Cases 58 and 59). A small dural-based mass is present posteriorly in Case 386-1 (*arrow*).

Vasular congestion of the meninges can cause an enhancement pattern similar to meningitis, as illustrated by Case 386-2. The filling defect within the lumen of the superior sagittal sinus (*arrow*) represents thrombus and is analagous to the "delta sign" or "empty triangle sign" of dural sinus thrombosis originally described on postcontrast CT scans. (See case 647 for another MR example of this finding.) Abnormally intense enhancement reflecting venous congestion is commonly seen with the dura in cases of sagittal sinus thrombosis. Occasionally abnormal leptomeningeal enhancement is also noted, as in the right pariental region of Case 386-2.

Leptomeningeal enhancement may be seen overlying acute cerebral infarcts (see Cases 484 and 485), with a pattern closely resembling the above cases. A third vascular etiology for meningeal enhancement is the Sturge Weber syndrome, illustrated in Case 770.

Contrast enhancement at the cerebral surface may also represent cortical pathology. Compare the images on this page to Cases 401 to 403.

Case 387

5-year-old girl who suffered a seizure after
admission for viral meningitis.
(coronal, noncontrast scan; SE 2500/90)

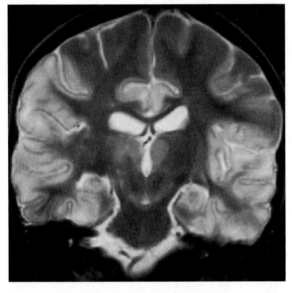

Encephalitis and Cerebral Infarction

Case 388

3-month-old boy, six weeks after
pneumococcal meningitis.
(coronal, noncontrast scan; SE 800/16)

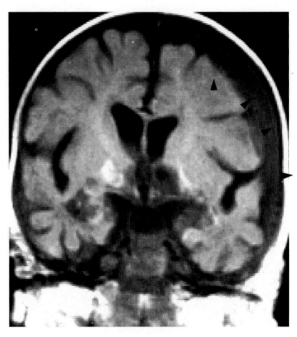

Subdural Effusion
(and deep hemispheric infarcts)

Meningeal inflammation may extend to the cerebral parenchyma, causing localized or generalized cerebritis. In many cases, encephalitis and meningitis are concurrent. Another mechanism of parenchymal damage associated with meningitis is subacute cerebral infarction, due to spasm or occlusion of arteries or veins traversing the infected subarachnoid space.

In Case 387, abnormally high signal intensity and swelling involve extensive areas of the cortical surface bilaterally. A gyriform pattern of superficial contrast enhancement often accompanies this appearance (see Case 403).

A different pattern of cerebral involvement is seen in Case 388. Areas of parenchymal damage are present in the region of the hypothalamus, basal ganglia, and medial temporal lobes. (T1-shortening in the affected regions may reflect residual subacute blood products or early dystrophic

calcification.) This appearance can result from the basal accumulation of thick exudates in meningitis, with spread of infection to the inferior surface of the brain. Arteritis and/or thrombophlebitis involving basal vessels may also cause hypothalamic and deep hemispheric lesions in cases of meningitis.

The subdural fluid collection over the left frontal region in Case 388 *(arrowheads)* was found to be a sterile effusion. Subdural effusions are common in bacterial meningitis, particularly in cases due to *Haemophilus influenzae*, the leading cause of meningitis in the United States. The effusions typically contain large amounts of protein but few cells. Their appearance is nonspecific and often indistinguishable from subdural empyemas (compare to Cases 392 and 393).

DIFFERENTIAL DIAGNOSIS:
MILIARY ENHANCEMENT IN THE BASAL GANGLIA

Case 388-1

10-year-old boy being treated for a PNET, now presenting with impaired consciousness.
(axial, postcontrast scan; SE 700/17)

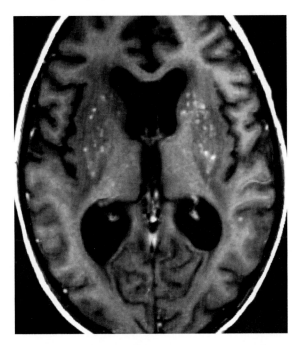

Encephalitis Secondary to Streptococcal Meningitis

Case 388-2

35-year-old woman presenting with headaches.
(axial, postcontrast scan; SE 600/15)

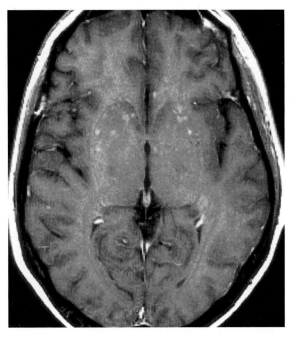

Carcinomatous Encephalitis
(metastatic carcinoma of the breast)

Case 388-1 illustrates miliary encephalitis developing as a consequence of streptococcal meningitis in an immunosuppressed patient. The predominance of lesions in the basal ganglia may reflect hematogenous seeding to these well-perfused nuclei, comparable to the presumably bloodborne distribution of metastatic disease in Case 388-2.

Alternatively, ganglionic infection may reflect direct extension of basal meningitis. Organisms can ascend along the Virchow-Robin spaces accompanying lenticulostriate arteries into the base of the brain. This route of spread is characteristic of cryptococcal meningitis, with small "gelatinous pseudocysts" developing in the same distribution as the enhancing foci of Case 388-1. Ascending infection from the skull base may account for the deep hemispheric involvement in some patients with viral encephalitis (see

Cases 395 and 396). Ganglionic lesions in the setting of meningitis may also represent sterile infarcts, as discussed in Case 388.

Cerebral involvement by multiple tiny metastases as in Case 388-2 is sometimes termed "carcinomatous encephalitis." Enhancement of such lesions produces a miliary pattern that resembles disseminated infection, vasculitis, or noninfectious inflammatory processes (e.g., multiple sclerosis or sarcoidosis). In some cases, numerous tiny metastases do not enhance significantly and are detected only as a finely granular texture within the basal ganglia and/or cerebral cortex, best appreciated on T2-weighted images.

Ventricular enlargement in Case 388-1 probably represents a combination of radiation effect and low grade communicating hydrocephalus.

Case 389A

49-year-old man with AIDS and
systemic CMV infection.
(axial, noncontrast scan; SE 2500/25)

Case 389B

Same patient.
(sagittal, postcontrast scan; SE 600/20)

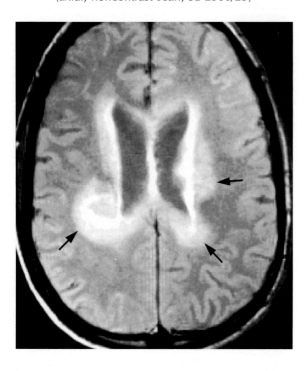

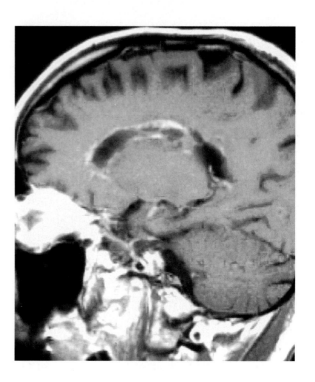

Bacterial, fungal, viral, or parasitic infections may involve the ventricular lining. Fungal or viral ventriculitis most commonly occurs in immunosuppressed patients, as in this case. Bacterial ventriculitis may develop in previously healthy individuals when organisms are introduced through trauma or surgery. Pyogenic ventriculitis may also accompany a cerebral abscess (see Case 411).

Case 389A demonstrates the thick rind of subependymal inflammation and edema associated with ventriculitis. (Compare to the periventricular edema in Cases 652 and 653.) The inflammatory process is beginning to "bud" or extend away from the ventricular system into the deep white matter of both hemispheres *(arrows)*.

Intraventricular sedimentation levels may occur in cases of ventriculitis, representing cells, proteinaceous material, and/or leakage of contrast material from inflammed ependyma or choroid plexus. The visualization of intracranial sedimentation levels requires a period of limited head movement prior to a CT or MR scan. A patient who is actively shaking his or her head will disperse sediment and make detection more difficult.

Prominent ependymal/subependymal enhancement is seen in Case 389B. Postcontrast scans may also highlight inflammatory septations and loculations within the ventricular chambers. Such adhesions can cause focal cysts or generalized hydrocephalus.

Cytomegalovirus (CMV) is recognized as a cause of intrauterine encephalitis and ventriculitis but is rarely associated with cerebritis in healthy adults. Patients with AIDS or other immunodeficiency states are susceptible to infection by opportunistic pathogens, and CMV encephalitis and ventriculitis may be encountered in such cases.

Case 390

79-year-old woman presenting with confusion.
(coronal, postcontrast scan; SE 600/15)

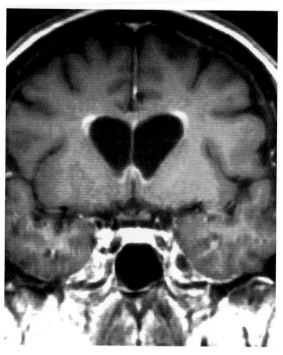

Systemic Lymphoma

Case 391

76-year-old man presenting with a seizure.
(coronal, postcontrast scan; SE 600/15)

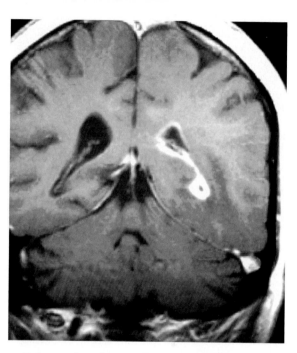

Subependymal Spread of Malignant Glioma

Enhancing ventricular margins may be caused by subependymal tumor as well as by inflammatory processes. Case 390 is an example of ependymal/subependymal metastasis from a systemic neoplasm. Melanoma and carcinomas of the breast and lung can cause a similar appearance.

Primary CNS tumors may involve ventricular margins through direct extension or by CSF seeding and colonization. The malignant glioma in Case 391 was centered more anteriorly in the left temporal lobe, with the medial portion of the tumor reaching the temporal horn and spreading posteriorly along its margin.

Primary CNS lymphoma may also arise near ventricular borders and extend subependymally (see Cases 319 and 320). Medulloblastomas and germinomas are among the primary intracranial tumors that frequently demonstrate CSF-borne metastases along ventricular or meningeal surfaces.

Ependymal/subependymal enhancement is occasionally seen in patients with noninfectious inflammatory disease (e.g., sarcoidosis).

Case 392A

15-year-old boy presenting with fever, decreased
mental status, and a history of sinusitis.
(coronal, postcontrast scan; SE 600/15)

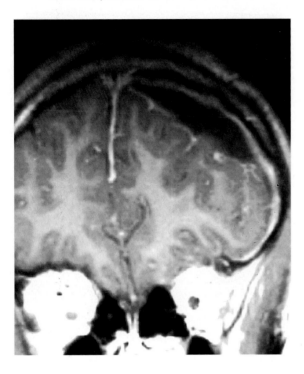

Case 392B

Same patient.
(axial, noncontrast scan; SE 2800/90)

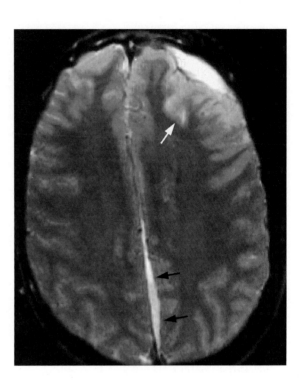

Sinusitis may cause intracranial infection by direct extension across the skull base or by septic thrombophlebitis traversing otherwise intact bone. Epidural and/or subdural abscesses may result.

Subdural fluid collections are present in the left frontal region and posterior interhemispheric fissure (*black arrows*, Case 392B) in this case. An area of cerebral edema is seen deep to the frontal collection (*white arrow*, Case 392B). Enhancement along the margin of the left frontal empyema is minimal in Case 392A.

The distinction between a sterile subdural effusion associated with meningitis (see Case 388) and a subdural empyema is best made by the clinical condition of the patient. Patients with even large subdural effusions are often remarkably well, while patients with even small subdural empyemas are usually remarkably ill. The relative amount of contrast enhancement within the membranes of the subdural collection is an inexact index of the degree of infection. In general, membranes surrounding subdural empy-

emas tend to enhance more than those bordering subdural effusions, but Case 392A demonstrates the unreliability of this criterion.

The narrow subdural collection adjacent to the posterior falx in Case 392B is typical of subdural empyemas. These abscesses are often very thin (although surprisingly extensive) and easily overlooked as symptoms begin. Involvement of the interhemispheric fissure and the tentorial surface is common. Convexity subdural empyemas are more easily detected by MR than by CT due to the absence of artifact from adjacent bone and the availability of the coronal scan plane.

Subdural empyemas are often considered to be a surgical emergency. The course in nonoperated cases can lead to rapid morbidity and mortality. One or more reexplorations may be necessary to remove persistent or recurrent loculations of subdural infection. The boy in this case underwent several craniotomies for recurrent empyemas. He eventually recovered completely.

DIFFERENTIAL DIAGNOSIS:
THICKENING AND ENHANCEMENT OF THE TENTORIUM

Case 393

15-year-old boy presenting with fever and
decreased mental status.
(coronal, postcontrast scan; SE 600/15)

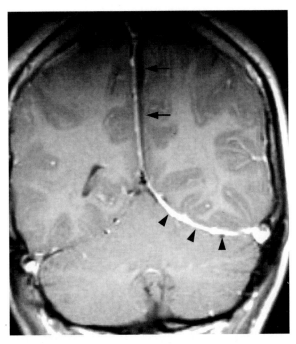

Inflammatory Meningeal Thickening
(associated with subdural empyema)

Case 394

17-year-old boy after a craniotomy (and multiple
lumbar punctures) for medulloblastoma.
(sagittal, postcontrast scan; SE 600/15)

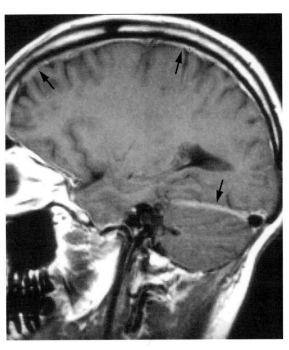

Dural Hyperemia
(due to intracranial hypotension)

The differential diagnosis of thick dural enhancement includes inflammatory disease (e.g., pyogenic meningitis, tuberculosis, fungal infections such as coccidioidomycosis, cysticercosis, and sarcoidosis), meningeal tumor (e.g., en plaque meningioma, carcinomatosis, seeding from a primary CNS malignancy, lymphoma, and leukemia), and vascular congestion or hyperemia (e.g., secondary to recent surgery, dural sinus thrombosis, or intracranial hypotension).

Case 393 again illustrates the subtle appearance of an interhemispheric subdural empyema *(arrows)*, which is associated with asymmetrical thickening of the tentorium of the left *(arrowheads)*.

In Case 394, abnormal tentorial enhancement *(lower arrow)* is part of a more generalized process including convexity dura *(upper arrows)*. Uniform dural thickening as seen here can be noted shortly after craniotomy or shunt placement and is often surprisingly diffuse. The rapid occurrence and widespread nature of this finding suggest a reactive phenomenon, probably reflecting an increase in dural blood volume.

A similar appearance is encountered in patients with intact skulls who experience low intracranial pressure due to spinal loss of CSF (after lumbar puncture or spontaneously). Such patients characteristically present with positional headaches (worse when upright). MR scans typically demonstrate abnormal inferior sagging of the brainstem and posterior fossa structures (see Case 463).

It is important to recognize that uniform dural thickening can be a normal consequence of craniotomy and/or lumbar punctures in patients with cranial or spinal neoplasms or infection. The finding does not necessarily imply recurrent or persistent tumor or meningitis.

Case 395

33-year-old man presenting with progressive somnolence.
(coronal, noncontrast scan; SE 600/16)

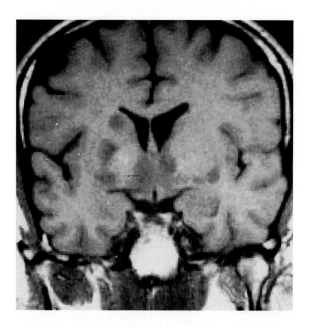

Case 396

9-year-old boy presenting with fever and lethargy.
(axial, noncontrast scan; SE 3000/80)

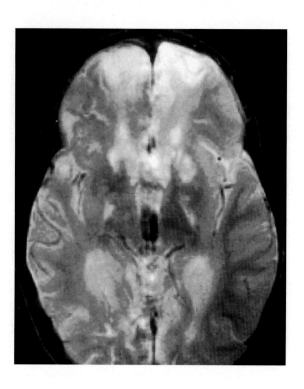

The MR appearance of viral encephalitis is widely variable, reflecting the age of the patient and the specific infectious agent.

Infants and young children often demonstrate panencephalitis. Herpes simplex virus type 2 is particularly likely to cause such widespread infection in a neonate (see Case 403).

Older children and adults often present with more localized involvement by viral encephalitis. Although any area of the brain may be affected, deep hemisphere regions near the skull base are often most severely involved.

The scans above illustrate this appearance. In Case 395, zones of edema with mass effect and prolonged T1 values are present in the hypothalamus and basal ganglia bilaterally. Case 396 demonstrates similar bilateral deep hemispheric involvement in association with more superficial lesions in the frontal lobes. (The low signal intensity within the third ventricle is due to CSF pulsations.)

Another possible etiology for inflammatory lesions near the third ventricle is the extension of basal meningitis into the hypothalamus (see Cases 388 and 388-1). Bacterial or fungal pathogens (e.g., cryptococcus) may ascend along prominent Virchow-Robin spaces accompanying penetrating arteries at the base of the brain to present at the hypothalamic level. Sarcoidosis may similarly spread from the suprasellar region into the brain to cause bilateral hypothalamic lesions.

Infants sometimes present with inflammation localized to the cerebellum. Several viruses (e.g., varicella and adenovirus) may cause such acute cerebellitis, which is often complicated by hydrocephalus and brainstem compression.

Case 397

60-year-old woman with a three-day history of worsening aphasia and memory loss.
(axial, noncontrast scan; SE 2500/90)

Case 398

35-year-old man presenting with fever and a two-day history of increasing aphasia.
(axial, noncontrast scan; SE 2500/100)

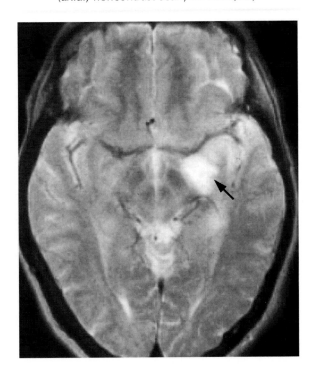

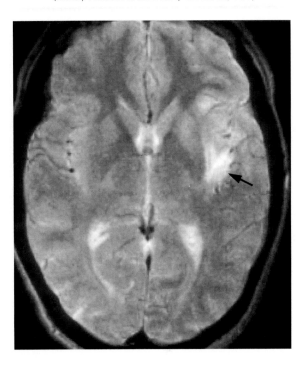

Adult encephalitis due to herpes simplex virus (type 1) typically begins in the medial anterior temporal and posterior-inferior frontal lobes. Early scan findings are limited to subtle edema and mass effect in these locations, much better demonstrated by MR than by CT. Bilateral involvement occurs in about one third of cases.

In Case 397, the very high signal intensity of the left uncus *(arrow)* is clearly pathological. Although the appearance is nonspecific, the characteristic location in the medial temporal lobe suggests herpes encephalitis in the appropriate clinical context. The diagnosis was confirmed by biopsy, and the patient made a good recovery on antiviral therapy.

As herpes encephalitis progresses, patchy hemorrhage and abnormal contrast enhancement are common. Small hemorrhages within the edematous tissue may be appar-

ent on MR scans as zones of T1- and/or T2-shortening. A rare alternative cause of rapidly progressive edema and patchy hemorrhage in the temporal lobe is thrombosis of the transverse sinus with venous infarction.

Case 398 demonstrates an area of high signal intensity extending superiorly from the temporal lobe into the hemisphere *(arrow)*. Involvement of the insula and white matter lateral to the lenticular nucleus is characteristic of herpes encephalitis (see Case 401). Edema sharply marginating the lateral border of the lenticular nucleus should suggest this diagnosis. Occasionally an embolic infarction affecting only the cortical distribution of the middle cerebral artery can present a similar appearance.

Gliomatosis cerebri may involve the frontal and temporal lobes unilaterally or bilaterally, resembling the MR appearance of herpes encephalitis (see Case 107).

DIFFERENTIAL DIAGNOSIS:
MASS EFFECT AND EDEMA INVOLVING THE MEDIAL TEMPORAL LOBE

Case 399

4-year-old boy presenting with seizures.
(axial, noncontrast scan; SE 2500/90)

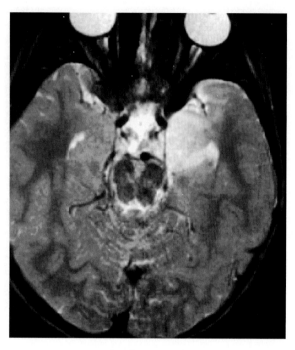

Low Grade Astrocytoma

Case 400

72-year-old man with a several month history of
memory loss and partial complex seizures.
(coronal, noncontrast scan; RSE 3500/119)

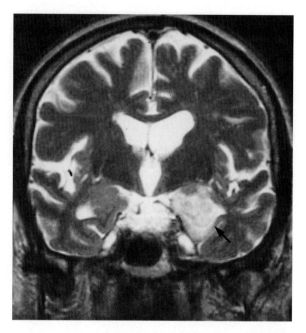

Limbic Encephalitis

The uncus is a characteristic site for herpes encephalitis, but other pathologies may also be encountered in this location.

Low or intermediate grade gliomas frequently involve the medial portion of the temporal lobe, as in Case 399. (See also Cases 69, 71, 78 and 102.) The MR features of glial tumors and localized encephalitis may be identical, with variably defined margins and infiltration. Contrast enhancement in either entity may be minimal or striking.

A relatively acute clinical context often distinguishes viral encephalitis from a long-standing mass lesion. However, occasional adult cases of herpes encephalitis present with a surprisingly long history of smoldering dysfunction; the diagnosis should still be considered in such cases if scan findings are suggestive.

Limbic encephalitis is a rare paraneoplastic disorder in which cerebral inflammation is associated with a systemic tumor, most frequently oat cell carcinoma of the lung. The presence of antineuronal nuclear antibodies within the CSF of affected patients presumably indicates the etiology of this cerebritis. Predilection for the medial temporal lobes mimics herpes encephalitis, but no viral inclusions are present in affected tissue. Bilateral involvement is common with frequent marked asymmetry, as was true in Case 400. Contrast enhancement may be absent or extensive, probably reflecting differing phases of inflammation.

Symptoms of limbic encephalitis may precede evidence of the primary neoplasm. The course of the disorder is usually more gradual than that of herpes encephalitis, evolving over weeks to months.

The clinical presentation, histological pattern, and antibody studies in Case 400 were all characteristic of limbic encephalitis. However, despite a thorough work-up, an associated tumor has not been identified.

Case 401

61-year-old man with a two-week history
of increasing confusion.
(axial, postcontrast scan; SE 900/20)

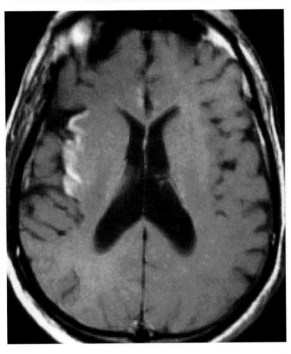

Herpes Encephalitis

Case 402

25-year-old Filipino man presenting with
mild aphasia and right hemiparesis.
(axial, postcontrast scan; SE 600/15)

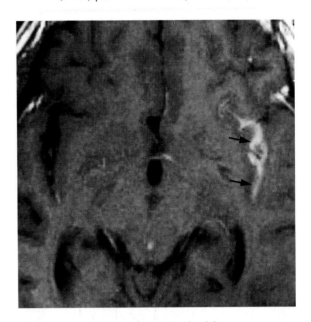

Tuberculous Meningitis

Superficial contrast enhancement may represent cortical or meningeal pathology, or a combination of the two.

Case 401 illustrates intense, gyriform enhancement of insular cortex involved by herpes encephalitis. (Compare to the gyriform enhancement seen in subacute infarcts such as Cases 485 and 486.) Involvement of the insula is characteristic of this disorder and should suggest the diagnosis. Edema and enhancement of the cingulate gyrus are also common and distinctive features of encephalitis due to herpes.

The superficial enhancement in Case 402 is meningeal in origin. Enhancing tissue fills the left sylvian cistern (compare to the normal right side), surrounding vascular structures. Fungal or granulomatous meningitis often localizes to a small portion of the subarachnoid space, as illustrated here. (Compare to the more extensive tuberculous meningitis in Case 386).

Cisternal or sulcal enhancement on MR scans is often more easily detected and more extensive than appreciated on CT studies. The absence of masking artifact from the adjacent calvarium, multiplanar display, and the higher sensitivity to small amounts of contrast material contribute to the advantage of MR in cases of enhancing superficial pathology.

Case 403

One-month-old girl presenting with fever
and seizures.
(coronal, postcontrast scan; SE 600/15)

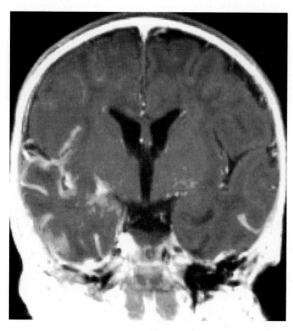

Herpes Encephalitis
(type 2)

Case 404

64-year-old man presenting with fever
and obtundation.
(axial, postcontrast scan; SE 600/15)

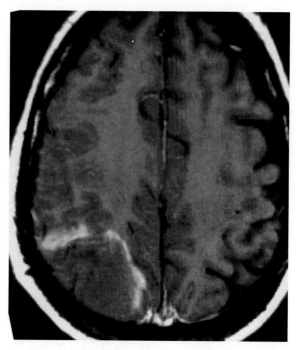

Presumed Pyogenic Cerebritis

The MR spectrum of cerebritis includes a wide range of pathogens and patterns. Neonatal encephalitis due to herpes simplex type 2 is typically diffuse and devastating, as illustrated in Case 403. Initial multifocal or symmetrical cerebral edema with loss of gray/white discrimination evolves to a phase of intense, gyriform contrast enhancement, as seen above. Rapid loss of parenchymal volume leads to generalized or patchy encephalomalacia, dystrophic calcification, and secondary ventricular enlargement (see Case 702).

No organism was cultured from CSF or brain biopsy in Case 404. However, the patient recovered on broad-spectrum antibiotics, and a presumptive diagnosis of pyogenic cerebritis was made.

Pyogenic or fungal cerebritis may initially present as a nonspecific region of edema and swelling similar to that seen in viral encephalitis. Patchy contrast enhancement is more common than the gyriform pattern typical of herpes encephalitis in Case 403.

Case 404 demonstrates a prominent band of enhancement at the margin of inflammation in the right parietal region. This peripheral zone represents the brain's attempt to contain the infection. Peripheral enhancement typically precedes the development of a true abscess capsule by days or weeks. Clues that a particular lesion is still in the cerebritis stage (i.e., lacks an organized capsule) include nonvisualization of the capsule on precontrast scans (see Cases 405-408) and progressive diffusion of contrast material into the center of the lesion on postcontrast images.

Case 405

62-year-old woman presenting with headaches
and confusion.
(sagittal, noncontrast scan; SE 600/17)

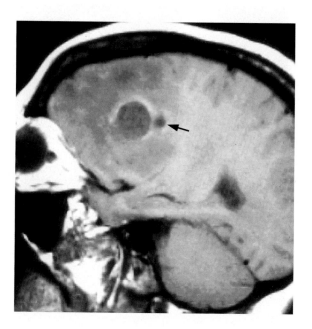

Case 406

13-year-old boy, one year after resection of a fourth
ventricular medulloblastoma, now presenting
with increasing ataxia and facial weakness.
(sagittal, noncontrast scan; SE 550/20)

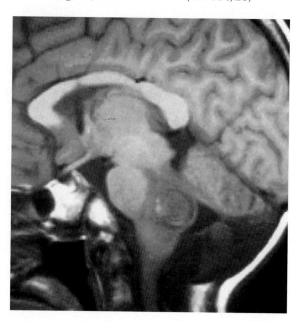

Cerebral abscesses are characterized by three distinct zones of signal abnormality on MR scans. Centrally, a necrotic cavity often demonstrates long T1 and T2 values. This feature is more obvious in Case 405 than in Case 406, where the abscess content is relatively isointense due to the presence of cells and/or protein. Peripherally, a zone of extensive edema surrounds the lesion. This area is well seen in both of the above cases as an amorphous region of reduced signal intensity.

Separating the abscess cavity from surrounding edema is the abscess capsule, which can often be identified as a discrete structure on noncontrast MR images. The capsule is typically smoothly rounded in shape and uniform in thickness. It may appear to be unilaminar or bilaminar.

Segments of the abscess capsule often demonstrate shortening of both T1 and T2. As a result, all or part of the capsule may be seen as a high signal intensity rim on T1-weighted sequences and as a low intensity rim on T2-weighted series. This appearance does not correlate well with the presence of blood products in the wall of the abscess. Other etiologies (e.g., the presence of free radicals produced by activated macrophages) have been suggested as the source of the paramagnetic effect.

The abscess capsule is well defined in each of the above cases as a uniformly thin and round layer of distinct signal intensity, with some areas of T1-shortening. These features are all useful in distinguishing abscesses from necrotic cerebral neoplasms. The wall of a tumor rarely demonstrates T1-shortening and is usually thicker, less uniform, and less round than the capsule of an abscess.

A small satellite or "daughter" abscess is present at the posterior margin of the main abscess in Case 405 *(arrow)*. This "budding" morphology is characteristic of inflammatory disease (see Case 389) but can occasionally be mimicked by a tumor.

Case 407

8-year-old boy presenting with increasing
headaches and vomiting.
(axial, noncontrast scan; SE 2800/90)

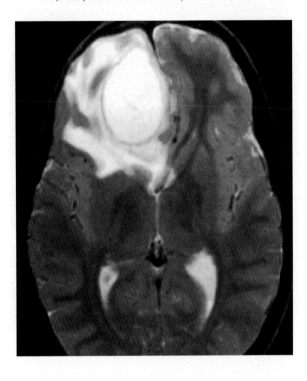

Case 408

13-year-old boy presenting with ataxia
and facial weakness.
(axial, noncontrast scan; SE 2500/90)

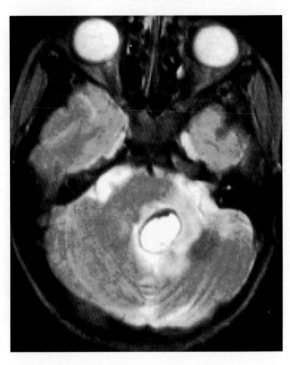

(same patient as Case 406)

The capsule of an abscess is usually defined on T2-weighted scans as a thin and round zone of isointensity or low signal intensity separating surrounding edema from the central cavity. The wall of many abscesses is uniformly thin, as in Case 407. In other cases, irregular thickening of tissue is encountered along portions of the abscess capsule (as seen anteriorly in Case 408), but the overall morphology remains suggestive of the correct diagnosis.

As discussed on the preceding page, T1- and T2-shortening within the wall of a cystic lesion favor the possibility of inflammatory origin.

Many abscesses can be aspirated with CT or MR guidance and/or followed to resolution by serial scans during antibiotic therapy. Repeated drainage may be necessary. Enhancement of the abscess capsule often persists for weeks or months during successful treatment.

Case 409

45-year-old man presenting with a seizure.
(axial, noncontrast scan; SE 2800/90)

Case 410

37-year-old woman presenting with
increasing ataxia.
(axial, noncontrast scan; SE 2500/90)

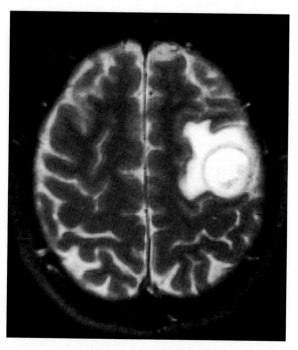

Glioblastoma Multiforme

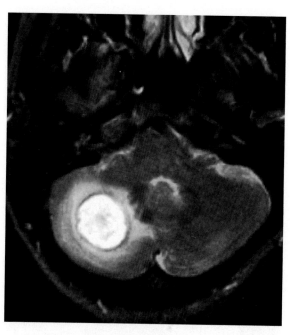

Metastatic Melanoma

Uniformly thin and spherical rims are characteristic of cerebral abscesses. However, a variety of tumors can present a similar appearance. The margin of some gliomas is surprisingly round and regular, as in Case 409. Similarly, occasional metastases are centrally necrotic with a uniform rim of surrounding viable tissue, demonstrated in Case 410.

Cerebral abscesses should be considered in the differential diagnosis of each of these cases. The absence of T1-shortening within the rim of the mass on short TR spin echo images can help to distinguish thin-walled neoplasms from abscesses.

Case 410 is a reminder that metastases are a possibility whenever cerebellar masses are encountered in adults. Hemangioblastoma is another cause for a cystic cerebellar neoplasm in this age group. However, the absence of large vessels and the lack of contact with the pial surface in Case 410 would argue against the diagnosis of hemangioblastoma (see Cases 136-140).

Case 411

62-year-old woman presenting with
headaches and confusion.
(coronal, postcontrast scan; SE 600/15)

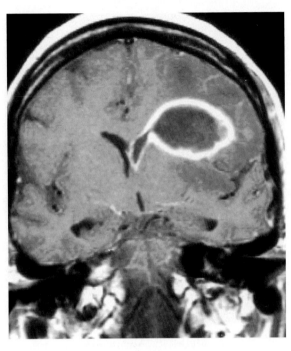

(same patient as Case 405)

Case 412

8-year-old boy presenting with increasing
headaches and vomiting.
(coronal, postcontrast scan; SE 600/15)

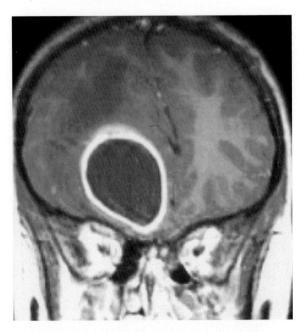

(same patient as Case 407)

The capsule of an abscess enhances intensely, demonstrating the same features of uniform thinness and round contour seen on noncontrast scans. The appearance of the above cases is typical.

Slight thickening and irregularity of the capsule as seen here is well within the spectrum of observed abscess morphologies. Occasional pyogenic abscesses develop a thicker and more irregular capsule, which resembles the periphery of a high grade glioma or metastasis. Fungal abscesses may also demonstrate thick-walled, loculated, or semisolid morphology.

The lesion in Case 411 has reached the margin of the lateral ventricle. Associated ependymal enhancement indicates ventriculitis (see Case 389).

The relatively poor inflammatory response of deep hemispheric white matter may cause the capsule of an abscess to be less developed along the medial wall than along the superficial margin. When present, this feature can help to distinguish an abscess from a tumor.

Abscesses (or cavitating tumors) occasionally rupture into the ventricular system. This event can cause dramatic clinical deterioration (from dissemination of infection) or improvement (from reduction of mass effect).

The inferior portion of the abscess in Case 412 "points" toward the cribriform plate. A history of old trauma was retrospectively obtained, and a fracture of the cribriform plate was identified at surgery as a likely route of infection.

DIFFERENTIAL DIAGNOSIS:
CEREBRAL MASS WITH A THIN, ENHANCING WALL

Case 413

52-year-old man presenting with headaches
and left hemiparesis.
(coronal, postcontrast scan; SE 600/15)

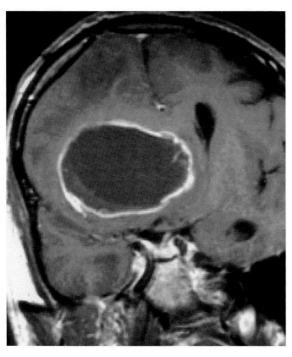

Glioblastoma Multiforme

Case 414

70-year-old woman presenting with ataxia
and confusion.
(coronal, postcontrast scan; SE 700/15)

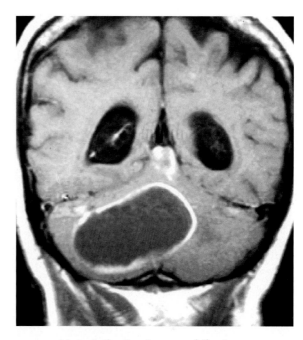

Metastatic Carcinoma of the Lung

Cases 413 and 414 demonstrate that the enhancing rim of some primary and metastatic tumors is quite uniform and may mimic the capsule of an abscess. The lack of precontrast T1-shortening in the margin of the lesion can help to distinguish such tumors, together with the clinical context. In any event, an abscess should remain the first diagnostic consideration when a thin-walled cystic lesion is encountered.

In Case 414, a second lesion involving the superior vermis raises the possibility of metastatic disease. Areas of high signal intensity projecting inferior to the tentorium bilaterally represent phase misregistration artifact from the transverse sinuses (see discussion of Case 17).

Extensive frontal edema and subfalcial herniation are present in Case 413, comparable to Case 412.

Case 415A

33-year-old man presenting with a seizure.
(axial, noncontrast scan; SE 2800/90)

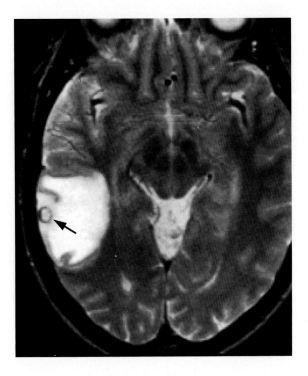

Case 415B

Same patient.
(axial, postcontrast scan; SE 600/15)

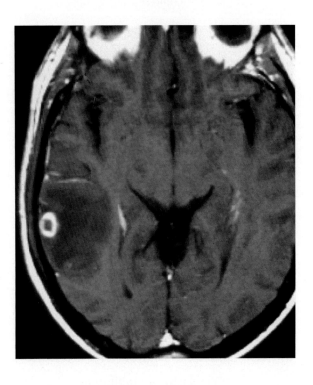

Cysticercosis is the most important parasitic infection of the CNS in this hemisphere. The disease occurs when man serves as an intermediate host for the larval form of the pork tapeworm, *Taenia solium.*

Cysts of cysticercosis may present as solitary lesions or clustered aggregates. "Racemose cysts" are commonly found in the suprasellar, sylvian, or cerebellopontine angle cisterns. Intraventricular cysts are common in all ventricles and may blend with surrounding spinal fluid while obstructing the ventricular system.

Typical parenchymal cysts measure about one centimeter in diameter, as seen in this case *(arrow)*. A small nodule may be visible along the perimeter of the cyst, representing the scolex of the parasite.

The cyst wall in Case 415A is well defined by extensive surrounding edema. Intense peripheral enhancement of the lesion is demonstrated in Case 415B. Enhancement becomes smaller and more solid as cysts degenerate and involute.

Contrast enhancement is observed when cysticerical larvae have incited a host response. Since living larvae are immunologically invisible and do not provoke cerebral edema or enhancement, the presence of these features usually implies larval death. In fact, edema and contrast enhancement may be correlates of successful treatment of cysticercosis.

An enhancing granulomatous stage follows the cystic form of parenchymal cysticercosis. A solitary lesion in this stage may resemble primary or metastatic tumors. Cysticercosis should also be included (along with tuberculosis and other potentially "miliary" infections) in the differential diagnosis of multiple focal enhancing lesions in an adult (see Cases 353 and 354).

Calcification is the final result of the host's response to the death of the larva. This appearance marks the end of the granulomatous phase in cysticercal infection. Lesions of variable activity (e.g., nonenhancing, enhancing, and calcified) may be seen in the same patient.

Case 416

15-year-old girl previously treated for disseminated
suprasellar germinoma.
(axial, noncontrast scan; SE 2500/90)

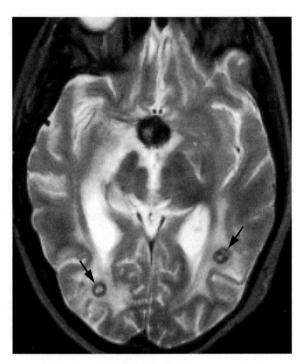

Candida Abscesses

Case 417

14-year-old Mexican boy presenting with seizures.
(axial, noncontrast scan; SE 2500/90)

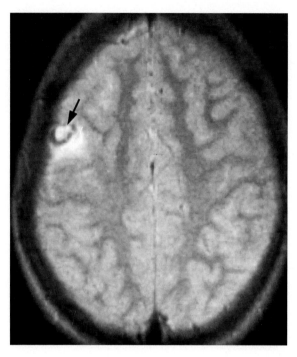

Cysticercosis

As discussed in Cases 407 and 408, the capsules of pyogenic abscesses are usually identifiable as isointense to low intensity structures on T2-weighted MR scans. Fungal and parasitic abscesses also present this appearance, as seen above.

The patient in Case 416 developed systemic candidiasis in association with immunosuppression. The low intensity rims of the fungal abscesses in the occipital lobes *(arrows)* are well outlined by surrounding edema. (A calcified mass is present at the site of the original germinoma in the suprasellar region.) Compare the lesions in Case 416 to the appearance of cavernous angiomas in Cases 629 and 630.

The cysticercosis cyst in Case 417 presents a similar appearance. Again, the wall of the lesion is visible as a rim of low signal intensity, separating the cyst content from reactive edema.

Compare the size and morphology of the above lesions to Cases 422 and 423.

Case 418

37-year-old man with AIDS, presenting
with headaches.
(sagittal, noncontrast scan; SE 600/15)

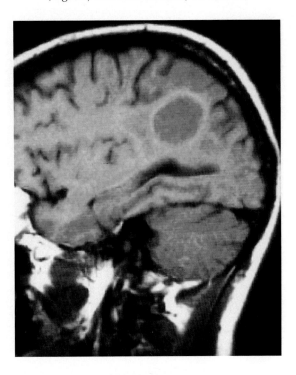

Case 419

44-year-old man with a history of AIDS,
presenting with left hemiparesis.
(axial, noncontrast scan; SE 2800/90)

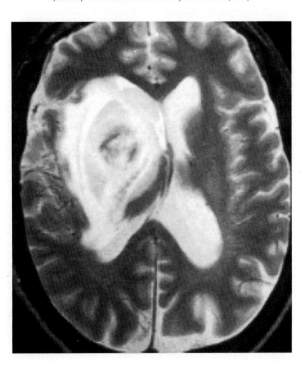

Intracranial masses are reported in over 20% of AIDS patients. Toxoplasmosis usually ranks as the most common etiology, followed by primary CNS lymphoma (see Cases 311-324). The disease is caused by *Toxoplasma gondii,* an environmentally common protozoan that produces mild or subclinical infection in immunocompetent individuals.

Toxoplasmosis usually presents as multiple lesions of variable size and depth. Solitary masses are found in about 20% of cases. Lesions are most commonly located within the basal ganglia or near the gray/white matter junction. Individual masses may appear solid or demonstrate central necrosis. Hemorrhage is common.

The subcortical lesion in Case 418 has a uniformly smooth and thin rim of mild T1-shortening that strongly suggests an abscess cavity (compare to Cases 405 and 406). Case 421 presents a postcontrast scan of the same patient, illustrating the expected correlation with peripheral enhancement.

The deep mass in Case 419 is another of the many potential appearances of cerebral toxoplasmosis in AIDS patients. Patchy zones of T2-shortening are present within the lesion, outlined by extensive surrounding edema. Case 420 presents a postcontrast view of the same mass.

Like primary CNS lymphoma, toxoplasmosis may also involve the corpus callosum.

Case 420

44-year-old man presenting with left hemiparesis.
(axial, postcontrast scan; SE 600/15)

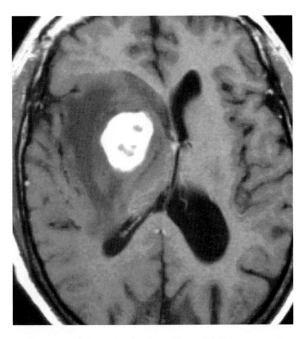

(same patient as Case 419)

Case 421

37-year-old man presenting with headaches.
(axial, postcontrast scan; SE 600/15)

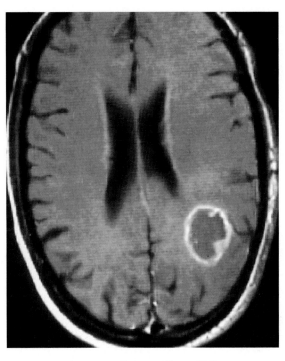

(same patient as Case 418)

Contrast enhancement within cerebral lesions of toxoplasmosis may be solid or peripheral. Neither pattern is specific: the broad spectrum of morphology seen in cerebral toxoplasmosis is overlapped by many other pathologies. Multiloculated abscesses are uncommon in toxoplasmosis and should raise alternate diagnostic possibilities (e.g., tuberculosis or fungal disease).

The hemispheric masses in the cases above could equally well represent primary CNS lymphoma (see Cases 317-320) or other opportunistic pathogens (e.g., fungi). Because of the high incidence of toxoplasmosis in patients with AIDS, antibiotic therapy is often begun empirically when masses are discovered. Biopsy is reserved for nonresponding lesions.

Cerebral toxoplasmosis may wax and wane over several months in response to courses of antimicrobial therapy. Treatment usually causes regression of toxoplasmosis within weeks but does not eradicate the pathogen. When treatment is discontinued (e.g., due to toxicity), recurrence is expected.

Toxoplasmosis and primary CNS lymphoma are among the pathologies to be considered when multiple ganglionic lesions are discovered. Mucormycosis can cause extensive ganglionic edema (usually with little contrast enhancement) in immunocompromised patients or intravenous drug users. Venous infarction due to thrombosis of the internal cerebral vein should also be included in the differential diagnosis.

Case 422

38-year-old man with AIDS presenting with
fever and lethargy.
(sagittal, postcontrast scan; SE 600/17)

Case 423

70-year-old woman presenting with confusion.
(axial, postcontrast scan; SE 600/15)

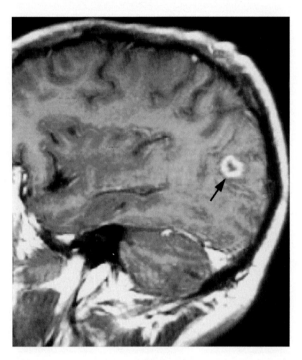

Toxoplasmosis

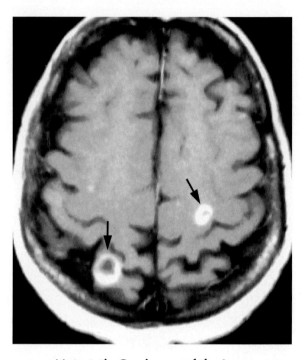

Metastatic Carcinoma of the Lung

Small, rim-enhancing masses like Case 422 are commonly seen in toxoplasmosis. While this appearance is entirely compatible with the diagnosis, it is not specific.

Cysticercosis, candidiasis, and tuberculosis may also present in this manner (see Cases 415 and 416). Case 423 illustrates that metastatic nodules can mimic the same morphology.

Case 424

26-year-old woman.
(axial, postcontrast scan; SE 600/15)

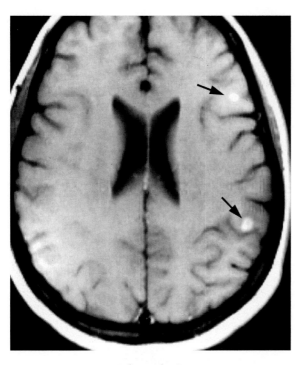

Tuberculosis

Case 425

62-year-old woman.
(coronal, postcontrast scan; SE 600/15)

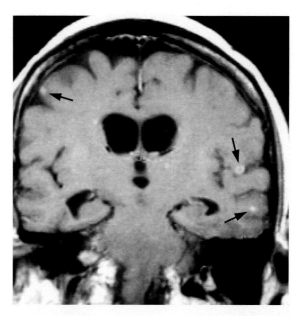

Metastatic Carcinoma of the Breast

As discussed on the preceding page, both inflammatory and neoplastic processes can cause nodules of contrast enhancement at the cortical surface. Tuberculosis should be considered among infectious etiologies, as illustrated in Case 424. Fungal and parasitic infections (e.g., toxoplasmosis and cysticercosis) may present similarly.

Multiple small enhancing superficial nodules can also represent metastatic tumor, either hematogenous parenchymal foci or CSF-borne leptomeningeal deposits. Case 425 demonstrates the former mechanism.

Vascular lesions (e.g., subacute cortial infarcts), small peripheral aneurysms due to vasculitis, and multiple sclerosis are included in this differential diagnosis. Compare the above scans to Cases 490 and 491.

Case 426

26-year-old man presenting with bilateral sensory disturbances, initially suggesting multiple sclerosis. (axial, noncontrast scan; SE 2500/90)

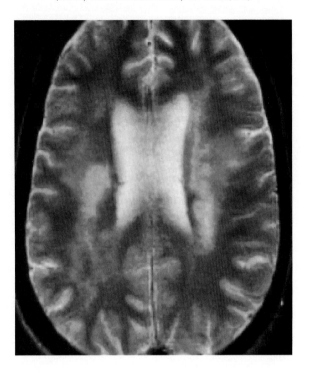

Case 427

33-year-old man with a history of AIDS. (axial, noncontrast scan; SE 2800/90)

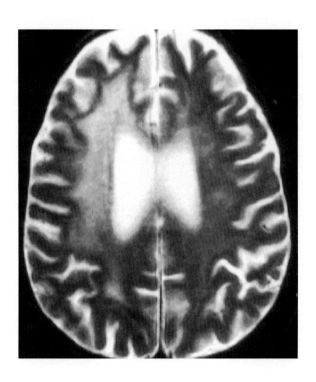

Most of the cerebral masses seen in patients with AIDS are well demonstrated by CT scans. MR is helpful to characterize lesions or detect additional masses that are more easily biopsied than those apparent on a CT study.

An additional imaging advantage of MR in AIDS is the detection of subtle white matter disease. Infection of glial and macrophage-derived cells by the human immunodeficiency virus (HIV) or by an opportunistic pathogen (e.g., CMV) can cause extensive leukoencephalopathy with little or no CT abnormality.

A CT scan in Case 426 was negative. The MR study documents large areas of signal abnormality throughout midhemispheric white matter. This soft, symmetrical pattern of bihemispheral white matter pathology is a common finding in HIV encephalitis. CMV can also cause this appearance.

Case 427 illustrates that white matter involvement by HIV encephalitis may be strikingly unilateral. The affected region of the right centrum semiovale demonstrates the same hazy quality seen bilaterally in Case 426.

Extension into the corpus callosum can occur with either unilateral or bilateral disease. A similar combination of hemispheric and callosal lesions in a patient with AIDS can be caused by progressive multifocal leukoencephalopathy.

In both of the above cases, the ventricles and sulci are abnormally large for the patient's age. This is a common finding on cerebral scans of patients with AIDS and may be the only apparent abnormality.

Cranial CT and MR scans in AIDS patients may also demonstrate sinusitis, multicystic enlargement of the parotid glands, and cervical adenopathy. These findings support the diagnosis in the appropriate clinical context.

Case 428A

26-year-old man presenting with "loss of muscle control."
(axial, noncontrast scan; SE 2500/45)

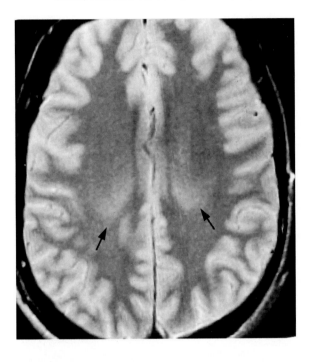

Case 428B

Same patient.
(axial, noncontrast scan; SE 2500/90)

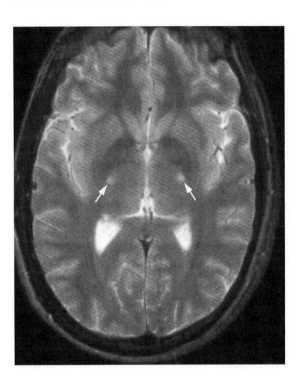

Amyotrophic lateral sclerosis (ALS) is an idiopathic degenerative disorder of upper and lower motor neurons. The clinical presentation is characterized by progressive dysfunction of the corticospinal tracts.

MR scans may be surprisingly negative in the presence of major neurological impairment. Other ALS patients demonstrate bihemispheral abnormality extending from the motor cortex to the brainstem.

In Case 428A, vague areas of increased signal intensity are seen at the junction of the centrum semiovale and the corona radiata bilaterally *(arrows)* This appearance reflects loss of myelin and increased water content along the course of the motor axons originating from the frontoparietal cortex. Compare this appearance to that of HIV encephalitis in Cases 426 and 427.

Signal abnormality within the corticospinal tract becomes increasingly concentrated and better defined as it passes inferiorly into the hemisphere. Case 428B illustrates strikingly sharp and symmetrical foci of abnormal intensity within the posterior limb of the internal capsule bilaterally *(arrows)*.

This finding should be correlated with ascending and descending extension along the corticospinal tracts to suggest the diagnosis of ALS. Other etiologies can cause symmetrical foci of abnormal signal limited to the level of the internal capsule (see Cases 429 and 430). Progressive multifocal leukoencephalopathy has been reported to produce unilateral or bilateral zones of abnormal intensity within the corticospinal tracts, resembling the appearance of ALS. Wallerian degeneration can also cause signal abnormality along the course of the corticospinal tract, as illustrated in Case 541-1.

Some cases of ALS demonstrate reduced signal intensity within involved cortex on T2-weighted images. This finding is typically uniform and laminar but localized, often affecting the precentral gyrus. The low cortical intensity may reflect an increased concentration of minerals associated with neuronal degeneration.

The above patient is younger than the average age at presentation of ALS, which is near 50. The disease is usually progressive and fatal.

DIFFERENTIAL DIAGNOSIS:
SYMMETRICAL HIGH SIGNAL FOCI NEAR THE POSTERIOR LIMBS OF THE INTERNAL CAPSULES ON T2-WEIGHTED IMAGES

Case 429

15-year-old girl presenting with headaches.
(axial, noncontrast scan; SE 3000/90)

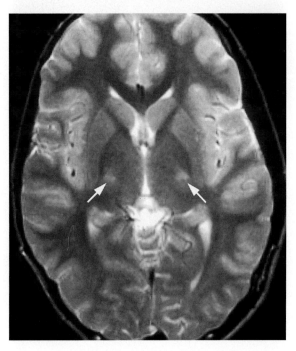

Normal Variant (Corticospinal Tract)

Case 430

46-year-old man with a history of alcoholism,
now presenting with obtundation.
(axial, noncontrast scan; SE 2500/70)

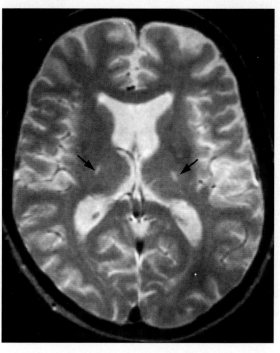

Extrapontine Myelinolysis
(same patient as Case 375)

A small area of a relatively high signal intensity may be seen within the posterior limb of the internal capsule on T2-weighted scans as a normal variant. This focal zone of relatively long T2 values occupies the posterior portion of the posterior limb and is bilaterally symmetrical *(arrows,* Case 429). The finding has been ascribed to relatively lower myelin density in the region of large axons constituting the corticospinal tract.

Clues to distinguish this incidental variant from bilateral capsular pathology (as in Case 428) include (1) relative isointensity of the variant on long TR, short TE images, on which true capsular lesions are usually well appreciated and (2) lack of contiguous extension of the abnormality to adjacent sections (see discussion of Case 428).

The symmetrical foci of signal abnormality in Case 430 *(arrows)* are caused by osmotic myelinolysis affecting the lateral portions of the thalami. Extrapontine myelinolysis occurs in the same clinical context as central pontine myelinolysis (see Case 375) and may be found in association with or independent of brainstem disease. Symmetrical hemispheric involvement may include the basal ganglia and/or thalami.

As illustrated on the preceding page, amyotrophic lateral sclerosis often causes small, symmetrical lesions within the posterior limb of the internal capsule. However, the paired abnormalities of ALS can be followed caudally into the cerebral peduncles and pons, unlike the findings in the above cases.

Case 431

28-year-old woman presenting with left
homonymous hemianopsia.
(axial, postcontrast scan; SE 600/15)

Case 432

43-year-old woman presenting with aphasia.
(coronal, noncontrast scan; SE 2500/90)

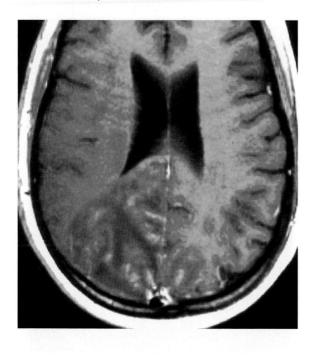

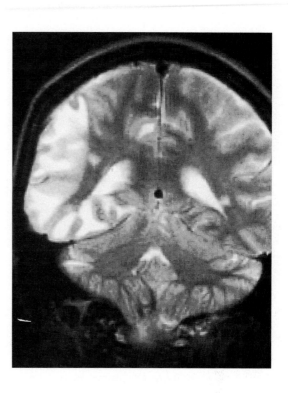

Systemic lupus erythematosus (SLE) may present a wide variety of MR appearances. Scans in many patients with clinically definite disease are normal. In other cases, nonspecific atrophy is seen, with or without a history of steroid treatment.

Focal parenchymal lesions may take two very different forms. Cases 431 and 432 illustrate large zones of cortical and subcortical edema. Overlying superficial contrast enhancement is present in Case 431. This appearance is typical of acute lupus cerebritis. The pattern is nonspecific, resembling encephalitis of other etiologies or subacute infarction (compare to granulomatous angiitis in Case 503). Such lesions are often rapidly and completely reversible, with no clinical or MR residual.

Another common pattern of parenchymal abnormality on MR scans of patients with SLE is seen in Case 433. Multiple small foci of signal abnormality are present in subcortical and deep hemispheric white matter. These lesions usually do not enhance with contrast material and may represent old, burned-out inflammatory foci or small infarcts secondary to vasculitis. This appearance is also nonspecific (see Cases 433-436).

Whether lesions are extensive, as in the above cases, or focal as in Case 433, the combination of cortical and subcortical involvement can be a clue to the diagnosis of a connective tissue disorder. In a younger patient, this same pattern of multifocal, patchy, and partially reversible lesions would raise the question of a mitochondrial encephalomyopathy (see Case 447).

Antiphospholipid antibodies are often present in patients with SLE, and infarcts due to coagulopathy probably account for many of the cerebral lesions in such cases.

Case 433

54-year-old woman presenting with vague complaints and a high sedimentation rate.
(axial, noncontrast scan; SE 2500/45)

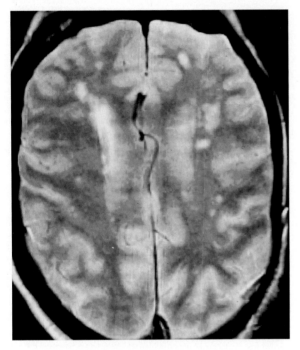

Systemic Lupus Erythematosus

Case 434

34-year-old woman presenting with bilateral spasticity of arms and legs.
(axial, noncontrast scan; SE 2500/45)

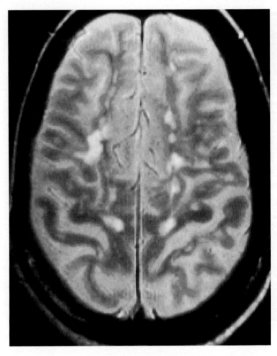

Multiple Sclerosis

A number of pathologies can involve subcortical white matter. Relatively large lesions in this location may be seen in progressive multifocal leukoencephalopathy, acute disseminated encephalomyelitis, multiple sclerosis, cerebral metastases, arterial or venous infarction, and tuberous sclerosis (see Cases 335, 336, 361-372, 644, and 760-763).

Smaller foci of subcortical signal abnormality may likewise arise in a variety of contexts. As discussed on the preceding page and illustrated in Case 433, systemic lupus erythematosus may involve subcortical white matter in this manner.

Case 434 demonstrates that the lesions of multiple sclerosis are often not confined to the periventricular regions. The association of small to medium-sized subcortical signal abnormalities with cerebral atrophy in Case 434 could equally well be seen in a case of long-standing lupus cerebritis.

Shearing injuries (diffuse axonal injury) can likewise present as multiple subcortical foci of high signal intensity on T2-weighted images (see Case 572). Multifocal infarction should also be included in the differential diagnosis (see Case 573).

DIFFERENTIAL DIAGNOSIS (CONTINUED):
SMALL FOCI OF SUBCORTICAL SIGNAL ABNORMALITY

Case 435

53-year-old woman presenting with fatigue
and myalgias.
(axial, noncontrast scan; SE 2800/90)

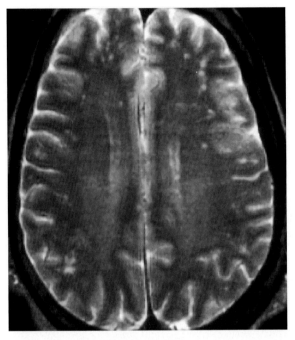

Lyme Disease

Case 436

58-year-old woman presenting with hilar
adenopathy.
(axial, noncontrast scan; SE 2800/90)

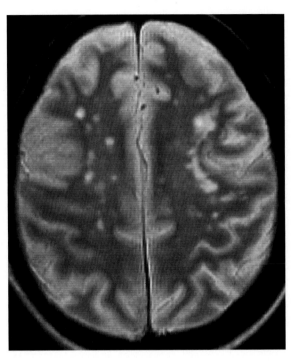

Sarcoidosis

Lyme disease, due to infection by the spirochete *Borrelia burgdorferi*, is among the inflammatory disorders that have been associated with multiple small, subcortical lesions on MR studies. Case 435 illustrates a patient with clinically definite Lyme disease and no other known explanation for the foci of long T2 in subcortical white matter. However, as emphasized here and on the preceding page, this is a nonspecific appearance.

Neurological presentations of Lyme disease also include meningitis and cranial neuritis (especially optic neuritis and Bell's palsy). Postcontrast scans may demonstrate abnormal enhancement of meninges and/or involved nerves.

Parenchymal involvement by sarcoidosis can closely mimic multiple sclerosis. Foci of signal abnormality may be found in periventricular regions or in subcortical white matter, as in Case 436. Localized contrast enhancement may occur.

Sarcoidosis may also present as meningeal disease, usually taking the form of uniform dural thickening (resembling Case 394). Associated meningeal enhancement may

help to distinguish the parenchymal lesions of sarcoidosis from multiple sclerosis. Focal involvement of the hypothalamus and/or pituitary infundibulum is a third form of intracranial sarcoidosis, which should be included in the differential diagnosis of Cases 225 and 226. Finally, like Lyme disease, sarcoidosis can present as a cranial neuritis (most often of nerves II and VII).

Another inflammatory disorder that may cause multiple small foci of signal abnormality is Behçet disease. This multisystem immune-mediated vasculitis presents clinically with the triad of oral and genital ulceration and ocular inflammation. Some of the cerebral lesions in such cases may demonstrate focal contrast enhancement.

Miliary subcortical metastases should also be considered in the differential diagnosis on these pages. Postcontrast scans with high contrast dose and/or magnetization transfer suppression may demonstrate confirmatory enhancement. Many focal, subcortical metastases do not significantly prolong T2 values and are poorly seen on noncontrast images.

Case 437

10-month-old girl examined because of
diffuse hypotonia.
(sagittal, noncontrast scan; SE 600/20)

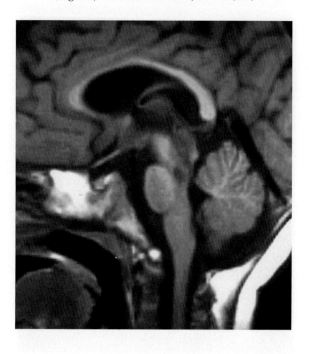

Case 438

1-year-old boy presenting with truncal
instability and nystagmus.
(axial, noncontrast scan; SE 3000/90)

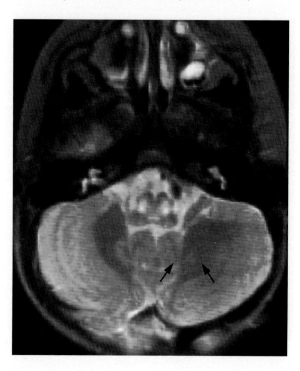

Leigh's disease (also called subacute necrotizing encephalomyelopathy) is a metabolic disorder caused by deficiency in one of the enzymes necessary for oxidative metabolism within mitochondria (e.g., cytochrome *c* oxidase, pyruvate carboxylase, and pyruvate dehydrogenase). Infants with this disease typically present during the first two years of life with ataxia, nystagmus, dystonia, and/or motor weakness. High levels of pyruvate and lactic acid are present in the serum and spinal fluid of affected individuals.

Brainstem lesions are found on MR scans in the majority of children with Leigh's disease. Case 437 demonstrates typical involvement of the dorsal midbrain and pons, with abnormally low signal intensity and moderate mass effect surrounding the aqueduct. Brainstem lesions are usually strikingly symmetrical on axial images, with high signal intensity on T2-weighted scans. Paired lesions are seen at the medullary level in Case 438 *(arrows)*.

All levels of the brainstem can be involved separately or simultaneously in Leigh's disease. Associated spinal cord lesions are common.

Case 439

1-year-old boy presenting with hypotonia
and ataxia.
(axial, noncontrast scan; SE 3000/90)

Case 440

10-month-old girl presenting with hypotonia.
(axial, noncontrast scan; SE 3000/90)

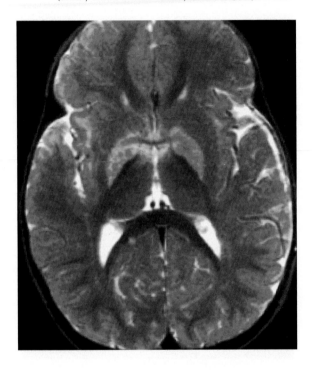

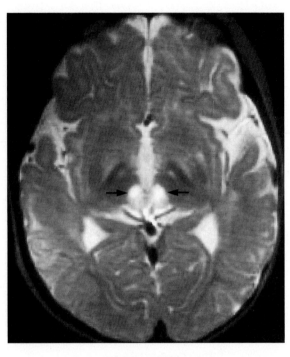

(same patient as Case 437)

The basal ganglia often demonstrate symmetrical signal abnormality in Leigh's disease, usually accompanying brainstem lesions but occasionally in isolation. The lenticular nuclei are commonly involved, with the globus pallidus particularly affected. Case 439 illustrates this pattern.

In Case 440, prominent symmetrical lesions are present within the thalami *(arrows)*. The pathological findings in Leigh's disease resemble those of Wernicke's encephalopathy in adults, which frequently demonstrates thalamic involvement.

The ganglionic and brainstem lesions of Leigh's disease usually do not enhance with contrast material.

Case 441

1-month-old boy presenting with hypotonia.
(axial, noncontrast scan; SE 3000/75)

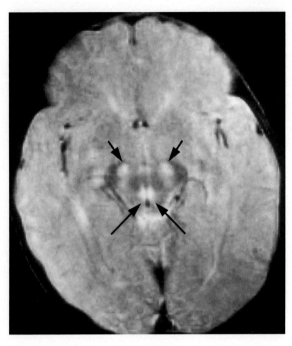

Leigh's Disease

Case 442

8-year-old boy presenting with bilateral
hearing loss.
(axial, noncontrast scan; SE 2900/30)

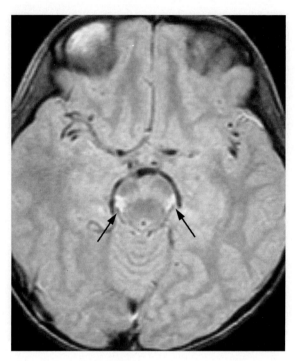

Adrenoleukodystrophy
(same patient as Case 380)

Paired, bilateral brainstem foci of signal abnormality are characteristic of Leigh's disease, as seen in Case 441. Lesions within the cerebral peduncles *(short arrows)* accompany the more typical involvement of the tegmentum *(long arrows)* in this instance.

Demyelinating and dysmyelinating disorders can also cause symmetrical zones of abnormal signal intensity within the brainstem, reflecting involvement of specific tracts. The ascending auditory pathways are often affected by adrenoleukodystrophy, as illustrated in Case 442. The bilateral foci of high signal intensity along the lateral margin of the brainstem represent the lateral lemnisci, which carry auditory in-

formation from the cochlear nuclei to the inferior colliculi. More rostral involvement of the auditory pathways (inferior colliculus, brachium of the inferior colliculus, and medial geniculate body) can be demonstrated in many cases.

Sites of active brainstem dysmyelination in adrenoleukodystrophy may demonstrate intense contrast enhancement, unlike the lesions of Leigh's disease. The usual age at presentation also distinguishes between these disorders: adrenoleukodystrophy typically presents between 5 and 10 years of age, while Leigh's disease becomes apparent during infancy.

DIFFERENTIAL DIAGNOSIS:
SYMMETRICAL LESIONS OF THE GLOBUS PALLIDUS IN A CHILD

Case 443

1-year-old boy presenting with hypotonia
and ataxia.
(axial, noncontrast scan; SE 2800/90)

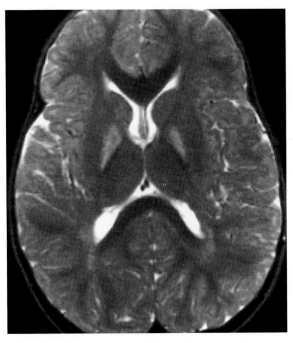

Leigh's Disease

Case 444

6-year-old boy presenting with abnormal gait.
(axial, noncontrast scan; SE 2500/90)

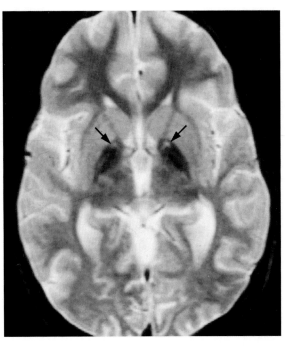

Hallervorden-Spatz Disease

Symmetrical lesions within the basal ganglia suggest an anoxic, toxic, or metabolic etiology. Carbon monoxide poisoning and other impairments of oxidative phosphorylation typically present with bilateral abnormality in the globus pallidus (see Case 554). As discussed previously, Leigh's disease is included in this category, illustrated by Case 443.

In Case 444, the bilateral abnormality is one of *low* signal intensity within the globi pallidi on a T2-weighted scan. This degree of T2-shortening should not be seen in a child. The smaller zones of higher signal intensity within the darker background have been described as an "eye of the tiger" appearance *(arrows)*.

These features are all characteristic of Hallervorden-Spatz disease, a metabolic disorder that causes degeneration of neurons in the globus pallidus and may also involve the substantia nigra. Associated deposition of pigments and/or metals probably accounts for the observed T2-shortening. Most patients with this disease experience progressive motor dysfunction and spasticity as children or adolescents, with subsequent development of dementia.

The proportion of "dark" and "bright" areas within the globus pallidus on the T2-weighted scans may vary from patient to patient, with the stage of disease in a given patient, and with field strength: at low fields, high signal intensity may predominate on T2-weighted images.

The differential diagnosis of abnormally low signal intensity within the globus pallidus (and substantia nigra) of a child on T2-weighted scans includes hypothyroidism. A similar appearance can be seen in adults with Wilson's disease (accompanied by *high* intensity within the putamen).

Amino acidopathies (e.g., methylmalonic acidemia) and mitochondrial encephalomyopathies other then Leigh's disease can also present with bilateral lesions of the globus pallidus in children. Symmetrical lesions predominantly involving the putamen would raise consideration of other toxic/metabolic etiologies such as Wilson's disease and methanol ingestion.

Unilateral or bilateral zones of T2-prolongation within the globus pallidus may be seen in neurofibromatosis type 1 (see Cases 764 and 765).

Case 445

56-year-old woman with chronic hepatitis.
(sagittal, noncontrast scan; SE 600/20)

Case 446

64-year-old man with a history of alcoholism.
(coronal, noncontrast scan; SE 700/15)

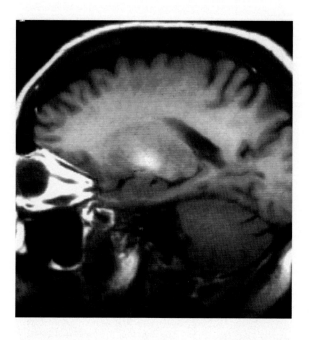

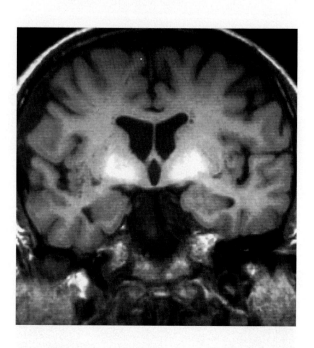

A number of metabolic disorders can cause symmetrical lesions of the basal ganglia and thalami in adults as well as in children. Wernicke's encephalopathy (due to thiamine deficiency) resembles Leigh's disease pathologically and in anatomical distribution. Symmetrical lesions occur in the medial thalami, along the walls and floor of the third ventricle, and within the periaqueductal region of the midbrain. In addition (and in contrast to Leigh's disease), the mamillary bodies are characteristically involved, demonstrating signal abnormality, contrast enhancement, and/or atrophy as the disorder progresses.

Wilson's disease, or "hepatolenticular degeneration," is an autosomal recessive disorder caused by low levels of ceruloplasmin, a serum protein that transports copper. Abnormal copper deposition occurs in the deep cerebral and cerebellar nuclei (particularly in the lenticular nucleus), as well as in the liver. Symmetrical involvement of the caudate nucleus, putamen, globus pallidus, thalamus, rostral brainstem, and dentate nucleus may be seen in variable combinations. High signal intensity and eventual atrophy of the putamen are typically apparent on T2-weighted scans.

A rare cause of symmetrically increased signal intensity within the basal ganglia of adults on T2-weighted scans is Creutzfeldt-Jakob disease (spongiform encephalopathy). The finding can be a clue to the etiology of a rapidly progressive dementia. See Cases 455 and 456 for discussion of basal ganglia changes in Huntington's disease.

More common than any of these disorders is symmetrical signal abnormality within the basal ganglia due to chronic hepatic disease, as illustrated in Cases 445 and 446. T1-shortening may be seen within the globus pallidus (as above), putamen, and other deep nuclei in various hepatocerebral syndromes, including alcoholic cirrhosis. The high signal intensity in these regions on noncontrast T1-weighted images is probably due to the deposition of paramagnetic minerals. (CT scans and T2-weighted images in such cases are usually normal.) The finding has been reported to resolve following liver transplantation.

An appearance similar to the above images may be seen in patients who are receiving total parenteral nutrition. Deposition of manganese is believed to be a key factor in this setting. Idiopathic calcification of the basal ganglin can also cause symmetrical T1-shortening.

MITOCHONDRIAL ENCEPHALOMYOPATHIES

Case 447A

16-year-old girl presenting with a stroke.
(axial, noncontrast scan; SE 2500/30)

Case 447B

Same patient.
(axial, noncontrast scan; SE 2500/90)

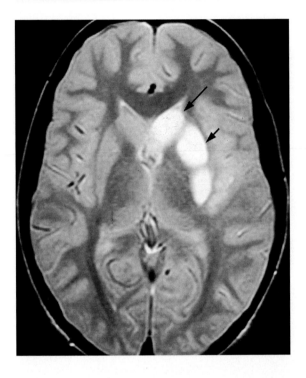

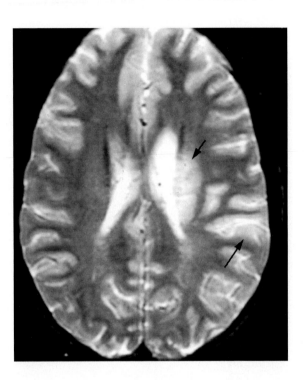

A number of systemic disorders with prominent neurological components are caused by abnormalities in oxidative metabolism within mitochondria. These multisystem diseases are characterized pathologically by the presence of "ragged red fibers" in muscle biopsies. Among the clinical syndromes in this category are Kearn's-Sayre syndrome, mitochondrial myopathy, MERRF or MERRLA (*m*yoclonus, *e*pilepsy, *r*agged *r*ed *f*ibers, and *l*actic *a*cidosis), and MELAS (*m*itochondrial myopathy, *e*ncephalopathy, *l*actic *a*cidosis, and *s*troke-like episodes).

MR findings in patients with mitochondrial encephalopathies are variable. Some cases demonstrate bilateral signal abnormality within the basal ganglia and brainstem, as illustrated on previous pages in Leigh's disease. Scans in other patients evidence diffuse, symmetrical T2 prolongation throughout cerebral white matter, resembling a leukodystrophy. Still other cases present with stroke-like lesions, illustrated by Case 447.

In most cases of MELAS, areas of cerebral infarction are seen bilaterally, with predilection for the posterior portions of the hemispheres. The infarcts often do not conform precisely to major arterial distributions. Subcortical involvement is common. Lesions may appear and disappear, sug-gesting a reversible insult. These features together with multiplicity of infarction in space and time should suggest the possibility of mitochondrial encephalomyopathy in a young patient.

Case 447 is somewhat unusual in that a single acute infarct is demonstrated involving portions of the distribution of the left middle cerebral artery. The caudate nucleus (*long arrow,* Case 447A) and putamen (*short arrow,* Case 447A) are edematous, with additional zones of signal abnormality within the corona radiata and inferior parietal cortex (*short* and *long arrows,* Case 447B). The subsequent clinical evaluation of this patient documented lactic acidosis and ragged red fibers on muscle biopsy.

Other pathologies that can resemble the MR appearance of mitochondrial encephalomyopathies are hypertensive encephalopathy (see Case 464) and systemic lupus erythematosus (see Cases 431 and 432). Type 1 neurofibromatosis may present with patchy areas of signal abnormality in the basal ganglia similar to some cases of mitochondrial disease (see Cases 764 and 765).

See Case 482 for discussion of the differential diagnosis of infarction in children and young adults.

Case 448A

8-year-old girl, four years after surgery and radiation therapy for a right occipital ependymoma, now presenting with left homonymous hemianopsia.
(axial, noncontrast scan; SE 2500/90)

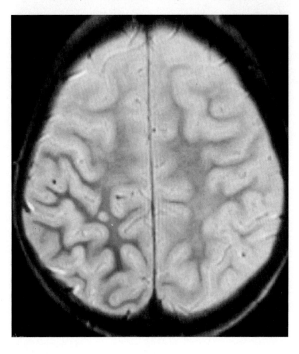

Case 448B

Same patient.
(sagittal, postcontrast scan SE 600/15)

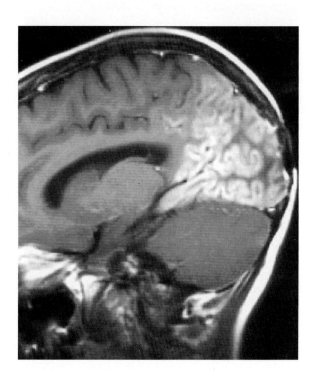

A spectrum of MR changes may be seen following cerebral radiation. Alterations can range from mild, generalized atrophy to the focal mass lesions of radiation necrosis (see Case 449). Intermediate patterns may be encountered with localized or multifocal abnormalities that are not mass-like.

Endothelial cells are among the most radiosensitive tissues in the brain. Damage to small vessels may lead to the deposition of calcium and other minerals.

Case 448 illustrates the development of microangiography within a radiation field. Low signal intensity suggesting mild mineralization is present throughout white matter of the right parietooccipital region in Case 448A. Subcortical iron accumulation in an area of recent infarction may contribute to this appearance. Mineralizing microangiography is often associated with a coarser pattern of multifocal calcifications near the gray/white matter junction.

The postcontrast scan in Case 448B demonstrates gyriform enhancement, compatible with small vessel compromise causing subacute cortical ischemia. Recent or subclinical seizure activity would be another possible explanation for the striking cortical enhancement involving several vascular distributions.

Some cases of radiation microangiopathy respond to steroid therapy, while others are progressive. The patient illustrated here recovered almost completely within one month.

Other patterns of abnormality occurring after radiation therapy include diffuse white matter damage (see Case 517) and the development of "hemorrhagic radiation vasculopathy" resembling scattered cavernous angiomas (see discussion of Cases 629 and 630).

Case 449A

28-year-old man, two years after surgery and radiation therapy for medulloblastoma of the right cerebellar hemisphere, now presenting with recurrent ataxia.
(coronal, noncontrast scan; SE 600/15)

Case 449B

Same patient.
(coronal, postcontrast scan; SE 600/15)

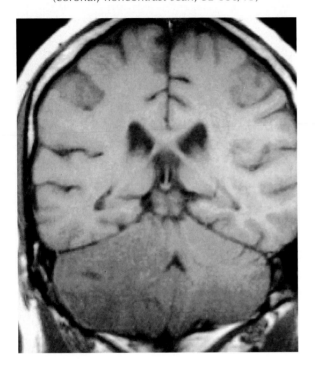

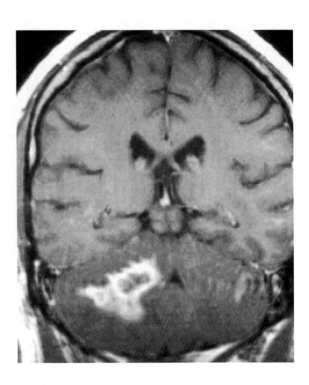

Necrosis of brain tissue due to radiation damage may present years after treatment as an enlarging mass stimulating recurrence of neoplasm. The morphology, contrast enhancement, and associated edema of such lesions can be indistinguishable from a tumor on MR images. In many cases a combination of radiation necrosis and recurrent tumor is present. Low metabolic activity within the lesion demonstrated by positron emission tomography or single photon emission CT supports the possibility of radiation necrosis, but some recurrent tumors are also hypometabolic.

In Case 449A, poorly defined edema and mass effect are seen within the right cerebellar hemisphere. Following contrast injection, confluent central enhancement is apparent. (Compare Case 449B to the peripheral, gyriform enhancement in Case 448B.)

Since adult hemispheric medulloblastomas may demonstrate indistinct or shaggy margins of enhancement, the appearance in Case 449B is compatible with recurrent tumor. However, at surgery the mass was found to consist entirely of radiation necrosis.

Case 450

22-year-old woman presenting with seizures.
(coronal, noncontrast scan; SE 2800/90)

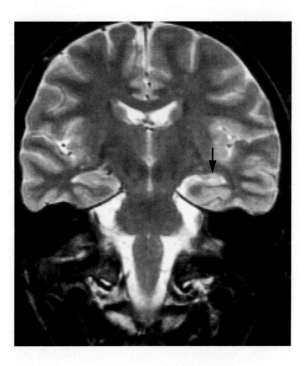

Case 451

40-year-old woman with seizures.
(coronal, noncontrast scan; partition from
three-dimensional T1-weighted GRE sequence)

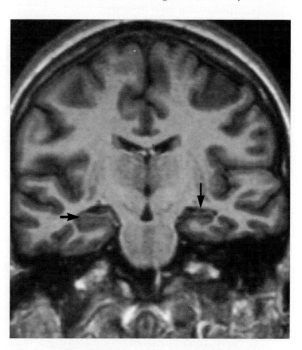

Magnetic resonance imaging is routinely used to screen for structural lesions of the brain in patients with seizures.

A second goal of MR scans in the context of epilepsy is careful assessment of the hippocampal formations. Many patients suffer from seizures of temporal lobe origin that are associated with neuronal loss and gliosis of the ipsilateral hippocampus. The etiology of such hippocampal "sclerosis" is not well established, but the relationship to subsequent seizures is strong. As a result, resection of the anterior temporal lobe may be recommended to epileptic patients whose seizures are correlated with structural changes in the hippocampus. Current studies indicate that seizures can be controlled or reduced by surgery in the majority of such cases.

Traditional reference to this entity as "mesial temporal sclerosis" should probably be replaced by the more specific name of "hippocampal sclerosis." The benign degenerative changes in this syndrome are largely confined to the hippocampus. More generalized abnormality in the medial temporal region should suggest an alternative diagnosis (see Cases 452 and 453).

The hippocampal formations are well visualized in cross section on thin, coronal scans that are angled so as to be perpendicular to the long axis of the temporal lobe. Hippocampal sclerosis may present two major features on such studies. A focal area of long T2 values may be directly demonstrated within the hippocampus, as seen on the left in Case 450 *(arrow)*. On thick sections partial volume of the temporal horn, enlarged due to hippocampal atrophy, may contribute to perceived hippocampal brightness.

More reliable is the demonstration of reduced hippocampal volume. Thin, oblique coronal images (at approximately the level of the red nucleus) will provide several sections over which the bulk of the left and right hippocampus can be visually compared and/or measured. Case 451 demonstrates convincing atrophy of the left hippocampal formation *(long arrow)* as compared to the right *(short arrow)*.

DIFFERENTIAL DIAGNOSIS:
FOCAL SIGNAL ABNORMALITY IN THE MEDIAL TEMPORAL LOBE OF A PATIENT WITH SEIZURES

Case 452

2-year-old boy with myoclonic seizures.
(coronal, noncontrast scan; SE 3000/90)

Case 453

10-year-old boy with temporal lobe seizures.
(coronal, non-contrast scan; SE 3000/45)

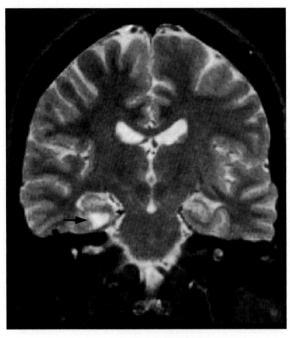

Low Grade Astrocytoma

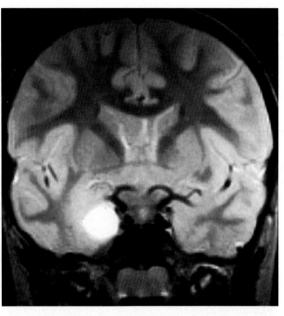

Ganglioglioma

Awareness of mesial temporal sclerosis as a potential diagnosis in epileptic patients may confuse the interpretation of small mass lesions in the medial temporal lobe. In each of the above cases, an incorrect diagnosis of benign sclerosis was made at an outside institution.

Signal abnormality in true mesial temporal sclerosis should be localized to the hippocampus (with possible involvement of subjacent collateral white matter) and associated with hippocampal atrophy. In Case 452, the small lesion is clearly inferior to the hippocampus (see Cases 77 and 78 for other examples of focal gliomas). Case 453 demonstrates mass effect throughout the medial temporal region, excluding the diagnosis of hippocampal sclerosis.

Case 454A

78-year-old woman presenting with tremor,
rigidity, and akinesia.
(axial, noncontrast scan; SE 2800/45)

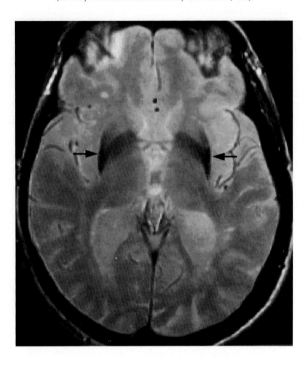

Case 454B

Same patient.
(axial, noncontrast scan; SE 2800/90)

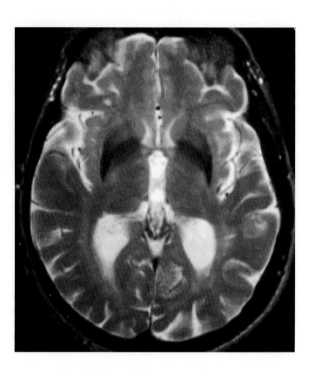

MR scans in most patients with Parkinson's disease demonstrate only atrophy and nonspecific age-related changes. Careful attention to the midbrain may demonstrate abnormal thinning of the pars compacta of the substantia nigra, a relatively high signal intensity band interposed between the lower signal intensity of the pars reticulata anteriorly and the red nucleus posteriorly on T2-weighted scans. This thinning correlates with the pathological loss of dopaminergic neurons in the substantia nigra, which is the primary cause of the disease.

Some patients with severe or drug-resistant Parkinson's disease and others with "Parkinson's plus" syndromes (e.g., striatonigral degeneration, Shy Drager syndrome, and progressive supranuclear palsy) may show abnormally prominent low signal intensity within the basal ganglia on long TR images. Case 454 demonstrates this finding. The globus pallidus is unusually dark bilaterally, even allowing for the patient's age. More important and specific is the prominent low intensity within the posterior and lateral portions of the putamen bilaterally (*arrows,* Case 454A). This signal loss likely reflects susceptibility effects due to degenerative deposition of pigment and/or metals, especially iron.

Susceptibility effects are less prominent on MR scans performed at lower field strengths. On such studies, symmetrically *increased* signal intensity may be seen in the putamen on T2-weighted scans of patients with Parkinson's syndromes. This appearance presumably reflects neuronal loss and gliosis, analogous to changes that typically occur in Wilson's disease.

The above patient was clinically categorized as having uncomplicated but severe Parkinson's disease, which proved to be unresponsive to therapy with dopamine agonists.

Case 455

61-year-old man presenting with dementia.
(coronal, noncontrast scan; SE 800/20)

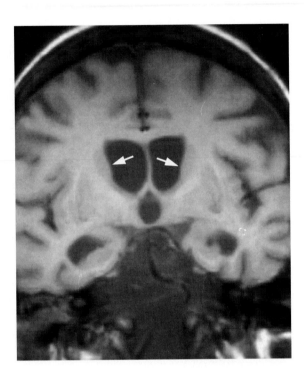

Case 456

57-year-old woman presenting with choreoathetosis and confusion.
(coronal, noncontrast scan; SE 600/20)

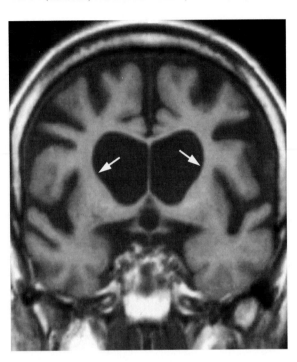

The normal caudate head bulges into the lateral aspect of the frontal horn to cause a medially convex margin. Atrophy of the caudate nucleus in advanced Huntington's disease causes this curvature to flatten or reverse, as seen above *(arrows)*. The putamen may also be severely atrophic in patients with this disorder. Associated ventricular and sulcal enlargement is often present.

On long TR images of patients with Huntington's disease the caudate nucleus and putamen may demonstrate either high or low signal intensity, depending on the predominance of neuronal loss and gliosis versus degenerative deposition of minerals and pigment. The signal intensity of these structures also depends to some extent on field

strength, with low intensity due to susceptibility effects more prominent at higher fields. Huntington's disease should be considered among the degenerative and metabolic disorders producing symmetrical signal abnormality within the basal ganglia.

The characteristic CT/MR finding of caudate atrophy is a late development in Huntington's disease and is not seen in presymptomatic carriers. Positron emission tomography can identify abnormal caudate metabolism before atrophy appears on CT or MR scans. A genetic marker for Huntington's disease has also been found and may enable screening of individuals at risk for inheriting this autosomal dominant disorder.

CEREBRAL ATROPHY

Case 457

75-year-old man presenting with dementia.
(sagittal, noncontrast scan; SE 700/17)

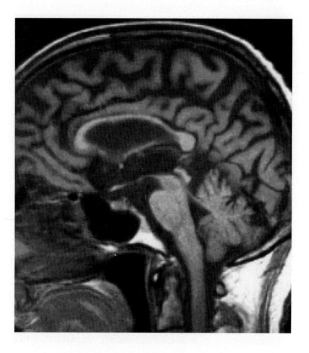

Case 458

65-year-old woman presenting with a TIA.
(axial, noncontrast scan; SE 2500/90)

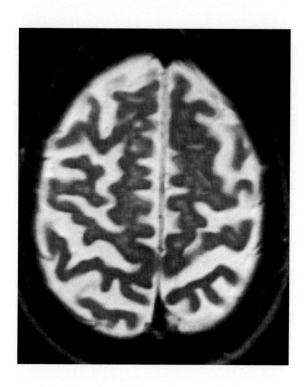

Cerebral atrophy is demonstrated on CT and MR scans by diffuse enlargement of ventricles and subarachnoid spaces. The relative degree of ventricular and sulcal enlargement is usually similar. Disproportionate prominence of the ventricular component raises the question of hydrocephalus (see Cases 656 to 658).

A number of conditions may cause enlargement of cerebral sulci resembling atrophy. Alcoholic "atrophy" is common, possibly due to nutritional or hydration factors as well as to direct effects of ethanol. In some patients the enlarged sulci return to a more normal size after successful treatment.

Other circumstances associated with abnormal enlargement of cerebral sulci include malnutrition (e.g., anorexia nervosa), high doses of exogeneous or endogeneous steroids, multiple sclerosis, lupus cerebritis, AIDS, chronic renal disease, radiation therapy, prior head trauma, anoxia, and presenile dementing disorders. When a young patient presents with enlarged sulci, these possibilities should be considered.

Localized atrophy of the hippocampal formation, amygdala, and temporal lobe is characteristic of Alzheimer's disease, the major cause of dementia in this country. Affected patients usually demonstrate enlargement of the temporal horns and subarachnoid spaces (e.g., hippocampal fissure) in the medial temporal region. Conversely, absence of temporal lobe atrophy argues against the diagnosis of Alzheimer's disease as an explanation for dementia. Evidence of medial temporal volume loss is more useful than generalized measures of atrophy in separating patients with Alzheimer's disease from cognitively normal patients of the same age.

The diagnosis of Pick's disease may be suggested when localized frontal atrophy is associated with prominent atrophy of the inferior and middle temporal gyri. Classic Pick's disease demonstrates strikingly thin gyri separated by gaping sulci in the frontal and temporal lobes. However, these "knife-like" gyri are not present in all cases. Furthermore, most cases with gross pathology suggesting Pick's disease are found to represent Alzheimer's disease microscopically.

Case 459

7-year-old boy presenting with ataxia.
(sagittal, noncontrast scan; SE 800/17)

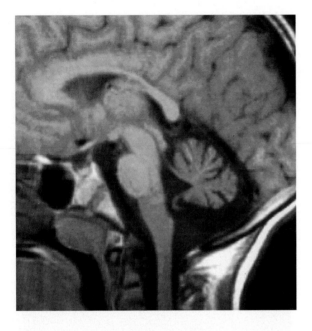

Case 460

14-year-old girl with a long history of seizures
and dilantin therapy.
(coronal, noncontrast scan; SE 3000/80)

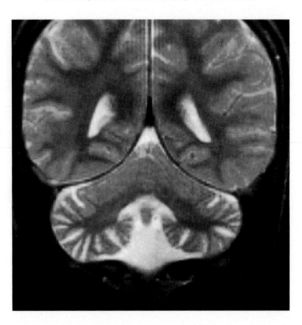

A number of familial syndromes (e.g., olivopontocerebellar degeneration and Marie's ataxia) may cause cerebellar degeneration with or without brainstem atrophy. The cause of the severe cerebellar atrophy in Case 459 has not been established. Friedrich's ataxia, which may present at this age, usually includes spinal cord involvement, with less prominent cerebellar findings.

Acquired cerebellar atrophy may be associated with alcohol abuse, paraneoplastic syndromes, and the phenytoin/seizure combination, as in Case 460. Alcoholic cerebellar atrophy primarily involves the superior vermis and is often more impressive than related symptoms.

Case 461

59-year-old man presenting with ataxia.
(sagittal, noncontrast scan; SE 800/16)

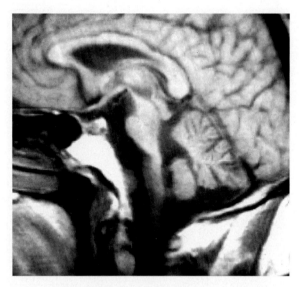

Olivopontocerebellar Degeneration

Case 462

44-year-old man presenting with gait abnormality.
(axial, noncontrast scan; SE 2500/90)

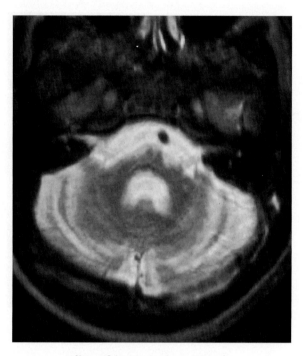

Idiopathic Brainstem Atrophy

Atrophy of the brainstem usually occurs in association with cerebellar atrophy, as in Case 461. The midbrain in this patient is normal in size. However, the bulk of the pons is markedly reduced. A characteristically flat and angular contour replaces the normally convex ventral margin. The prepontine cistern and fourth ventricle are large. Associated atrophy of the cerebellum and medulla is present, due to degeneration of tracts passing through the middle and inferior cerebellar peduncles.

This combination of morphological features is helpful in establishing the diagnosis of olivopontocerebellar degen-

eration, which is clinically nonspecific. T2-weighted MR scans may demonstrate increased signal intensity involving transverse pontine tracts, with sparing of ascending and descending fiber bundles. Olivopontocerebellar degeneration is among the "Parkinson's plus" syndromes that are often correlated with abnormal T2-shortening in the lenticular nucleus (see Case 454).

The relatively isolated brainstem atrophy in Case 462 is rare. The cross section of the brainstem at the pontomedullary junction is tiny, with marked enlargement of the prepontine cistern and fourth ventricle.

SPONTANEOUS INTRACRANIAL HYPOTENSION

Case 463A

40-year-old woman presenting with severe postural headaches.
(sagittal, noncontrast scan; SE 600/15)

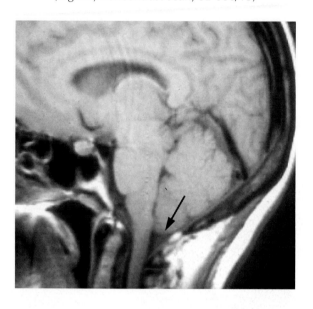

Case 463B

Same patient.
(axial, postcontrast scan; SE 800/15)

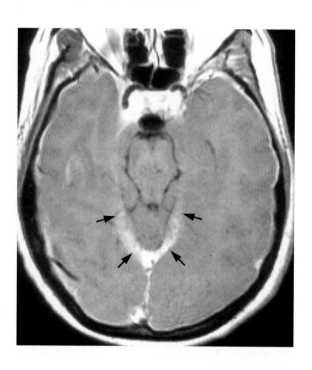

Some patients present with postural headaches (worse when standing) due to low intracranial pressure caused by loss of fluid from the spinal subarachnoid space. The CSF leakage may be spontaneous (e.g., due to rupture of a root sleeve cyst) or posttraumatic (e.g., following lumbar puncture).

When contrast-enhanced MR scans are performed in such cases, diffuse dural thickening and enhancement may be demonstrated (see Case 394). This finding probably represents an increase in dural blood volume resulting from the low intracranial pressure. The uniform dural thickening can be misinterpreted as meningeal pathology causing the patient's symptoms.

Sagittal scans such as Case 463A provide an important clue to the correct diagnosis. The brainstem and cerebellum sag inferiorly, reflecting the low pressure within the spinal subarachnoid space. The ventral margin of the pons is flatter than normal, the cerebellar tonsils approach the foramen magnum *(arrow)*, and the fourth ventricle

looks narrowed in anteroposterior dimension. These findings are all reversible when the cause of low spinal fluid pressure is corrected.

Case 463B demonstrates thick enhancement of the tentorium *(arrows)* and the convexity dura. Crowding of tissue at the tentorial hiatus resembles the appearance of a Chiari II hindbrain malformation (compare to Case 717). Unusually prominent signal loss from CSF pulsation ventral to the brainstem reflects the obstruction of more dorsal incisural CSF pathways by the caudal displacement of the brain.

Additional potential MR findings in cases of intracranial hypotension include unusually prominent enhancement of choroid plexus, enlarged dural veins, and subdural effusions.

The etiology of intracranial hypotension in this case was not established. Symptoms gradually improved over a period of several weeks.

Case 464A

11-year-old girl presenting with headaches and impaired vision, found to be severely hypertensive.
(axial, noncontrast scan; SE 2800/90)

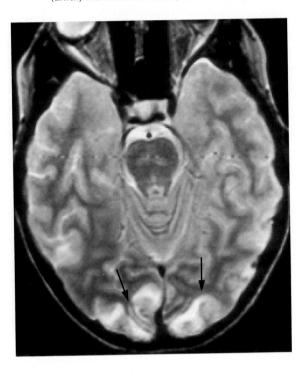

Case 464B

Same patient.
(axial, noncontrast scan; SE 2800/90)

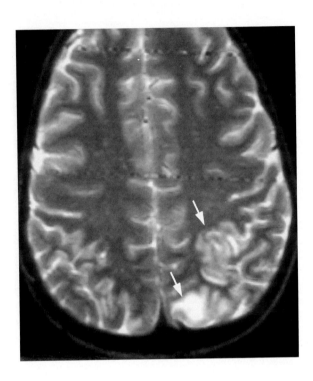

Severe hypertension may be associated with patchy or coalescent areas of edema in cerebral and cerebellar white matter. Involvement of both periventricular and subcortical regions has been noted, with lesions most common in the parietooccipital regions. Case 464 illustrates typical lobulated subcortical edema involving the occipital lobes and correlating with the patient's impaired vision.

This appearance has been encountered in spontaneous hypertension, uremia, and eclampsia. In each of these circumstances, the clinical and MR findings have been shown to be potentially reversible, presumably representing transient edema due to leakage of plasma across a compromised blood/brain barrier. The relative cortical sparing illustrated in this case argues against frank infarction. (Compare the above scans to Cases 476 and 477.)

Transient areas of patchy edema in white matter of the parietooccipital regions can also be seen in transplant patients with cyclosporin toxicity (see Case 465). Lupus cerebritis (see Cases 431 and 432) and mitochondrial encephalomyopathies (see Case 447) can cause a similar appearance.

White matter edema in uremia, malignant hypertension, and eclampsia may coalesce to produce diffuse cerebral swelling and increased intracranial pressure. These entities should be considered in the differential diagnosis of swollen hemispheres along with superior sagittal sinus thrombosis, pseudotumor cerebri, and Reye's syndrome. Head trauma, anoxia, and encephalitis may present a similar appearance but are usually evident clinically.

The syndrome of benign intracranial hypertension or "pseudotumor cerebri" may be considered in young patients with papilledema and symptoms of elevated intracranial pressure. Apart from a few specific associations (e.g., hypervitaminosis A, tetracycline toxic reaction) the cause of the syndrome is undefined and controversial. It is characterized by the typical clinical picture in the absence of specific intracranial pathology. In such patients, CT or MR scans serve the primary purpose of excluding a mass lesion, hydrocephalus, or venous thrombosis. The secondary finding of small ventricles suggesting cerebral swelling is seen in a minority of cases.

Case 465A

58-year-old woman with a history of cardiac transplantation, presenting with a seizure.
(axial, noncontrast scan; SE 2800/90)

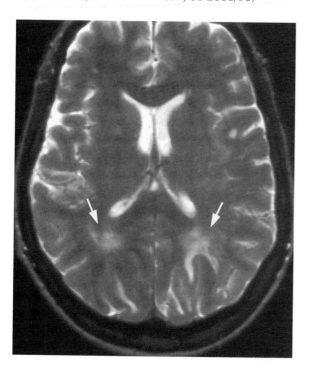

Case 465B

Same patient.
(axial, noncontrast scan; SE 2800/90)

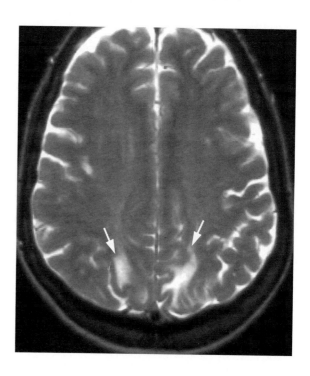

Patients receiving cyclosporin A after organ transplantation may present with symptoms of neurological toxicity, including seizures and confusion. MR studies in such cases have demonstrated reversible zones of nodular or scalloped subcortical edema. The parietal and occipital lobes are most commonly affected. Cerebellar edema has been noted in some cases.

The MR pattern of cyclosporin toxicity resembles the findings in hypertensive encephalopathy (compare Case 465 to Case 464.) The subcortical predominance of edema, multifocality, and usual absence of contrast enhancement may also mimic progressive multifocal leukoencephalopathy in an immunosuppressed patient (see Cases 367-371).

The mechanism of reversible white matter edema in cyclosporin toxicity has not been established. Some form of endothelial injury is likely. Associated hypertension is usually not high enough to implicate loss of autoregulation, which is believed to underlie hypertensive encephalopathy.

Neurotoxicity from cyclosporin may present within days (or even hours) after the initiation of treatment.

REFERENCES

Abdollah A, Tampieri D, Melanson D: Wilson's disease: Computed tomography and magnetic resonance imaging findings. *Can Assoc Radiol J* 42:130-134, 1991.

Aisen AM, Gabrielsen TO, McCune WJ: MR imaging of systemic lupus erythematosus involving the brain. *AJNR* 6:197-202, 1985.

Aisen AM, Martel LW, Gabrielsen TO, et al: Wilson's disease of the brain: MR imaging. *Radiology* 157:137-142, 1985.

Allard JC, Tilak S, Carter AP: CT and MR of MELAS syndrome. *AJNR* 9:1234-1238, 1988.

Angelini L, Nardocci N, Rumi V, et al: Hallervorden-Spatz disease: clinical and MR study of 11 cases diagnosed in life. *J Neurol* 239-417-425, 1992.

Ashdown BC, Tien RD, Felsberg GJ: Aspergillosis of the brain and paranasal sinuses in immunocompromised patients: CT and MR imaging findings. *AJR* 162:155-159, 1994.

Ashtari M, Barr WB, Schaul N, Bogerts B: Three-dimensional fast low-angle shot imaging and computerized volume measurement of the hippocampus in patients with chronic epilepsy of the temporal lobe. *AJNR* 12:941-947, 1991.

Balakrishnan J, Becker PS, Kumur AJ, et al: Acquired immunodeficiency syndrome: correlation of radiologic and pathologic findings in the brain. *Radiographics* 10:201-215, 1990.

Bale JF, Anderson RD, Grose C: Magnetic resonance imaging of the brain in childhood herpesvirus infections. *Pediatr Infect Dis J* 6:644-647, 1987.

Ball WS Jr, Prenger EC, Ballard ET: Neurotoxicity of radio/chemotherapy in children: pathologic and MR correlation. *AJNR* 13:761, 1992.

Barboriak DP, Provenzale JM, Boyko OB: MR diagnosis of Creutzfeldt-Jakob disease: significance of high signal intensity of the basal ganglia. *AJR* 162:137-140, 1994.

Bargallo N, Berenguer J, Tomas X, et al: Intracranial tuberculosis: CT and MRI. *Eur J Radiol* 3:123-128, 1993.

Barkovich AJ, Good WV, Koch TK, Berg BO: Mitochondrial disorders: analysis of their clinical and imaging characteristics. *AJNR* 14:1119-1138, 1993.

Barkovich AJ, Lindan CE: Congenital cytomegalovirus infection of the brain: imaging analysis and embryologic considerations. *AJNR* 15:703-715, 1994.

Barloon TJ, Yuh WTC, Knepper LE, et al: Cerebral ventriculitis: MR findings. *J Comput Assist Tomogr* 14:272-275, 1990.

Bazan C III, Rinaldi MG, Rauch RR, Jinkins JR: Fungal infections of the brain. *Neuroimaging Clin N Amer* 1:57-88, 1991.

Becker LE: Infections of the developing brain. *AJNR* 13:537-549, 1992.

Becker LE: Lysosomes, peroxisomes, and mitochondria: function and disorder: *AJNR* 13:609-620, 1992.

Bell CL, Partington C, Robbins M, et al: Magnetic resonance imaging of central nervous system lesions in patients with lupus erythematosus. *Arthritis Rheum* 34:437-441, 1991.

Braffman BH, Gussman RI, Goldberg HI, et al: MR imaging of Parkinson disease with spin-echo and gradient-echo sequence. *AJNR* 9:1093-1099, 1988.

Broderick DF, Wippold FJ, Clifford DB, et al: White matter lesions and cerebral atrophy in MR images in patients with and without AIDS dementia complex. *AJR* 161:177-181, 1993.

Bronen RA: Epilepsy: the role of imaging. *AJR* 159:1165-1174, 1992.

Bronen RA, Cheung G, Charles JT, et al: Imaging findings in hippocampal sclerosis: correlation with pathology. *AJNR* 12:933-940, 1991.

Brooks BS, King DW, el Gammal T, et al: MR imaging in patients with intractable complex partial seizures. *AJR* 154:577-583, 1990.

Brunberg J, Kanal E, Hirsch W, Van Thiel DH: Chronic acquired hepatic failure: MR imaging of the brain at 1.5 T. *AJNR* 12:909-914, 1991.

Burke JW, Podrasky AE, Bradley WG Jr: Meninges: benign postoperative enhancement on MR images. *Radiology* 174:99, 1990.

Callebaut J, Dormant D, Dubois B, et al: Contrast-enhanced MR imaging of tuberculous pachymeningitis cranialis hypertrophica: case report. *AJNR* 11:821-822, 1990.

Cendes F, Leproux F, Melanson D, et al: MRI of amygdala and hippocampus in temporal lobe epilepsy. *J Comput Assist Tomogr* 16:206-210, 1993.

Chamberlain MC, Nichols SL, Chase CH: Pediatric AIDS: comparative cranial MRI and CT scans. *Pediatr Neurol* 7:357-362, 1992.

Chanalet S, Gense de Beaufort D, Greselle JF, et al: Clinical and radiological aspects of extracerebral empyemas: 39 cases. *Neuroradiology* 33 (suppl):225-228, 1991.

Chang KH, Cho SY, Hesselink JR, et al: Parasitic diseases of the central nervous system. *Neuroimaging Clin N Amer* 1:159-178, 1991.

Chang KH, Han MH, Kim HS, et al: Delayed encephalopathy after acute carbon monoxide intoxication: MR imaging features and distribution of cerebral white matter lesions. *Radiology* 184:117-122, 1992.

Chang K-H, Han M-H, Roh J-K, et al: Gd-DTPA-enhanced MR imaging in intracranial tuberculosis. *Neuroradiology* 238:340-344, 1991.

Chang KH, Han MH, Roh JK, et al: Gd-DTPA-enhanced MR imaging of the brain in patients with meningitis: comparison with CT. *AJNR* 11:69-76, 1990.

Chang KH, Lee JH, Han MH, Han MC: The role of contrast-enhanced MR imaging in the diagnosis of neurocysticersosis. *AJNR* 12:509-512, 1991.

Chapelon C, Zisa JM, Piette JC, et al: Neurosarcoidosis: signs, course and treatment in 35 confirmed cases. *Radiology* 179:887, 1991.

Chen JC, Hardy PA, Kucharczyk W, et al: MR of human postmortem brain tissue: correlative study between T2 and assays of iron and ferritin in Parkinson and Huntington disease. *AJNR* 14:275-282, 1993.

Chrysikopoulos HS, Press GA, Grafe MR, et al: Encephalitis caused by human immunodeficiency virus: CT and MR imaging manifestations with clinical and pathologic correlation. *Radiology* 175:185-191, 1990.

Cohen WA, Maravilla KR, Gerlach R, et al: Prospective cerebral MR study of HIV seropositive and seronegative men: correlation of MR findings with neurologic, neuropsychologic, and cerebrospinal fluid analysis. *AJNR* 13:1231-1240, 1992.

Constine L, Konski A, Ekholm S, et al: Adverse effects of brain irradiation correlated with MR and CT. *Int J Radiat Oncol Biol Phys* 13:88, 1987.

Cooper SD, Brady MB, Williams JP, et al: Neurosarcoidosis: evaluation using CT and MRI. *J Comput Assist Tomogr* 12:96-99, 1988.

Cox J, Murtagh FR, Wilfong A, Brenner J: Cerebral aspergillosis: MR imaging and histopathologic correlation. *AJNR* 13:1489-1492, 1992.

Curnes JT, Laster DW, Ball MR, et al: Magnetic resonance imaging of radiation injury to the brain. *AJNR* 7:389-394, 1986.

D'Aprile P, Gentile MA, Carella A: Enhanced MR in the acute phase of Wernicke encephalopathy. *AJNR* 15:591-593, 1994.

Davenport C, Dillon WP, Sze G: Neuroradiology of the immunosuppressed state. *Rad Clin North Am* 30:611-638, 1992.

Davidson HD, Steiner RE: Magnetic resonance imaging of infections of the central nervous system. *AJNR* 6:499-504, 1985.

Davis PC, Hoffman JC Jr, Braun IF, et al: MR of Leigh's disease (subacute necrotizing encephalomyelopathy). *AJNR* 8:71-75, 1987.

De Castro CC, Hesselink JR: Tuberculosis. *Neuroimaging Clin N Amer* 1:119-139, 1991.

De Haan J, Grossman RI, Civitello L, et al: High-field magnetic resonance imaging of Wilson's disease. *J Comput Assist Tomogr* 11:132-135, 1987.

Del Brulto OH, Zenbeno MA, Salgado P, et al: MR imaging of cysticercotic encephalitis. *AJNR* 10:518, 1989.

De Leon MJ, Golomb J, George AE, et al: The radiologic prediction of Alzheimer disease: the atrophic hippocampal formation. *AJNR* 14:897-906, 1993.

Demaerel Ph, Wilms G, Robberecht W, et al: MRI of herpes simplex encephalitis. *Neuroradiology* 34:490-493, 1992.

Digre KB, Varner MV, Osborn AG, Crawford S: Cranial magnetic resonance imaging in severe pre-eclampsia versus eclampsia. *Arch Neurol* 50:399-406, 1993.

DiRocco A, Molinari S, Stollman AL, et al: MRI abnormalities in Creutzfeldt-Jakob disease. *Neuroradiology* 35:584-585, 1993.

Donnal JF, Heinz ER, Burger PC: MR of reversible thalamic lesions in Wernicke syndrome. *AJNR* 11:893-894, 1990.

Dooms GC, Hecht S, Brant-Zawadski M, et al: Brain radiation lesions: MR imaging. *Radiology* 158:149-156, 1986.

Drayer BP: Basal ganglia: significance of signal hypointensity on T2-weighted MR images. *Radiology* 173:311-312, 1989.

Drayer BP: Imaging of the aging brain. Part II. Pathologic conditions. *Radiology* 166:797-806, 1988.

Drayer BP, Olanow W, Burger P, et al: Parkinson plus syndrome: diagnosis using high field MR imaging of brain iron. *Radiology* 159:493-498, 1986.

Duguid JR, DeLa Paz R, DeGroot J: Magnetic resonance imaging of the midbrain in Parkinson's disease. *Ann Neurol* 20:744-747, 1986.

Ekholm S, Simon JH: Magnetic resonance imaging and the acquired immunodeficiency syndrome dementia complex. *Acta Radiol* 28:227-230, 1988.

Enzmann D, Chang Y, Augustyn G: MR findings in neonatal herpes simplex encephalitis type II. *J Comput Assist Tomogr* 14:453-457, 1990.

Falcone S, Quencer RM, Bowen B, et al: Creutzfeldt-Jakob disease: Focal symmetrical cortical involvement demonstrated by MR imaging. *AJNR* 13:403-406, 1992.

Fazekas F, Chawluk JB, Alavi A, et al: MR signal abnormalities at 1.5 T in Alzheimer's dementia and normal aging. *AJNR* 8:421-426, 1987.

Fernandez RE, Rothberg M, Ferencz G, et al: Lyme disease of the CNS: MR imaging findings in 14 cases. *AJNR* 11:479-481, 1990.

Fishman RA, Dillon WP: Dural enhancement and cerebral displacement secondary to intracranial hypotension. *Neuroradiology* 43:609-611, 1993.

Fitz CR: Inflammatory diseases of the brain in childhood. *AJNR* 13:551-567, 1992.

Flowers CH, Mafee MF, Crowell R, et al: Encephalopathy in AIDS patients: evaluation with MR imaging. *AJNR* 11:1235-1245, 1990.

Friedman D, Flanders A, Tartaglino L: Contrast-enhanced MR imaging of idiopathic hypertrophic craniospinal pachymeningitis. *AJR* 160:900-901, 1993.

Galluci M, Bozzao A, Splendiani A, et al: Follow-up in Wernicke's encephalopathy. *Neuroradiology* 33 (suppl) :594-595, 1991.

Galluci M, Bozzao A, Splendiani A, et al: Wernicke encephalopathy: MR findings in five patients. *AJNR* 11:887-892, 1990.

Galluci M, Cardona F, Arachi M, et al: Follow-up MR studies in Hallervorden-Spatz disease. *J Comput Assist Tomogr* 14:118-120, 1990.

Gee GT, Bazan C III, Jinks JR: Miliary tuberculosis involving the brain: MR findings. *AJR* 159:1075-1076, 1992.

George AE, DeLeon MV, Kalnin A, et al: Leukoencephalopathy in normal and pathologic aging. 2. MRI of brain lucencies. *AJNR* 7:567-570, 1986.

Gertz HJ, Henkes H, Cervos-Navarro J: Creutzfeldt-Jakob disease: correlation of MRI and neuropathologic findings. *Neurology* 38:1481-1482, 1988.

Geyer CA, Sartor KH, Prensky AJ, et al: Leigh disease (subacute necrotizing encephalomyelopathy): CT and MR in five cases. *J Comput Assist Tomogr* 12:40-44, 1988.

Gibby WA, Stecker MM, Goldberg HI, et al: Reversal of white matter edema in hypertensive encephalopathy. *AJNR* 10:578, 1989.

Ginier BL, Porier VC: MR imaging of intraventricular cysticercosis. *AJNR* 13:1247-1248, 1992.

Goodin DS, Rowley HA, Olney RK: Magnetic resonance imaging in amyotrophic lateral sclerosis. *Ann Neurol* 23:418-420, 1988.

Grafe MR, Press GA, Berthofy DP, et al: Abnormality of the brain in AIDS patients: correlation of postmortem MR findings with neuropathology. *AJNR* 11:905-911, 1990.

Grattan-Smith JD, Harvey AS, Desmond PM, Chow CW: Hippocampal sclerosis in children with intractable temporal lobe epilepsy: detection with MR imaging. *AJR* 161:1045-1048, 1993.

Greco A, Steiner R: Magnetic resonance imaging in neurosarcoidosis. *Magn Reson Imaging* 5:15-21, 1987.

Gupta RK, Jena A, Sharma A: MR imaging of intracranial tuberculomas. *J Comput Assist Tomogr* 12:280-285, 1988.

Haimes AB, Zimmerman RD, Morgello S, et al: MR imaging of brain abscesses. *AJNR* 10:279-291, 1989.

Hanner JS, Li KCP, Davis GL: Acquired hepatocerebral degeneration: MR similarity with Wilson disease. *J Comput Assist Tomogr* 12:1076-1077, 1988.

Harris GJ, Pearlson GD, Peyser CE, et al: Putamen volume reduction on magnetic resonance imaging exceeds caudate changes in mild Huntington's disease. *Ann Neurol* 31:69-75, 1992.

Harris TM, Edwards MK: Meningitis. *Neuroimaging Clin N Amer* 1:39-56, 1991.

Hawkins CP, McLaughlin JE, Kendall BE, McDonald WI: Pathological findings correlated with MRI in HIV infection. *Neuroradiology* 35:264-268, 1993.

Hayes WS, Sherman JL, Stern BJ, et al: MR and CT evaluation of intracranial sarcoidosis. *AJNR* 8:841-848, 1987.

Hecht-Leavitt C, Grossman R, Curran W, et al: MR of brain radiation injury. *AJNR* 8:427, 1987.

Heckmann JM, Eastman R, Handler L, et al: Leigh disease (subacute necrotizing encephalomyelopathy): MR documentation of the evolution of an acute attack. *AJNR* 14:1157-1159, 1993.

Heinz E, Heinz T, Radtke R, et al: Efficacy of MR vs. CT in epilepsy. *AJNR* 9:1123, 1988.

Heinz R, Ferris N, Lee EK, et al: MR and positron emission tomography in the diagnosis of surgically correctable temporal lobe epilepsy. *AJNR* 15:1341-1348, 1994.

Ho VB, Fitz CR, Chuang SH, Geyer CA: Bilateral basal ganglia lesions: pediatric differential considerations. *Radiographics* 13:269-292, 1993.

Holland BA, Perrett LV, Mills CM: Meningovascular syphilis: CT and MR findings. *Radiology* 158:439-442, 1986.

Huber SJ, Chakeres DW, Paulson GW, Khanna R: Magnetic resonance imaging in Parkinson's disease. *Arch Neurol* 47:735-737, 1990.

Huber SJ, Shuttleworth EC, Christy JA, et al: Magnetic resonance imaging in dementia of Parkinson's disease. *J Neurol Neurosurg Psychiatr* 52:1221-1227, 1989.

Inoue E, Hori S, Narumi Y, et al: Portal-systemic encephalopathy: presence of basal ganglia lesions with high signal intensity on MR images. *Radiology* 179:551-555, 1991.

Jack CR, Petersen RC, O'Brien PC, Tangalos EG: MR-based hippocampal volumetry in the diagnosis of Alzheimer's disease. *Neurology* 42:183, 1992.

Jackson GD, Berkovic SF, Duncan JS, Connelly A: Optimizing the diagnosis of hippocampal sclerosis using MR imaging. *AJNR* 14:753-762, 1993.

Jarvik JG, Hesselink JR, Kennedy C, et al: Acquired immunodeficiency syndrome: magnetic resonance patterns of brain involvement with pathologic correlation. *Arch Neurol* 45:731-736, 1988.

Jensen MC, Brant-Zawadzki M: MR imaging of the brain in patients with AIDS: value of routine use of IV gadopentetate dimeglumine. *AJR* 160:153-157, 1993.

Jordan J, Enzmann DR: Encephalitis. *Neuroimaging Clin N Amer* 1:17-38, 1991.

Kaufman WM, Sivit CJ, Fitz CR, et al: CT and MR evaluation of intracranial involvement in pediatric HIV infection: a clinical-imaging correlation. *AJNR* 13:949-957, 1992.

Kendall BE: Disorders of lysosomes, peroxisomes, and mitochondria. *AJNR* 13:621-653, 1992.

Ketonen L, Oksanen U, Kuuliala I: Preliminary experience of magnetic resonance imaging in neurosarcoidosis. *Neuroradiology* 29:127-129, 1987.

Kieburtz KD, Ketonen L, Zettelmaier AE, et al: Magnetic resonance imaging findings in HIV cognitive impairment. *Arch Neurol* 47:643-645, 1990.

Koci TM, Chiang F, Chow P, et al: Thalamic extrapontine lesions in central pontine myelinolysis. *AJNR* 11:1229-1233, 1990.

Kodama T, Numagredri Y, Gella FE, et al: Magnetic resonance imaging of limbic encephalitis. *Neuroradiology* 33:520-523, 1991.

Kovanen J, Erkinjuntti T, Iivanainen M, et al: Cerebral MR and CT imaging in Creutzfeldt-Jakob disease. *J Comput Assist Tomogr* 9:125-128, 1985.

Krageloh-Mann I, Grodd W, Niemann G, et al: Assessment and therapy monitoring of Leigh disease by MRI and proton spectroscopy. *Pediatr Neuro* 8:60-64, 1992.

Kuhn MJ, Mikulis DJ, Ayoub DM, et al: Wallerian degeneration after cerebral infarction: evaluation with sequential MR imaging. *Radiology* 172:170-182, 1989.

Kulisevsky J, Pugol J, Balanzo J: Pallidal hyperintensity on magnetic resonance imaging in cirrhotic patients: clinical correlations. *Hepatology* 16:1382-1388, 1992.

Kulisevsky J, Ruscalleda J, Grau JM: MR imaging of acquired hepatocerebral degeneration. *AJNR* 12:527-528, 1991.

Kupfer M, Zee CS, Colleti PM, et al: MRI Evaluation of AIDS-related encephalopathy: toxoplasmosis vs lymphoma. *Magn Reson Imaging* 8:51-57, 1990.

Lacomis D, Koshbin S, Schick RM: MR imaging of paraneoplastic limbic encephalitis. *J Comput Assist Tomogr* 14:115-117, 1990.

Lee BCP: Magnetic resonance imaging of metabolic and primary white matter disorders in children. *Neuroimaging Clin N Amer* 3:267-289, 1993.

Lester JW, Carter MP, Reynolds TL: Herpes encephalitis: MR monitoring of response to acyclovir therapy. *J Comput Assist Tomogr* 12:941-943, 1988.

Lexa FJ, Grossman RI: MR of sarcoidosis of the head and spine: spectrum of manifestations and radiographic response to steroid therapy. *AJNR* 15:973-982, 1994.

Littrup PJ, Gebarski SS: MR imaging of Hallervorden-Spatz disease. *J Comput Assist Tomogr* 9:491, 1985.

Lotz J, Hewlett R, Alheit B, Bowen R: Neurocysticercosis: correlative pathomorphology and MR imaging: *Neuroradiology* 30:35-41, 1988.

Mamelak AN, Kelly WM, Davis RL, Rosenblum ML: Idiopathic hypertrophic cranial pachymeningitis. *J Neurosurg* 79:270-276, 1993.

Martinez HR, Rangel-Guerra R, Elizondo G, et al: MR imaging in neurocysticercosis: a study of 56 cases. *AJNR* 10:1011-1019, 1989.

Mathews VP, Alo PL, Glass JD, et al: AIDS-related CNS cryptococcosis: radiologic-pathologic correlation. *AJNR* 13:1477-1486, 1992.

Mathews VP, Smith RR, Bognanno JR, et al: Gd-DTPA-enhanced MR of meningitis: initial clinical experience. *AJNR* 10:1290, 1989.

Medina L, Chi TL, DeVivo DC, Hilal SK: MR findings in patients with subacute necrotizing encephalomyelopathy (Leigh syndrome): correlation with biochemical defect. *AJNR* 11:379-384, 1990.

Miller DH, Kendall BE, Barter S, et al: MRI in central nervous system sarcoidosis. *Neurology* 38:378-383, 1988.

Mirowitz S, Sartor K, Gado MG, et al: Focal signal-intensity variations in the posterior internal capsule: normal MR findings and distinction from pathologic findings. *Radiology* 172:535-539, 1989.

Mirowitz SA, Westric TJ: Basal ganglial signal intensity alterations: reversal after discontinuation of parenteral manganese administration. *Radiology* 185:525-526, 1992.

Moser FG, Hilal SK, Abrams G, et al: MR imaging of pseudotumor cerebri. *AJNR* 9:39-46, 1988.

Naidu SB, Moser HW: Value of neuroimaging on metabolic diseases in affecting the CNS. *AJNR* 12:413-416, 1991.

Nazer H, Brismar J, Al-Kawi MZ, et al: Magnetic resonance imaging of the brain in Wilson's disease. *Neuroradiology* 35:130-133, 1993.

Neils EW, Lukin R, Tomsick TA, Tew JM: Magnetic resonance imaging and computerized tomography scanning of herpes simplex encephalitis: report of two cases. *J Neurosurg* 67:592-594, 1987.

Offenbacher H, Fazekas F, Schmidt R, et al: MRI in tuberculous meningoencephalitis: report of four cases and review of the neuroimaging literature. *J Neurol* 238:340-344, 1991.

Olsen WL, Longo FM, Mills CM, Norman D: White matter disease in AIDS: findings at MR imaging. *Radiology* 169:445-448, 1988.

Osborn RE, Byrd SE: Congenital infections of the brain. *Neuroimaging Clin N Amer* 1:105-118, 1991.

Pannullo SC, Reich JB, Krol G, et al: MRI changes in intracranial hypotension. *Neurology* 43:919-926, 1993.

Pastakia B, Polinsky R, DiChiro G, et al: Multiple system atrophy (Shy-Drager syndrome): MR imaging. *Radiology* 159:499-505, 1986.

Pearl GS, Anderson RE: Creutzfeldt-Jakob disease: high caudate signal on magnetic resonance imaging. *South Med J* 82:1177-1180, 1989.

Post MJD: Neuroimaging in various stages of human immunodeficiency virus infections. *Curr Opin Radiol* 2:73-79, 1990.

Post MJD, Berger JR, Duncan R, et al: Asymptomatic and neurologically symptomatic HIV-seropositive subjects: results of long-term MR imaging and clinical follow-up. *Radiology* 188:727-733, 1993.

Post MJD, Berger JR, Quencer HM: Asymptomatic and neurologically symptomatic HIV-seropositive individuals: prospective evaluation with cranial MR imaging. *Radiology* 178:131-139, 1991.

Post MJD, Levin BE, Berger JR, et al: Sequential cranial MR findings of asymptomatic and neurologically symptomatic HIV + subjects. *AJNR* 13:359-370, 1992.

Post MJD, Tate LG, Quencer RM, et. al: CT, MR and pathology in HIV encephalitis and meningitis. *AJNR* 9:469-476, 1988.

Press GA, Weindling SM, Hesselink JR, et al: Rhinocerebral mucor-mycosis: MR manifestations. *J Comput Assist Tomogr* 12:744-749, 1988.

Pujol JA, Pujol J, Graus F, et al: Hyperintense globus pallidus on T1-weighted MRI in cirrhotic patients is associated with severity of liver failure. *Neurology* 43:65-69, 1993.

Rafto Se, Milton WJ, Galetta SL, et al: Biopsy-confirmed CNS Lyme disease: MR appearance at 1.5 T. *AJNR* 11:482, 1990.

Rajshekhar V, Haran RP, Prakash S, Chandy MJ: Differentiating soli-tary small cysticercus granulomas and tuberculomas in patients with epilepsy. *J Neurosurg* 78:402-406, 1993.

Ramsey RG, Geremia GK: CNS complications of AIDS: CT and MR findings. *AJR* 151:449-454, 1988.

Rhee RS, Kumasaki DY, Sarwar M, et al: MR imaging of intra-ventricular cysticercosis. *J Comput Assist Tomogr* 11:598, 1987.

Riccio TJ, Hesselink JR: Gd-DTPA-enhanced MR of multiple crypto-coccal brain abscesses. *AJNR* 10:565-566, 1989.

Rosen L, Phillipo S, Enzmann DR: Magnetic resonance imaging in MELAS syndrome. *Neuroradiology* 32:168, 1990.

Rosenblum JD, Kim T, Ramsey RG: Neuroradiologic evaluation of complications of AIDS: a review. *Postgrad Radiol* 10:245-262, 1990.

Rovira MJ, Post MJD, Bowen BC: Central nervous system infections in HIV-infected persons. *Neuroimaging Clin N Amer* 1:179-200, 1991.

Rusinek H, DeLeon MJ, George AE, et al: Alzheimer disease: mea-suring loss of cerebral gray matter with MR imaging. *Radiology* 178:109-114, 1991.

Rutledge JN, Hilal SK, Silver AJ, et al: Study of movement disorders and brain iron by MR. *AJNR* 8:397-411, 1987.

Sandhu FS, Dillon WP: MR demonstration of leukoencephalopathy associated with mitochondrial encephalopathy: case report. *AJNR* 12:385-379, 1991.

Savoiardo M, Halliday WC, Nardocci N, et al: Hallervorden-Spatz dis-ease: MR and pathologic findings. *AJNR* 14:155-162, 1993.

Savoiardo M, Strada L, Girotti F, et al: MR imaging in progressive supranuclear palsy and Shy-Drager syndrome. *J Comput Assist Tomogr* 13:555-560, 1989.

Savoiardo M, Strada L, Girotti F, et al: Olivopontocerebellar atrophy: MR diagnosis and relationship to multisystem atrophy. *Radiol-ogy* 174:693-696, 1990.

Schaffert DA, Johnsen SD, Johnson PC, et al: Magnetic resonance imaging in pathologically proven Hallervorden-Spatz disease. *Neurology* 39:440-442, 1989.

Schoeman J, Hewlett R, Donald P: MR of childhood tuberculous meningitis. *Neuroradiology* 30:473, 1988.

Schroth G, Gawehn J, Thron A, et al: Early diagnosis of herpes sim-plex encephalitis by MRI. *Neurology* 37:179-183, 1987.

Schroth G, Kretzschmar K, Gawehn J, Voight, K: Advantages of mag-netic resonance imaging in the diagnosis of cerebral infections. *Neuroradiology* 29:120-126, 1987.

Schroth G, Wichmann W, Valavanis A: Blood-brain-barrier disruption in acute Wernicke encephalopathy: MR findings. *J Comput As-sist Tomogr* 15:1059-1061, 1991.

Schwaighofer BW, Hesselink JR, Healy ME: MR demonstration of re-versible brain abnormalities in eclampsia. *J Comput Assist To-mogr* 13:310-312, 1989.

Schwartz RB, Jones KM, Kalina P, et al: Hypertensive encephalopa-thy: findings on CT, MR imaging and SPECT imaging in 14 cases. *AJR* 159:379-383, 1992.

Seltzer S, Mark AS, Atlas SW: CNS sarcoidosis: evaluation with contrast-enhanced MR imaging. *AJNR* 12:1227-1233, 1991.

Sethi KD, Adams RJ, Loring DW, et al: Hallervorden-Spatz syndrome:

clinical and magnetic resonance imaging correlations. *Ann Neurol* 24:692-694, 1988.

Shaw DWW, Cohen WA: Viral infections of the CNS in children: im-aging features. *AJR* 160:125-133, 1993.

Shen W-C, Cheng T-Y, Lee S-K, et al: Disseminated tuberculomas in spinal cord and brain demonstrated by MRI with gadolinium-DTPA. *Neuroradiology* 35:213-215, 1993.

Sherman JL, Stern BJ: Sarcoidosis of the CNS: comparison of unen-hanced and enhanced MR images. *AJNR* 11:915-923, 1990.

Shogry MEC, Curnes JT, Mamillary body enhancement on MR as the only sign of acute Wernicke encephalopathy. *AJNR* 15:172-174, 1994.

Silbergleit T, Junck L, Gebarski S, Hatfield MK: Idiopathic intracra-nial hypertension (pseudotumor cerebri): MR imaging. *Radiol-ogy* 170:207-210, 1989.

Smith AS, Meisler DM, Tomsak RL, et al: High signal periventricular lesions in patients with sarcoidosis: neurosarcoidosis or multiple sclerosis? *AJNR* 10:898-891, 1989.

Starkstein SE, Brandt J, Bylsma F, et al: Neuropsycological correlates of brain atrophy in Huntington's disease: a magnetic resonance imaging study. *Neuroradiology* 34:487-489, 1992.

Stern MB, Braffman BH, Skolnick BE, et al: Magnetic resonance im-aging in Parkinson's disease and parkisonian syndromes. *Neurol-ogy* 39:1524-1526, 1989.

Sugita K, Ando M, Makino M, et al: Magnetic resonance imaging of the brain in congenital rubella virus and cytomegalovirus infec-tions. *Neurorad* 33:239-242, 1991.

Suss RA, Maravilla KR, Thompson J: MR imaging of intracranial cys-ticercosis: comparison with CT and anatomopathologic features. *AJNR* 7:235-242, 1986.

Sze G, Brant-Zawadzki M, Norman D, Newton TH: The neuroradiol-ogy of AIDS. *Semin Roentgenol* 22(1):42-53, 1987.

Sze G, Zimmerman RD: Magnetic resonance imaging of infec-tious and inflammatory disease. *Rad Clin North Am* 26:839-860, 1988.

Teitelbaum GP, Otto RJ, Lin M, et al: MR imaging of neurocysticer-cosis. *AJNR* 10:709-718, 1989.

Thuomas KA, Acquilonius SM, Bergstrom K, Westermark K: Mag-netic resonance imaging of the brain in Wilson's disease. *Neuro-radiology* 35:134-141, 1993.

Tien RD, Chu PK, Hesselink JR, et al: Intracranial crytocroccosis in immunocompromised patients: CT and MR findings in 29 cases. *AJNR* 12:283-289, 1991.

Tien RD, Felsberg GJ, Compi de Castro C, et al: Complex partial seizures and mesial temporal sclerosis: evaluation with fast spin-echo MR imaging. *Radiology* 189:835-842, 1993.

Tien RD, Felsberg GJ, Ferris NJ, Osumi AK: The dementias: correla-tion of clinical features, pathophysiology, and neuroradiology. *AJR* 161:245-255, 1993.

Tien RD, Felsberg GJ, Osumi AK: Herpesvirus infections of the CNS: MR findings. *AJR* 161:167-176, 1993.

Tishler S, Williamson T, Mirra SS, et al: Wegener granulomatosis with meningeal involvement. *AJNR* 14:1248-1252, 1993.

Truwit CL, Denaro CP, Lake JR, DeMarco T: MR imaging of revers-ible cyclosporin A-induced neurotoxicity. *AJNR* 12:651-659, 1991.

Tsuchiya K, Makita K, Furui S, et al: Contrast-enhanced magnetic resonance imaging of sub- and epidural empyemas. *Neuroradi-ology* 34:494-496, 1992.

Tsuruda JS, Kortman KE, Bradley WG, et al: Radiation effects in ce-rebral white matter: MR evaluation. *AJNR* 8:431-438, 1987.

Tuite M, Ketonen L, Kieburtz K, Handy B: Efficacy of gadolinium in MR brain imaging of HIV infected patients. *AJNR* 14:257-263, 1993.

Valk PE, Dillon WP: Review article. Radiation injury of the brain. *AJNR* 12:45-62, 1991.

Valk J, Van der Knapp MS: Toxic encephalopathy. *AJNR* 13:747-760, 1992.

Van der Knapp MS, Valk J: The MR spectrum of peroxisomal disorders. *Neuroradiology* 33:30-37, 1991.

Wehn SM, Heinz ER, Burger PC, Boyko OB: Dilated Virchow-Robin spaces in cryptococcal meningitis associated with AIDS: CT and MR findings. *J Comput Assist Tomogr* 13:756-762, 1989.

Weingarten K, Barbut D, Filippi C, Zimmerman RD: Acute hypertensive encephalopathy: findings on spin-echo and gradient-echo MR imaging. *AJR* 162:665-670, 1994.

Weingarten K, Zimmerman RD, Becker RD, et al: Subdural and epidural empyemas: MR imaging. *AJNR* 10:81-87, 1989.

Whiteman MLH, Post MJD, Bowen BC, Bell MD: AIDS-related white matter diseases. *Neuroimaging Clin N Amer* 3:331-359, 1993.

Williams DW III, Elster AD, Kramer SI: Neurosarcoidosis: Gadolinium-enhanced MR imaging. *J Comput Assist Tomogr* 14:704, 1990.

Wood BP: Children with acquired immune deficiency syndrome. *Invest Radiol* 27:964-970, 1992.

Wrobel CJ, Meyer S, Johnson RH, Hesselink JR: MR findings in acute and chronic coccidioidmycosis meningitis. *AJNR* 13:1241-1245, 1992.

Yuh WTC, Drew JM, Rizzo M, et al: Evaluations of pachymeningitis by contrast-enhanced MR imaging: a patient with rheumatoid disease. *AJNR* 11:1247-1248, 1990.

Zee C-S, Segall HD, Boswell W, et al: MR imaging of neurocysticercosis. *J Comput Assist Tomogr* 12:927-934, 1988.

Zimmerman RD, Becker RD, Devinsky O, et al: Magnetic resonance features of cerebral abscesses and other intracranial inflammatory lesions. *Acta Radiol* (Suppl) 369:754, 1986.

Zimmerman RD, Weingarten K: Neuroimaging of cerebral abscesses. *Neuroimaging Clin N Amer* 1:1-16, 1991.

CHAPTER 9

Infarction and Anoxia

Case 466

14-month-old girl presenting with a one-day
history of hemiparesis.
(sagittal, noncontrast scan; SE 600/15)

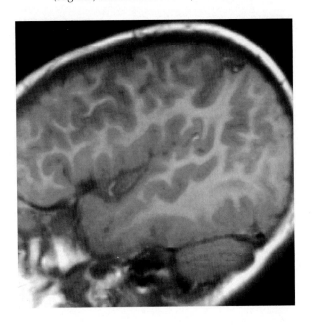

Case 467

73-year-old woman presenting one day
after the acute onset of confusion.
(sagittal, noncontrast scan; SE 600/17)

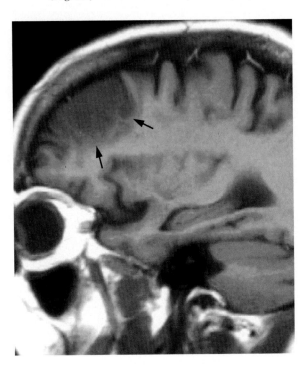

The MR appearance of cerebral infarction evolves over time. The rate and nature of these changes are characteristic and may be used to identify an initially ambiguous lesion.

Standard spin echo scans are usually normal within the first few hours after infarction. The rapid development of edema within infarcted cortex soon causes prolongation of T1 and T2 values and associated swelling. These findings are usually perceptible on standard spin echo images within 6 to 10 hours after the onset of a clinical deficit.

Demonstration of unequivocal tissue abnormality by MR scans in cases of cerebral infarction precedes definite CT demonstration by several hours. Even earlier MR evidence of acute cerebral infarction can be accomplished by diffusion and/or perfusion imaging, or by evidence of reduced flow in major vessels (see Cases 482 and 483).

The pattern of ischemic edema in an area of recent infarction is often gyriform, as seen in Case 466. (See Case 484 for another example.) Cortex throughout the distribution of the middle cerebral artery is thicker and darker than the normal gray matter at the frontal and occipital poles. This "super normal" appearance reflects the longer T1 values and mild mass effect caused by cortical edema. CT scans at this early stage of infarction would demonstrate blurring of the normal gray/white matter interface by developing edema and indistinct sulcal markings reflecting mild gyral swelling.

In other cases a zone of ischemic edema appears confluent or solid. This morphology may mimic a mass lesion (compare Case 467 to Case 63). Clues to the correct diagnosis include the clinical context of an acute neurological event and the peripherally based, often wedge-shaped involvement of tissue extending to the termination of a vascular distribution.

Case 468

34-year-old woman, one day after the
onset of left hemiparesis.
(axial, noncontrast scan; SE 2800/90)

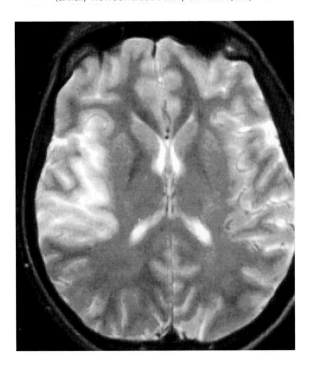

Case 469

2-month-old boy, twelve hours after the
onset of right hemiparesis.
(axial, noncontrast scan; SE 3000/90)

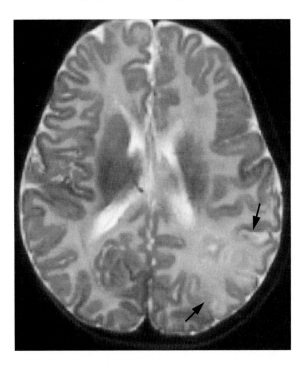

Case 468 presents the T2-weighted equivalent of the pattern demonstrated in Case 466. Cortical edema within a recent infarct is seen as a gyriform increase in signal intensity in the right sylvian region. Involved cortex is thickened or swollen, although there is no overall mass effect. (A similar lesion is presented as Case 473.)

The MR demonstration of gyral edema may clarify the etiology of ambiguous zones of low attenuation on CT studies. However, a gyriform pattern of signal abnormality can be noted in nonvascular lesions (see Cases 74 and 75).

Ischemic cortical edema in infants may be much less obvious on T2-weighted scans than in older children or adults. The normal high water content of immature white matter provides little contrast to overlying edema within ischemic gray matter. Careful attention is required to recognize cortical infarction in infants as an area of *reduced* cortical definition. Conversely, preservation of a normally defined cortical ribbon is reassuring evidence that the watery appearance of underlying white matter does not represent edema from an arterial occlusion.

In Case 469, infarcted cortex of the left parietal lobe is "washed-out" or partially "erased" as compared with other areas of the brain *(arrows)*. This finding is most apparent at the depths of sulci in the affected region. (The tops of gyri are normally better perfused than the depths of sulci in the neonatal period.)

The demonstration of ischemic edema does not necessarily imply cerebral infarction. MR has documented many cases of reversible prolongation of T1 and T2 values correlating with transient clinical deficits in patients who have suffered temporary vascular insults.

Case 470

3-year-old boy, two days after the onset
of right hemiparesis and aphasia.
(axial, noncontrast scan; SE 3000/75)

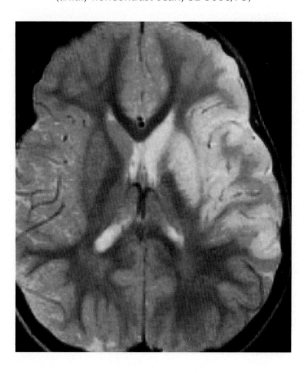

Case 471

60-year-old man presenting with the acute
onset of confusion three days earlier.
(axial, noncontrast scan; SE 3000/90)

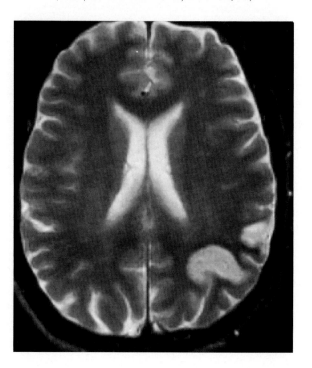

Infarction within the distribution of the middle cerebral artery (MCA) may present variable morphology, depending on the extent of cortical involvement and the presence or absence of ganglionic components.

When the main trunk of the MCA is occluded, a zone of midhemisphere infarction develops. (A similar pattern may occur with occlusion of the internal carotid artery when the ipsilateral anterior cerebral artery is well-perfused from the anterior communicativity artery.) The anterior and posterior margins of the infarct reflect the anatomical and physiological extent of collateral flow from the anterior and posterior cerebral arteries. The lesion often has a trapezoidal shape based laterally, as seen on axial or coronal images. If the occlusion compromises the origins of the lenticulostriate arteries, deep nuclei will also be involved.

In Case 470, gyriform cortical edema is present through-out the territory of the anterior division of the MCA. In addition, uniform high signal intensity is seen throughout the putamen and caudate head. (Compare to the normal demonstration of the caudate nucleus and frontal horn on the right side.) These nuclei are supplied by lenticulostriate branches arising from the horizontal or M-1 segment of the MCA. Occlusion of this segment (e.g., by embolus, dissection, or arteritis) produces a combination of cortical and ganglionic infarction.

Other patients may present with cortical infarcts limited to the distribution of a single branch of a major vessel. Case 471 illustrates a small infarct involving the territory of the angular artery, one branch of the posterior division of the MCA. Characteristic gyriform morphology of localized cortical edema should suggest infarction even when a lesion is very focal.

DIFFERENTIAL DIAGNOSIS:
SUPERFICIAL EDEMA WITHIN THE MCA DISTRIBUTION

Case 472

41-year-old woman presenting with a seizure.
(axial, noncontrast scan; SE 3000/30)

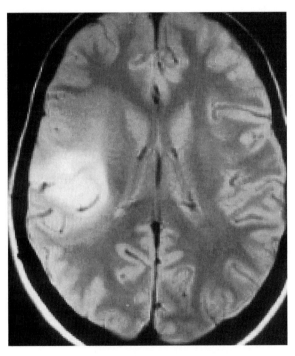

Low Grade Astrocytoma

Case 473

42-year-old man presenting with right hemiparesis.
(axial, noncontrast scan; SE 3000/30)

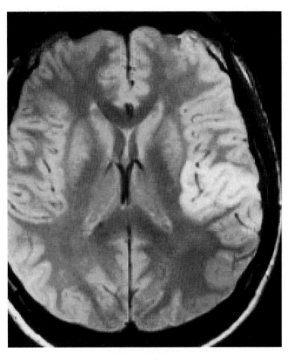

MCA Infarct

An important characteristic of cerebral infarcts is their conformity to vascular distributions. However, mass lesions or inflammatory processes can also occur within the territory of a single cortical artery, as demonstrated in Case 472. (Compare also to localized perisylvian edema caused by herpes encephalitis in Case 398.)

The glioma in Case 472 has a mass-like contour, which is distinct from the characteristic gyriform pattern of edema due to infarction in Case 473. This difference in morphology often helps to categorize lesions localized within an arterial distribution.

However, as illustrated in Case 467 (and also in Case 530), recent infarcts may cause zones of confluent edema and mass effect. Conversely, gyriform patterns of edema are occasionally seen in infiltrating neoplasms (see Cases 74 and 75).

Contrast enhancement is often diagnostic when the clinical context and noncontrast scans are ambiguous. Acute or subacute infarction may be associated with arterial, pial, and/or gyriform enhancement (see Cases 482-486). Tumor enhancement patterns are usually more mass-like or heterogeneous (see Cases 95-98).

When the plane of a scan passes parallel to a sulcus or cistern, a vague area of CSF-like signal intensity is seen. The posterior portion of the sylvian cistern commonly causes this appearance on axial images, potentially mimicking pathology in this region. Such pseudo-infarctions lack mass effect, are usually present at only one level, and are unimpressive on long TR, short TE spin echo images.

Other locations at which partial imaging of sulci and cisterns may mimic focal infarction include the circular sulcus/external capsular area, the lateral suprasellar cistern/hypothalmic region, the calcarine sulcus/medial occipital lobe, and the horizontal fissure/posterior cerebellar hemisphere (see Cases 526 and 527).

Case 474

37-year-old man presenting with sudden
disorientation.
(axial, noncontrast scan; SE 2500/45)

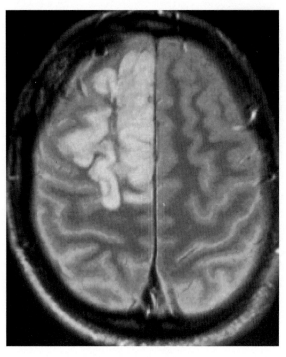

Low Grade Astrocytoma
(recurrent)

Case 475

28-year-old woman presenting with acute
confusion.
(axial, noncontrast scan; SE 2500/100)

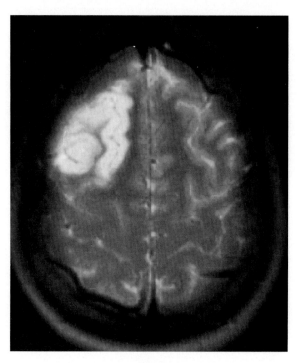

Infarct
(anterior division, MCA)

Although gyriform cortical edema is characteristic of recent infarction, other pathologies can cause a similar appearance. Superficial cerebral edema may develop secondary to overlying meningeal disease (meningitis or meningeal carcinomatosis; see Case 537). Alternatively, encephalitis may involve cerebral cortex and provoke associated edema (see Cases 401 and 403).

Case 474 demonstrates that tumors can also present a gyriform morphology. The pattern of cortical edema in this case is compatible with infarction, but the lesion crosses the cortical watershed between the anterior and middle cerebral arteries. This lack of conformity to a single arterial territory should raise consideration of nonvascular etiologies (or multifocal embolic infarction). An old right frontal craniotomy flap confirms a nonvascular diagnosis.

The subacute infarction in Case 475 demonstrates characteristic cortical edema with relative sparing of subcortical white matter. (Compare this appearance to the reversed pattern of subcortical edema with cortical sparing in Cases 367-371.) The lesion is confined to the distribution of the anterior division of the middle cerebral artery. The medial margin of the infarct defines the watershed with the anterior cerebral artery (see Case 486). This anatomical boundary has been displaced medially by swelling of the involved tissue.

Mass effect develops during the first week following cerebral infarction, most commonly after a few days have elapsed. If the patient is first scanned at this time and the clinical context is ambiguous, the possibility of a neoplasm may be raised on CT studies. MR scans can resolve the issue by demonstrating characteristic gyriform edema and/or laminar necrosis (see Case 478) within subacute infarction.

INFARCTION IN THE DISTRIBUTION OF THE POSTERIOR CEREBRAL ARTERY

Case 476

41-year-old woman presenting ten days
postpartum and one day after a CVA.
(axial, noncontrast scan; SE 2800/90)

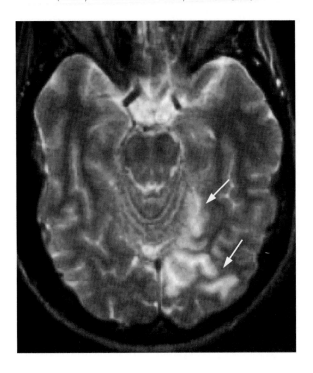

Case 477

2-year-old girl with a history of congenital heart
disease and recent change in mental status.
(axial, noncontrast scan; SE 3000/90)

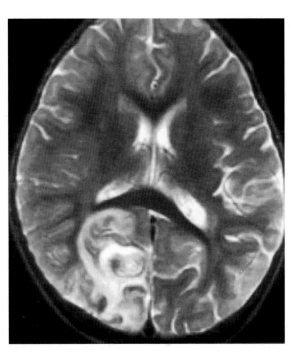

The posterior cerebral artery (PCA) supplies the medial temporal lobe, the tentorial surface of the temporal and occipital lobes, the occipital pole, and a variably extensive band of the parasagittal parietooccipital lobes. The superior and lateral extent of this distribution reflects variations in size of the anterior and middle cerebral arteries.

Thalamo-perforating branches arise from the proximal PCA (as well as from the posterior communicating artery). For this reason, thalamic infarction is often associated with infarcts of the medial temporal and occipital lobes.

Acute infarction in Case 476 has caused cortical edema within portions of the left PCA distribution. The medial margin of the lesion is sharply defined by the tentorium and falx. The lateral margin is more irregular, reflecting the watershed with the posterior division of the middle cerebral artery.

Hemorrhage is frequently present within PCA infarcts, as seen in Case 477. Areas of T1- and T2-shortening due to blood products may be superimposed on the overall background of long T1 and T2 values within the infarct. The combination of subtotal involvement of the PCA territory with hemorrhagic components can cause diagnostic confusion. Cerebral infarction should be considered whenever a puzzling occipital lesion is encountered.

The infarction in Case 476 proved secondary to embolization from dissection of the left vertebral artery, possibly related to the recent delivery (see Case 547). Another important diagnostic consideration when cerebral symptoms develop postpartum is dural sinus thrombosis (see Cases 642-648).

In Case 477, early ischemic edema is also seen within cortex of the posterior temporal and inferior parietal regions bilaterally. This tissue is supplied by the posterior division of the middle cerebral artery.

See Cases 479, 539, and 543 for other examples of infarction involving the PCA distribution. Also compare the above scans to the appearance of hypertensive encephalopathy in Case 464 and cyclosporin toxicity in Case 465.

Case 478

69-year-old woman, three days after the
acute onset of confusion.
(sagittal, noncontrast scan; SE 800/20)

Case 479

74-year-old woman, with a four day history of
worsening homonymous hemianopsia.
(sagittal, noncontrast scan; SE 600/15)

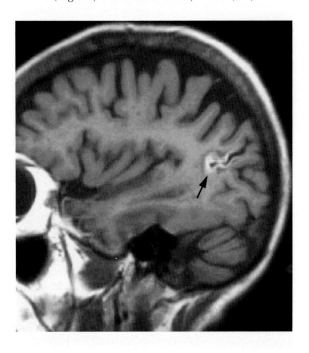

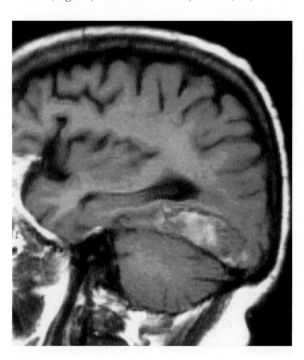

Zones of T1-shortening often develop within subacute infarcts, helping to localize and characterize the lesions. Case 478 illustrates a ribbon of high signal intensity following the contour of involved cerebral cortex *(arrow)*. This gyriform pattern may be due to petechial hemorrhage and/or biochemical changes caused by laminar necrosis (e.g., protein denaturation). CT scans in such cases usually do not demonstrate high attenuation values in the area of T1-shortening, and the MR finding does not by itself contraindicate anticoagulation. Compare the morphology of precontrast T1-shortening as in Case 478 to the gyriform enhancement of subacute infarction illustrated in Cases 485 and 486.

Less commonly, recent ischemic infarcts become frankly hemorrhagic, either spontaneously or following therapy with anticoagulants. Dissolution of a cerebral embolus may predispose to hemorrhagic infarction by allowing reperfusion of damaged vessels. Multifocal hemorrhagic infarcts suggest an embolic source such as subacute bacterial endocarditis.

Case 479 demonstrates extensive T1-shortening due to subacute hemorrhage within an occipital infarct. As mentioned in Case 477, hemorrhage is a particularly common component of infarction in the distribution of the posterior cerebral artery.

Case 480

64-year-old woman presenting with ataxia,
nausea and vomiting.
(axial, noncontrast scan; SE 2800/90)

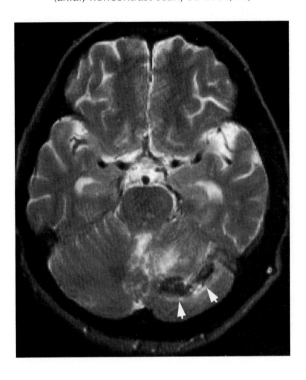

Case 481

79-year-old woman with known atrial fibrillation,
two days after the acute onset of confusion.
(axial, noncontrast scan; SE 2800/45)

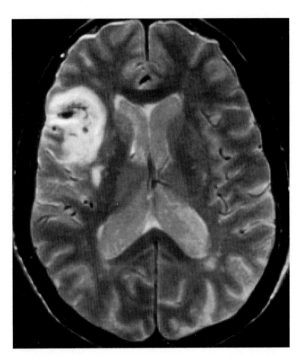

Low signal intensity on T2-weighted images is a characteristic feature of acute or early subacute intracerebral hemorrhage (see discussion of Cases 555-558). This finding may add complexity to the MR appearance of recent infarcts, as illustrated above.

In Case 480, a major portion of the cerebellar infarct has become hemorrhagic *(arrows)*. The patchy morphology of this low signal zone favors hemorrhagic transformation of infarction rather than spontaneous hematoma (compare to Case 556) or bleeding into an underlying neoplasm (compare to Case 562).

The complex lesion in Case 481 is nonspecific. The combination of hemorrhage and mass effect simulates a tumor (compare to Cases 112 and 562). However, the clinical context and localization of the lesion within the territory of the anterior division of the middle cerebral artery suggest the correct diagnosis. CT scanning might be considered to

prove that the focal areas of low signal intensity represent hemorrhage rather than calcification.

It is important to remember that hemorrhage within cerebral infarcts can mimic other causes of atypical hematomas. Conversely, the presence of an edematous zone surrounding an intracerebral hematoma within a vascular distribution does not assure a diagnosis of hemorrhagic infarction.

Chronic atrial fibrillation is known to be associated with an increased risk of stroke, which can be reduced by anticoagulation. The small focus of high signal abnormality posterior to the main lesion in Case 481 probably represents an additional infarct of undetermined age.

Venous pathology (e.g., dural sinus thrombosis) should also be considered as the etiology of hemorrhagic cerebral infarction.

Case 482

16-year-old girl, one day after the rapid development of aphasia and hemiparesis.
(axial, postcontrast scan; SE 800/18)

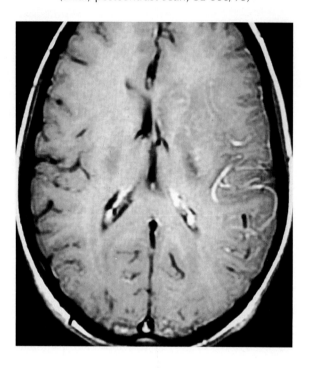

Case 483

72-year-old woman, one day after the onset of aphasia.
(axial, postcontrast scan; SE 600/15)

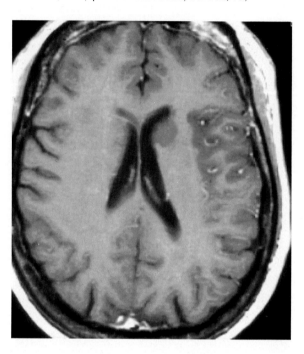

Rapid blood flow through normal cerebral arteries causes a lack of signal or "flow void" on routine spin echo images. Slower flow, whether in normal veins or abnormal arteries, is often associated with intraluminal enhancement on postcontrast scans.

Abnormal contrast enhancement within major arteries may be the earliest sign of cerebral infarction on standard MR studies. This finding depends on the presence of slow antegrade or retrograde collateral perfusion of the affected vascular territory. Abnormal arterial enhancement may persist for several days, disappearing as more normal flow velocities are reestablished in the obstructed distribution.

Both of the above cases demonstrate abnormal enhancement of middle cerebral artery branches supplying the left hemisphere. (Compare this finding to the normal lack of arterial enhancement over the right hemisphere in each case.) In both cases, evidence of early parenchymal change

is present, with edema causing swelling and reduced signal intensity of sylvian cortex and deep hemisphere nuclei.

Increasingly sophisticated pulse sequences are becoming available, offering excellent flow compensation with routine demonstration of arterial enhancement. However, this successful rephasing of normal arterial flow may decrease conspicuity of reduced arterial velocities in an area of cerebral infarction.

A cerebrovascular accident is a young patient should suggest the possibility of an embolic source (see also Case 476). Leading causes include spontaneous dissection of the carotid or vertebral arteries or posttraumatic lesions of these vessels (e.g., pseudoaneurysm). Cardiac emboli or coagulopathy should also be considered. The patient in Case 482 was found to have a mitochondrial encephalomyopathy (MELAS; see Case 447) that is associated with stroke-like events.

Case 484

55-year-old woman presenting with acute
weakness of the right leg.
(coronal, postcontrast scan; SE 900/20)

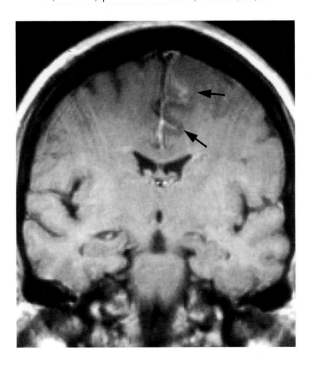

Case 485

2-year-old girl with suspected cerebral emboli.
(coronal, postcontrast scan; SE 600/15)

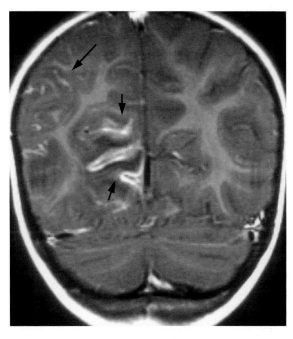

(same patient as Case 477)

In Case 484, the cortical ribbon in the medial posterior left frontal region is abnormally prominent, with thickening and T1-prolongation indicating edema *(arrows)*. A thin layer of contrast enhancement is present in the overlying meninges.

This combination of features may be observed early in the course of cerebral infarction (day one or two). The phase of superficial pial enhancement is interposed between (and often superimposed on) the periods of arterial enhancement and gyral enhancement. It is important to recognize that this pattern may occur within the MR spectrum of a vascular event, since the appearance could otherwise be interpreted as meningeal disease (e.g., meningitis or meningeal carcinomatosis) with secondary cortical edema.

Parenchymal contrast enhancement in cerebral infarcts is usually confined to gray matter. Several morphologies may be encountered. The most characteristic pattern is band-like, tubular, or gyriform enhancement as seen in the right occipital region of Case 485 *(short arrows)*. More amor-phous patterns can occur (see Case 531), and solid enhancement is common when deep nuclei are involved. Ring-enhancing appearances are occasionally noted. In most cases, the enhancing lesion retains the peripherally based shape typical of a large infarct.

The occipital enhancement in Case 485 involves the gray matter ribbon, with sparing of the intervening sulcal/meningeal spaces. A different pattern with pial enhancement is present in the posterior parietal region *(long arrow)*. The latter finding represents a more recent infarct, which evolved to gyral enhancement over the subsequent two days.

Gyriform contrast enhancement is a familiar CT hallmark of subacute infarction, seen from the end of week one through week three or four. MR demonstration of this pattern begins a little earlier, often by day two or three following the clinical event. Reactive "luxury perfusion" (hyperperfusion with loss of autoregulation) and breakdown of the blood-brain barrier both contribute to this finding.

Case 486

55-year-old woman, nine days after the
acute onset of right leg paresis.
(coronal, postcontrast scan; SE 700/15)

Case 487

61-year-old man with decreased mental status.
(coronal, postcontrast scan; SE 600/15)

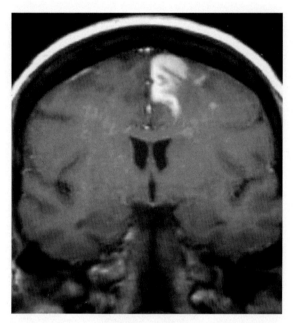

Subacute Infarction
(same patient as Case 484)

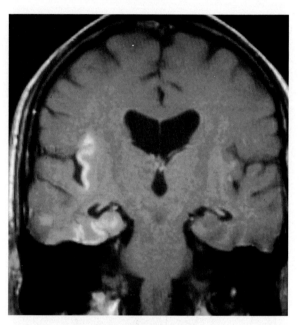

Herpes Encephalitis
(same patient as Case 401)

A gyriform pattern of contrast enhancement is characteristic but not specific for cerebral infarction. In an ambiguous clinical context, a differential diagnosis of this finding should be considered.

Case 486 demonstrates the typical evolution of contrast enhancement in a recent infarct from pial to gyral patterns. (Compare this image to the earlier scan of the same patient in Case 484.)

The infarction in Case 486 is localized to the distribution of the anterior cerebral artery (ACA). The ACA supplies a parasagittal band of tissue extending from the medial frontal lobe to the parietal vertex. (Compare the area involved by infarction in Case 486 to the spared territory in Case 475.) Included in this distribution is the medial portion of the motor cortex supplying the lower extremity, correlating with the leg weakness in this patient. Obstruction of the ACA may be caused by embolization, spasm following subarach-

noid hemorrhage, compression by a subfrontal mass, or marked subfalcial herniation.

Herpes encephalitis characteristically involves cortex of the temporal lobe and insula, as in Case 487. The resultant edema and enhancement following the cortical contour may mimic subacute cerebral infarction. The diagnosis of infarction in Case 487 is unlikely because the affected areas fall within more than one vascular distribution. The medial temporal lobe is supplied by the anterior choroidal and posterior cerebral arteries, while the insula is perfused by the middle cerebral artery.

Occasional tumors (usually gliomas) infiltrate cortex and can mimic the appearance of cerebral infarction (see Cases 74, 75, 474, and 475).

Gyriform contrast enhancement has also been reported in association with recent seizures. This finding is transient and usually does not conform to a vascular distribution.

Case 488

33-year-old woman with multiple neurological deficits one day following cardiac surgery.
(axial, noncontrast scan; SE 2500/28)

Case 489

50-year-old man admitted after a cardiopulmonary arrest.
(axial, noncontrast scan; SE 2800/90)

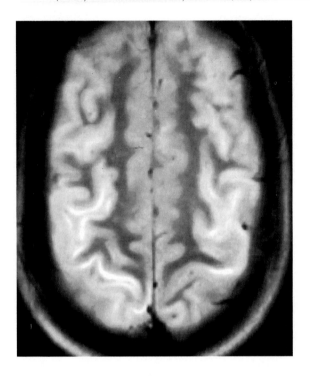

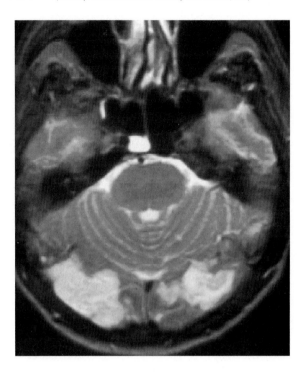

Infarction occurs along the margins of cerebral vascular territories when flow is impaired on both sides of the boundary. The cause may be generalized hypoperfusion, isolated vascular compromise, or a combination of both factors. For example, stenosis of an internal carotid artery may lead to infarction along the anterior/middle cerebral artery watershed during systemic hypotension.

The location of the cortical watersheds has been illustrated by the margins of the infarcts on preceding pages. Watershed infarcts are typically small, patchy lesions aligned along these same parasagittal boundaries. (The differential diagnosis of this parasagittal pattern includes venous infarction due to thrombosis of the superior sagittal sinus; see Cases 642-645.)

The above cases demonstrate unusually extensive, bihemispheral watershed infarcts reflecting severe hypoperfusion. In Case 488, symmetrical high signal intensity is present within gyri throughout the parasagittal zones of the anterior cortical arterial watershed. (Compare the location of the gyral edema in this case to Cases 475 and 484.) Laminar high signal intensity was apparent in the same distribution on T1-weighted scans.

Case 489 demonstrates a more confluent pattern of ischemic edema involving posterior watershed areas in the occipital lobes. (Compare the involved regions to Cases 476 and 477; also note that axial scans near the tentorium often include the inferior portion of the occipital lobes positioned posterior to the cerebellar hemispheres.) Again the bilateral symmetry of the lesions suggests a diffuse cerebral insult, and the localization to the watershed areas indicates a vascular etiology.

Mucosal thickening causes high signal intensity in the right sphenoid sinus in Case 489.

Case 490

50-year-old man admitted after
a cardiopulmonary arrest.
(axial, postcontrast scan; SE 600/15)

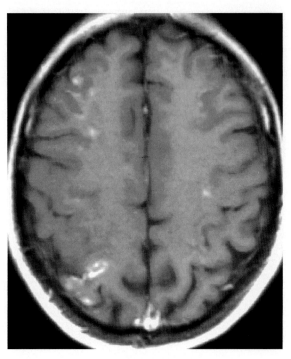

Subacute Watershed Infarcts
(same patient as Case 489)

Case 491

26-year-old woman complaining of scattered
parsthesias and unsteady gait.
(axial, post-contrast scan; SE 600/15)

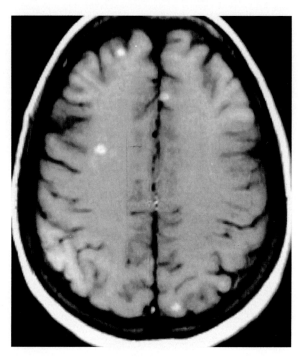

Multiple Sclerosis

Small areas of infarction often demonstrate focal enhancement, as seen in Case 490. Enhancement defining cortical infarcts is best demonstrated by MR scans, since the cerebral surface is not obscured by artifact from the adjacent calvarium as in CT studies. Postcontrast scans using magnetization transfer suppression are particularly helpful to detect and characterize subacute ischemic foci.

The appearance in Case 490 is nonspecific and could suggest inflammatory or metastatic disease. The correct diagnosis is supported by (1) the location of the lesions along the parasagittal zones of the cortical arterial watershed and (2) the pial and gyriform components of enhancement within some of the affected areas. Multifocal infarction may also be caused by multiple emboli, cerebral vasculitis (e.g., systemic lupus erythematosus), meningitis, or cortical venous thrombosis.

Case 491 demonstrates the multifocal contrast enhancement commonly noted in active demyelinating disease (see Cases 349-353). The enhancement of small plaques is typically solid, with progression to a ring-enhancing pattern as the lesions age and enlarge. The correct diagnosis is Case 491 is favored by the age of the patient, although other inflammatory etiologies should be considered (see Cases 422 and 424).

Cases 354, 423, and 425 present examples of cerebral metastases resembling the above scans.

Case 492

6-year-old boy with a history of a stroke as
an infant and developmental delay.
(coronal, noncontrast scan; SE 3000/90)

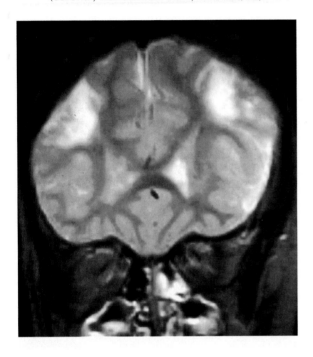

Case 493

61-year-old man with bilateral carotid stenosis.
(axial, noncontrast scan; SE 2500/28)

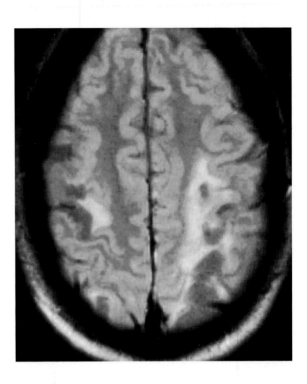

MR scans in the coronal plane display the parasagittal location of ischemic lesions involving the cortical watershed.
In Case 492, symmetrical zones at the junction of the distributions of the anterior and middle cerebral arteries demonstrate old encephalomalacia, characterized by tissue loss
and increased water content. This localization is comparable to the acute lesions in Case 488, suggesting a major
episode of hypoperfusion. The appearance contrasts with
the pattern of periventricular leukomalacia, as illustrated in
Cases 498-501.

In Case 493, old infarcts are identified along the cortical
watersheds of both cerebral hemispheres (see discussion of
Cases 540 and 541). The areas of involvement are somewhat larger than in Case 490, but the location within
parasagittal watershed zones is the same.

The distribution of multiple cerebral infarcts may help to
characterize underlying pathophysiology. Multiple infarcts
at scattered cortical locations independent of watershed
boundaries suggest multifocal occlusion of distal cerebral
arteries and raise the possibility of embolization, vasculitis,
or coagulopathy. On the other hand, multiple infarcts
aligned along watershed distributions as in Case 493 suggest generalized hypoperfusion rather than involvement of
individual cortical vessels.

Tissue damage from cortical watershed infarction is often most severe in the parietal regions (see Case 703). This
area represents the most distal supply zone of the major
cerebral arteries. A generalized reduction in perfusion
would be expected to most adversely affect parenchyma
that is furthest downstream, while more proximal territories might be relatively spared.

In term infants, this gradient of ischemic damage along
the (mature) cortical arterial watershed from anterior to
posterior may produce a clinical picture of spastic diplegia. Such clinical presentations may resemble the outcome
of periventricular leukomalacia, caused by hypoxic/isch-
emic insult to the immature brain (see Cases 498-501 and
Cases 703 and 704).

Case 494

59-year-old woman with occlusion of
the left internal carotid artery.
(axial, noncontrast scan; SE 2500/45)

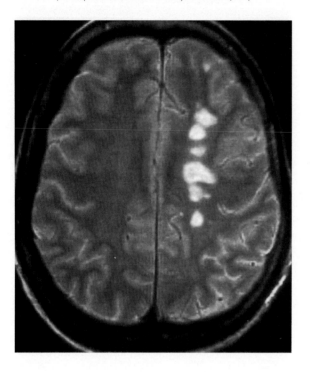

Case 495

45-year-old woman with high grade stenosis
of the right internal carotid artery.
(axial, noncontrast scan; SE 2800/90)

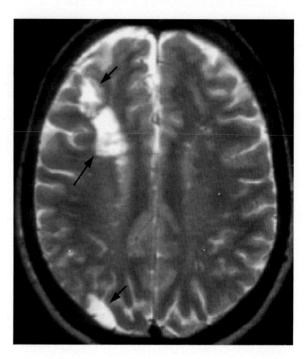

In addition to the cortical arterial watershed over the cerebral convexity, a watershed zone exists within each cerebral hemisphere. This area occurs at the junction of centrifugal perfusion from basal perforating arteries (e.g., lenticulostriate arteries) and centripetal perfusion from penetrating branches of the cortical vessels. The location of this intrahemispheric watershed moves peripherally during fetal development. At full term (and thereafter) the watershed region is within white matter of the centrum semiovale, slightly lateral and superior to the bodies of the lateral ventricles.

Reduced perfusion of one cerebral hemisphere may cause scattered infarction within the intrahemispheric watershed zone. Such infarcts may occur in isolation or accompany cortical lesions. While cortical watershed infarcts are frequently due to global hypoperfusion from cardiovas-cular impairment, intrahemispheric watershed infarction often reflects isolated disease of the ipsilateral internal carotid artery.

In Case 494, the parasagittal row of white matter lesions is strikingly unilateral. The appearance would be unusual for inflammatory disorders, and compromise of the ipsilateral internal carotid artery should be suspected. Examination of "flow void" within arteries at the skull base and/or MR angiography is indicated when lesions resembling unilateral multiple sclerosis are encountered.

Case 495 demonstrates the association of cortical watershed infarcts *(short arrows)* with intrahemispheric watershed infarction *(long arrow)*. The size and number of lesions in either category may be variable, but their position should raise consideration of watershed hemodynamics.

DIFFERENTIAL DIAGNOSIS:
UNILATERAL PREDOMINANCE OF WHITE MATTER LESIONS

Case 496

31-year-old woman presenting with right
arm weakness.
(axial, noncontrast scan; SE 2600/45)

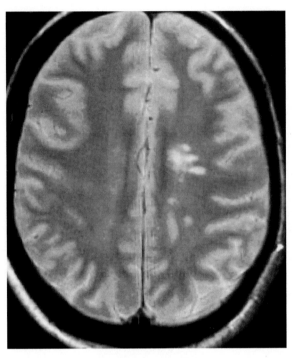

Multiple Sclerosis

Case 497

56-year-old man presenting with left-sided
headaches and right hemiparesis.
(axial, noncontrast scan; SE 2500/45)

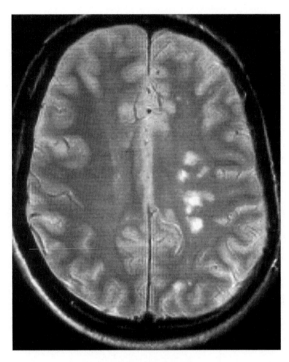

Watershed Infarction
(due to ICA dissection)

Hemispheric involvement by multiple sclerosis may be asymmetrical, as in Case 496. In some instances, multiple plaques are entirely unilateral.

Unilateral clustering of small lesions in the centrum semiovale should also raise the possibility of intrahemispheric watershed infarction. This diagnosis is favored by a parasagittal, band-like distribution of foci, as in Case 497.

Attention to the presence or absence of normal "flow void" within basal arteries and/or MR angiography can confirm the vascular etiology of white matter lesions in such cases.

The patient in Case 497 was found to have suffered a dissection of the left internal carotid artery at the skull base (see Cases 544 and 545).

Case 498

8-year-old boy presenting with a mildly spastic gait.
(axial, noncontrast scan; SE 3000/90)

Case 499

18-month-old girl with "cerebral palsy."
(coronal, noncontrast scan; SE 600/15)

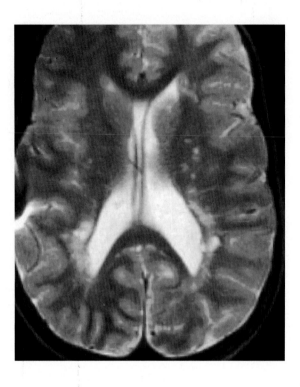

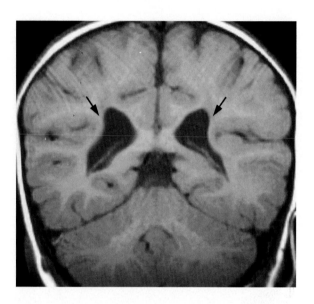

Periventricular leukomalacia (PVL) is a syndrome of multifocal damage within deep hemisphere white matter in premature infants. The etiology of PVL has traditionally been assumed to be a hypoxic/ischemic insult to the watershed zones of the developing brain. Other contributing factors (toxic, metabolic, and immune-mediated) have been suggested recently. The perinatal diagnosis of PVL is based on ultrasound studies, which demonstrate abnormal echogenicity and subsequent cyst formation in the periventricular regions.

White matter near the posterior bodies and trigones of the lateral ventricles is most frequently and most severely affected. Areas of focal periventricular necrosis frequently cavitate. They may persist as independent cysts surrounded by margins of scar tissue. Alternatively, they may become incorporated into the adjacent ventricular body, causing it to acquire an irregular or scalloped lateral margin.

Case 498 illustrates the former appearance. Multiple posterior periventricular foci of signal abnormality indicate sites of white matter necrosis. The posterior bodies of the

lateral ventricles are expanded due to the loss of adjacent parenchyma.

The areas of abnormal signal intensity in Case 498 are sharper, smaller, and closer to the ventricular border than the zones of slow myelination frequently seen in deep parietal white matter of young children (compare to Case 381). The multifocal and sharply defined morphology of the lesions combine with ventricular expansion to distinguish the overall appearance from adrenoleukodystrophy (see Case 380).

Loss of white matter volume is a hallmark of periventricular leukomalacia and may establish the diagnosis even when individual lesions are poorly defined. Case 499 demonstrates marked thinning of white matter which should normally separate the cortical sulci from the ventricular margin (arrows). Together with expansion of the posterior portions of the lateral ventricles, this abnormally deep invagination of lateral sulci suggests a hypoxic/ischemic insult before or early in the third trimester of fetal development.

PERIVENTRICULAR LEUKOMALACIA:
IRREGULAR VENTRICULAR CONTOURS

Case 500

3-year-old boy presenting with seizures
and spasticity.
(axial, noncontrast scan; SE 2800/45)

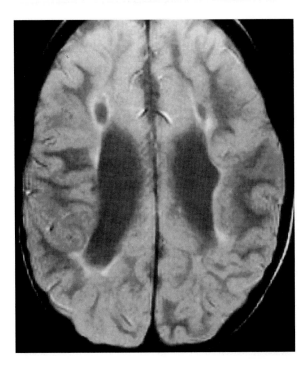

Case 501

18-month-old girl with "cerebral palsy."
(axial, noncontrast scan; SE 2800/90)

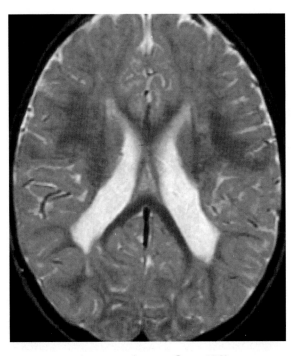

(same patient as Case 499)

The reactive capability of the immature brain is very limited. Parenchymal damage or any type leads to dissolution of tissue with minimal residual gliosis. As a result, PVL may present as a featureless loss of white matter volume (see Case 499). Alternatively, areas of focal necrosis within periventricular white matter may be incorporated into the adjacent ventricular chamber.

This process results in a typical morphology of the lateral ventricles, as illustrated in the above cases. The posterior portions of the ventricles are symmetrically expanded, reflecting overall loss of deep hemispheric white matter. In addition, the lateral margin of the ventricles is irregular or angular, due to loss and cavitation of subependymal parenchyma. Margins of gliosis may line the ventricular contour, as in Case 500.

The dilatation of the posterior portion of the lateral ventricles associated with PVL should be distinguished from the more rounded appearance of colpocephaly, a developmental malformation (see Cases 722 and 723).

The clinical presentation of spastic diplegia or "cerebral palsy" is a common manifestation of PVL. However, PVL (and presumed hypoxic/ischemic encephalopathy) accounts for only a small fraction of such cases. Many infants with "cerebral palsy" attributed to "birth asphyxia" are found to have congenital malformations of the brain such as neuronal migration disorders (see Cases 732-740).

Case 502

44-year-old woman with a history of recurrent
small strokes.
(axial, noncontrast scan; SE 2800/45)

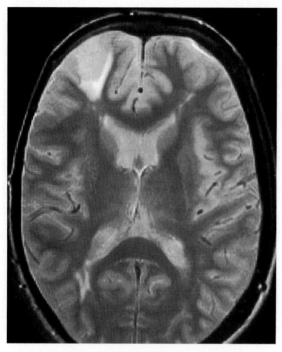

Antiphospholipid Antibody Syndrome
(positive lupus anticoagulant)

Case 503

45-year-old man presenting with decreased
level of consciousness.
(axial, noncontrast scan; SE 3000/45)

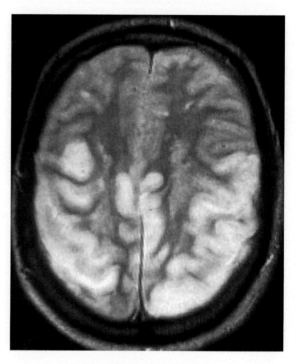

Granulomatous Angiitis

As discussed in Cases 492 and 493, multifocal infarction occurring simultaneously or over a period of time suggests a differential diagnosis including emboli, coagulopathy, and vasculitis.

The heart and carotid arteries are the most likely sources of multiple cerebral emboli. Paradoxical cardiac embolization may be due to congenital heart disease or pulmonary arteriovenous communication, as in the Osler-Weber-Rendu syndrome (hereditary hemorrhagic telangiectasia).

Case 502 is an example of multiple deep and superficial cerebral infarcts due to coagulopathy. The presence of the lupus anticoagulant (an antiphospholipid antibody) in vitro is a marker for a tendency toward thrombosis in vivo. This syndrome may also present clinically as recurrent thrombophlebitis, dural sinus thrombosis, or repeated fetal loss during pregnancy.

The widespread cortical abnormality in Case 503 is associated with swelling indicating active edema. This multifo-

cal pattern suggests the category of vasculitis and could be seen in association with entities such as meningitis (compare to Case 387), meningovascular sypilis, or systemic lupus erythematosus (see Cases 431 and 432).

Granulomatous angiitis is an idiopathic inflammatory disorder, affecting small cerebral arteries and veins. An alternative name for the disorder is "primary angiitis of the CNS" or PACNS. Associations with immunosuppression and herpes zoster have been suggested. The course of the disease is usually progressive and fatal. Granulomatous angiitis occasionally presents with multifocal or "miliary" enhancement on MR scans, presumably representing the scattered sites of vascular inflammation and/or focal ectasia.

Other etiologies of multifocal infarction include moya moya disease (see Case 546), watershed arterial infarction (see Cases 488-490), and venous infarction secondary to dural sinus thrombosis (see Cases 642-645).

Case 504

3-year-old boy adopted from Eastern Europe,
presenting with a stroke.
(axial, noncontrast scan; SE 2800/45)

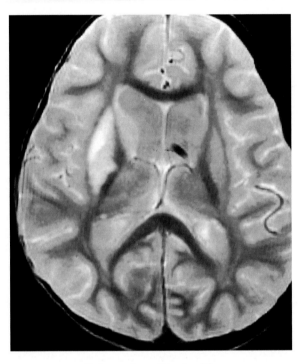

Tuberculous Meningitis

Case 505

6-year-old boy presenting with right hemiparesis.
(submentovertex display of noncontrast, three
dimensional, time-of-flight GRE sequence)

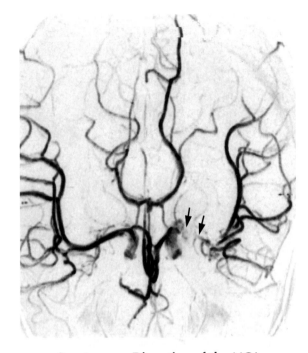

Spontaneous Dissection of the MCA

The lenticulostriate arteries supplying the basal ganglia arise from the horizontal or M-1 segment of the middle cerebral artery. When this vessel is compromised or occluded, the origins of the lenticulostriate arteries are obstructed. Since these perforating branches are end arteries without significant collateral anastomoses, their obstruction causes infarction within deep hemisphere nuclei.

Such ganglionic infarction may accompany infarction in the cortical distribution of the MCA (as in Cases 470, 482, and 483). Alternatively, infarction of the basal ganglia may be an isolated finding, as in Case 504.

In young patients, collateral flow across leptomeningeal anastomoses may prevent infarction of midhemisphere cortex despite complete occlusion of the MCA (or internal carotid artery). Ganglionic infarction may be the only manifestation of major arterial compromise in such cases.

Basal meningitis due to tuberculosis in Case 504 had caused focal inflammation and constriction of the MCA and its lenticulostriate branches. Confluent ischemic edema is

seen throughout the putamen; the caudate nucleus is spared. A shunt is present within the left frontal horn to decompress communicating hydrocephalus, another frequent complication of meningitis.

In Case 505, routine scans showed infarction involving the left caudate nucleus, putamen, and internal capsule. No accompanying cortical edema was present. The MR angiogram demonstrates severely reduced caliber of the proximal left middle cerebral artery *(arrows)*, affecting the origins of lenticulostriate arteries. Dissection of the middle cerebral artery occurs as an infrequent spontaneous event in both children and adults.

Sydenham's chorea has been reported with edema and contrast enhancement of the corpus striatum in children, potentially resembling ganglionic infarction. This syndrome, most commonly a sequela of streptococcal infection, is thought to be caused by immune-mediated cross reactivity.

Case 506

33-year-old woman presenting with acute
weakness of the left arm.
(axial, noncontrast scan; SE 2800/80)

Case 507

35-year-old woman who suddenly developed
left hemiparesis four days earlier.
(axial, noncontrast scan; SE 3000/80)

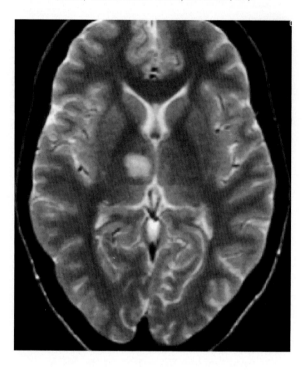

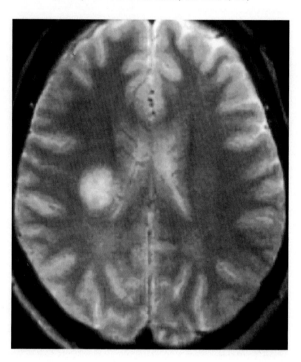

The basal ganglia, internal capsule, and corona radiata are largely supplied by lenticulostriate branches arising from the horizontal portion of the middle cerebral artery. Other contributions include medial lenticulostriate branches from the anterior cerebral artery, the anterior choroidal artery, and thalamo-perforating branches of the posterior cerebral artery (see Case 538).

Occlusion of these small perforating arteries may cause localized infarction within deep nuclei or periventricular white matter. Such lesions are often quite round and about one centimeter in diameter, as seen in the above cases. Deep hemisphere infarction may accompany extensive cortical ischemia or occur as an isolated event.

Many ganglionic/capsular infarcts are presumed to reflect atherosclerotic disease of small cerebral arteries. Other possible etiologies include arteritis (e.g., due to herpes zoster involving the basal cisterns as a complication of trigeminal neuritis). The etiology of infarction in the young adults above was not established (see discussion of Case 482).

Focal infarcts within the basal ganglia may be seen in children after head trauma. It has been suggested that the sharp angle of origin of the lenticulostriate arteries predisposes them to stretch injury and subsequent spasm. As discussed in Cases 504 and 505, ganglionic infarcts in children may also reflect large vessel disease or pathology within the basal cisterns.

DIFFERENTIAL DIAGNOSIS:
SMALL, ROUND, DEEP HEMISPHERE LESIONS

Case 508

51-year-old man.
(axial, noncontrast scan; SE 3000/90)

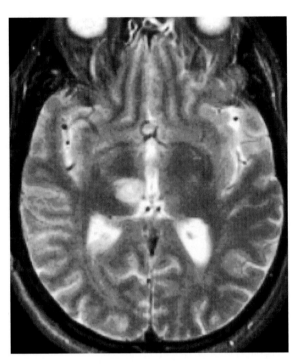

Metastatic Melanoma

Case 509

21-year-old woman with worsening
left hemiparesis.
(axial, noncontrast scan; SE 2500/45)

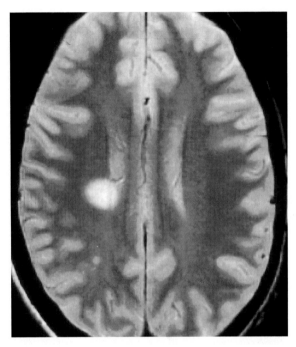

Multiple Sclerosis

The appearance of the small infarcts on the preceding page is nonspecific. The above cases emphasize the potential resemblence of neoplastic, inflammatory, and vascular lesions deep within the cerebral hemispheres.

As discussed in Chapter 1, metastatic disease typically involves subcortial portions of the brain. Case 508 illustrates that deep hemisphere metastases also occur. The faint visualization of a ring of internal architecture within the lesion would be unusual for a simple infarct and warrants further evaluation with contrast injection.

The lesion in Case 509 is comparable in size, shape, and location to Case 507. The diagnosis of demyelination can be established by a characteristic history, the presence of associated MR findings that are hallmarks for multiple sclerosis (see Chapter 7), or CSF analysis. A ring or target appearance resembling Case 508 is also commonly encountered in an intermediate stage of focal demyelination (see Cases 338-340).

Another cause of focal signal abnormality within the corona radiata, internal capsule, or brainstem is Wallerian degeneration (see Case 541-1).

Case 510

71-year-old woman with a history of hypertension.
(axial, noncontrast scan; SE 2500/28)

Case 511

89-year-old woman.
(axial, noncontrast scan; SE 2500/45)

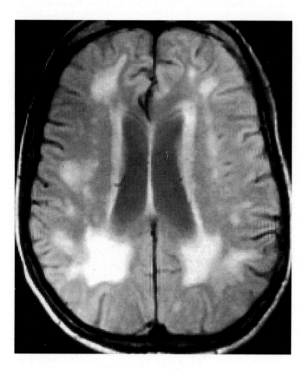

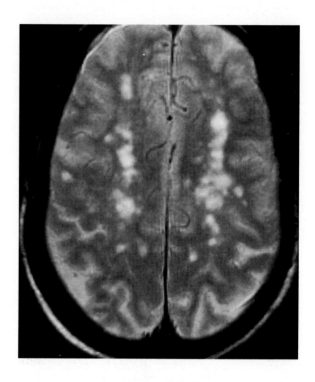

Multiple sites of focal and confluent signal abnormality are commonly seen in subcortical and periventricular white matter of patients with disease affecting small arteries. This pattern is frequently present in diabetic and/or hypertensive individuals and is routinely noted in elderly people. The lesions have been pathologically demonstrated to represent a spectrum ranging from atrophy to frank infarction.

Small, deep, cerebral infarcts are often called "lacunar infarcts," using the name that pathologists have given to tiny lesions found in the basal ganglia at autopsy. Large numbers of such infarcts have previously been suggested to be the cause of clinical "lacunar states," with components of dementia or pseudobulbar palsy. These correlations are controversial; the symptoms of patients with

multiple deep hemisphere infarcts may range from minimal to profound.

MR frequently demonstrates more ischemic foci than are visible on CT studies. In some cases these lesions are so large and numerous that they coalesce to form zones of ischemic leukoencephalopathy (see Cases 514 and 515).

The bilaterality and overall symmetry of the lesions in Cases 510 and 511 favor small arterial disease as the etiology. This pattern is distinct from intrahemispheric watershed infarction due to large vessel compromise (compare to Cases 494 and 497).

Like the plaques of demyelinating disease, ischemic white matter lesions are well-demonstrated by FLAIR (fluid-attenuated inversion recovery) pulse sequences.

Case 512

59-year-old woman presenting with left
body numbness.
(axial, noncontrast scan; SE 2500/45)

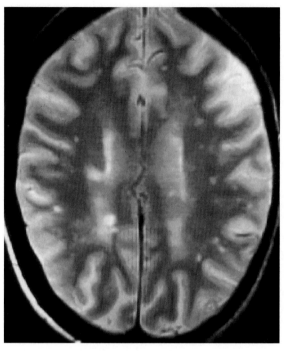

White Matter Infarcts
(associated with diabetes mellitus)

Case 513

38-year-old woman presenting with left
facial numbness.
(axial, noncontrast scan; SE 2500/45)

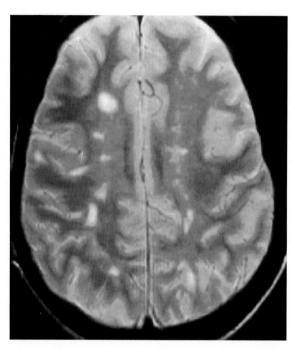

Multiple Sclerosis

Scattered infarcts in and near the corona radiata as in Case 512 may mimic the appearance of demyelinating plaques in multiple sclerosis, illustrated by Case 513. In both pathologies, periventricular lesions may be accompanied by more peripheral foci of signal abnormality in the centrum semiovale or subcortical white matter.

The periventricular plaques of multiple sclerosis are often elliptical in morphology, with the long axis perpendicular to the ventricular margin (see discussion of Cases 329 and 330). Deep hemisphere infarcts tend to be more rounded or angular in shape. However, this distinction is often difficult, as seen in the above cases.

Prolongation of T1 is usually apparent within established plaques of multiple sclerosis (see Cases 327 and 328). Low signal intensity on T1-weighted scans is usually less impres-

sive and less well defined in zones of focal ischemic change.

Associated clinical clues (e.g., a history of prior optic neuritis) or scan findings (see Cases 343-346) may also help to establish the diagnosis of multiple sclerosis when periventricular lesions are ambiguous. Patient age can assist in separating demyelinating disease from deep hemisphere infarcts, but substantial overlap in the incidence of these pathologies occurs between ages 45 and 65.

Sarcoidosis may cause multifocal white matter lesions similar to the above cases (see Case 436). Intrahemispheric watershed infarction due to large vessel disease should also be considered in the differential diagnosis (see Cases 494 and 497).

Case 514

82-year-old woman presenting with dementia.
(axial, noncontrast scan; SE 2500/90)

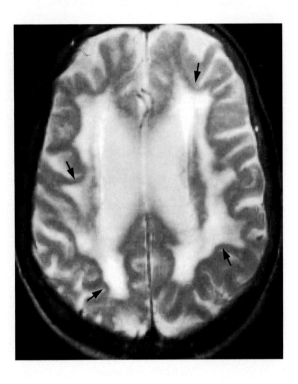

Case 515

81-year-old woman presenting with confusion.
(axial, noncontrast scan; SE 3000/45)

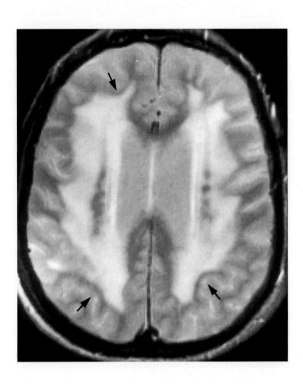

The spectrum of ischemic white matter changes extends from focal lesions such as Case 507 through multifocal patterns such as Cases 510-512 to the confluent, diffuse signal abnormality seen above. This common finding in elderly patients represents generalized microvascular white matter disease or "ischemic leukoencephalopathy." Pathological studies demonstrate hyalinization of arterioles in such cases.

Involvement may be limited to periventricular regions near the frontal horns and trigones or may extend diffusely throughout the centrum semiovale, as in Cases 514 and 515. No associated mass effect is present, and no enhancement is seen on postcontrast scans.

There is relative sparing of subcortical "U" fibers (*arrows;* compare to Case 378), which receive a dual blood supply from recurrent loops and penetrating branches of cortical arteries. The corpus callosum is also usually spared, as seen above. The latter feature has been attributed to callosal sup-

ply from short arterioles that are not as susceptible to the vascular changes developing with age as longer penetrating vessels.

Microvascular white matter disease may present a pattern of scattered, patchy signal abnormality resembling a leukoencephalopathy such as PML (see Cases 367-371). Clues to the correct diagnosis include the general symmetry of ischemic cerebral involvement and the predominant location in midhemisphere and deep hemisphere regions. By contrast, PML frequently affects subcortical white matter and often demonstrates less symmetry than is seen in Cases 514 and 515.

White matter changes in elderly patients correlate clinically with impairment of fine motor control, diminished reflexes, gait abnormality, and an increased incidence of falls. There is little relationship to reduced cognitive ability, which is better correlated with ganglionic lesions and temporal lobe atrophy (see Cases 457 and 458).

DIFFERENTIAL DIAGNOSIS:
DIFFUSE WHITE MATTER DAMAGE IN AN ADULT

Case 516

50-year-old woman with a long history
of diffuse spasticity.
(axial, noncontrast scan; SE 2800/25)

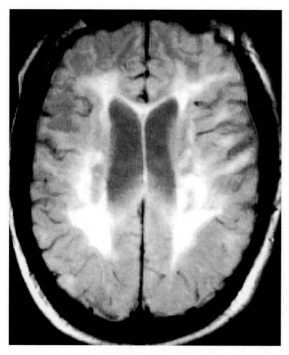

Multiple Sclerosis

Case 517

65-year-old man with a history of carcinoma
of the lung.
(axial, non-contrast scan; SE 2500/90)

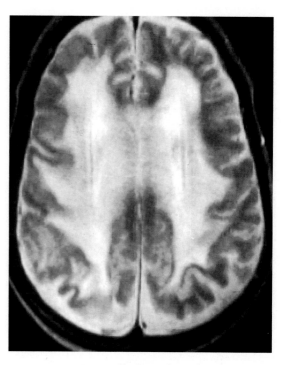

Postradiation Change

Widespread injury to cerebral white matter is most commonly the result of aging and presumed ischemic change, as illustrated on the preceding page. However, any severe leukoencephalopathy can lead to confluent alteration of CT attenuation values and MR signal intensity within the centrum semiovale.

Case 516 illustrates extensive, multifocal white matter involvement in severe multiple sclerosis. In an older patient and in an ambiguous clinical context, demyelinating disease can be distinguished from ischemic white matter changes by involvement of subcortical "U" fibers and the corpus callosum in the former disorder. These regions are typically spared from ischemic change, as discussed previously.

Radiation therapy can cause diffuse abnormality of cerebral white matter. (See Cases 448 and 449 for other possible presentations of radiation change.) Such alterations

may be seen at any age. In adults, the extent of radiation damage as depicted by MR and its clinical significance appear to increase with patient age at the time of treatment.

Some cases of carbon monoxide poisoning result in extensive damage to white matter indistinguishable from Cases 514 to 517. In such instances, initial recovery from an anoxic insult is followed by rapid deterioration after several weeks or months due to delayed postanoxic leukoencephalopathy. Mitochondrial encephalomyopathies (see Case 447) can also lead to an appearance resembling the above scans.

Compare the diffuse acquired white matter disease in Cases 514 through 517 with the leukodystrophies due to abnormal formation of myelin in Cases 377 and 380, and contrast this appearance with the multifocal pattern of inflammatory and neoplastic diseases such as Cases 371 and 372.

Case 518

82-year-old woman presenting with dementia.
(axial, noncontrast scan; SE 3000/90)

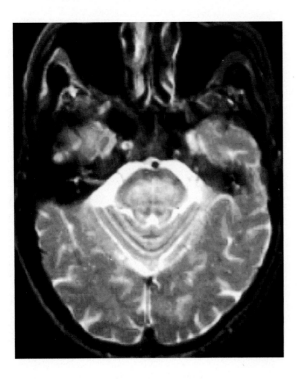

Case 519

38-year-old man presenting with the acute onset
of right hemiparesis and hemianesthesia.
(axial, noncontrast scan; SE 3000/90)

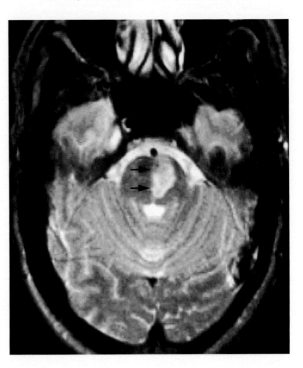

MR is valuable for confirming and localizing the clinical diagnosis of brainstem ischemia. CT scans may fail to define recent brainstem infarcts, since they are often small and their subtle attenuation changes are obscured by interpetrous artifact.

Small arterial disease affecting the brainstem is usually most apparent at the rostral pontine level. Case 518 is a typical example, with multiple hazy foci of increased signal intensity clustered centrally. Scans through the cerebral hemispheres in such cases usually demonstrate associated lacunar infarcts in the basal ganglia and periventricular white matter, comparable to Cases 510 and 511. Patients with this MR appearance may have surprisingly minimal symptoms.

Case 519 illustrates a focal brainstem infarct. Such lesions are usually larger, better defined, and less symmetrical than the generalized ischemic changes seen in Case 518. A sharp medial margin of the lesion at the anatomical midline is apparent *(arrows)*. This feature is common in brainstem infarcts and may help to distinguish them from demyelinating foci, central pontine myelinolysis, and other brainstem pathologies.

The status of the basilar artery is of interest in cases of brainstem ischemia. Reduced lumen size and absence of normal "flow void" may be noted (see Case 543). However, most localized brainstem infarcts are caused by small vessel disease involving the pontine perforating arteries. In the above cases, the basilar artery appears normal.

DIFFERENTIAL DIAGNOSIS:
HIGH SIGNAL FOCI WITHIN THE BRAINSTEM ON T2-WEIGHTED IMAGES

Case 520

35-year-old woman presenting with acute ataxia.
(axial, noncontrast scan; SE 2800/90)

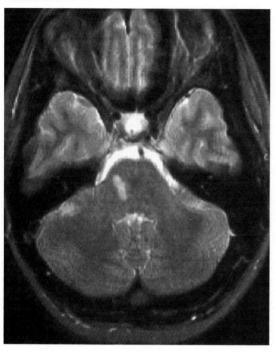

Brainstem Infarct

Case 521

45-year-old woman complaining of dizziness.
(axial, noncontrast scan; SE 2800/90)

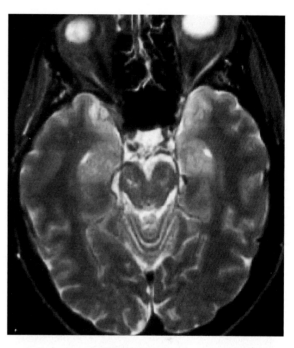

Midbrain Cysts
(normal variant)

Case 520 is another example of a typical brainstem infarct. The lesion is smaller than Case 519 but is similarly eccentric and well-defined.

Small cysts of developmental origin are occasionally found within the cerebral peduncles, as in Case 521. These tiny CSF collections have been described as prominent perivascular spaces, analogous to similar structures in the sublenticular areas (see Case 705) or cerebral hemispheres (see Case 334). They may be unilateral or bilateral, producing a vague haze of focally increased signal intensity or a clearly defined cystic zone. Their characteristic location within the ventral midbrain and the absence of associated symptoms distinguish these developmental variants from brainstem infarcts, most of which occur more caudally. (The lack of visualization of the basilar artery in the interpeduncular region of Case 521 is due to a congenitally low bifurcation.)

Small brainstem infarcts may resemble involvement by

multiple sclerosis (see Case 358). The clinical setting and associated lesions usually distinguish between these pathologies. Demyelinating plaques in the brainstem tend to be rounder than focal infarcts.

Brainstem metastases can present a similar appearance and should be considered in the appropriate context (see Case 357). Wallerian degeneration may cause a focal area of signal abnormality resembling brainstem infarction on axial images (see Case 541-1). Associated encephalomalacia within the ipsilateral cerebral hemisphere is apparent in such cases, and the lesion can be followed in continuity across several levels of anatomy as it courses along a fiber tract.

Central pontine myelinolysis may also produce abnormal signal intensity within the brainstem, as discussed in Cases 375 and 376. The characteristic clinical context and symmetrical central involvement of the pons usually establish the diagnosis of this disorder.

Case 522

9-year-old boy presenting with the acute
onset of ataxia.
(axial, noncontrast scan; SE 2500/90)

Case 523

73-year-old woman presenting with nausea
and ataxia.
(axial, noncontrast scan; SE 2500/45)

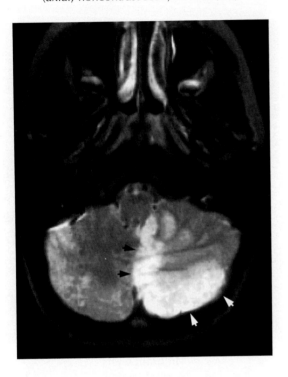

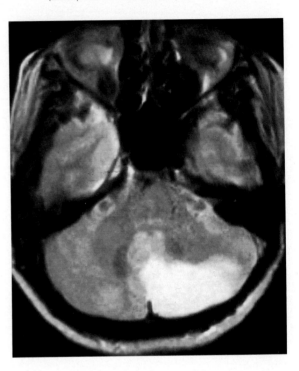

Infarction of the cerebellum may cause confusing lesions in the posterior fossa. In many cases the diagnosis can be made by recognizing the distribution of a major cerebellar artery.

The posterior inferior cerebellar artery (PICA) supplies (1) a broad rim of peripheral cerebellar hemisphere along the occipital inner table (*white arrows*, Case 522) and (2) a parasagittal strip of medial hemisphere and inferior vermis extending posteriorly from the fourth ventricle (*black arrows*, Case 522). Infarction in the PICA distribution is suggested when a cerebellar lesion demonstrates a scythe-like configuration, with a curving peripheral crescent of involved hemisphere linked to a parasagittal band that borders the midline. Incomplete infarction in the PICA territory may cause abnormal signal intensity in either the peripheral or the parasagittal component of the distribution.

In Case 523, the predominant hemispheric involvement and the early mass effect present a more spherical morphology. The lesion could be confused with a tumor. However, the peripheral base and the suggestion of a parasagittal component favor PICA infarction.

Early ischemic edema is seen within the lateral portion of the right cerebellar hemisphere in Case 522. This boy was found to have spontaneous dissection of a vertebral artery, with multiple secondary emboli to the basilar system. Symptoms associated with dissection of carotid or vertebral arteries are more commonly due to secondary embolization than to hypoperfusion from luminal compromise.

Case 524

55-year-old man with a four-day history of vertigo.
(coronal, postcontrast scan; SE 600/15)

Case 525

42-year-old man presenting with dizziness.
(coronal, postcontrast scan; SE 600/15)

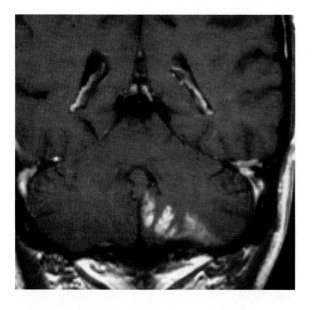

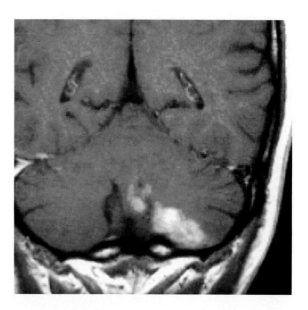

The localization of a cerebellar lesion within a major arterial distribution may be more easily appreciated on coronal or sagittal scans than on axial images.

The PICA supply to the inferior surface of the cerebellar hemisphere is clearly displayed in the coronal plane, as seen above. Case 524 illustrates the cerebellar equivalent of gyriform enhancement as discussed in Cases 485 and 486. The frond-like morphology of enhancing gray matter within cerebellar folia is peripherally based and falls within the distribution of the left PICA, supporting a diagnosis of subacute infarction.

Enhancement of the subacute PICA infarct in Case 525 is more solid and amorphous. However, the localization within a vascular distribution again suggests the correct diagnosis.

In both of these cases, the medial margin of the lesion is sharply defined at the midline. This respect for an anatomical boundary helps to place otherwise ambiguous cerebellar lesions in the vascular category.

Case 526

24-year-old woman presenting with the
acute onset of ataxia.
(axial, noncontrast scan; SE 2800/90)

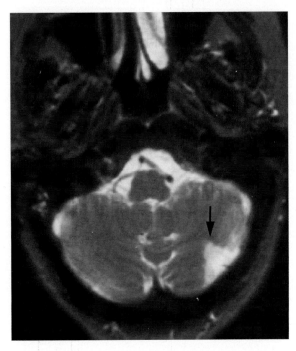

Infarction Within the PICA Distribution

Case 527

37-year-old woman with a history of seizures.
(axial, noncontrast scan; SE 2800/90)

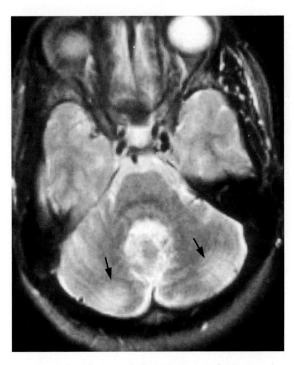

Partial Volume of the Horizontal Fissures

Cerebellar infarction may involve only peripheral portions of a major arterial distribution. Case 526 is an example of this pattern. The small area of superficially based edema within the left cerebellar hemisphere *(arrow)* is due to distal occlusion of a branch of the PICA.

Infarction is the most likely cause of acute cerebellar signs in a young adult. This possibility should be considered (along with labyrinthine disease) when young patients present with vertigo or ataxia.

Case 527 demonstrates mild cerebellar atrophy, likely associated with long-term dilantin therapy (see Case 460). Atrophy causes enlargement of the great horizontal fissures, which are mildly oblique to the plane of axial MR images. As a result, partial volume of CSF within the fissures may cause a focal area of long T1 and T2 values at the margin of the cerebellar hemispheres. This appearance is bilateral in Case 527 *(arrows)*, aiding identification. However, a small amount of head tilt may cause the finding to be unilateral, potentially resembling a small PICA infarct. Correlation with sagittal and coronal scans is helpful in ambiguous cases (see Cases 591 and 614 for additional examples).

DIFFERENTIAL DIAGNOSIS:
FOCAL LESION WITHIN THE LATERAL MEDULLA

Case 528

85-year-old woman presenting with nausea, vertigo, dysphagia, and left facial numbness.
(axial, noncontrast scan; SE 2500/90)

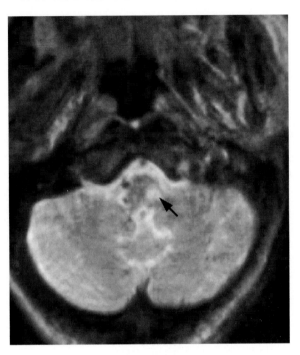

PICA Infarct

Case 529

39-year-old woman presenting with diplopia.
(axial, noncontrast scan; SE 3000/90)

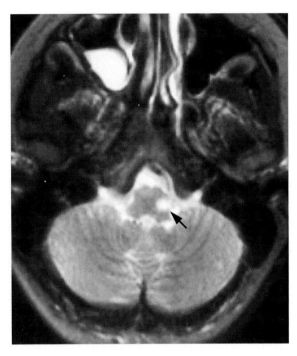

Multiple Sclerosis

Magnetic resonance imaging is more sensitive than CT for demonstrating the brainstem consequences of PICA occlusion. The lateral aspect of the medulla is often infarcted in such cases, correlating with the clinical picture of Wallenberg's syndrome.

Case 528 is a typical example. The lack of apparent cerebellar infarction in this case may reflect either partial occlusion with sparing of hemispheric trunks or good leptomeningeal collateral perfusion of the hemispheric territory. The latter situation is common, with high flow anastomoses between the inferior vermian branch of the PICA and the superior vermian branch of the superior cerebellar artery.

Multiple sclerosis can involve all levels of the brainstem (see Cases 355-358 for additional examples). The lesion in Case 529 is nonspecific but should raise the question of demyelinating disease. Clinical context will usually distinguish this possibility from medullary infarction in a young adult, which is often due to dissection of the vertebral artery.

Focal signal abnormality may develop within the lateral medulla when the olive is disconnected from afferent tracts by lesions of the pontine tegmentum or contralateral cerebellum. This transsynaptic degeneration occurs weeks to months after the inciting lesion, which is most commonly a hematoma. Such "hypertrophic olivary degeneration" includes vacuolization of neurons and hypertrophy of astrocytes, causing focal swelling as well as prolongation of T1 and T2. The resulting medullary lesion may mimic a subacute infarct, demyelinating plaque, or small mass. The presence of coexisting pathology and the typical clinical presentation with palatal myoclonus and dysarthria help to establish the diagnosis.

A retention cyst is present in the right maxillary sinus in Case 529.

Case 530

75-year-old man presenting with ataxia and
decreasing level of consciousness.
(axial, noncontrast scan; SE 2500/90).

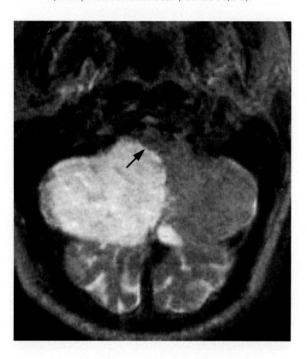

Case 531

45-year-old woman with a week-long history of
incoordination and right hemihypesthesia.
(coronal, postcontrast scan; SE 600/15)

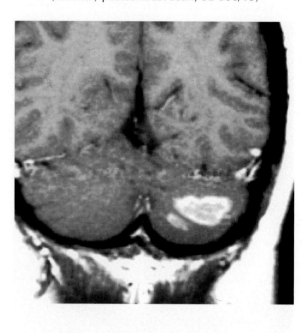

The linear margins emphasized in Cases 524 and 525 can
be an important clue to the diagnosis of PICA infarction.
However, subacute cerebellar infarcts may demonstrate
convex borders mimicking mass lesions.

In Case 530, the convex margins and homogeneous texture of the lesion resemble an intraaxial neoplasm. The medial margin of the infarct represents the anatomical midline
but is bowed contralaterally by edema. Mass effect within
the infarcted region causes mild flattening of the right posterolateral aspect of the medulla *(arrow)*.

Tissue swelling from cerebellar infarction may lead to
life-threatening pressure on the brainstem. Acute decompression is required in such cases, similar to the urgent
evacuation of large cerebellar hematomas.

Contrast enhancement in Case 531 is more central and
less frond-like than the characteristic patterns of Cases 524
and 525. This solid-appearing morphology is nonspecific
but does occur within the spectrum of cerebellar infarction.
Clinical correlation and follow-up scans may be necessary
to establish the diagnosis.

Case 532

40-year-old woman presenting with tinnitus.
(axial, noncontrast scan; SE 3000/75)

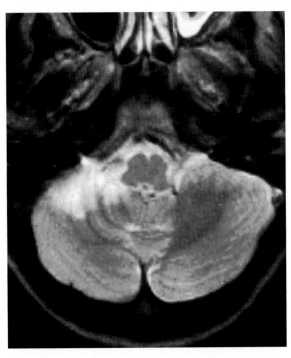

Infarction in the Distribution of the AICA

Case 533

24-year-old woman presenting with right
facial numbness.
(axial, noncontrast scan; SE 2200/90)

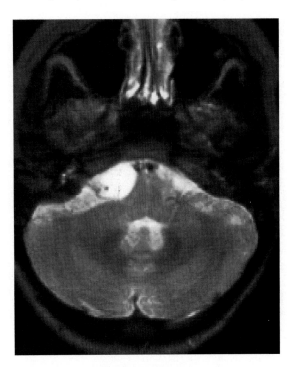

Epidermoid Cyst

Infarction in the distribution of the anterior inferior cerebellar artery (AICA) is infrequent, reflecting the normally good collateral flow to this region. When an AICA infarct is encountered as in Case 532, the appearance may mimic other intraaxial or extraaxial pathologies.

The AICA supplies the anterolateral portion of the cerebellar hemisphere, immediately posterior and lateral to the medulla. This distribution fills in the gap left by the crescent-shaped PICA territory supplying the medial and posterior cerebellar surface. Compare the involved region in Case 532 with the spared region of the left cerebellar hemisphere in Case 522.

A clue to the diagnosis in Case 532 is the finger-like or serrated medial margin of the lesion caused by ischemic edema widening individual folia. This layered edema reflects the parallel structure of cerebellar cortex, contrasting with the more curvilinear organization of gyriform edema within cerebral convolutions. (See Case 536 for another example of layered edema in cerebellar infarction.)

The epidermoid cyst in Case 533 is clearly extraaxial, with displacement and deformity of the brainstem and middle cerebellar peduncle. An arachnoid cyst might be considered in the differential diagnosis (see Cases 693-695), but the suggestion of heterogeneous signal intensity within the lesion would be unusual. A predominantly cystic schwannoma or meningioma could present a similar appearance.

Mucosal thickening is present in the left maxillary sinus in Case 532.

Case 534

9-year-old boy presenting with the acute
onset of ataxia.
(sagittal, noncontrast scan; SE 600/20)

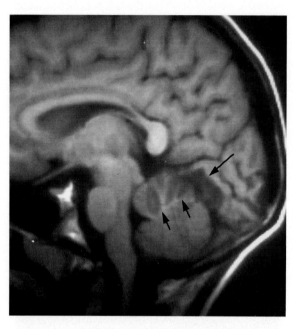

(same patient as Case 522)

Case 535

60-year-old woman presenting with headaches.
(axial, noncontrast scan; SE 2500/90)

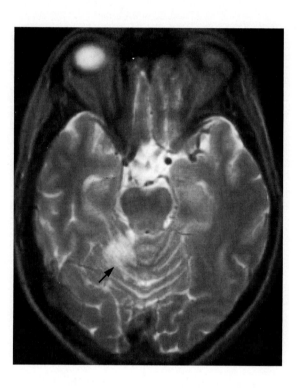

The superior cerebellar artery (SCA) supplies the superior portion of the cerebellar hemisphere and vermis. Infarction in the distribution of this vessel usually involves the hemisphere but may spare the vermis due to collateral circulation from the inferior vermian arteries.

The above cases illustrate the variable medial/lateral extent of SCA infarction. In Case 534, a midsagittal scan demonstrates cortical edema within folia of the superior vermis *(short arrows)*. In Case 535, the midline SCA territory is spared, and infarction is limited to a small portion of the superior cerebellar hemisphere on the right *(arrow)*.

Cerebellar infarcts may accompany lesions in the occipital lobes when embolization has occurred within the vertebrobasilar system. Ischemic occipital edema is present in Case 534 *(long arrow;* see also Case 539). A careful search for cerebellar lesions can help to suggest vertebrobasilar emboli when ambiguous occipital pathology is encountered.

Cerebellar watershed infarction is infrequent. Such lesions are usually intrahemispheric, occurring within the corpus medullaris at the junction of the PICA, AICA, and SCA territories. Cystic encephalomalacia is occasionally seen in this location in children, possibly reflecting intrauterine or perinatal vascular insufficiency of the watershed zone.

Case 536

24-year-old man presenting with the acute
onset of ataxia.
(axial, noncontrast scan; SE 2500/90)

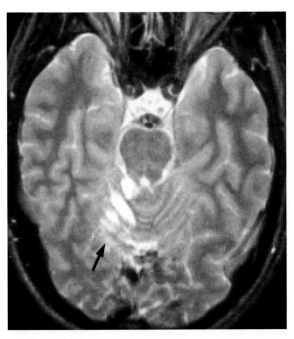

SCA Infarct

Case 537

60-year-old woman presenting with unsteady gait.
(axial, noncontrast scan; SE 3000/90)

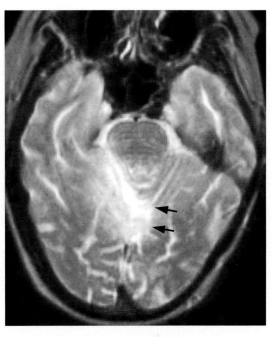

Leptomeningeal Metastasis
(from carcinoma of the breast)

The small region of high signal intensity involving the superior right cerebellar hemisphere in Case 536 *(arrow)* represents infarction within the distribution of the superior cerebellar artery. The straight, diagonal lateral margin of the lesion is a hallmark of infarction in the SCA territory, which is bounded laterally by the tentorium.

The medial margin of SCA infarcts is variable and less distinct, depending on collateral flow patterns. A mildly serrated pattern of edema following the orientation of folia is characteristic of subacute cerebellar infarction (compare to Case 532).

Meningeal seeding of intracranial tumors or systemic neoplasms often affects the superior cerebellar surface (see Cases 160-162 for additional examples). This pattern resembles the preferential deposition of superficial siderosis in the same region under conditions of chronic subarachniod hemorrhage (see Case 591). Both phenomena may reflect patterns of CSF flow and stagnation, with subarach-

noid cells or hemorrhage preferentially bathing superior cerebellar tissue.

The zone of signal abnormality in Case 537 corresponds approximately to the SCA distribution. However, the extension across midline *(arrows)* would be atypical for a vascular etiology.

Postcontrast scans in both of the above cases might show a gyriform pattern of parallel, enhancing bands. In Case 536 the enhancement would represent ischemic cortex. In Case 537 a similar morphology could be produced by enhancing layers of meningeal tumor within cerebellar sulci (see Cases 160B, 161, and 162).

Case 537 also illustrates that pathologies other than SCA infarction can be marginated by the tentorium. A subdural empyema or chronic hematoma along the inferior surface of the tentorium could resemble the overall morphology of the above cases.

Case 538

72-year-old man who suddenly became
unresponsive.
(axial, noncontrast scan; SE 2500/90)

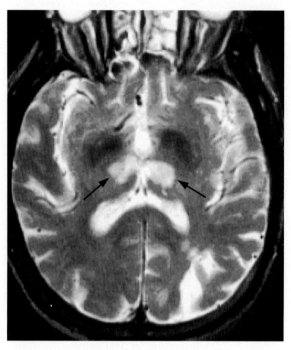

Embolic Occlusion of the Distal Basilar Artery

Case 539

9-year-old boy presenting with the
acute onset of ataxia.
(axial, noncontrast scan; SE 2500/90)

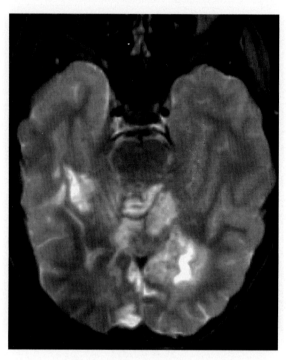

**Multiple Emboli from Dissection
of a Vertebral Artery**

The pattern of bithalamic infarction in Case 538 *(arrows)* is characteristic of small arterial compromise near the tip of the basilar artery. Perforating branches arise near the basilar bifurcation (and from the posterior communicating and proximal posterior cerebral arteries) to supply the diencephalon. Pathology affecting these vessels at the level of the suprasellar and interpeduncular cisterns may cause a characteristic pattern of symmetrical thalamic infarction. Such "thalamotuberal" infarcts may also occur unilaterally due to asymmetrical occlusion or spasm of anterior thalamo-perforating arteries.

Bithalamic infarction in Case 538 was due to embolic occlusion of the distal basilar artery. A similar appearance could be seen following subarachnoid hemorrhage from a basilar tip aneurysm complicated by vasospasm and/or surgery. A mass involving the retrosellar region could produce a comparable image by encasement or compression of perforating basilar branches.

In addition to basilar tip infarction, symmetrical signal abnormality within the thalami may be due to Wernicke's encephalopathy, Leigh's disease (see Case 440), extrapontine myelinolysis (see Case 430), bithalmic glioma crossing the massa intermedia, or deep venous thrombosis.

Case 539 illustrates multiple temporooccipital and cerebellar lesions caused by embolization within the territory of the basilar artery. Infarction should be considered along with metastases or inflammatory foci when scattered lesions are encountered throughout the basilar artery distribution. This appearance can be due to a single shower of emboli or reflect recurrent embolization from a proximal source of thrombus. Dissections of the vertebral or basilar artery are a primary consideration when this pattern is encountered.

A small infarct at the lateral margin of the left occipital lobe is present in Case 538.

Case 540

51-year-old woman, two years after a
right hemisphere stroke.
(axial, noncontrast scan; SE 3000/30)

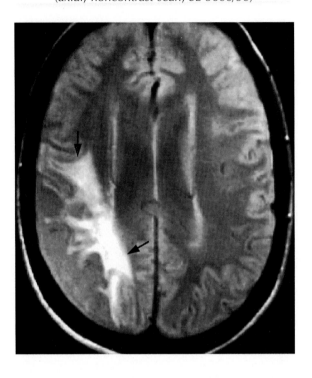

Case 541

26-year-old women with a life-long history
of seizures and mild right hemiparesis.
(axial, noncontrast scan; SE 2500/28)

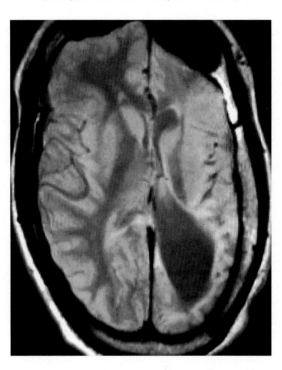

Spin echo scans with long TR and short TE values typically demonstrate two zones of signal abnormality within old cerebral infarcts. Case 540 illustrates this characteristic appearance. (See Case 493 for another example.)

Scar tissue along the interface between the affected area and normal parenchyma causes a margin of high signal intensity *(arrows)*. This border zone is typically irregular and of variable thickness. The more peripheral portion of the infarcted region is homogeneous and comparable to CSF in intensity. This region may be microcystic and/or grossly cavitated, with variable communication to the subarachnoid space.

Volume loss usually accompanies the altered signal intensity of old infarcts, with expansion of adjacent portions of the ventricular system. No enhancement is seen after contrast injection.

Case 541 is an example of the Dyke-Davidoff-Masson syndrome of cerebral hemiatrophy with hemicranial hypertrophy (see also Cases 672 and 769). A cerebrovascular ac-

cident in infancy has caused reduced parenchymal volume throughout the distribution of the left middle cerebral artery. Scarring is present in the posterior portion of the hemisphere, where localized volume loss is indicated by expansion of the ventricular trigone.

The reduced hemisphere volume in Case 541 has led to ipsilateral changes in calvarial morphology, demonstrating the interrelationship of brain growth and skull contour. The involved hemicranium is small, with eccentric falx position. The skull is thickened on the side of cerebral atrophy. An additional typical finding is asymmetrical enlargement of ipsilateral sinuses and air cells.

More focal areas of intrauterine or perinatal infarction may present as localized regions in which the volume of individual cerebral gyri is markedly reduced. Subsequent development of the remainder of the brain may crowd the shrunken gyri, creating an appearance of secondary polymicrogyria.

Case 541-1A

48-year-old man, one year after severe
head trauma.
(axial, noncontrast scan: SE 2400/80)

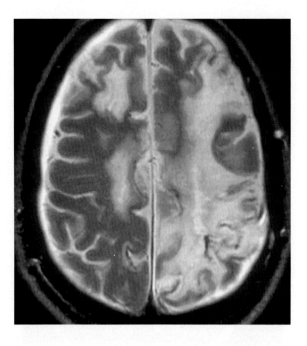

Case 541-1B

Same patient.
(axial, noncontrast scan; SE 2400/80)

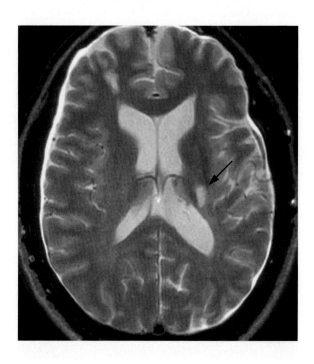

The phrase "Wallerian degeneration" is used to describe degeneration of an axon secondary to injury to the body (or more proximal axon) of a nerve cell. When tissue damage involves a group of neurons that serves as the source of a major fiber tract, the aggregate degeneration of clustered axons may become apparent on CT and MR scans. This finding is most commonly noted after cerebral infarction, although other causes of cortical injury can produce the same appearance.

MR studies have shown biphasic intensity changes during Wallerian degeneration. An initial period of T2-shortening within the fiber tract is possibly related to predominance of hydrophobic myelin lipids. This is followed by permanent prolongation of T2 reflecting cell death and gliosis. Accompanying volume loss of the affected tract is often apparent.

Case 541-1B demonstrates a focal zone of signal abnormality at the junction of the posterior corona radiata and the posterior limb of the internal capsule. This "lesion" represents the cross-section of axonal degeneration along the corticospinal tract, which begins in the area of frontoparietal encephalomalacia shown in Case 541-1A. High signal intensity within this tract could be followed sequentially across every section of the scan, with an increasingly compact area at more inferior levels (see the next page).

Areas of T2-shortening within the left parietal lesion in Case 541-1A are probably due to old blood products in a zone of previous contusion. Small subdural hygromas are present bilaterally.

Case 541-1C

Same patient.
(axial, noncontrast scan; SE 2400/80)

Case 541-1D

Same patient.
(axial, noncontrast scan; SE 2400/80)

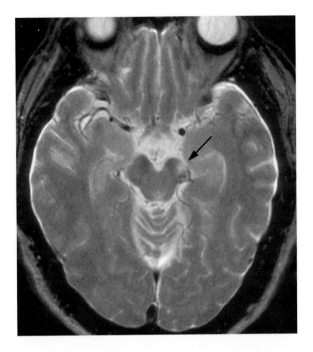

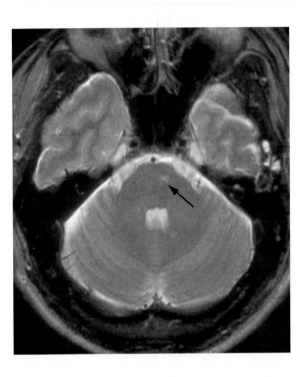

Abnormal signal intensity along the left corticospinal tract continues caudally in these images. Lower sections documented extension of Wallerian degeneration into the pyramid of the medulla.

The cross-sectional appearance of Wallerian degeneration on any one axial image resembles focal infarction within the corona radiata, internal capsule, or brainstem. (Compare the above scans to Cases 506, 507, 519, and 520.)

However, the continuity of the finding across adjacent levels establishes the diagnosis. Coronal scans confirm the cephalocaudal course of the tract degeneration in such cases.

Involvement of the corticospinal tract by Wallerian degeneration is analagous to the MR findings in some cases of amyotrophic lateral sclerosis, illustrated in Case 428.

Case 542

59-year-old woman presenting with left
hemisphere TIAs.
(axial, noncontrast scan; SE 2500/90)

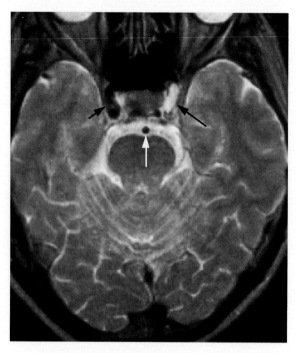

Left Internal Carotid Artery Occlusion

Case 543

67-year-old man presenting with transient
diplopia and ataxia.
(axial, noncontrast scan; SE 2800/90)

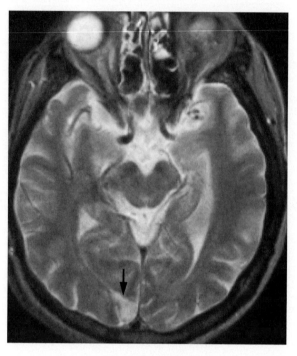

Basilar Artery Stenosis

The characteristic appearance of rapidly flowing blood on routine spin echo MR scans is an absence of signal intensity or "flow void." When this expected lack of signal is replaced by measurable intraluminal intensity, slow flow or thrombus should be suspected. (See the discussion of arterial enhancement in Cases 482 and 483.)

In Case 542, high signal within the left supraclinoid internal carotid artery *(long black arrow)* contrasts with the normal "flow void" of the right paraclinoid internal carotid artery *(short black arrow)* and rostral basilar artery *(white arrow)*. The left parasellar internal carotid artery was found to be completely occluded at angiography.

Case 543 demonstrates conspicuous absence of the expected "flow void" of the basilar artery within the interpeduncular cistern. A small infarct at the right occipital pole *(arrow)* is the only evidence of secondary infarction in this case. However, fluctuating symptoms of basilar ischemia led to angiography, which demonstrated high grade stenosis of the mid-basilar artery.

Congenitally low bifurcation of the basilar artery can cause an appearance similar to Case 543 (see Case 521 for an example). This anatomical variant can be easily recognized by following the course of the posterior cerebral arteries to or from the basilar artery.

The signal intensity of intraluminal thrombus is variable. Arterial ("white") thrombi are often isointense to cerebral parenchyma. Venous ("red") thrombi containing more erythrocytes may demonstrate T1- and T2-shortening.

Reduced caliber of patent arteries at the skull base is another MR sign of vascular compromise. This finding may be associated with extracranial or intracranial stenoses (see discussion of Moya Moya disease in Case 546).

Case 544

58-year-old man with a two-day history of
left neck pain, now presenting with TIAs.
(axial, noncontrast scan; SE 2500/45)

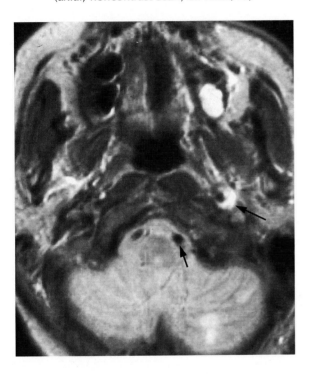

Case 545

47-year-old man presenting with a three-day
history of left neck pain and mild aphasia.
(axial, noncontrast scan; SE 2500/45)

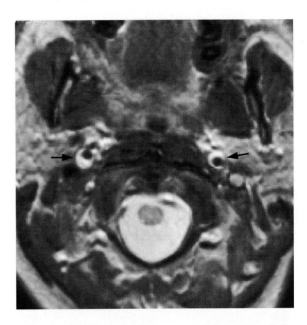

Spontaneous dissections of cervical arteries tend to occur in young to middle-aged adults (mean age 45 years). The internal carotid arteries are involved four times more commonly than the vertebral arteries.

MR can diagnose arterial dissection by direct demonstration of the intramural hematoma. Scans perpendicular to the long axis of an artery define crescentic thickening of the vessel wall, eccentrically narrowing the lumen at the level of dissection.

In Case 544, an intramural hematoma involving the left internal carotid artery at the skull base *(long arrow)* is seen as a high intensity crescent along the lateral wall of the vessel. (Compare this appearance to the normal wall thickness of the distal vertebral artery; *short arrow.*) The right internal carotid artery was severely narrowed due to an old dissection. Small cerebellar infarcts are present on the left, and a retention cyst is seen in the left maxillary sinus.

Case 545 illustrates bilateral dissection of the internal carotid arteries near the junction of the cervical and petrous

segments *(arrows)*. The patient could not recall a history of right-sided neck pain or right hemisphere symptoms.

About 25% of patients with dissection of one internal carotid artery or vertebral artery are found to have coexisting dissection of a second cervical vessel. Unusually tortuous or coiled arteries seem to be prone to this pathology. When a single spontaneous carotid or vertebral artery dissection occurs, the risk of recurrence (usually in a different neck artery) is reported to be 5% to 10%.

Spontaneous or posttraumatic dissections of the internal carotid artery commonly extend to the petrous segment. The dissection itself is usually associated with headache and a partial Horner's syndrome. Neurological deficits often reflect secondary cerebral embolization (see Cases 476 and 539).

Intracranial extension of carotid or vertebral artery dissections carries the risk of subarachnoid hemorrhage. Dissections of the distal vertebral arteries are particularly prone to present in this manner and should be considered among the causes of hemorrhage within the posterior fossa.

Case 546A

9-year-old boy presenting with bihemispheral TIAs.
(axial, noncontrast scan; SE 600/15)

Case 546B

Same patient.
(noncontrast scan; axial partition from three
dimensional GRE sequence)

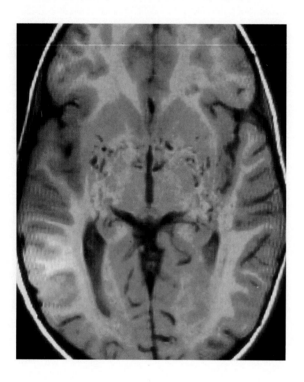

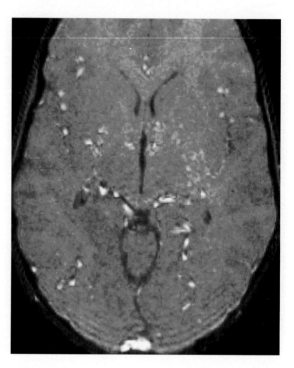

Moya moya disease is a syndrome of progressive, idiopathic occlusion of major cerebral arteries at the skull base. The supraclinoid internal carotid arteries and proximal anterior, middle, and posterior cerebral arteries are commonly involved. Gradually worsening stenosis of these vessels causes hypertrophy of collateral channels. Prominent among these are perforating branches such as the lenticulostriate arteries. Angiography in such cases demonstrates a "cloud" or "puff" of small collateral arteries at the base of the brain, described historically by the Japanese phrase "moya moya."

The diagnosis of moya moya disease is suggested on routine MR images by: (1) absence or reduced caliber of "flow voids" within the proximal middle, anterior, and posterior cerebral arteries; (2) abnormal prominence of low signal foci within the basal ganglia, representing hypertrophied lenticulostriate collaterals; and (3) evidence of hemispheric ischemia.

Case 546A illustrates the appearance of hypertrophied, transganglionic collateral vessels. The small diameter, slight

tortuosity, and sublenticular concentration of these channels should distinguish them from lacunar infarcts. (Compare also to the miliary lesions in Cases 388-1 and 388-2.)

Flow sensitive gradient echo sequences can be used to confirm the vascular nature of such foci. Case 546B demonstrates high flow within small vessels throughout the ganglionic region bilaterally. Case 548 provides a three dimensional representation of the same examination.

The diagnosis of idiopathic arterial occlusion at the base of the brain (i.e., moya moya disease) should be made only after other possible etiologies are excluded. Basal meningitis, sickle cell disease, Down syndrome, neurofibromatosis, tumors such as meningiomas, and radiation therapy may all be associated with stenosis or occlusion of basal vessels.

The ischemic symptoms in this case are typical for the pediatric presentation of moya moya disease. Adolescents and adults with this syndrome may present with intracerebral or subarachnoid hemorrhage due to rupture of hypertrophied collateral arteries.

Case 547

41-year-old woman presenting with cerebellar and occipital infarcts ten days postpartum. ("chin-up" AP display of noncontrast, three dimensional, time-of-flight GRE sequence)

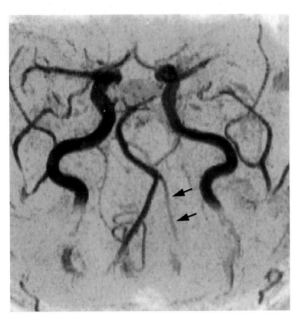

(same patient as Case 476)

Case 548

9-year-old boy presenting with bihemispheral TIAs. (submentovertex display of noncontrast, three dimensional, time-of-flight GRE sequence)

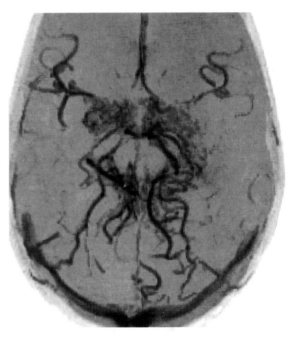

(same patient as Case 546)

MR angiography can effectively supplement routine studies in patients suffering from cerebral ischemia. The preferred technique at a given center (two dimensional vs. three dimensional, time-of-flight vs. phase contrast) is less important than the substantial contribution that any of these methods can make to patient management.

Case 547 demonstrates poor flow in the distal left vertebral artery (arrows). The curvature of the basilar artery suggests that the dominant vertebral artery should be on the left (which is also statistically more common). Even if the left vertebral artery were congenitally of the size demonstrated in Case 547, it should exhibit stronger flow characteristics. A subsequent catheter angiogram confirmed dissection of the proximal left vertebral artery, which had served as the source of embolic infarction.

MR angiography of the vertebrobasilar system is very helpful in assessing elderly patients with suspected brainstem ischemia. The noninvasive documentation of severe arterial stenosis can clarify ambiguous or intermittent symptoms and support a decision to begin anticoagulation.

Case 548 is the three-dimensional MR angiogram of the patient presented in Case 546. The diagnosis of moya moya disease is established by demonstrating the reduced caliber of major cerebral arteries (e.g., the M-1 segments of the middle cerebral arteries) and a "cloud" of collateral flow through the base of the brain.

See Case 505 for another example of MR angiography in the context of cerebral vascular disease.

Case 549

7-year-old boy with decreased level of consciousness one day after abdominal surgery. (sagittal, noncontrast scan; SE 600/15)

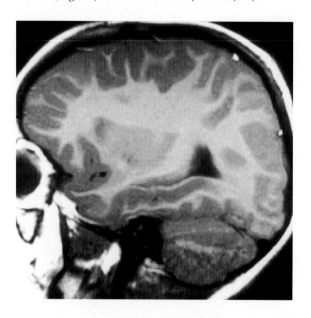

Case 550

4-month-old boy three days after resuscitation for "sudden infant death syndrome." (sagittal, noncontrast scan; SE 600/15)

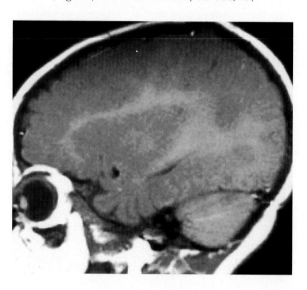

Cerebral anoxia may cause edema leading to prolongation of T1 and T2 values and swelling within involved regions. Gray matter is usually more severely affected than white matter, although holohemispheric patterns with diffuse white matter edema may be encountered (see Case 574).

Gray matter damage in anoxia may involve cortex, deep hemisphere nuclei, or both. This variability is probably due to differing combinations of hypoxia and hypoperfusion, as well as variable severity of the anoxic injury.

Another factor in the MR presentation of cerebral anoxia is the time elapsed from the insult. Scans in the first few days after an anoxic episode are characterized by progressively increasing swelling and signal abnormality, which

may eventually cause effacement of sulci and ventricles. Later examinations may demonstrate a rapid transition (often within days) to a pattern of parenchymal loss with secondary expansion of ventricles and subarachnoid spaces.

In Case 549, the cortical gray matter is abnormally well defined due to swelling and prolongation of T1. The appearance closely resembles that of acute infarction (compare to Case 466) but involves multiple arterial distributions.

By contrast, cortical definition is diffusely blurred in Case 550. Severe edema has developed in the several days since the profound insult, extending into subcortical white matter and effacing overlying subarachnoid spaces.

Case 551

2-week-old girl.
(axial, noncontrast scan; SE 600/15)

Case 552

1-day-old girl.
(coronal, noncontrast scan; SE 600/15)

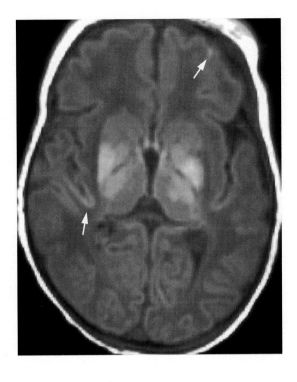

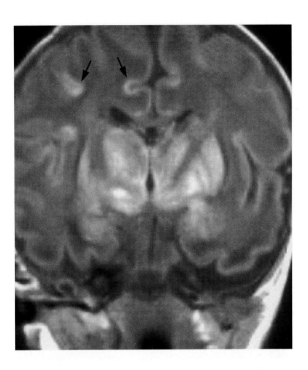

High signal intensity is commonly seen subacutely on T1-weighted scans in gray matter damaged by cerebral anoxia. Petechial hemorrhage may contribute to this appearance, but other biochemical changes (such as protein denaturation, myelin breakdown products, and/or calcification) probably play a role.

As discussed on the preceding page, MR findings of cerebral anoxia may be seen in the basal ganglia, cortical gray matter, or both. Severe neonatal anoxia usually damages the deep gray nuclei, with typical involvement of the globus pallidus, posterior putamen, and ventrolateral thalamus. Less severe anoxia often affects watershed regions of cortex and white matter, with relative sparing of the corpus striatum and thalamus. In the above infants, confluent signal abnormality throughout the deep nuclei dominates the presentation. However, smaller areas of T1-shortening within gyri *(arrows)* are also present in each case.

The internal capsule is well outlined as a spared zone between the putamen and thalamus in Case 551 and between the caudate and lenticular nuclei in Case 552. This is the reverse of the normal pattern within the newborn brain on T1-weighted scans: the region of the posterior limb

of the internal capsule should be the "brightest" structure visible. The lateral portions of the thalamus are most severely involved in Case 551, as is usual. In both cases, the columns of the fornix are prominently affected.

Contrast enhancement is common within cerebral cortex or nuclei following an anoxic insult. Enhancement of the cortical ribbon may resemble the gyriform pattern seen in subacute cerebral infarction, except that several arterial distributions are involved. Such enhancement may persist for hours or days after contrast injection. This stain indicates severe cortical injury and resembles the appearance in some cases of infantile encephalitis (see Case 403).

Neonatal "anoxia" is probably a multifactorial insult, with components of hypoxia, hypercarbia, acidosis, and hypotension. The newborn brain is actually quite resistant to hypoxia per se, but cerebral autoregulation and cardiac function are significantly impaired under hypoxic conditions. The resulting hypoperfusion is probably more responsible for cerebral damage than the initiating hypoxia. Because ischemia plays a key role in the pathophysiology, this neonatal insult is often called "hypoxic/ischemic encephalopathy" or HIE.

Case 553A

14-year-old boy resuscitated after near hanging.
(axial, noncontrast scan; SE 3000/75)

Case 553B

Same patient.
(axial, noncontrast scan; SE 3000/75)

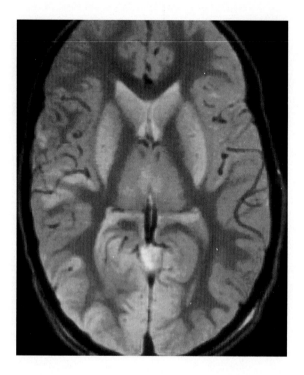

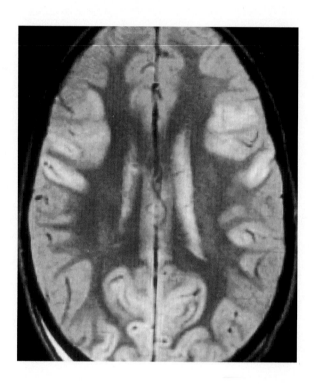

Like the T1-weighted scans in Cases 549-552, T2-weighted images may demonstrate ganglionic and/or cortical injury due to cerebral anoxia. The presence of edema causing swelling and increased signal intensity is the most common finding in either region. Alternatively, infants may develop uniform T2-shortening throughout the corpus striatum and thalamus several days after a severe anoxic insult.

In Case 553A, homogeneously increased signal intensity is present throughout the lenticular nuclei, caudate nuclei, and thalami. Accompanying symmetrical zones of gyral edema are seen bilaterally in Case 553B, predominantly involving frontal and occipital cortex.

Anoxic changes within the basal ganglia may be very subtle on MR scans performed within a day or two of the insult. Similarly, MR evidence of cortical anoxia may be limited to an inconspicuous layer of long T2 values at the base of the gray matter ribbon. CT examinations sometimes demonstrate convincing low attenuation changes in patients whose MR studies are equivocal. This diagnostic disparity is frequently noted in infants.

Scans of newborns who have experienced severe anoxia may also demonstrate signal abnormality within white matter tracts that are myelinated or myelating (and therefore metabolically active) at birth. The corticospinal tracts and the optic radiations are frequently affected.

As discussed in Chapter 8, a variety of metabolic disorders can cause symmetrical abnormalities of the basal ganglia resembling anoxia in pediatric patients (see Cases 439, 440, 443, 444, and 447).

Case 554A

17-year-old woman.
(coronal, noncontrast scan; SE 2500/70)

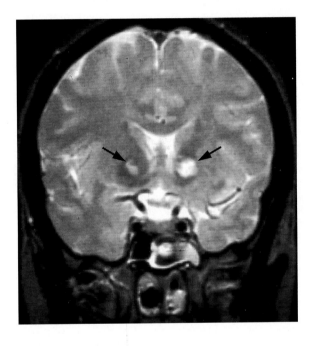

Case 554B

Same patient.
(axial, noncontrast scan; SE 2500/70)

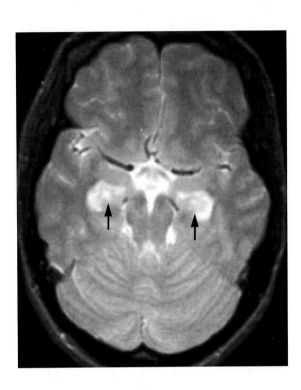

Carbon monoxide poisoning characteristically leads to necrosis of the globus pallidus. Typical bilateral lesions in this location are demonstrated in Case 554A *(arrows)*. The central high intensity areas suggest cytotoxic edema. The more peripheral zone of low intensity may simply represent a background of normal T2-shortening in pallidal tissue. (Compare to the appearance of Hallervorden-Spatz disease in Case 444.)

Other processes that may cause pallidal necrosis include barbiturate intoxication, cyanide poisoning, hydrogen sulfide poisoning, hypoglycemia, hypoxia (e.g., drug overdose), and hypotension. Leigh's disease (subacute necrotizing encephalomyelopathy; see Cases 439-441) may demonstrate symmetrical foci of signal abnormality in the basal ganglia, usually in children and commonly associated with brainstem involvement. Myelinolysis related to electrolyte disorders (see Case 430) may affect the basal ganglia symmetrically or asymmetrically. Unilateral or bilateral zones of

signal abnormality in the globus pallidus may also be noted in neurofibromatosis type 1 (see Cases 764 and 765).

Symmetrical foci of T2 prolongation can occur within the posterior limb of the internal capsule (e.g., adjacent to the globus pallidus) in amyotrophic lateral sclerosis (see Case 428). Wilson's disease may be associated with T2 prolongation in the lenticular nuclei despite the deposition of metals. The scan findings of methanol intoxication are usually seen within the putamen, often including hemorrhagic necrosis.

Hypoxia due to carbon monoxide poisoning can affect susceptible tissue outside of the globus pallidus. Case 554B illustrates edema and swelling within gray matter of the hippocampal formations *(arrows)*. Neurons of the hippocampus are known to be vulnerable to anoxic injury. This susceptibility has been suggested as the basis for mesial temporal sclerosis, illustrated in Cases 450 and 451.

REFERENCES

Amerenco P, Kase CS, Rosengart A, et al: Very small (border zone) cerebellar infarcts. *Brain* 116:161-186, 1993.

Amerenco P, Rosengart A, DeWitt, et al: Anterior inferior cerebellar artery territory infarcts: mechanisms and clinical features. *Arch Neurol* 50:154-161, 1993.

Anderson CM, Saloner D, Lee RE, et al: Assessment of carotid artery stenosis by MR angiography: comparison with x-ray angiography and color-coded Doppler ultrasound. *AJNR* 13:989-1003, 1992.

Anson JA, Heiserman JE, Drayer BP, Spetzler RF: Surgical decisions on the basis of magnetic resonance angiography of the carotid arteries: *Neurosurgery* 32:335-343, 1993.

Bacharach JM, Stanson AW, Lie JT, Nichols Da: Imaging spectrum of thrombo-occlusive vascular disease associated with antiphospholipid antibodies. *Radiographics* 13:417-423, 1993.

Baenziger O, Martin E, Steinlin M, et al: Early pattern recognition in severe perinatal asphyxia: a prospective MRI study. *Neuroradiology* 35:437-442, 1993.

Baker LL, Stevenson DK, Enzmann DR: End-stage periventricular leukomalacia: MR evaluation. *Radiology* 168:809-816, 1988.

Barkhof F, Valk J: "Top of the basilar" syndrome: a comparison of clinical and MR findings. *Neuroradiology* 30:293, 1988.

Barkovich AJ: MR and CT evaluation of profound neonatal and infantile asphyxia. *AJNR* 13:959-972, 1992.

Barkovich AJ, Truwitt CL: Brain damage from perinatal asphyxia: correlation of MR findings with gestational age. *AJNR* 11:1087-1096, 1990.

Bell DA, Davis WL, Osborn AG, Harnsberger HR: Bithalamic hyperintensity on T2-weighted MR: vascular causes and evaluation with MR angiography. *AJNR* 15:893-899, 1994.

Biller J, Adams HP Jr, Dunn V, et al: Dichotomy between clinical findings and MR abnormalities in pontine infarction. *J Comput Assist Tomogr* 10:379-385, 1986.

Birbamer G, Aichner F, Felber S, et al: MRI of cerebral hypoxia. *Neuroradiology* (suppl):53-55, 1991.

Braffman BH, Zimmerman RA, Trojanowski JQ, et al: Brain MR: pathologic correlation with gross and histopathology. I. Lacunar infarction and Virchow-Robin spaces. *AJNR* 9:621-638, 1988.

Brant-Zawadzki M, Fein G, Van Dyke C, et al: MR imaging of the aging brain: patchy white-matter lesions and dementia. *AJNR* 6:675-682, 1985.

Brant-Zawadzki M, Weinstein P, Bartkowski H, Moseley M, et al: MR imaging and spectroscopy in clinical and experimental cerebral ischemia: a review. *AJNR* 8:39-48, 1987.

Brown JJ, Hesselink JR, Rothbrock JF, et al: MR and CT of lacunar infarcts. *AJNR* 9:477-481, 1988.

Bryan RN: Imaging of acute stroke. *Radiology* 177:615-616, 1990.

Bryan RN, Levy LM, Whitlow WD, et al: Diagnosis of acute cerebral infarction: comparison of CT and MR imaging. *AJNR* 12:611-620, 1991.

Bui LN, Brant-Zawadzki M, Verghese P, Gillan G: Magnetic resonance angiography of craniocervical dissection. *Stroke* 24:126-131, 1993.

Chang KH, Han MH, Kim HS, et al: Delayee encephalopathy after acute carbon monoxide intoxication: MR imaging features and distribution of cerebral white matter lesions. *Radiology* 184:117-122, 1992.

Chien D, Kwong KK, Gress DR, et al: MR diffusion imaging of cerebral infarction in humans. *AJNR* 13:1097-1102, 1992.

Cordes M, Henkes H, Roll D, et al: Subacute and chronic cerebral infarctions: SPECT and gadolinium-DTPA-enhanced MR imaging. *J Comput Assist Tomogr* 13:567-571, 1989.

Cormier PJ, Long ER, Russell EJ, et al: MR imaging of posterior fossa infarctions: vascular territories and clinical correlations. *Radiographics* 12:1079-1096, 1992.

Crain MR, Yuh WTC, Greene GM, et al: Cerebral ischemia: evaluation with contrast-enhanced MR imaging. *AJNR* 12:631-640, 1991.

Cross PA, Atlas SW, Grossman RI: MR evaluation of brain iron in children with cerebral infarction. *AJNR* 11:341-348, 1990.

D'Aprile P, Farchi G, Pagliarulo R, Carella A: Thrombotic thrombocytopenic purpura: MR demonstration of reversible brain abnormalities. *AJNR* 15:19-20, 1994.

Demaerel P, Casaer P, Casteels-Van Daele M, et al: Moyamoya disease: MRI and MR angiography. *Neuroradiology* 33(suppl):50-52, 1991.

Desai SP, Rees C, Jinkins JR: Paradoxical cerebral emboli associated with pulmonary arteriovenous shunts: report of three cases. *AJNR* 12:355-359, 1991.

Dewitt LD, Kistler JP, Miller DC: NMR-neuropathologic correlation in stroke. *Stroke* 18:342-351, 1987.

Dharker, SR, Mittal RS, Bhargava N: Ischemic lesions in basal ganglia in children after minor head injury. *Neurosurgery* 33:863-865, 1993.

Dietrich RB, Bradley WG Jr: Iron accumulation in the basal ganglia following severe ischemic-anoxic insults in children. *Radiology* 168:203-206, 1980.

Elster AD: MR contrast enhancement brainstem and deep cerebral infarctions. *AJNR* 12:1127-1132, 1991.

Elster AD, Moody DM: Early cerebral infarction: Gadopentetate dimeglumine enhancement. *Radiology* 177:627-632, 1990.

Elster AD, Richardson DN: Focal high signal on MR scans of the midbrain caused by enlarged perivascular spaces: MR-pathologic correlation. *AJNR* 11:1119-1122, 1990.

Erkinjuntti T, Ketonen L, Sulkava R, et al: Do white matter changes on MRI and CT differentiate vascular dementia from Alzheimer's disease? *J Neurol Neurosurg Psychiatr* 50:37-42, 1987.

Flodmark O, Lupton B, Li D, et al: MR imaging of periventricular leukomalacia in childhood. *AJNR* 10:111-118, 1989.

Fox AJ, Bogousslavsky J, Carey LS, et al: Magnetic resonance imaging of small medullary infarctions. *AJNR* 7:229-234, 1986.

Friedman DP: Abnormalities of the posterior inferior cerebellar artery: MR imaging findings. *AJR* 160:1257-1263, 1993.

Fujisawa I, Asato R, Nishimura K, et al: Moyamoya disease: MR imaging. *Radiology* 164:103-106, 1987.

Fujita N, Hirabuki N, Fujii K, et al: MR imaging of middle cerebral artery stenosis and occlusion: value of MR angiography. *AJNR* 15:335-342, 1994.

Goldberg HI, Grossman RI, Gomori JM, et al: Cervical internal carotid artery hemorrhage: diagnosis using MR. *Radiology* 158:157-162, 1986.

Greenan TJ, Grossman RI, Goldbert HI: Cerebral vasculitis: MR imaging and angiographic correlation. *Radiology* 182:65-72, 1992.

Harris KG, Tran DD, Sickels WJ, Cornel SH: Diagnosing intracranial vasculitis: the roles of MR and angiography. *AJNR* 15:317-330, 1994.

Hecht-Leavitt C, Gomori JM, Grossman RI, et al: High field MRI of hemorrhagic cortical infarction. *AJNR* 7:581-586, 1986.

Heier L: White matter disease in the elderly: vascular etiologies. *Neuroimaging Clin N Amer* 2:441-461, 1992.

Heinz ER, Yeates AE, Djang WT: Significant extracranial carotid stenosis: detection on routine cerebral MR images. *Radiology* 170:843-848, 1989.

Heiserman JE, Drayer BP, Keller PJ, Fram EK: Intracranial vascular occlusion: evaluation with three dimensional time-of-flight MR angiography. *Radiology* 185:667-673, 1992.

Hershey LA, Modic MT, Greenough G, et al: Magnetic resonance imaging in vascular dementia: *Neurology* 37:29-36, 1987.

Horowitz AL, Kaplan R, Sarpel G: Carbon monoxide toxicity: MR imaging in the brain. *Radiology* 162:787-788, 1987.

Horowitz SH, Zito JL, Donnarumma R, et al: Clinical-radiographic correlations within the first five hours of cerebral infarction. *Acta Neurol Scan* 86:207-214, 1992.

Ida M, Mizunuma K, Hata Y, Tada S: Subcortical low intensity in early cortical ischemia. *AJNR* 15:1387-1393, 1994.

Imakita S, Nishimura T, Naito H, et al: Magnetic resonance imaging of cerebral infarction: time course of Gd-DTPA enhancement and CT comparison. *Neuroradiology* 30:372-378, 1988.

Imakita S, Nishimura T, Naito H, et al: Magnetic resonance imaging of human cerebral infarction: enhancement with Gd-DTPA. *Neuroradiology* 29:422-429, 1987.

Johnson BA, Heiserman JE, Drayer BP, Keller PJ: Intracranial MR angiograpnhy: its role in the integrated approach to brain infarction. *AJNR* 15:901-908, 1994.

Jungreis CA, Kanal E, Hirsch WL, et al: Normal perivascular spaces mimicking lacunar infarction: MR imaging. *Radiology* 169:101-104, 1988.

Katz BH, Quencer RM, Kaplan JO, et al: MR imaging of intracranial carotid occlusion. *AJNR* 10:345-350, 1989.

Keeney SE, Adcock EW, McArdle CB: Prospective observations of 100 high-risk neonates by high field (1.5 Tesla) magnetic resonance imaging of the central nervous system: II. Lesions associated with hypoxic-ischemic encephalopathy. *Pediatrics* 87:431-438, 1991.

Kienzie GD, Bregar RK, Chun RWM, et al: Sydenham chorea: MR manifestations in two cases. *AJNR* 12:73-76, 1991.

Kitajima M, Korogi Y, Shimomura O, et al: Hypertropic olivary degeneration: MR imaging and pathologic findings. *Radiology* 192:539-543, 1994.

Knepper L, Biller J, Adams HP Jr, et al: MR imaging of basilar artery occlusion. *J Comput Assist Tomogr* 14:32-35, 1990.

Kuhn MJ, Mikulis DJ, Ayoub DM, et al: Wallerian degeneration after cerebral infarction: evaluation with sequential MR imaging. *Radiology* 172:179-183, 1989.

Lane JL, Flanders AE, Doan HT, Bell RD: Assessment of carotid artery patency in routine spin-echo MR imaging of the brain. *AJNR* 12:819-826, 1991.

Lang E, Lang C, Huk W, Neundorfer B: Magnetic resonance imaging of dorsolateral medullary infarction in Wallenberg syndrome. *Neuroradiology* 36:269-270, 1994.

Laster RE Jr, Acker JD, Halford HH III, Nauert TC: Assessment of MR angiography versus arteriography for evaluation of cervical carotid bifurcation disease. *AJNR* 14:681:688, 1993.

Lazar EB, Russel EJ, Cohen BA, et al: Contrast-enhanced MR of cerebral arteritis: intravascular enhancement related to flow stasis within areas of focal arterial ectasia. *AJNR* 13:271-276, 1992.

Lisovoski F, Rosseaux P: Cerebral infarction in young people: a study of 148 patients with early cerebral angiography. *J Neurol Neurosurg Psychiatry* 34:576-579, 1991.

Litt AW, Eidelman EM, Pinto RS, et al: Diagnosis of carotid artery stenosis: comparison of 2DFT time-of-flight MR angiography with contrast angiography in 50 patients. *AJNR* 12:149-154, 1991.

Lundblom N, Katevuo K, Kumo M, et al: T1 in subacute and chronic brain infarctions: time-dependent development. *Invest Radiol* 27:673-680, 1992.

Marshall VG, Bradley WG, Marshall CE, et al: Deep white matter infarction: correlation of MR imaging and histopathologic findings. *Radiology* 167:517-522, 1988.

Matthews VP, King JC, Elster AD, Hamilton CA: Cerebral infarction: effects of dose and magnetization transfer saturation at gadolinium-enhanced MR imaging. *Radiology* 190:547-552, 1994.

McArdle CB, Richardson CJ, Hayden CK, et al: Abnormalities of the neonatal brain: MR imaging. Part II. Hypoxic-ischemic brain injury. *Radiology* 163:395-404, 1987.

Milandre L, Rumeau C, Sangla I, et al: Infarction in the territory of the anterior inferior cerebellar artery: report of five cases. *Neuroradiology* 34:500-503, 1992.

Miller DH, Ormerod IEC, Gibson A, et al: MR brain scanning in patients with vasculitis: differentiation from multiple sclerosis. *Neuroradiology* 29:226-231, 1987.

Miyashita K, Naritomi H, Sawada T, et al: Identification of recent lacunar lesions in cases of multiple small infarctions by magnetic resonance imaging. *Stroke* 19:834-839, 1988.

Mueller DP, Yuh WTC, Fisher DJ, et al: Arterial enhancement in acute cerebral ischemia: clinical and angiographic correlation. *AJNR* 14:661-668, 1993.

Nabatame H, Fujimoto N, Nakamura K, et al: High intensity areas on noncontrast T1-weighted MR images in cerebral infarction. *J Comput Assist Tomogr* 14:521-526, 1990.

Provenzale JM, Heinz ER, Ortel TL, et al: Antiphospholipid antibodies in patients without systemic lupus erythematosis: neuroradiologic findings. *Radiology* 192:531-537, 1994.

Pulpeiro JR, Cortes JA, Macarron J, et al: MR findings in primary antiphospholipid syndrome. *AJNR* 12:452-453, 1991.

Quint D, Spickler E: Magnetic resonance demonstration of vertebral artery dissection. Report of two cases. *J Neurosurg* 72:964-967, 1990.

Regli L, Regli F, Maeder P, Bogousslavski J: Magnetic resonance imaging with gadolinium contrast in small deep (lacunar) cerebral infarcts. *Arch Neurol* 50:175-180, 1993.

Revel MP, Mann M, Brugieres P, et al: MR appearance of hypertrophic olivary degeneration after contralateral cerebellar hemorrhage. *AJNR* 12:71-72, 1991.

Salomon A, Yeates AE, Burger PC, Heinz ER: Subcortical arteriosclerotic encephalopathy: brain stem findings with MR imaging. *Radiology* 165:625-629, 1987.

Schouman-Claeys E, Henry-Feugeas M, Roset F, et al: Periventricular leukomalacia: correlation between MR imaging and autopsy findings during the first 2 months of life. *Radiology* 189:59-64, 1993.

Seibert JJ, Miller SF, Kirby RS, et al: Cerebrovascular disease in symptomatic and asymptomatic patients with sickle cell anemia: screening with duplex transcranial doppler US—correlation with MR imaging and MR angiography. *Radiology* 189:457-466, 1993.

Shimosegawa E, Inugami A, Okudera T, et al: Embolic cerebral infarction: MR findings in the first 3 hours after onset. *AJR* 160:1077-1082, 1993.

Shoemaker EI, Lin Z-S, Rae-Grant AD, Little B: Primary angiitis of the central nervous system: unusual MR appearance. *AJNR* 15:331-334, 1994.

Shuaib A, Lee D, Pelz D, et al: The impact of magnetic resonance imaging on the management of acute ischemic stroke. *Neurology* 42:816-818, 1992.

Silverman CS, Brenner J, Murtagh FR: Hemorrhagic necrosis and vascular injury in carbon monoxide poisoning: MR demonstration. *AJNR* 14:168-170, 1993.

Simmons Z, Biller J, Adams HP, et al: Cerebellar infarction: Comparison of computed tomography and magnetic resonance imaging. *Ann Neurol* 19:291-293, 1986.

Simonson TM, Yuh WTC, Hindman BJ, et al: Contrast MR of the brain after high-perfusion cardiopulmonary bypass. *AJNR* 15:3-8, 1994.

Sue DE, Brant-Zawadzki MN, Chana J: Dissection of cranial arteries in the neck: correlation of MRI and arteriography. *Neuroradiology* 34:273-278, 1992.

Takahashi S, Higano S, Ishii K, et al: Hypoxic brain damage: cortical laminar necrosis and delayed changes in white matter at sequential MR imaging. *Radiology* 189:449-456, 1993.

Takanashi J, Sugita K, Ishii M, et al: Moyamoya syndrome in young children: MR comparison with adult onset. *AJNR* 14:1139-1142, 1993.

Tardy B, Page Y, Convers P, et al: Thrombotic thrombocytopenic purpura: MR findings. *AJNR* 14:489-490, 1993.

Truwit CL, Barkovich AJ, Koch TK, Ferriero DM: Cerebral palsy: MR findings in 40 patients. *AJNR* 13:67-78, 1992.

Truwit CL, Kucharczyk J: Reversible cerebral ischemia. *Neuroimaging Clin N Amer* 2:577-595, 1992.

Uchino A, Hasuo K, Uchida K, et al: Olivary degeneration after cerebellar or brain stem haemorrhage: MRI. *Neuroradiology* 35:335-338, 1993.

Virapongse C, Mancuso A, Quisling R: Human brain infarcts: Gd-DTPA-enhanced MR imaging. *Radiology* 161:785-794, 1986.

Warach S, Chien D, Li W, et al: Fast magnetic resonance diffusion-weighted imaging of acute human stroke. *Neurology* 42:1717-1723, 1992.

Warach S, Li W, Ronthal M, Edelman RR: Acute cerebral ischemia: evaluation with dynamic contrast-enhanced MR imaging and MR angiography. *Radiology* 182:41-47, 1992.

Wentz KY, Röther J, Schwartz A, et al: Intracranial vertebrobasilar system: MR angiography. *Radiology* 190:105-110, 1994.

Wolpert SM, Bruckmann H, Greenlee R, et al: Neuroradiologic evaluation of patients with acute stroke treated with recombinant tissue plasminogen activator. *AJNR* 14:3-13, 1993.

Yamada I, Matsushima Y, Suzuki S: Childhood moyamoya disease before and after encephalo-duro-arterio-syanangiosis: an angiographic study. *Neuroradiology* 34:318-322, 1992.

Yamada I, Matsushima Y, Suzuki S: Moyamoya disease: diagnosis with three-dimensional time-of-flight MR angiography. *Radiology* 184:773-778, 1992.

Yuh WTC, Crain MR, Loes DJ, et al: MR imaging of cerebral ischemia: findings in the first 24 hours. *AJNR* 12:621-629, 1991.

Zeiss J, Brinker RA: MR imaging of cerebral hemiatrophy. *J Comput Assist Tomogr* 12:640-643, 1988.

Zimmerman RA, Gill F, Goldberg HI, et al: MRI of sickle cell cerebral infarction. *Neuroradiology* 29:232-1987.

CHAPTER 10

Hemorrhage, Trauma, and Vascular Lesions

Case 555

83-year-old woman with a history of a CVA
two days before admission.
(sagittal, noncontrast scan; SE 600/17)

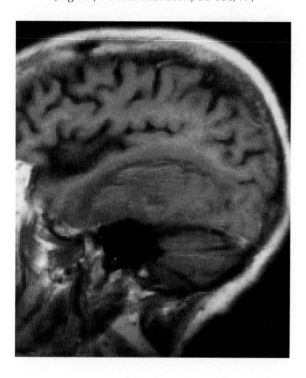

Case 556

69-year-old woman, two days after the
acute onset of aphasia.
(axial, noncontrast scan; SE 2800/90)

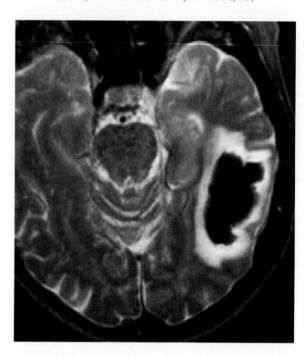

The appearance of recent intracranial hemorrhage is more complicated and time-dependent on MR scans than on CT studies. A sequence of changes in signal intensity reflects progressive oxidation and breakdown of blood products.

Acute intracerebral hematomas usually present as nearly isointense masses on T1-weighted scans. Mild prolongation of T1 may be present, causing slightly decreased signal intensity within the lesion. In Case 555, a large hematoma in the middle cranial fossa is slightly lower in intensity than adjacent parenchyma. A rim of edema helps to define the perimeter of the hemorrhage.

T2-weighted images of acute hematomas typically demonstrate very low signal intensity, as in Case 556. This signal loss reflects selective T2 relaxation enhancement due to magnetic field inhomogeneity produced when deoxyhemoglobin is compartmentalized within erythrocytes. The combination of isointensity on T1-weighted scans and markedly low signal intensity on T2-weighted images is characteristic of an acute hematoma. (See Cases 616 and 617 for additional examples.)

Hyperacute intracerebral hematomas may present a less distinctive MR appearance. Such fresh hemorrhages represent a solution of nonparamagnetic oxyhemoglobin. Their MR behavior resembles that of proteinaceous fluid, with prolongation of T1 and T2. Hyperacute hematomas can therefore mimic other homogeneous cystic or solid masses.

"Spontaneous" lobar hemorrhages in elderly patients are often due to amyloid angiopathy. In younger adults, spontaneous intraparenchymal hemorrhages tend to occur in the basal ganglia, thalamus, pons, and cerebellum, often correlating with a history of systemic hypertension and angiopathic changes of small arteries.

Hematomas usually displace more tissue than they destroy. They often have a better long-term prognosis than cerebral infarctions causing equal initial deficits.

Case 557

33-year-old man with a history of hypertension, five
days after admission with acute hemiparesis.
(sagittal, noncontrast scan; SE 600/17)

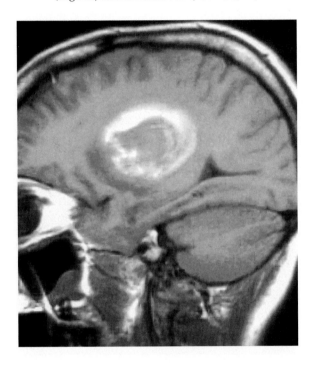

Case 558

63-year-old man, one month after presentation
with acute ataxia.
(axial, noncontrast scan; SE 2800/45)

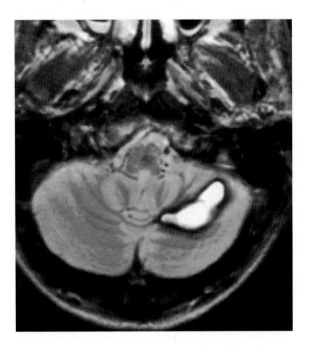

The MR appearance of intracerebral hemorrhage on T1-weighted scans changes during the first week of age. Prominent T1-shortening usually begins near the periphery of the lesion, gradually extending toward the center over a period of days to weeks. This alteration in signal intensity reflects the oxidation of deoxyhemoglobin to methemoglobin, which acts as a paramagnetic agent shortening T1.

The thick rind of high signal intensity surrounding an isointense center in Case 557 is a typical presentation for an early subacute hematoma on a T1-weighted scan. A follow-up scan with the same parameters after an additional week showed uniformly high signal intensity throughout the lesion.

Cell lysis and watery dilution of blood products accompanies the oxidation of intracerebral hematomas, progressing inward from the periphery of the lesion. The combination of these events converts the initially low signal intensity of acute hematomas on T2-weighted scans to high signal intensity over a period of weeks. Case 558 illustrates this transformation. Case 561 presents a hematoma midway through this transition.

The rim of low signal intensity surrounding the lesion in Case 558 is due to the accumulation of old blood products (mainly hemosiderin) within macrophages at the perimeter of the organizing hematoma. This intracellular debris causes selective T2 relaxation enhancement. The presence of a low intensity rim on T2-weighted scans implies that a hematoma has reached the late subacute or chronic stage. (The absence of surrounding edema also suggests that the hemorrhage is not a recent event.) Note that the relative position of the high and low signal components of the late subacute hematoma in Case 558 is reversed from the acute hematoma in Case 556.

About 10% to 15% of spontaneous and/or hypertensive hematomas occur in the posterior fossa. They may involve the cerebellum or the brainstem, usually the pons. Cerebellar hemorrhages often originate near the dentate nucleus, as in Case 558. It is important to distinguish between cerebellar and brainstem hematomas in patients with symptoms of brainstem compromise, since the former may be evacuated with life-saving results.

Case 559

58-year-old woman presenting with altered
mental status.
(sagittal, noncontrast scan; SE 600/20)

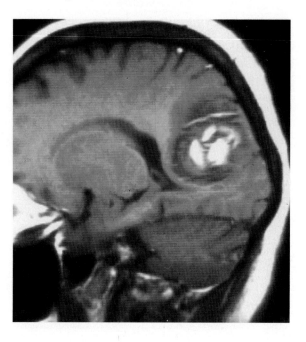

Case 560

63-year-old woman presenting with
acute confusion.
(axial, noncontrast scan; SE 3000/90)

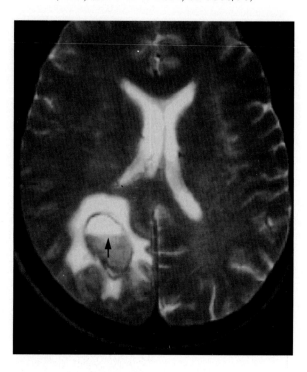

The concentric zones of evolving signal intensity illustrated in Cases 555-558 are typical of most spontaneous intracerebral hematomas. However, idiopathic hemorrhages occasionally present more complex morphologies. These heterogeneous patterns may resemble the appearance of secondary bleeding within a preexisting structural lesion (see Cases 616-619).

The multinodular morphology and central concentration of T1-shortening in Case 559 are unusual for a simple intracranial hematoma. However, this lesion was followed to resolution, with no evidence of underlying pathology or systemic disease after two years of observation.

Case 560 demonstrates a sedimentation level *(arrow)* within the blood-filled cavity, in turn surrounded by a rim of edema. The level represents a hematocrit phenomenon,

with cellular elements of extravasated blood settling to the dependent portion of the cavity. Deoxyhemoglobin within these cells causes reduced signal intensity. The supernatant demonstrates the expected high intensity of aqueous fluid.

The presence of a sedimentation level implies that the content of a cavity is liquid. This appearance can reflect hemorrhage into a preexisting cavity (see Case 214). However, a spontaneous hemorrhage may also present in this manner if impaired clotting mechanisms prevent coagulation. The presence of a sedimentation level within an intracerebral hemorrhage is therefore a clue to coagulopathy as a precipitating cause of bleeding. The patient in Case 560 was receiving coumadin and was found to have a significantly prolonged clotting time.

DIFFERENTIAL DIAGNOSIS:
HEMORRHAGIC MIDHEMISPHERE MASS

Case 561

33-year-old hypertensive man, five days
after a CVA.
(axial, noncontrast scan; SE 3000/80)

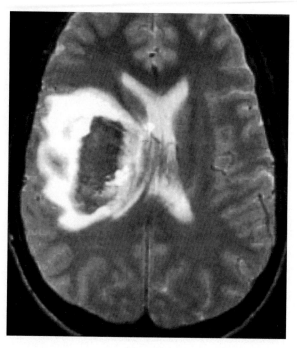

Spontaneous Intracerebral Hematoma
(same patient as Case 557)

Case 562

89-year-old woman presenting with a two-day
history of worsening confusion.
(axial, noncontrast scan; SE 2500/90)

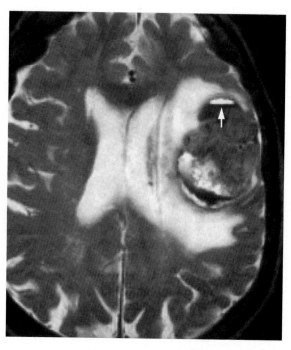

Hemorrhage into a Glioblastoma

The discovery an intracerebral hematoma should be followed by critical assessment of its location and morphology. The diagnosis of spontaneous hemorrhage is reserved for hematomas occupying typical sites and demonstrating no unusual features.

Case 561 presents the characteristic appearance of an early subacute intracerebral hematoma. Although a core of homogenous T2-shortening remains, a broadening perimeter of the lesion evidences high signal intensity (compare to Case 556). After another week or two, the entire center of the lesion would be expected to demonstrate high intensity on a T2-weighted sequence (see Case 558).

Areas of T2-shortening due to hemorrhage are also present within the mass in Case 562. However, the internal architecture of this lesion is much more complex than the hematoma of Case 561. A sedimentation level is seen within a small cyst anteriorly *(arrow)*, while the midportion of the lesion appears to represent solid tissue. A cystic or necrotic zone of high signal intensity is present posteromedially.

This high degree of structure and heterogeneity strongly suggests an underlying mass with secondary hemorrhage.

The spontaneous hematoma in Case 561 is centered in the superior ganglionic region, while the lesion of Case 562 arises more peripherally. (Note that edema is predominantly lateral in Case 561 and predominantly medial in Case 562.) A superficial location of intracerebral hemorrhage should raise the suspicion of an underlying structural lesion, trauma, coagulopathy, or vasculopathy (such as amyloid angiopathy in older patients).

Cocaine use should be considered among the etiologies of spontaneous intracerebral hemorrhage in young patients. Such hematomas may originate from underlying vascular lesions (aneurysms or arteriovenous malformations) that bleed due to cocaine-induced hypertension.

Hemorrhage into a tumor is one mechanism by which mass lesions may present acutely, simulating a CVA (see also Case 9).

Case 563

4-day-old girl, born at 36-weeks' gestation.
(sagittal, noncontrast scan; SE 550/20)

Case 564

5-day-old boy, born at 33-weeks' gestation.
(axial, noncontrast scan; SE 3000/90)

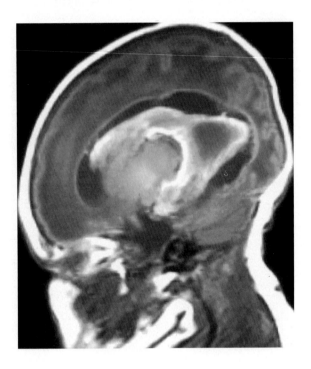

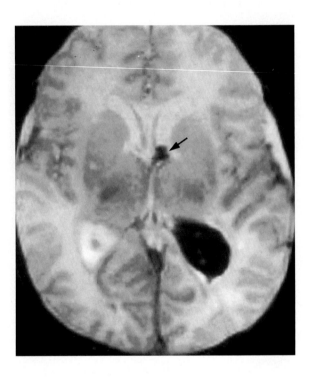

Hemorrhage commonly arises from fragile vessels in the periventricular germinal matrix of premature newborns. Hematomas may remain confined to the subependymal region or rupture into the ventricular system, often causing secondary hydrocephalus.

Cribside ultrasound (using the open fontanelles as acoustic windows) is the procedure of choice for following the initial course of such infants. CT or MR scans of neonatal intraventricular hemorrhage may be performed in ambiguous or complicated cases.

In Case 563, a hemorrhagic cast of the lateral ventricle was formed at the time it filled with blood. This clot now resides within a larger CSF space caused by consequent hydrocephalus. The predominant high signal intensity of the intraventricular thrombus indicates the presence of methemoglobin and suggests that the hemorrhagic event occurred several days earlier.

Case 564 illustrates prominent T2-shortening within intraventricular thrombus filling the trigone of the left lateral ventricle. Both deoxyhemoglobin and intracellular methemoglobin may cause this appearance; the former is associated with an isointense appearance on T1-weighted scans (see Case 555), while the latter produces T1-shortening. In either case the intraventricular hemorrhage is clearly recent and likely perinatal. A tiny clot at the foramen of Monro, as seen on the left in Case 564 *(arrow)*, is occasionally an isolated clue to recent intraventricular hemorrhage.

In adults, hematomas in the posterior fossa or basal ganglia may rupture into the fourth, third, or lateral ventricles. The ventricles may be grossly expanded by thrombus. Alternatively, the intraventricular hematoma may cause obstructive hydrocephalus.

Case 565

39-year-old man with a history of an old stroke.
(axial, noncontrast scan; SE 3000/45)

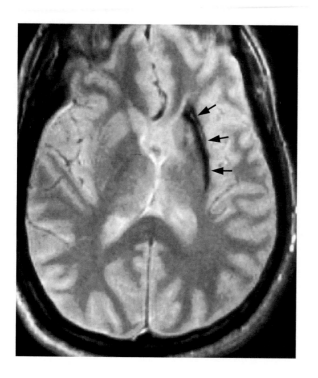

Case 566

47-year-old man, one year after
a left hemisphere CVA.
(coronal, noncontrast scan; GRE 200/13)

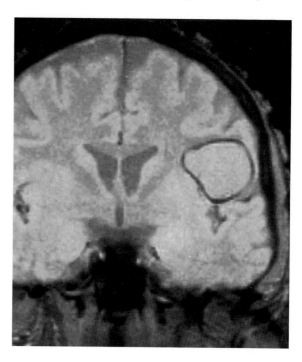

As discussed in Case 558, a characteristic MR feature of cerebral hemorrhage is the signature of T2-shortening left at the site of bleeding. Breakdown products accumulated by macrophages at the perimeter of organized hematomas cause prominent low signal intensity on long TR spin echo images. Focal signal loss remains as a hallmark of prior hemorrhage even after the lesion has been completely resorbed. (This is strictly true only in areas of normal brain involved by hemorrhage; hemosiderin-laden macrophages within hemorrhagic neoplasms may gain abnormal vascular access and leave the region.)

In Case 565, T2-shortening causes low signal intensity along the margins of an old hematoma in the region of the left putamen *(arrows)*. This finding suggests a spontaneous hemorrhage that has been resorbed, leaving a hemosiderin-lined cleft (compare to Case 633). An appearance similar to Case 565 would be the likely endpoint of the subacute hematoma illustrated in Cases 557 and 561.

Rarely an old hematoma cavity persists and fills with fluid rather than collapsing as in Case 565. Case 566 illustrates such a "hematic cyst." The rim of low signal intensity identifies a period of hemorrhage in the history of the current lesion. The fluid within the cyst differs in signal intensity from CSF and is likely proteinaceous, but there is no evidence of mass effect or edema to suggest an inflammatory or malignant lesion.

Gradient echo images (which lack 180-degree refocusing RF pulses) are more sensitive than spin echo sequences to susceptibility effects caused by paramagnetic blood breakdown products. For this reason, gradient echo sequences may be helpful in characterizing hemorrhagic lesions. Such sequences are particularly useful in screening for suspected small angiomas, hemorrhagic metastases, or shearing injuries (see Cases 570-572).

Case 567A

12-year-old boy presenting one day after a seizure, with a history of minor head trauma.
(axial, noncontrast scan; SE 2800/90)

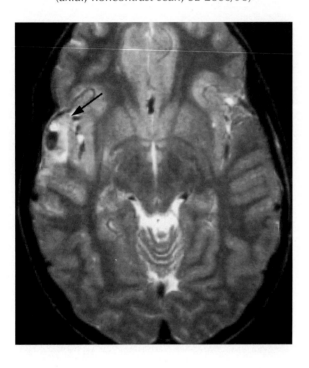

Case 567B

Same patient, three weeks later.
(coronal, noncontrast scan; SE 600/15)

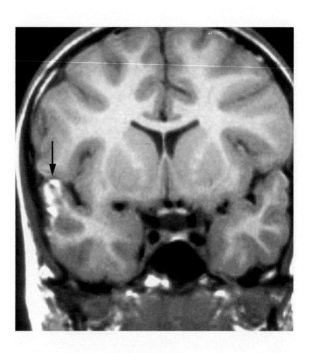

Posttraumatic intracerebral hemorrhages are often superficial lesions, reflecting bruising of the cortical surface against the adjacent calvarium. Common locations include the inferior frontal lobe, the anterior temporal lobe, and the occipital pole. The mechanism of injury may involve direct impact or recoil. As a result, evidence of parenchymal damage should be sought both immediately beneath and directly opposite a skull fracture or scalp injury.

The small lesion in Case 567 represents localized contusion of the superior temporal gyrus. The initial scan demonstrates central low signal intensity due to deoxyhemoglobin, with a surrounding rim of high intensity edema *(arrow, Case 567A)*. A T1-weighted scan at this same time showed only a small zone of mildly reduced signal intensity. This initial appearance is nonspecific; hemorrhage within a small neoplasm could not be excluded.

The follow-up scan (Case 567B) demonstrates characteristic evolution, which establishes the diagnosis of cerebral contusion. Edema and mass effect have subsided. T1-shortening has developed, with a gyriform contour following the cortical convolutions. This ribbon-like distribution of subacute hemorrhage is commonly seen within zones of contusion, resembling the pattern of T1-shortening in subacute infarction or anoxia (compare to Case 478).

Cerebral contusion may be much more extensive than the focal hemorrhage in this case. Scans may also demonstrate the development or dramatic enlargement of posttraumatic intracerebral hemorrhages occurring hours or days after injury. This phenomenon should be suspected in any trauma patient whose condition deteriorates or fails to improve as expected.

"Posttraumatic" hemorrhages occurring in atypical locations must be carefully evaluated. Such hematomas may represent an initial cerebral event leading to trauma, or posttraumatic hemorrhage into a preexisting structural lesion.

Surprisingly minor head trauma may be associated with serious cerebral injury. For example, a simple fall from the standing position can cause extensive intracranial hemorrhage in elderly patients.

DIFFERENTIAL DIAGNOSIS:
SUPERFICIAL FOCI OF HEMORRHAGIC "STAINING"

Case 568

48-year-old woman.
(axial, noncontrast scan; SE 2800/45)

Case 569

64-year-old man.
(axial, noncontrast scan; SE 2800/45)

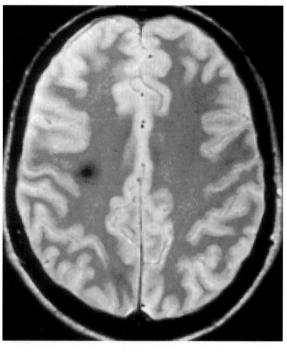

Old Contusion

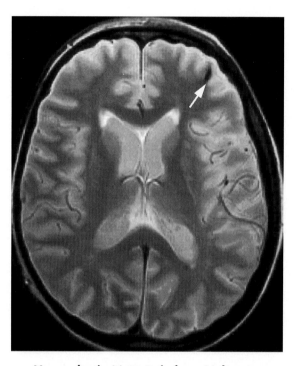

Hemorrhagic Metastasis from Melanoma

One or more areas of localized low signal intensity near the cerebral surface on long TR spin echo images (or on gradient echo images maximizing susceptibility effects) may be seen in several different clinical contexts. This finding suggests hemorrhagic foci, with short T2 values due to acute (deoxyhemoglobin) or chronic (hemosiderin) blood products.

Trauma may cause one or more superficial hemorrhages representing cortical contusion, as in Cases 567 and 568. Alternatively, subcortical axonal damage (shearing injuries; see Cases 570-572) may contain hemorrhage, which is more apparent on MR studies than on CT scans. A third potential cause of posttraumatic cerebral hemorrhages is dural sinus thrombosis (see Cases 642-645).

However, superficial hemorrhagic lesions are not necessarily traumatic, even when multiple. Small hemorrhagic masses should also be considered in the differential diagnosis. Metastases commonly occur near the gray-white matter junction. If such lesions are small and contain blood products, they may present as superficial low signal foci, illustrated in Case 569. In addition to metastases from vascular primary tumors, leukemia may present in this manner, with multiple hemorrhagic chloromas.

The differential diagnosis of small, multifocal intracerebral hemorrhages also includes coagulopathy, arteritis, amyloid angiopathy, and moya moya disease. Multiple cavernous angiomas could present a similar appearance on T2-weighted or gradient echo sequences (see Cases 627-630).

Case 570

10-year-old boy presenting with behavioral problems one year after an automobile accident.
(axial, noncontrast scan; SE 3000/80)

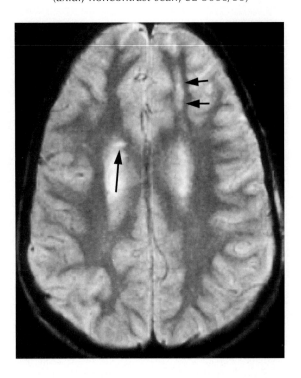

Case 571

30-year-old man admitted one week earlier after a fall.
(axial, noncontrast scan; SE 2500/90)

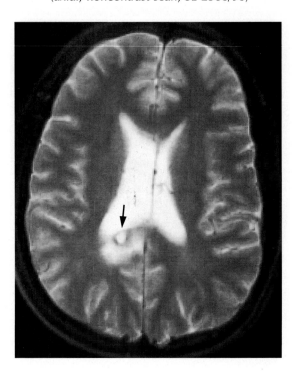

The superiority of MR over CT for defining white matter pathology as emphasized in Chapter 7 extends to the demonstration of shearing injuries. These foci of axonal disruption are usually invisible on CT examination; occasionally, associated hemorrhages are apparent. MR scans are much more sensitive to small sites of injury within white matter of the cerebral hemispheres and posterior fossa.

Shearing injuries occur in approximately 40% of patients with severe head trauma, most commonly in the frontal and temporal lobes. They may range from millimeters to centimeters in size. The majority are bland but up to 25% are hemorrhagic. Focal hemorrhage within these lesions can be demonstrated by MR scans using gradient echo sequences to highlight the magnetic susceptibility effects of blood products.

In Case 570, a parasagittal band of signal abnormality reflects injury within white matter of the left frontal lobe *(short arrows)*. A smaller focus of abnormal signal in the right minor forceps *(long arrow)* represents a second site of axonal damage.

The corpus callosum is a common location for shearing injury. The splenium is most frequently involved, as in Case 571 *(arrow)*. A small amount of hemorrhage is present within the lesion, seen as a low intensity zone of shortened T2. Shearing injury to the corpus callosum is often associated with intraventricular hemorrhage, which can be a CT clue to the diagnosis.

Callosal lesions correlate strongly with the presence of diffuse axonal injury ("DAI") of the cerebral hemispheres and primary brainstem injury, which usually involves the posterolateral portions of the midbrain and pons. (Secondary brainstem injury after head trauma is often the result of transtentorial herniation, with caudal displacement of the brainstem stretching the penetrating branches of the basilar artery and leading to infarction and/or hemorrhage.)

Although MR is more sensitive than CT for demonstrating hemorrhagic or nonhemorrhagic shearing injuries, microscopically documented axonal damage is often undetected by either modality.

DIFFERENTIAL DIAGNOSIS:
MULTIPLE FOCI OF SIGNAL ABNORMALITY IN PERIPHERAL WHITE MATTER

Case 572

39-year-old woman presenting with
neuropsychological deficits nine months
after an automobile accident.
(axial, noncontrast scan; SE 3000/90)

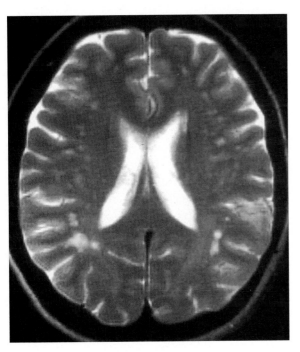

Shearing Injuries

Case 573

56-year-old woman with a history of
hypertension and TIAs.
(axial, noncontrast scan; SE 2500/90)

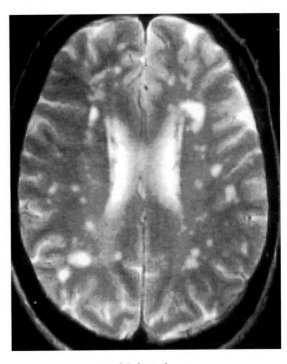

Multiple Infarcts

Axonal injury is common near interfaces between tissues of different consistency. Shearing forces develop in such locations when rotation/acceleration imparts different velocity and momentum to parenchyma on each side of the tissue boundary.

The junction between gray and white matter of the cerebral convexity is a frequent site of "shear strain" and axonal injury, as illustrated in Case 572. Shearing injury is often correlated with significant persistent neuropsychological deficits. MR scans can establish the diagnosis in such cases, while CT studies are usually negative.

The spectrum of multifocal infarction may include peripheral hemispheric lesions, as in Case 573. Close analysis usually demonstrates overall sparing of subcortical "U" fibers (see discussion of Cases 514 and 515). In addition, deeper lesions in the centrum semiovale or corona radiata are almost always found in association with superficial foci.

A variety of inflammatory processes may also cause multiple small areas of signal abnormality within peripheral white matter of the cerebral hemispheres. Examples include demyelinating disease, collagen vascular disease, sarcoidosis, and Lyme disease (see Cases 433-436). Multiple sclerosis in particular may present with a combination of callosal and subcortical lesions that can resemble diffuse axonal injury.

Case 574A

30-year-old woman scanned several days after a shunt for obstructive hydrocephalus and previous cardiopulmonary arrest.
(coronal, noncontrast scan; SE 800/17)

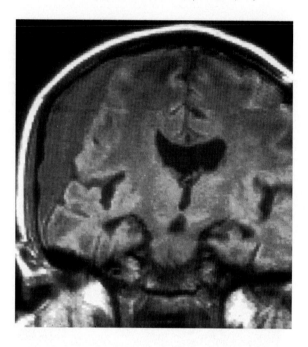

Case 574B

Same patient, seven days later.
(coronal, noncontrast scan; SE 1000/17)

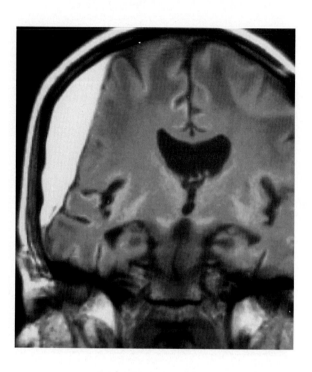

As discussed in Cases 555 to 558, the MR appearance of hemorrhage is a complex function of many variables. In general, acute intracerebral or extracerebral hematomas are isointense or slightly lower in signal intensity than cerebral parenchyma on T1-weighted images.

In Case 574A, a T1-weighted coronal scan clearly documents a subdural collection overlying the right hemisphere. The signal intensity of the acute hematoma is intermediate between that of CSF and brain tissue. Abnormally low signal intensity throughout cerebral white matter reflects the history of severe anoxia and ischemia.

The signal intensity of the subdural hematoma in this case changed dramatically within one week, as seen in Case 574B. This evolution reflects the oxidation of deoxyhemoglobin to methemoglobin, with consequent T1-shortening (see Case 557).

The increase in signal intensity commonly seen on T1-weighted images of intracranial hemorrhages during the first week after bleeding contrasts with the CT pattern of immediate maximal attenuation. As a result, CT scans may be more characteristic than MR studies for diagnosis of acute intracranial hemorrhage, while MR scans are more specific than CT exams for the characterization of subacute or old hemorrhages.

Subdural hematomas may become very large, particularly in elderly patients. The presence of preexisting atrophy delays the onset of cerebral compression by an expanding collection. When the buffering capacity of enlarged CSF spaces has been exceeded, rapidly developing symptoms may lead to the discovery of a surprisingly thick hematoma.

The initial clinical presentation of patients with subdural hematomas can range from vague headache to generalized disorientation and confusion (see Case 575) to focal deficits mimicking an acute CVA (see Case 578). Hemiparesis may be contralateral or ipsilateral to the hematoma; the latter occurrence reflects brainstem displacement causing pressure on the contralateral cerebral peduncle. Elderly patients with subdural hematomas have a generally poorer prognosis than younger individuals.

Case 575

77-year-old man whose family reported
him to be increasingly forgetful.
(axial, noncontrast scan; SE 2800/90)

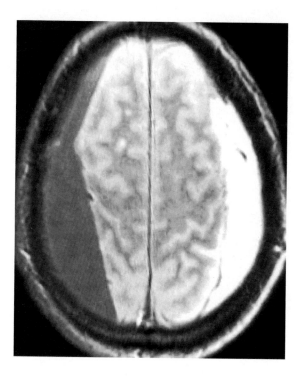

Case 576

30-year-old woman, ten days after a shunt for
obstructive hydrocephalus and previous
cardiopulmonary arrest.
(axial, noncontrast scan; SE 3000/80)

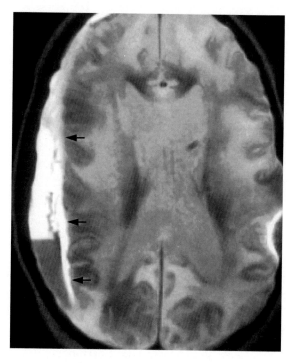

(same patient as Case 574)

The appearance of subdural hematomas on long TR spin echo images depends on the age and compartmentalization of blood products within the lesion. Case 575 illustrates the typical low signal intensity of an acute or early subacute subdural hematoma overlying the right hemisphere. A loculated chronic subdural hematoma is present on the left side. Comparison of the two collections demonstrates that lysis of cells, aqueous dilution, and removal of blood products from the extracerebral space convert the initially low intensity of fresh subdural hemorrhage on T2-weighted scans to the eventual high intensity appearance expected for a proteinaceous solution.

Two areas of subdural hemorrhage overlie the right hemisphere in Case 576. The thinner, medial component (*arrows*) demonstrates uniformly high signal intensity, as is commonly seen in chronic subdural hematomas (or hygromas) on T2-weighted scans. The larger lateral collection contains a sedimentation level with a dependent zone of T2-shortening. This combination of long and short T2 components suggests a subacute or chronic collection with sedimentation of cellular material.

Liquefaction of subdural hematomas usually occurs by two to three weeks of age. The presence of an earlier sedimentation level in Case 576 may reflect coagulapathy (compare to Case 560).

Heterogeneous signal intensity within subdural hematomas may also be caused by old clot surrounded by fresh blood, loculated plasma separated from red cells, or encysted spinal fluid from an associated arachnoid tear.

Approximately 25% of subacute and chronic subdural hematomas are bilateral, as in Case 575. Bilateral hematomas of equal size may cause symmetrical distortions of anatomy. This presence of balancing mass effect may be overlooked on CT studies if the hematomas themselves are nearly isodense. The MR scan in Case 575 clearly demonstrates compression of cerebral parenchyma, effacement of sulci, and medial displacement of several large cortical veins.

The cerebral hemispheres in Case 576 are diffusely abnormal, with edema throughout the white matter reflecting the history of anoxia.

DIFFERENTIAL DIAGNOSIS:
HOMOGENEOUS EXTRACEREBRAL "COLLECTION"

Case 577

53-year-old man presenting with headaches.
(sagittal, noncontrast scan; SE 500/15)

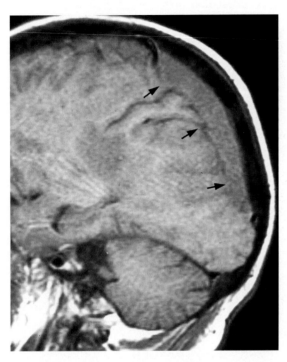

**Dural-Based Metastatic Carcinoma
of the Prostate**

Case 578

65-year-old man presenting with rapidly
developing hemiparesis.
(sagittal, noncontrast scan; SE 600/15)

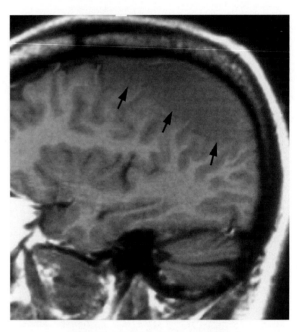

Chronic Subdural Hematoma

In Case 577, a homogeneous extracerebral "collection" causes displacement of the underlying hemisphere and cortical veins *(arrows)*. It is important to remember that epidural and/or subdural tumors can present in this manner, mimicking a subdural hematoma.

A clue to the diagnosis in Case 577 is abnormal signal intensity throughout the diploic space of the calvarium. Although dural-based metastases can occur without osseous involvement, associated skull lesions are often apparent (see Cases 25, 28, and 29). The low signal intensity throughout the vault in Case 577 (compare to the normal diploic space in Case 578) may reflect cellular infiltration, reactive sclerosis, or both.

The greater sphenoid wing is another frequent location of dural-based metastatic disease, especially from carcinomas of the prostate (see Case 59). Breast carcinoma is the most common tumor to present in this manner in women. An appearance comparable to Case 577 may be seen in children due to neuroblastoma or lymphoma.

Chronic subdural hematomas often demonstrate intermediate signal intensity on T1-weighted scans, as in Case 578. This appearance probably reflects the clearing of methemoglobin present during subacute stages, liquefaction, and aqueous dilution. Intermediate signal intensity may also represent an averaging of blood components of varying age. Rebleeding is common in subdural hematomas, contributing to their progressive enlargement. Recurrent hemorrhages may cause a layered or laminated appearance or simply add volume to a unilocular collection.

Postcontrast scans would clearly distinguish between the above lesions. Dural-based tumor typically demonstrates homogeneous enhancement (see Case 28 for a postcontrast scan of Case 577). The enhancement of subdural hematomas is usually limited to membranes that develop by about three weeks of age. Membrane enhancement is typically linear, adjacent to the cortical surface and along the inner table. Loculation of enhancing membranes occasionally presents a confusing appearance.

DIFFERENTIAL DIAGNOSIS:
EXTRACEREBRAL "COLLECTION" WITH HIGH SIGNAL INTENSITY ON T1-WEIGHTED SCANS

Case 579

82-year-old woman presenting after head trauma with seizures involving the left side of the body. (coronal, noncontrast scan; SE 600/15)

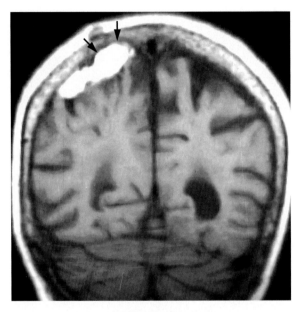

Convexity Lipoma

Case 580

80-old-woman presenting with dementia. (coronal, noncontrast scan; SE 600/17)

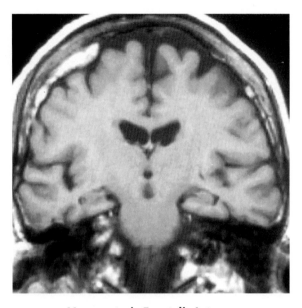

Hyperostosis Frontalis Interna

Subacute hemorrhage within the subdural space is the most common cause of a layered zone of short T1 values overlying the cerebral convexity. However, other conditions can mimic this appearance.

In Case 579, superficial high signal intensity is due to lipid protons within an unusual lipoma. Intracranial lipomas are more commonly encountered as midline lesions in the interhemispheric fissure or along the base of the brain (see Cases 252, 290, and 724-727). The long-standing mass in Case 579 has caused remodeling of the calvarium *(arrows)* and depression of underlying cortex. (The small nodule within subcutaneous tissue of the scalp was unrelated to the intracranial mass.) The lipoma was removed, and seizures did not recur.

Case 580 presents a normal variant, which should not be mistaken for a layer of subdural hemorrhage. Prominent thickening of the inner aspect of the skull frequently occurs in elderly patients. This widened bone appears dense or "hyperostotic" on x-rays or CT scans, but its MR appearance may be dominated by short T1 values presumed to

represent fatty marrow spaces. This finding is usually most prominent in the frontal region and is also characterized by a somewhat undulating inner margin. Bilaterality is usual, often with more symmetry than is seen above.

A similar pattern of layered high signal intensity may occur along the falx on T1-weighted scans of patients with calcified or ossified dural plaques. The short T1 values may reflect fatty marrow within bone or the effect of a calcium matrix on water protons. In any event, this normal variant frequently accounts for small or large areas of bright signal in the interhemispheric fissure on short TR scans. Such patches are characteristically very thin on coronal or axial images and are associated with calcification on CT scans or skull films.

Fat saturation pulse sequences would demonstrate reduced signal intensity of the "lesions" in each of the above cases, distinguishing them from subacute subdural hematomas. The presence of chemical shift artifact on long TR images can also help to identify lipomas (see Cases 252 and 726).

Case 581

17-year-old boy complaining of headaches
one week after a bicycle accident.
(sagittal, noncontrast scan; SE 700/17)

Case 582

2-month-old girl with suspected
"nonaccidental trauma."
(coronal, noncontrast scan; SE 3000/100)

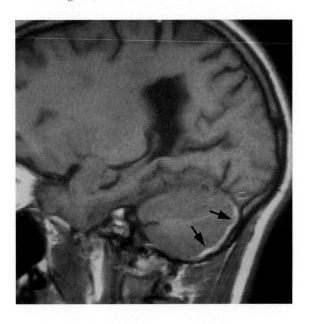

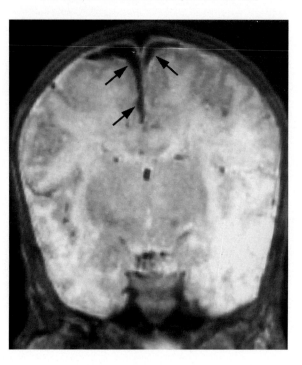

The increased attenuation of small acute or subacute subdural hematomas can be difficult to distinguish from the inner table on CT studies. MR offers two major advantages for detecting such lesions: (1) multiplanar display and (2) high contrast between subacute hematomas and adjacent bone.

As discussed in Case 574, the T1-shortening typically seen within subacute subdural hematomas makes these lesions conspicuous on T1-weighted images. In Case 581, a sagittal scan clearly defines a thin hematoma along the posterior margin of the posterior fossa *(arrows)*.

The demonstration of equally thin subdural hemorrhages adjacent to the posterior falx or tentorium can be an important clue to the diagnosis of child abuse ("nonaccidental trauma"). Posterior interhemispheric subdural hematomas are commonly seen in children subjected to shaking injuries and are a hallmark of the "battered child syndrome." The ability of MR to document variable age of multiple intracerebral and extracerebral hemorrhages is also useful in suggesting a history of repetitive injury.

In Case 582, a CT scan failed to demonstrate the acute subdural hematomas at the vertex due to partial volume artifact from the calvarium. The coronal projection and lack of bone artifact on the MR study clearly document the prognostically (and legally) important hemorrhages.

Interhemispheric clot characteristically demonstrates a flat medial margin along the falx and a variable thick lateral extension. (Compare to the subdural empyemas in Cases 392 and 393.)

The dilatation of the lateral ventricular trigone in Case 581 represented an old porencephalic cyst (see Cases 697 and 698).

EPIDURAL HEMATOMAS

Case 583

1-month-old girl who suffered a parietal
skull fracture one week earlier.
(sagittal, noncontrast scan; SE 600/15)

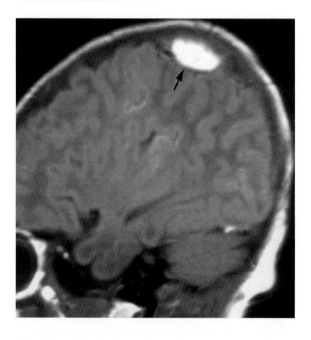

Case 584

3-day-old boy with abnormal findings on a
neonatal cranial ultrasound examination.
(sagittal, noncontrast scan; SE 600/15)

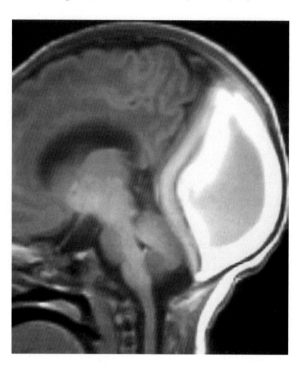

The dura functions as periosteum for the inner table and is tightly adherent to the skull. For this reason, hemorrhage accumulating between the calvarium and the dura remains relatively confined. An epidural hematoma acquires substantial thickness and a convex margin before sufficient pressure develops to strip the dura for further expansion. This biconvex or lentiform shape, as illustrated in Case 583, contrasts with the thin, crescentic morphology of most acute subdural hematomas (compare to Case 581).

Subdural hematomas often widen with time. Subacute or chronic subdural collections may demonstrate a medial margin that is straight or even convex (see Cases 574-576), resembling an epidural hematoma. The clinical context (e.g., association with skull fracture and rapidity of neurological deterioration) will usually distinguish between the two lesions.

Most supratentorial epidural hematomas are due to lacerations of branches from the middle meningeal artery at the point of skull fracture. Epidural hemorrhages may enlarge rapidly and warrant close observation in cases where emergency surgery is not performed. A "lucid interval" of several hours between trauma and the rapid onset of symptoms is a characteristic clinical feature. Small epidural hematomas in asymptomatic patients may resolve without surgery, as was true in Case 583.

Epidural hematomas in the posterior fossa are usually caused by venous bleeding from torn dural sinuses. As a result, they present less acutely and may have less characteristic morphology than supratentorial epidural hemorrhages. Regardless of shape, an extracerebral hematoma is established as epidural if it crosses the plane of the tentorium or falx.

The very large subacute epidural hematoma in Case 584 spans the plane of the tentorium (compare to Case 581). Axial images and MR angiography confirmed anterior displacement and compression of the superior sagittal sinus and torcular Herophili.

A source of the hemorrhage in Case 584 was not established. However, the child has done well, with follow-up scans demonstrating contraction of the hematoma to a small fraction of its original size.

Case 585

2-year-old boy presenting with bilateral
sixth nerve palsies.
(coronal, noncontrast scan; SE 600/15)

Case 586

16-year-old girl presenting with headaches,
one week after head trauma.
(axial, noncontrast scan; SE 3000/30)

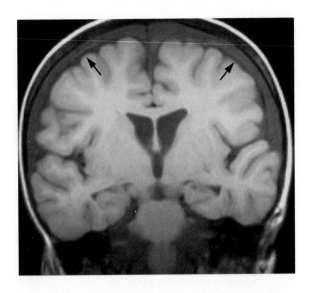

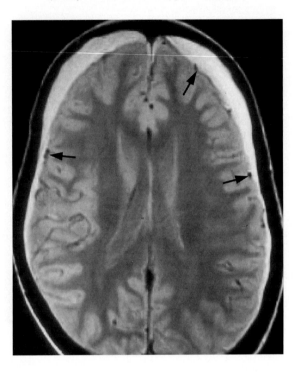

Some patients develop acute aqueous subdural collections following head trauma. These accumulations have been termed "subdural hygromas," because they usually contain clear or lightly colored cerebrospinal fluid. The fluid apparently gains access to the subdural space through an arachnoid tear. Subdural hygromas are most often seen in elderly patients and young children. Most of these collections remain small and resolve spontaneously.

Subdural hygromas are sometimes confused with widened subarachnoid spaces due to cerebral atrophy. These two processes are usually distinguishable on the basis of (1) cortical contour and gyral position and (2) signal intensity, especially on long TR spin echo images. As seen in the above cases, the margin of compressed cortex beneath a subdural collection is abnormally smooth, contrasting with the irregular outline of atrophic cortex reflecting widened sulci. The tips of cortical gyri seldom retract significantly from the inner table even in the presence of marked atrophy (see Cases 457 and 458). By contrast, the cortical surface is unequivocally displaced from the calvarium by subdural collections. Similarly, displacement of cortical veins from the inner table indicates subdural accumulation of fluid (*arrows* in Case 586).

The signal intensity of subdural hygromas is usually higher than that of subarachnoid or ventricular CSF due to the presence of increased protein content and/or cell count. Relative lack of signal loss from CSF pulsation may also contribute to this difference. The distinction between hygroma fluid and CSF is often best appreciated on long TR, short TE images such as Case 586.

The child in Case 585 is unusual in that the subdural hygromas have grown sufficiently large to increase intracranial pressure and cause sixth nerve palsies. Drainage of the collections demonstrated clear, golden fluid. The mild ventricular prominence in this case may reflect impairment of CSF circulation through convexity subarachnoid spaces, which are faintly seen as a line of lower signal intensity at the medial margin of the hygromas *(arrows)*.

Case 587

5-month-old boy.
(sagittal, noncontrast scan; SE 900/17)

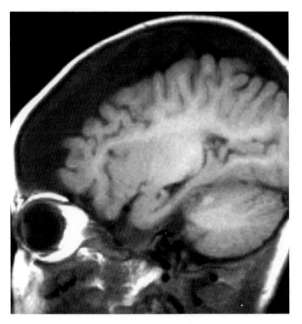

Subdural Hygroma

Case 588

79-year-old man.
(sagittal, noncontrast scan; SE 700/17)

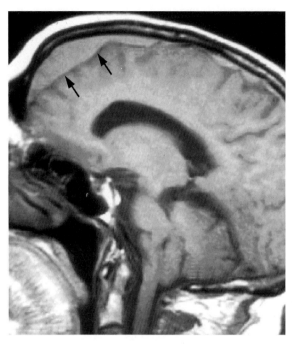

Chronic Subdural Hematoma

The distinction between a subdural hygroma and a chronic subdural hematoma may be difficult on CT scans, since both lesions demonstrate uniform low attenuation. When this distinction is clinically or legally important, MR can provide useful characterization.

The large subdural collection in Case 587 contains signal intensity that is very close to that of spinal fluid. (Compare to the temporal horn or the vitreous humor of the globe.) This appearance favors a subdural hygroma rather than a chronic subdural hematoma, which usually contains fluid that is higher in intensity than CSF (as in Case 588; see also Case 578).

Some subdural hygromas are found to contain traces of hemorrhage or increased levels of protein at surgery. Such collections demonstrate signal intensities that are somewhat higher than CSF on all pulse sequences (see Cases 585 and

586). Even these complicated hygromas are rarely as different from CSF signal intensity on T1-weighted images as the usual chronic subdural hematoma.

The signal intensity of the chronic hematoma in Case 588 has returned to a level intermediate between the acute and subacute stages illustrated in Case 574. Chronic subdural hematomas are often relatively isointense to cortex on T1-weighted scans. However, the interface between the extraaxial collection and the underlying brain is usually clearly defined by a combination of compressed subarachnoid space *(arrows),* displaced cortical veins (see Case 575), and/or subdural membranes.

The contrast between the signal intensity of the subdural collection in Case 588 and that of normal CSF would be less on T2-weighted images, where both would appear "bright."

Case 589

64-year-old woman, one week after hemorrhage
from an aneurysm at the PICA origin.
(sagittal, noncontrast scan; SE 600/17)

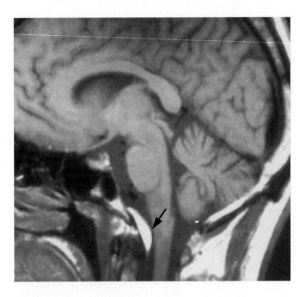

Case 590

74-year-old woman, two days after subarachnoid
hemorrhage of undetermined origin.
(sagittal, noncontrast scan; SE 750/20)

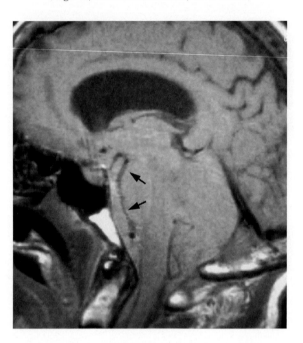

Magnetic resonance imaging is less sensitive than CT for the diagnosis of acute subarachnoid hemorrhage. A number of factors probably contribute to the inconspicuity of subarachnoid blood on MR scans. High oxygen tension within the CSF, spinal fluid pulsation, and averaging of subtle signal changes with the long T1 and T2 values of CSF have been suggested as possible causes.

On the other hand, MR can confirm the suspicion of subacute subarachnoid hemorrhage at a stage when the CT attenuation of cisterns has returned to near normal. In Case 589, the small area of T1-shortening along the posterior surface of the clivus (arrow) represents residual subacute thrombus. Similar remnants of clot may be found on MR scans adjacent to a ruptured aneurysm, helping to localize the site of bleeding.

MR scans in patients with extensive subarachnoid hemorrhage may demonstrate replacement of CSF spaces by altered signal intensity, as in Case 590. The prepontine cistern is filled with nearly isointense hemorrhage, surrounding and defining the lumen of the basilar artery (arrows).

This appearance is not specific. A similar pattern might be seen in meningeal carcinomatosis or exudative meningitis (see Case 385).

Several complications of subarachnoid hemorrhage may be more apparent on MR scans than the hemorrhage itself. Obstructive or communicating hydrocephalus may develop due to clot within the ventricular system or clogging of arachnoid granulations. Cerebral infarction may occur secondary to spasm of cerebral arteries, which typically develops a few days after hemorrhage and tends to be most severe in the areas of densest subarachnoid clot.

Parenchymal hematomas associated with subarachnoid hemorrhage may provide clues to the location of a ruptured aneurysm, which is the cause of subarachnoid hemorrhage in about 75% of cases. For example, a hematoma within the inferior portion of the septum pellucidum or the medial inferior frontal lobe suggests bleeding from an aneurysm of the anterior communicating artery.

See Case 1041 for an example of spinal subarachnoid hemorrhage.

Case 591A

65-year-old man with a history of multiple subdural hematomas, now presenting with bilateral hearing loss.
(axial, noncontrast scan; SE 2500/85)

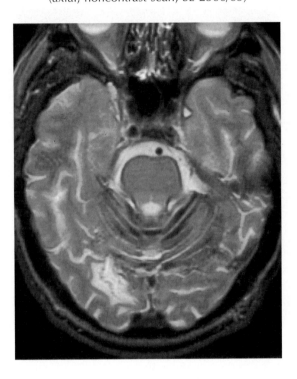

Case 591B

Same patient.
(coronal, noncontrast scan; SE 2500/85)

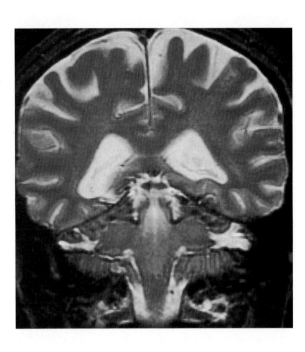

Case 591 demonstrates an unusual layer of low signal intensity along the surface of the cerebellum and brainstem. (Unrelated background findings include cerebral atrophy, cerebellar atrophy with gaping horizontal fissures, and a small area of encephalomalacia in the right occipital lobe.) This strikingly uniform outline of parenchymal contours is caused by subpial accumulation of old blood products, mainly hemosiderin.

Such "superficial siderosis" is seen in situations of chronic or repetitive subarachnoid hemorrhage. The source of bleeding may be a leaking vascular lesion (e.g., aneurysm or vascular malformation) or a spinal or intracranial neoplasm. Ependymomas of the spinal canal have been particularly frequently associated with intracranial siderosis (see Case 952). In about 50% of cases the etiology of superficial siderosis cannot be established, even at autopsy.

The meningeal surfaces of the posterior fossa are often most severely affected in cases of generalized siderosis. The superior aspect of the cerebellum is especially commonly involved. (Compare this localization to the preferential distribution of meningeal carcinomatosis, as discussed in Cases 160-162 and 537.)

Patients suffering from superficial siderosis frequently present with bilateral sensorineural hearing loss. The eighth cranial nerves are particularly susceptible to damage from the deposition of blood products on their surface. Cerebellar symptoms are usually absent, but ataxia has been noted in some cases.

Localized siderosis may occur anywhere over the cerebral convexity in proximity to a source of small, repeated subarachnoid hemorrhages. Examples include a long-standing neoplasm or an old operative site.

Fragile vessels within the membranes of chronic subdural hematomas frequently bleed. Although this mechanism probably contributes to the growth of such lesions, it is an unusual cause of cerebral siderosis.

Case 592

32-year-old woman presenting with headaches and a family history of subarachnoid hemorrhage.
(axial, noncontrast scan; SE 2800/45)

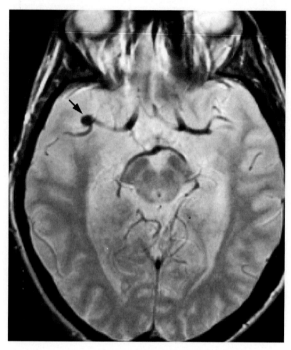

Aneurysm of the Middle Cerebral Artery

Case 593

67-year-old man with a history of TIAs.
(axial, noncontrast scan; SE 2800/45)

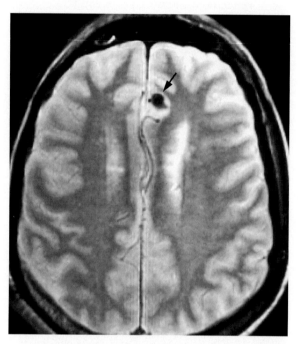

Aneurysm of the Pericallosal Artery

Small, patent aneurysms can be identified on spin echo MR studies as nodular expansions of "flow void" along the course of cerebral arteries. Such lesions are particularly well outlined by the high signal intensity of CSF on long TR sequences.

The genu or "trifurcation" region of the middle cerebral artery is one of the most common sites for intracranial aneurysms, illustrated in Case 592. Pericallosal artery aneurysms, as in Case 593, are less frequent. A single or "azygous" A-2 segment of the anterior cerebral artery was present in this case, with the aneurysm occurring at the bifurcation into paired pericallosal vessels.

Larger patent aneurysms may present more complicated appearances. Zones of slow flow or stasis within giant aneurysms can generate regions of variable intensity that may be difficult to distinguish from thrombus. Gradient echo sequences emphasizing flow-related enhancement help to separate these intraluminal components. Both slow flow and thrombus may be associated with enhancement on postcontrast MR scans.

Unruptured aneurysms can occasionally cause symptoms by embolization of thrombi formed within their lumens. It was not possible to clearly establish the source of the TIAs in Case 593.

Even "incidental" aneurysms in asymptomatic patients may be considered for surgery (or intraarterial occlusion with balloons or coils), depending on the aneurysm size and patient age. Population studies have estimated the risk of bleeding from unruptured aneurysms to be about 1% to 2% per year.

Aneurysms are occasionally found at sites distant from the circle of Willis. Peripheral aneurysms exhibit the same characteristics of extraaxial location and low signal intensity due to "flow void" as seen in conventional lesions. When such aneurysms are found, the possibility of mycotic, traumatic, or neoplastic origin should be considered.

MR is an excellent tool for noninvasive screening of patients with an increased risk of or concern about intracranial aneurysms. MR angiography is an important adjunct to routine imaging for this purpose (see Cases 600 and 601).

DIFFERENTIAL DIAGNOSIS:
FOCAL LOW SIGNAL INTENSITY NEAR THE SUPRACLINOID INTERNAL CAROTID ARTERY

Case 594

23-year-old man presenting with headaches.
(axial, noncontrast scan; SE 2800/45)

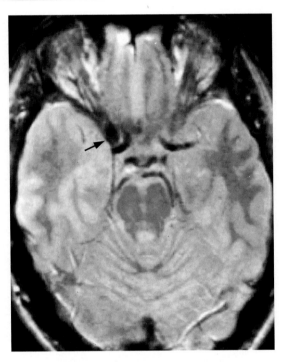

Pneumatized Anterior Clinoid Process

Case 595

54-year-old woman with a history of
subarachnoid hemorrhage.
(axial, noncontrast scan; SE 2800/90)

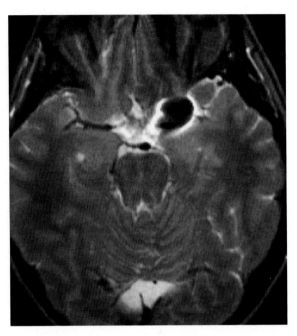

Metallic Artifact from an Aneurysm Clip

A large pneumatized or sclerotic anterior clinoid process may cause a focal zone of low signal intensity adjacent to the lumen of the internal carotid artery. Case 594 is an example of this appearance *(arrow)*, which may be accentuated on axial scans by a small amount of head tilt causing right/left asymmetry.

The anterior clinoid process may resemble a small, patent aneurysm in such instances. A similar "pseudoaneurysm" can occur in the region of the anterior communicating artery when partial volume of a prominent tuberculum sella is included on an axial scan.

Scans in the coronal plane will convincingly exclude or document an aneurysm in many cases. A flow-sensitive gradient echo sequence should settle the question when necessary.

The large area of low signal intensity in the left supraclinoid region of Case 595 is due to artifact caused by a metallic aneurysm clip. This appearance could be misinterpreted as indicating recurrence of a large, patent aneurysm.

Focal distortion of the magnetic field should be expected in proximity to any metallic device. More importantly, the possible ferromagnetic character of an aneurysm clip must be excluded before a patient who has had prior aneurysm surgery can be safely subjected to an MR study. There is substantial risk of torque or motion with consequent arterial injury if ferromagnetic aneurysm clips are brought into the magnetic field of an MR scanner.

Most currently manufactured vascular clips are produced from nonferromagnetic alloys to enable subsequent MR evaluation. Older clips are of variable composition. The manufacturer of a clip in question may be able to provide information about its magnetic properties.

Case 596

58-year-old woman presenting with bitemporal hemianopsia.
(coronal, noncontrast scan; SE 800/20)

Case 597

41-year-old woman with a parasellar lesion discovered on a CT scan.
(axial, noncontrast scan; SE 2800/45)

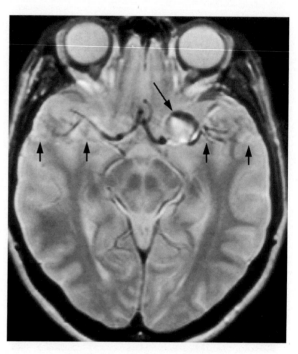

**Aneurysm of the Supraclinoid
Internal Carotid Artery**

**Aneurysm of the Supraclinoid
Internal Carotid Artery**

The circulation of blood within medium- and large-sized aneurysms is often complex, with lower flow velocities and less turbulence than is typically present within the lumen of smaller lesions. As a result, large aneurysms may demonstrate mixed intraluminal signal intensity on noncontrast scans and prominent enhancement on postcontrast images.

It may be difficult to distinguish between slowly flowing but patent components of the aneurysm and intraluminal thrombus on standard spin echo scans. Gradient echo sequences emphasizing flow-related enhancement are useful for demonstrating the patent portions of the lumen in such cases.

The midline suprasellar mass in Case 596 is nonspecific. Craniopharyngioma or other solid tumors should be considered in the differential diagnosis. Distortion of the optic chiasm *(arrows)* is comparable to other suprasellar masses and accounts for the patient's presenting symptoms. A characteristic rim of laminated T2-shortening on long TR images (such as in Case 604) or further evaluation by angiographic sequences could help to establish the diagnosis of aneurysm in this case.

The paraclinoid mass in Case 597 *(long arrow)* had been interpreted as a parasellar meningioma on an outside CT scan, which demonstrated uniform high attenuation and intense contrast enhancement. The band of pulsation artifact passing through the lesion on the MR study *(short arrows)* favors the alternative diagnosis of a large aneurysm. The mixture of signal intensities within the lumen reflects typically complex and slow flow. MR angiography and subsequent surgery demonstrated no intraluminal thrombus (see Case 601).

Aneurysms of the supraclinoid internal carotid artery (usually arising at the origin of the posterior communicating artery) are among the etiologies of a third nerve palsy. Fibers serving pupillary function are located near the surface of the third nerve and are typically affected by aneurysmal compression. (By contrast, the pupil is usually spared in third nerve palsies due to infarction.)

Case 598

50-year-old man who experienced subarachnoid
hemorrhage after head trauma.
(axial, noncontrast scan; SE 2500/30)

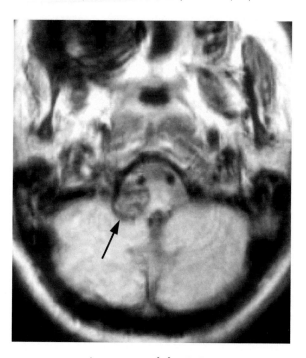

Aneurysm of the PICA

Case 599

81-year-old woman presenting with confusion.
(axial, noncontrast scan; SE 2800/45)

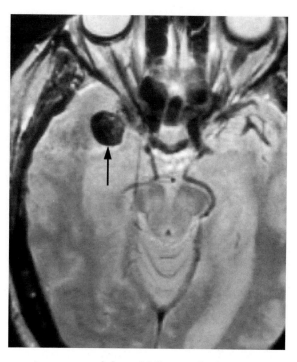

Aneurysm of the Middle Cerebral Artery

Thrombosed aneurysms present a variety of appearances on MR scans. The aneurysmal lumen may contain coarsely heterogeneous components with overall tissue-like signal intensity, as in Case 598. This pattern is difficult to distinguish from eddies of slow flow within a patent lumen, as in Cases 596 and 597. More generally, the lesion may resemble a soft tissue mass. (Compare Case 598 to the meningioma in Case 62.)

Alternatively, marked T2-shortening from intraluminal thrombus may cause very low signal intensity within an aneurysm, illustrated in Case 599. The prominent signal loss in such cases reflects the presence of paramagnetic blood products, which may be recent (deoxyhemoglobin) or old (hemosiderin). This appearance may blend with and/or mimic "flow void" within patent portions of the lumen.

In short, the patency of medium- and large-sized aneurysms is often difficult to judge on routine spin echo images. Flow-sensitive sequences are an important step in evaluating such cases.

Pulsation artifact is seen as a transverse band of mottled signal intensity passing through the aneurysms in Cases 597 and 599. This spatial mismapping of signal along the phase-encoding axis of the image is caused by pulsatile flow within the aneurysm and systolic/diastolic motion of its wall. The finding is most marked on long TR sequences without motion compensation. Pulsation artifact may be noted in association with both patent and thrombosed aneurysms. Its presence can be a useful clue to the vascular nature of an otherwise ambiguous mass.

Case 598 demonstrates that subarachnoid hemorrhage following head trauma should be carefully analyzed. In such cases the hemorrhage may reflect rupture of an underlying vascular lesion, with trauma following as a secondary event.

Extensive metallic artifact generated by dental apparatus is present in the region of the right maxilla in Case 598 (compare to Case 595).

Case 600A

44-year-old man presenting with headaches.
(axial, noncontrast scan; SE 2800/45)

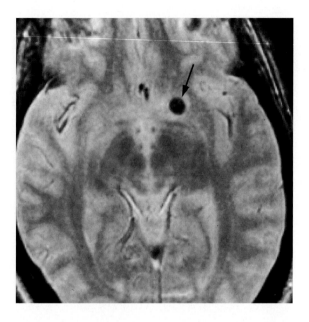

Case 600B

Same patient.
(AP projection of a three-dimensional,
time-of-flight GRE sequence)

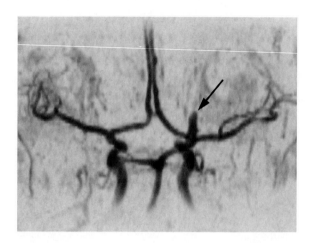

Flow-sensitive pulse sequences add substantial information to the MR evaluation of intracranial aneurysms. Both time-of-flight and phase-contrast techniques have proponents and advantages.

The fundamental goal of MR angiography in aneurysm cases is to demonstrate the patent portion of the lumen. Such documentation establishes the diagnosis and can guide the choice of therapeutic options.

The focal area of low signal intensity in the left suprasellar region of Case 600A suggests the lumen of a small, patent aneurysm, resembling Cases 592 and 593. However, the location of the lesion is a little higher than might be expected for typical aneurysms arising from the supraclinoid internal carotid artery or proximal middle cerebral artery.

The MR angiogram in Case 600B explains this appearance. An aneurysm does arise from the distal bifurcation of the left supraclinoid internal carotid artery (compare to the normal right side). It projects directly superiorly for a distance of about one centimeter, causing the dome to appear in isolation on higher axial sections.

Case 601A

41-year-old woman with a left parasellar lesion
demonstrated on a CT scan.
(axial, noncontrast scan; SE 2800/45)

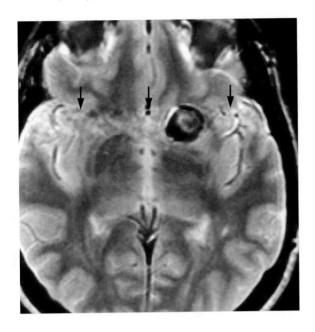

Case 601B

Same patient.
(AP projection of a three-dimensional,
time-of-flight GRE sequence)

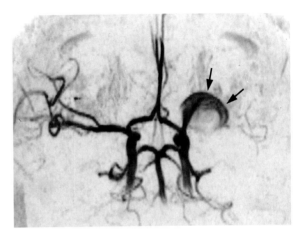

(same patient as Case 597)

The thick rind of low signal intensity at the perimeter of the lesion in Case 601A combines with the prominent band of pulsation artifact traversing the mass *(arrows)* to strongly suggest an aneurysm. However, it is unclear whether the intermediate signal intensity at the center of the lesion is due to slow flow or thrombus. Similarly, the peripheral zone of low intensity could either represent flow or a layer of clot with prominent T2-shortening.

Case 601B resolves these questions by demonstrating a "jet" of flow entering the neck of the aneurysm inferiorly and splashing against the opposite wall before swirling around the circumference of the dome *(arrows)*. This image clearly establishes luminal patency. Equally important, it defines the size and location of the aneurysm neck, which assists in planning treatment.

Compare this case to the thrombosed giant aneurysm in Case 635.

Case 602

59-year-old woman presenting with a third nerve palsy.
(sagittal, noncontrast scan; SE 600/17)

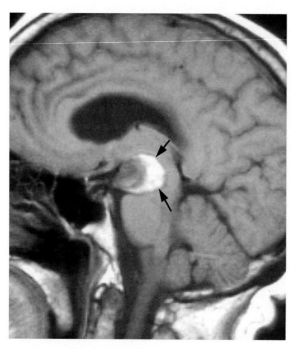

Thrombosed Aneurysm of the Basilar Artery

Case 603

76-year-old man with progressive aphasia and hemiparesis, referred for resection of a "brain tumor."
(coronal, noncontrast scan; SE 600/15)

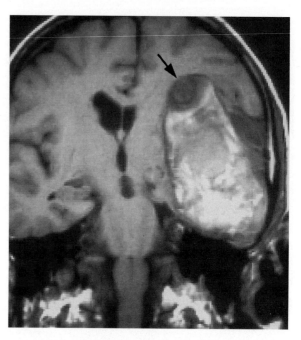

Predominantly Thrombosed Aneurysm of the Middle Cerebral Artery

---

Large aneurysms have been angiographically described as "giant" when their diameter reaches 2.5 cm. Giant aneurysms most commonly arise from the supraclinoid internal carotid artery or the middle cerebral artery. They often present as mass lesions, but hemorrhage is not as rare as previously believed.

The lumina of giant aneurysms are usually at least partially occupied by thrombus, which often has a lamellar or concentric appearance. The association of subarachnoid or intracerebral hemorrhage with a large, marble-like mass near the skull base is highly characteristic of a ruptured giant aneurysm.

Partially or completely thrombosed aneurysms present variable MR appearances, depending on the age of intraluminal clot and the parameters of the pulse sequence. On T1-weighted images, thrombosed aneurysms often demonstrate a mixture of isointensity and high signal zones, as in Case 602.

Craniopharyngioma might be considered in the differential diagnosis of this retrosellar lesion with T1-shortening (see Case 228), particularly since the CT scan of the mass demonstrated a peripheral shell of calcification (as is common in giant aneurysms). Characteristic morphology on long TR spin echo images (presented as Case 604) established the correct diagnosis.

Case 603 demonstrates that giant aneurysms can reach remarkable size through slow expansion, gradually deforming the surrounding brain. Here the midline shift is quite small for the size of the mass, attesting to its long-standing nature.

The coronal MR scan in Case 603 establishes that the middle fossa "tumor" is an extraaxial mass, filled with subacute thrombus. The appearance suggests a giant aneurysm of the middle cerebral artery. At angiography, the horizontal segment of the middle cerebral artery was draped over the top of the aneurysm. A small patent lumen was found, corresponding to the low-intensity zone at the dome of the lesion *(arrow)*.

Case 604

59-year-old woman presenting with diplopia.
(axial, noncontrast scan; SE 2500/28)

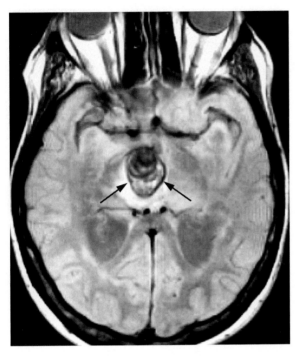

(same patient as Case 602)

Case 605

76-year-old man presenting with
aphasia and hemiparesis.
(axial, noncontrast scan; SE 3000/22)

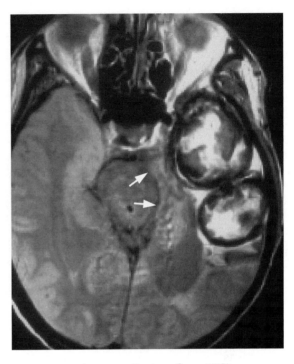

(same patient as Case 603)

On long TR spin echo images, the presence of T2-shortening due to blood products helps to characterize thrombosed giant aneurysms. The pattern of such zones of low signal intensity is variable. They may be strikingly lamellar, as in Case 604, or peripherally clumped, as in Case 605. In some cases, T2-shortening due to deoxyhemoglobin and/or intracellular methemoglobin occupies most of the lumen of a thrombosed aneurysm, mimicking "flow void" (see Case 635).

The benefit of combining MR planes and sequence weightings in analysis of vascular masses is apparent when the above images are compared to the preceeding page. In Case 604, the layered morphology of blood products on the long TR image distinguishes the lesion from other suprasellar pathologies, while the T1-weighted scan (Case 602) is indeterminate. By contrast, the coronal T1-weighted scan in Case 603 is more definitive than the long TR axial image in Case 605. On the latter scan, the high signal intensity of distorted cisterns surrounding the mass could be interpreted as edema, and blood products within the lesion could be attributed to intratumoral hemorrhage (compare to Case 562.)

The clinical presentation of patients with giant intracranial aneurysms often reflects the mass effect of the lesion, as in Case 603/605. The bilobed mass in the left sylvian region has caused uncal herniation *(arrows)*.

Contrast enhancement of giant aneurysms may take several forms. Occasionally the lumen is entirely patent. Intense enhancement of slowly flowing blood within such lesions may mimic a meningioma. Completely thrombosed giant aneurysms typically demonstrate a thin rim of surrounding enhancement due to adventitia or a capsule. Finally, many lesions present a combination or target-like appearance. A small, often eccentric lumen (such as in Case 603) is surrounded by a large zone of nonenhancing thrombus, which is in turn bordered by a rim of peripheral enhancement.

373

Case 606

25-year-old woman presenting with seizures.
(sagittal, noncontrast scan; SE 600/14)

Case 607

23-year-old man complaining of severe headaches.
(coronal, noncontrast scan; SE 600/15)

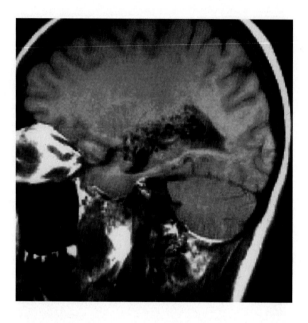

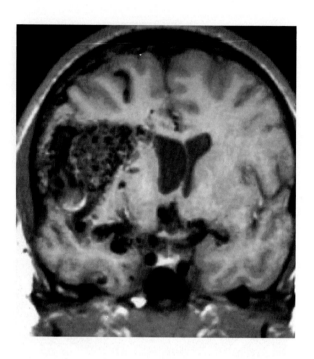

Uncomplicated arteriovenous malformations (AVMs) present on spin echo MR scans as tightly packed clusters of serpentine channels demonstrating "flow void." The contour of the lesions may vary from spherical to wedge-shaped, often based against the cerebral surface or the ventricular margin. The AVM in Case 606 follows the temporal horn, while the lesion in Case 607 is transcerebral.

High intensity components interspersed with "flow void" in AVMs may represent zones of slow flow, hemorrhage, and/or intervening parenchyma or scar tissue. Mass effect is unusual in the absence of associated hemorrhage. However, Case 607 demonstrates that some AVMs do contain sufficiently bulky vascular components to cause compression of adjacent structures. Encephalomalacia may be present due to old hemorrhage or to parenchymal damage arising from the pulsations or "steal" of the malformation.

Patients with AVMs commonly experience seizures, as in Case 606. Other frequent symptoms include headache (as in Case 607) and focal hemispheric deficits. Hemorrhage is the initial manifestation of a cerebral AVM in about 50% of cases (see Cases 616 and 617).

The high flow within the nidus, feeding arteries and draining veins of arteriovenous malformations can be demonstrated on angiographic gradient echo scans. Such sequences maximize the signal intensity of fresh spins entering the imaging volume while suppressing background signal through RF saturation of stationary tissue. As a result, flow appears "bright" against a dark background. (This contrast is often inverted photographically to provide three-dimensional displays of vascular anatomy that resemble the subtraction studies of catheter angiography; see Cases 600 and 601 for examples.) Phase-contrast angiography with variable velocity encoding may be useful to separately image slow flow components of an AVM.

Large vessels may be associated with intracranial tumors (see Cases 40, 41, 87, 88, 137, and 139), but the pattern is rarely as tightly interwoven as in AVMs.

Case 608

28-year-old man presenting with left superior quadrantanopsia.
(axial, noncontrast scan; SE 2500/45)

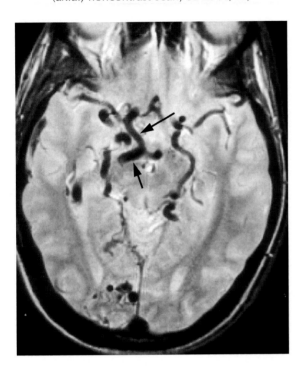

Case 609

23-year-old man presenting with headaches.
(axial, noncontrast scan; SE 2800/90)

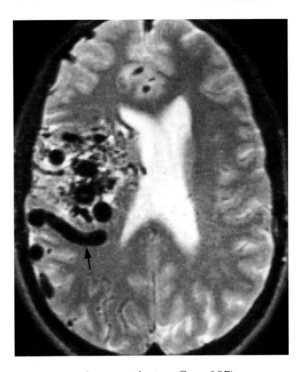

(same patient as Case 607)

Ectatic feeding arteries or draining veins may be prominent components of high flow AVMs. Case 608 illustrates hypertrophy of multiple arteries that supplied an extensive right hemisphere AVM, predominantly involving the occipital lobe. Note for example the gross enlargement of the right posterior communicating artery *(long arrow)* and the proximal posterior cerebral artery *(short arrow)*.

The large vessel at the posterior margin of the AVM in Case 609 *(arrow)* was angiographically proven to represent a varix draining the malformation.

One or more aneurysms are frequently found along the course of arteries feeding an AVM. They may cause large, rounded areas of "flow void" simulating varices within the malformation. The occurrence of such aneurysms is likely flow-related; they may thrombose spontaneously after the AVM is embolized or resected. Among patients who present with subarachnoid hemorrhage and are found to have aneurysms associated with AVMs, the aneurysm is the more frequent source of bleeding.

Areas of low signal intensity within arteriovenous malformations on MR scans may also be due to calcification, which is common within the walls of vascular channels or within dystrophic cerebral parenchyma. Zones of acute hemorrhage (containing deoxyhemoglobin) and/or hemosiderin accumulation from old hemorrhages may also contribute to low signal intensity on long TR spin echo images.

Case 610

14-month-old girl with a history of borderline
heart failure since infancy.
(axial, noncontrast scan; SE 2800/45)

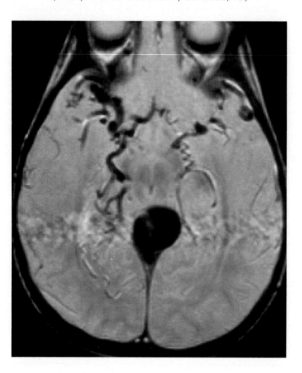

Case 611

2-month-old girl presenting with a rapidly
enlarging head and a cranial bruit.
(axial, noncontrast scan; SE 2500/90)

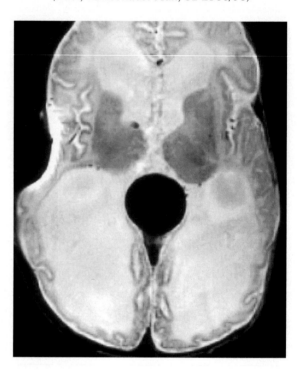

AVMs draining into the vein of Galen often contain direct arteriovenous fistulae. The associated high flow causes marked expansion of the receiving vein, traditionally misnamed as a vein of Galen "aneurysm."

Rapid and turbulent flow through the arterialized veins of a vascular malformation exceeds the rephasing capability of most nonangiographic MR sequences. The signal void within such structures usually persists after the injection of contrast material. In the above cases, the dilated vein of Galen is strikingly defined as a midline zone of absent signal. Other possible sources of signal loss (e.g., dense calcification or marked T2-shortening) are rarely as uniform, severe, and sharply marginated as seen here (but compare Case 611 to Case 617).

In Case 610, a band of pulsation artifact passes through the varix, comparable to the appearance of aneurysms such as Cases 597 and 599. Multiple hypertrophied feeding arteries are apparent near the circle of Willis.

High flow through a vein of Galen malformation may cause congestive heart failure in the neonatal period. Infants and older children with less severe arteriovenous shunts often present with hydrocephalus, as in Case 611. Venous hypertension may impair resorption of CSF, leading to communicating hydrocephalus. Alternatively, the mass effect of the varix may cause obstructive hydrocephalus by compressing the posterior third ventricle and aqueduct.

Secondary development of distal stenoses along the path of drainage through dural veins and sinuses is a common feature of high flow vascular malformations. This process may play an important role in the morphological and symptomatic progression or regression of vein of Galen "aneurysms."

When outflow obstruction develops in association with dural arteriovenous fistulae (e.g., those involving the transverse and sigmoid sinuses), a characteristic pattern of enlarged corkscrew venous collaterals is often apparent overlying the cerebellum or cerebral surface (see Case 612A).

Case 612A

62-year-old man presenting with left-sided
tinnitus and mild ataxia.
(axial, noncontrast scan; SE 2500/20)

Case 612B

Same patient.
(coronal, postcontrast scan; SE 570/15)

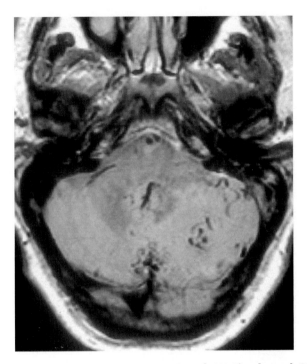

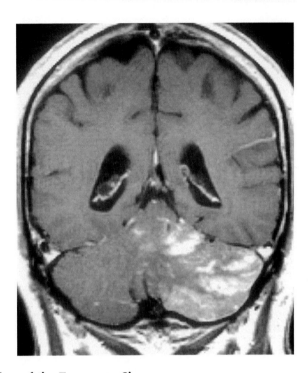

Dural AV Fistula and Occlusion of the Transverse Sinus

About 15% of intracranial vascular malformations are found within the dura. The most common locations for such lesions are the walls of major dural sinuses, especially the transverse sinus (as in the above example) and the cavernous sinus (see discussion of Case 796). Many dural vascular malformations are true arteriovenous fistulae, with direct shunting of blood from dural arteries into a venous compartment.

If the outflow of a dural AVM is not compromised, symptoms are often nonspecific and standard MR scans may demonstrate no associated parenchymal changes. A negative MR scan does not exclude the diagnosis of a dural vascular malformation.

However, many dural AVMs are accompanied by partial or complete occlusion of the receiving venous sinus. There is evidence that primary sinus thrombosis leads to subsequent development of a dural AVM in some cases. In other patients, a flow-induced vasculopathy causes progressive constriction of the initially patent sinus draining a dural fistula.

Restriction of venous outflow may cause severe symptoms and characteristic parenchymal changes on MR images. These findings are due to cortical venous drainage which develops as a collateral system when the dural sinuses are stenosed or occluded. Patients whose dural AVMs drain into cortical veins are at risk for venous infarction and/or intracranial hemorrhage.

Case 612A demonstrates typical findings of a dural AVM with restricted outflow. Multiple dilated, tortuous veins are seen as short, corkscrew-like "flow voids" within and on the surface of the left cerebellar hemisphere. Unlike the parenchymal AVMs in Cases 606-609, no hypertrophied feeding arteries or intracerebral nidus are associated with the scattered venous ectasia. Extensive edema is also present throughout the left cerebellum as a result of venous hypertension. Venous congestion and impaired parenchymal drainage are demonstrated by the parenchymal stain of abnormal enhancement throughout the left cerebellum in Case 612B.

A pattern of contrast enhancement resembling Case 612B is occasionally seen within the territory drained by a venous angioma when the stem vein is constricted or stenosed (see discussion of Cases 622 and 623).

Case 614A

31-year-old man presenting with seizures
and right hand weakness.
(sagittal, noncontrast scan; SE 600/17)

Case 614B

Same patient.
(coronal, noncontrast scan; SE 3000/90)

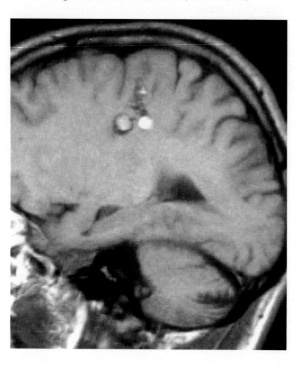

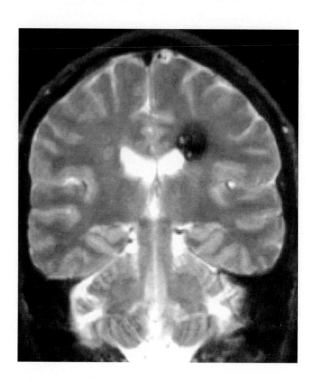

Thrombosed vascular malformations are often said to be "occult," meaning that they are not demonstrable by angiographic techniques. Such lesions are usually apparent on CT scans as small, high attenuation regions. Their CT density may be due to calcification, blood volume, and/or contrast enhancement.

Thrombosis of an AVM eliminates the characteristic flow patterns illustrated in Cases 606 to 611. However, the nidus of a malformation remains well-defined on MR scans as a zone of mixed signal abnormality reflecting blood products and calcification within the lesion.

Case 614A illustrates the typical MR appearance of a thrombosed vascular malformation. A multinodular lesion contains prominent components of T1-shortening, suggesting the presence of methemoglobin. Case 614B demonstrates low signal intensity within and surrounding the lesion due to local accumulation of hemosiderin from old microhemorrhages.

The periventricular region is a common location for patent or thrombosed vascular malformations. Some AVMs extend as a transcerebral band from the cortex to the ventricular margin.

The lesion in Case 614 was known to represent an AVM from angiographic studies demonstrating patency on an earlier admission. However, the appearance presented on the scans above is indistinguishable from that of a cavernous hemangioma (see Cases 627-630). For this reason, thrombosed AVMs and cavernous angiomas are sometimes discussed together as "occult cerebral vascular malformations" or "OCVMs."

Case 615A

20-year-old man presenting with seizures.
(sagittal, noncontrast scan; SE 500/25)

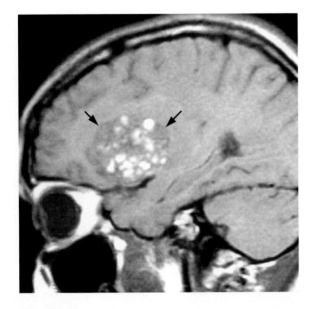

Case 615B

Same patient.
(coronal, postcontrast scan; SE 550/25)

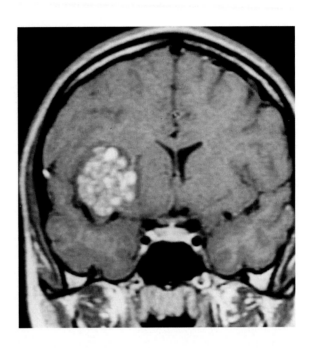

Occasional thrombosed AVMs are sufficiently large and mass-like to mimic a cerebral neoplasm. The overall contour of the lesion in Case 615 is approximately spherical. Multiple internal nodules of T1-shortening on the precontrast scan resemble the appearance of Case 614A. However, their distribution throughout a larger mass raises the question of hemorrhagic loculations, proteinaceous cysts, or even lipid material within a complex tumor such as an oligodendroglioma or teratoma (see Cases 111, 112, and 283-287).

On the postcontrast scan (Case 615B), tissue between the nodules enhances intensely. Again the possibility of neoplasm is raised. The relative lack of mass effect for the size of the lesion is a clue to the correct diagnosis, but longstanding, low grade tumors may also demonstrate this feature.

The mass was resected and proved to be an entirely thrombosed AVM.

Case 616

7-year-old boy presenting with a seizure
and headache after a fall.
(axial, noncontrast scan; SE 2800/90)

Case 617

43-year-old man experiencing the sudden
onset of right hemiparesis.
(axial, noncontrast scan; SE 2800/45)

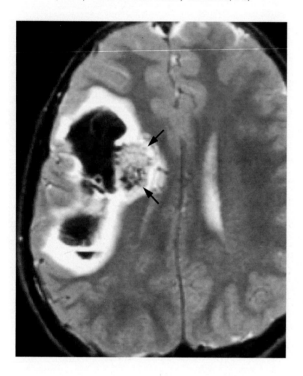

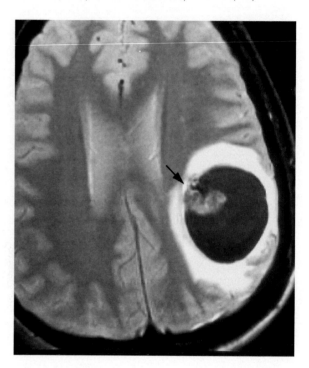

Hemorrhage is the most common presentation of AVMs, occurring in one third to two thirds of patients in most series. The majority of these hemorrhages are intracerebral rather than subarachnoid. CT and MR scans usually demonstrate both the hematoma and the responsible vascular malformation. Rarely a small AVM is destroyed at the time of rupture or compressed by the resulting hematoma.

Both of the above cases demonstrate acute intracerebral hematomas (compare to Case 556). Very low central signal intensity due to intracellular deoxyhemoglobin is surrounded by a thick collar of high intensity representing reactive edema.

In Cases 616 and 617 an area of tissue with distinctly different architecture is apparent at the margin of hemorrhage *(arrows)*. This feature strongly suggests a preexisting structural lesion as the source of bleeding. Although neoplasm could be considered, the reticular or racemose morphology of the tissue nodules and epidemiological factors in these young patients favor the diagnosis of vascular malformations.

The annual risk of bleeding from an unruptured AVM is estimated to be about 2% to 4% per year. For this reason, treatment by embolization, surgery, and/or radiation is recommended for most patients. The choice of modality is influenced by the size and location (i.e., resectibility) of the malformation, as well as the age and symptoms of the patient.

Once an AVM has bled, the annual risk of new hemorrhage initially rises to 5% to 15% per year. Many surgeons choose to attempt resection of a malformation that has "declared itself" by an episode of hemorrhage. The space created by evacuation of an adjacent hematoma often aids excision.

Case 618

11-year-old girl presenting with a visual
field deficit.
(axial, noncontrast scan; SE 2800/90)

Case 619

66-year-old man presenting with personality
change and right hemiparesis.
(axial, noncontrast scan; SE 2500/90)

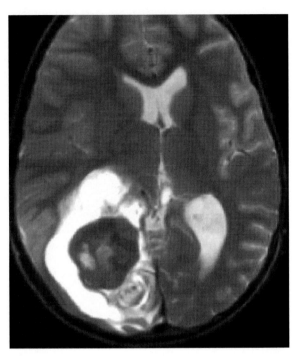

Ependymoma

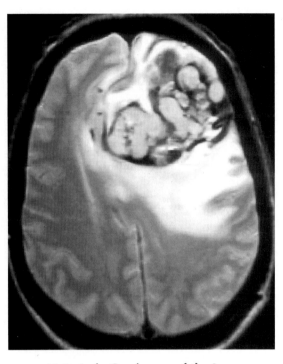

Metastasic Carcinoma of the Lung

As illustrated on the preceding page, intracerebral hemorrhage from AVMs may result in a complex pattern of thrombus, edema, and nodular tissue representing the malformation itself.

Hemorrhagic primary or metastatic tumors such as Cases 618 and 619 can present a similar appearance. (See also Cases 90 and 562.) The pattern of T2-shortening due to blood products may vary from uniform, as in Case 618, to multinodular as in Case 619.

Several MR features can help to distinguish a hemorrhagic neoplasm from bleeding due to rupture of a vascular malformation. Edema surrounding cerebral tumors is often more extensive and irregular than the uniform rind encircling benign hematomas. (Compare the above cases to the scans on the preceding page.) More importantly, blood products are found within the substance of a hemorrhagic neoplasm, contrasting with the usual eccentricity of hematomas seen adjacent to the nidus of a vascular malformation.

Case 620

28-year-old woman complaining of headaches.
(sagittal, noncontrast scan; SE 600/20)

Case 621

42-year-old woman presenting with dizziness.
(axial, noncontrast scan; SE 2800/90)

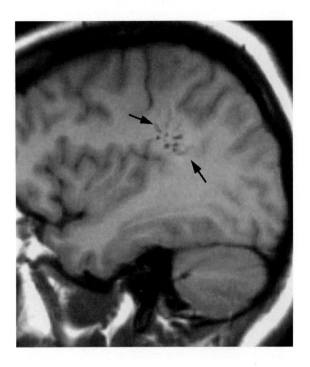

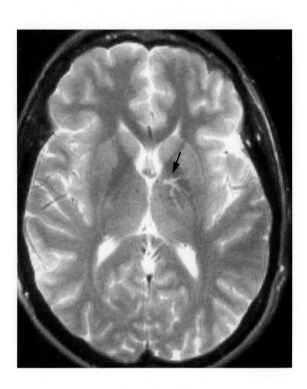

Venous angiomas have a characteristic morphology that is often recognizable on CT and MR scans. The lesion has two components: (1) a group of radially oriented tributary veins converging like spokes of an umbrella to a central point and (2) a single, abnormally large draining vein formed at the confluence of the tributaries and following an aberrant route through cerebral parenchyma.

The above cases illustrate the appearance of the converging tributary channels, seen in cross section (Case 620) or parallel to the scan plane (Case 621).

Blood flow within venous angiomas is slow. As a result, these vascular anomalies usually demonstrate fluid-like signal intensity rather than "flow void." For the same reason, venous angiomas characteristically enhance with contrast material (see Case 623). In fact, they may be visible only on postcontrast studies.

Venous angiomas are most often incidental anomalies rather than threatening "malformations." They are infrequently associated with seizures. Clinically significant bleeding is uncommon in the absence of outflow obstruction; a possibly increased incidence in cerebellar lesions is controversial.

Small hemorrhages localized to the vicinity of a venous angioma are probably more frequent. The common occurrence of cavernous angiomas adjacent to venous malformations has suggested that organization of small hemorrhages from a venous angioma may play a role in formation of some cavernous lesions.

Case 622

6-year-old girl presenting with seizures.
(sagittal, noncontrast scan; SE 600/15)

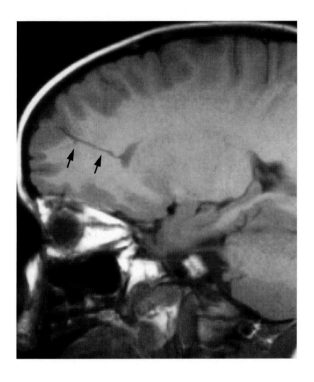

Case 623

48-year-old woman being evaluated for
demyelinating disease.
(coronal, postcontrast scan; SE 600/15)

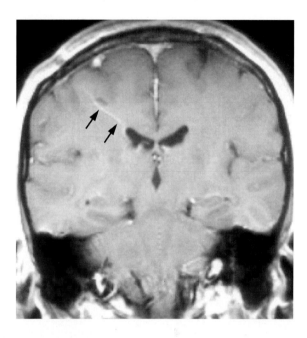

The typically aberrant, transparenchymal course of the major stem vein within a venous angioma is demonstrated in the above cases *(arrows)*. This channel emerges from the confluence of radially oriented tributary vessels and traverses broad regions of parenchyma to reach the cerebral surface or the ventricular margin. The central vein of the angioma usually terminates by merging with the normal venous system in one of these locations. Even when tributary veins are inconspicuous, the dilated and anomalously located stem of a venous angioma is highly characteristic.

In Cases 622 and 623, long segments of stem veins are visualized because they are parallel to the scan plane. The central channels of other venous angiomas may intersect the plane of the scan perpendicularly or at oblique angles, resulting in circular or elliptical cross sections (see Case 625).

As mentioned earlier, slow flow within venous angiomas results in obvious contrast enhancement, demonstrated in Case 623. Lack of enhancement within a vascular channel should raise doubt about the diagnosis of venous angioma.

Stenosis of the stem vein of a venous angioma may predispose to hemorrhage within its watershed. Such constriction typically occurs at the site where a stem vein penetrates the dura. A vague haze of contrast enhancement throughout the parenchyma drained by the angioma can be a clue to stasis caused by partial outflow obstruction. (A similar appearance may be caused by venous sinus occlusion in association with a dural arteriovenous fistula, often accompanied by a number of distended and tortuous parenchymal veins; see Case 612.)

Enhancement along the course of a prior shunt tube or ventriculostomy catheter can simulate the transcerebral stem vein of a venous angioma in patients with a recent history of hydrocephalus.

Case 624

28-year-old man presenting with vague
paresthesias.
(axial, noncontrast scan; SE 3000/80)

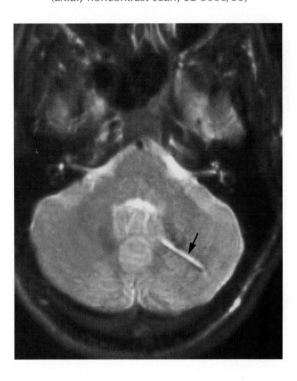

Case 625

11-year-old girl being evaluated for personality
changes.
(axial, noncontrast scan; SE 2800/90)

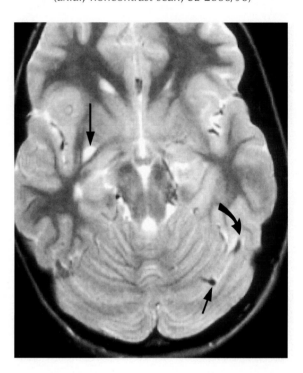

Venous angiomas may occur within the brainstem and are commonly encountered in the cerebellum. The majority of these anomalies are found incidentally, although the frequency of hemorrhage has been reported to exceed that of supratentorial angiomas.

Cases 624 and 625 demonstrate that the morphology of cerebellar venous angiomas is comparable to their cerebral counterparts. Large stem veins characteristically traverse the cerebellar hemispheres to reach the fourth ventricle or the pial surface. The direction of flow in such transcerebellar channels may be either centripetal or centrifugal.

In Case 624, a long segment of the central vein runs within the plane of the scan. High intensity within the large vein is due to successful rephasing of the signal from slowly flowing protons. This recovery of signal (i.e., avoidance of "flow void") is mainly due to refocusing features of current spin echo pulse sequences, designed to reduce mismapping of CSF signal from pulsating cisterns. Rephasing can also be seen on "even echoes" of nonrefocused spin echo sequences.

Case 625 demonstrates the appearance of a venous angioma oriented perpendicular to the scan plane. Even slow flow that crosses the plane of a scan results in signal loss on routine spin echo images. The small circle of low intensity in Case 625 *(short arrow)* could be followed across multiple adjacent sections to demonstrate the tubular morphology of a vascular channel.

Large cortical veins are normally present near the tentorium *(curved arrow,* Case 625). These prominent vessels drain the inferior surfaces of the temporal and occipital lobes, passing through or near the tentorial dura to reach the transverse sinus. Their location immediately adjacent to the tentorium distinguishes such normal veins from parenchymal components of a vascular malformation.

A small sublenticular cyst is present on the right side of Case 625 *(long arrow;* see Case 705).

Case 626A

16-year-old girl presenting with seizures.
(axial, postcontrast scan; SE 700/15)

Case 626B

Same patient.
(axial, postcontrast scan; SE 700/15)

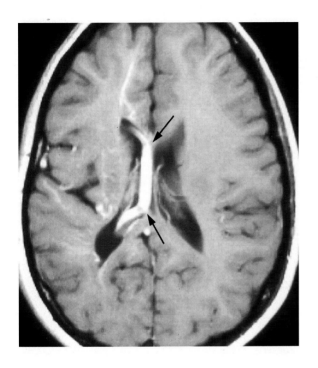

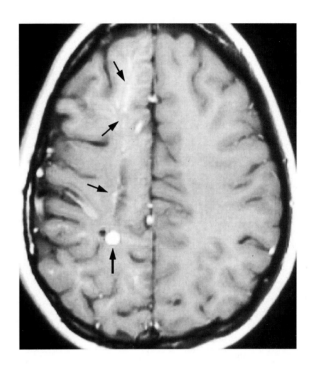

Occasional venous malformations are large and complex. The presence of two or three "heads" (i.e., systems of radial tributaries converging to a central stem) is relatively common. Anomalous venous drainage of an entire hemisphere, as in Case 626, is much rarer.

The above scans demonstrate abnormally large, contrast-filled veins throughout much of the white matter of the right cerebral hemisphere. These aberrant medullary channels receive flow from radially oriented tributaries *(thin arrows,* Case 626B) and drain centrally to a greatly enlarged ventricular vein *(arrows,* Case 626A). This vein subsequently courses superiorly through the parietal lobe (*thick arrow,* Case 626B) to reach the convexity.

Such cases emphasize that venous angiomas are best considered to represent anomalies of cerebral venous development. However aberrant their morphology, they provide functional venous drainage from major zones of cerebral parenchyma. Resection of these "lesions" may lead to venous infarction. In symptomatic cases with a history of hemorrhage, the size and location of a venous angioma must be considered to judge the advisability of resection.

Case 627

43-year-old man with headaches and multiple high attenuation lesions discovered on a CT scan.
(sagittal, noncontrast scan; SE 800/17)

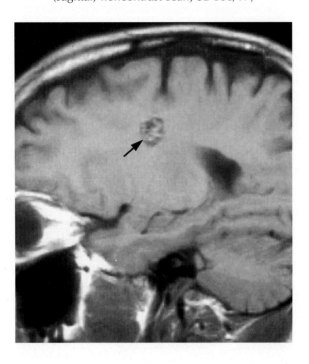

Case 628

45-year-old woman, with a long-standing diagnosis of brainstem glioma.
(axial, noncontrast scan; SE 2500/30)

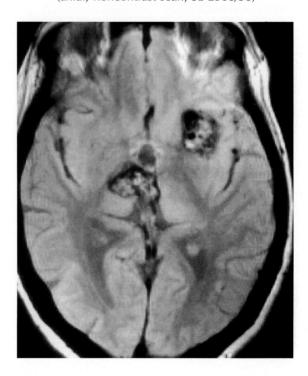

Cavernous hemangiomas or "angiomas" are collections of sinusoidal vascular spaces without intervening neuroglial tissue. Although well-recognized pathologically as one of the major categories of cerebral vascular malformations, these lesions have been difficult to diagnose prior to CT scanning. Their frequent demonstration on CT and MR studies requires recognition and distinction from other masses. Cavernous angiomas are angiographically "occult" and account for the majority of so-called "cryptic" vascular malformations.

The MR appearance of cavernous angiomas is highly characteristic. An aggregate, multinodular or "popcorn" morphology with prominent central zones of T1-shortening is surrounded by a characteristic rind of T2-shortening. Septations and focal areas of additional T2-shortening are often seen within the lesion.

Cavernous angiomas may range in size from a few millimeters to several centimeters in diameter. Any region of the brain may be affected. A diagnostically helpful characteristic of cavernous angiomas is frequent multiplicity, with oc-

casional familial incidence. Ambiguous lesions are commonly accompanied by other more typical angiomas.

Case 627 illustrates the characteristic architecture of a small cavernous angioma. (Note that a hemorrhagic metastasis like Case 8 can present a similar appearance.) The larger masses in Case 628 demonstrate the common multiplicity of these lesions: a brainstem angioma in the same patient is presented as Case 637.

Thrombosed or low flow AVMs may have a similar MR appearance (see Case 614). Mixed vascular malformations containing several histological patterns are common, particularly the combination of venous angioma and cavernous angioma (see discussion of Cases 620 and 621).

Thrombosed aneurysms may present with a heterogeneous combination of signal intensities resembling that of cavernous angiomas. However, the morphology of such lesions is often lamellar or concentric (see Case 604), in contrast to the nodular or "honeycomb" architecture of most cavernous malformations (see also Cases 635 and 636).

Case 629

38-year-old woman presenting with a long
history of seizures.
(coronal, noncontrast scan; SE 3000/90)

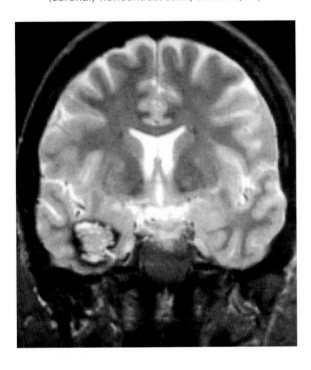

Case 630

23-year-old man presenting with seizures.
(coronal, noncontrast scan; SE 3000/90)

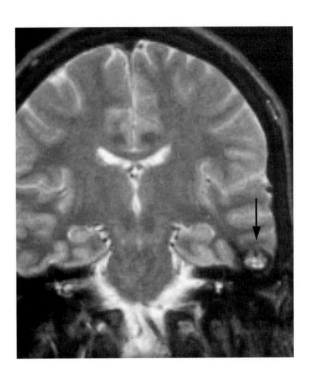

The perimeter of cavernous angiomas is usually outlined by a prominent zone of low signal intensity on T2-weighted images, as seen above. This rind of T2-shortening is attributable to an accumulation of hemosiderin from old hemorrhages.

Cavernous angiomas are commonly found in the temporal lobes, where they represent an important cause of seizures (as in Cases 629 and 630). These lesions are among the most common structural abnormalities encountered in patients with temporal lobe epilepsy. (See also Case 78 and Cases 450-453.) The absence of reactive edema and mass effect argues against neoplasm in such cases.

Calcification may also contribute to low signal intensity within and surrounding cavernous angiomas. The walls of cavernous channels within the malformations are often thickened, with secondary calcification or even ossification.

Serial scans have documented progressive enlargement of some cavernous angiomas, presumably due to recurrent small hemorrhages with subsequent organization and recanalization of thrombus. Such events are usually subclinical. Angiomas are occasionally implicated as the source of major parenchymal hematomas.

Lesions resembling the MR appearance of cavernous angiomas may develop within the brain after radiation therapy. Such foci likely represent small, organizing hemorrhages secondary to radiation-induced vascular injury.

DIFFERENTIAL DIAGNOSIS:
TEMPORAL LOBE FOCUS OF LOW SIGNAL INTENSITY

Case 631

23-year-old woman presenting with a first seizure.
(coronal, noncontrast scan; SE 3000/25)

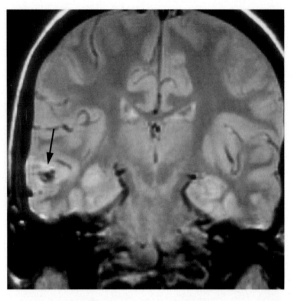

Low Grade Astrocytoma

Case 632

48-year-old man complaining of severe headaches.
(axial, noncontrast scan; SE 2500/45)

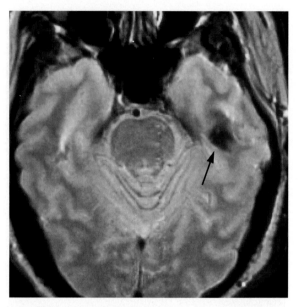

Partial Volume of Normal Arcuate Eminence

The appearance of small cavernous angiomas may be dominated by the T2-shortening of associated hemosiderin. Nodular areas of low signal intensity within cerebral parenchyma on long TR images are a common manifestation of these lesions.

The above cases demonstrate that such an appearance is not specific for cavernous malformations. The low grade glioma in Case 631 was shown by CT to be densely calcified. (Calcification may cause localized signal loss by physical replacement of protons and by susceptibility effects that accelerate proton relaxation.) Although the resultant appearance resembles a cavernous angioma, the perimeter of high signal intensity would be unusual (compare to Cases 629 and 630) and should suggest an alternative diagnosis.

Case 632 presents the MR equivalent of a well-known CT pseudolesion. The superior semicircular canal causes a bump on the superior surface of the temporal bone. Axial scans passing along the inferior surface of the temporal lobe may partially include this "arcuate eminence," causing the spurious appearance of a calcified parenchymal lesion. Minor right/left asymmetry and mild head tilt can accentuate this finding. Since the inferior portion of the temporal lobe is a common location for cavernous angiomas, a coronal scan is appropriate for further evaluation when an appearance similar to Case 632 is encountered on an axial study.

Relatively high signal intensity of gray matter in the medial temporal regions bilaterally in Case 631 is artifactual.

DIFFERENTIAL DIAGNOSIS:
SMALL CEREBRAL LESIONS WITH RIMS OF LOW SIGNAL INTENSITY

Case 633

56-year-old woman with a distant history of CVA.
(axial, noncontrast scan; SE 2500/45)

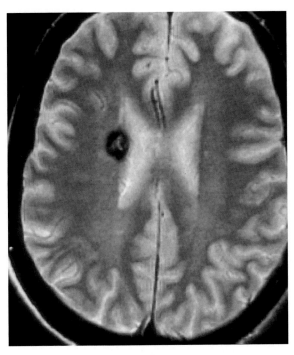

Old Hematoma

Case 634

64-year-old woman with a known hypernephroma.
(axial, noncontrast scan; SE 2800/45)

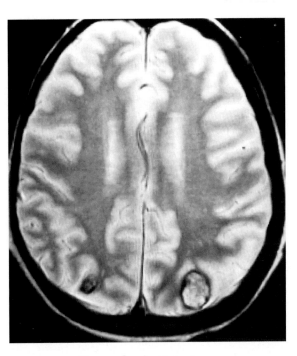

Hemorrhagic Metastases

The hemosiderin rim that is characteristic of cavernous angiomas is not specific for this diagnosis. As discussed previously, the organization of spontaneous parenchymal hematomas leads to a layer of hemosiderin-containing macrophages at the perimeter of the lesion. This "stain" persists indefinitely and may be demonstrated on subsequent MR studies or at autopsy.

Case 633 is an example of this occurrence. Since the region of the basal ganglia and corona radiata is a common location for both cavernous angiomas (see Case 627) and spontaneous intracerebral hemorrhage (see Case 557), a hemosiderin-lined lesion in this area may represent either pathology.

Case 634 illustrates that hemorrhage into neoplasms may mimic the MR presentation of cavernous angiomas. Like angiomas, vascular metastases may contain blood products and demonstrate a rim of low signal intensity on T2-weighted scans. As discussed in Chapter 1, metastases may incite little or no surrounding edema. Multiplicity is a common feature of both metastatic disease and cavernous angiomas. For these reasons, careful attention to clinical context and follow-up examinations are appropriate before the diagnosis of "multiple cavernous angiomas" is accepted. The lesions in Case 634 enlarged rapidly on subsequent scans.

DIFFERENTIAL DIAGNOSIS:
PARASELLAR MASS CONTAINING BLOOD PRODUCTS

Case 635

54-year-old woman presenting with diplopia
and pressure in the right eye.
(axial, noncontrast scan; SE 2800/45)

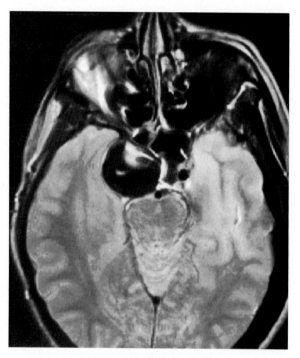

Thrombosed Aneurysm

Case 636

62-year-old woman presenting with a
right visual field deficit.
(axial, noncontrast scan; SE 3000/30)

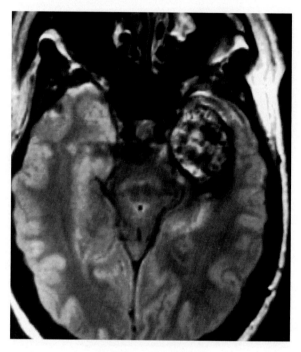

Cavernous Angioma

Both aneurysms and cavernous angiomas can present as masses in the medial portion of the middle cranial fossa. Both lesions may demonstrate components of T1-shortening and T2-shortening due to focal accumulation of blood products.

However, the internal architectures of these two pathologies are usually distinct. Thrombus within the lumen of an aneurysm often has a marbled or laminated morphology, illustrated by Case 635 (see also Cases 604 and 605). The structure of a cavernous angioma is characteristically more reticulated, with a "honeycomb" or "mulberry" texture, as is apparent in Case 636.

The low signal intensity occupying most of the lumen of the giant aneurysm in Case 635 represents T2-shortening due to deoxyhemoglobin (and/or intracellular methemoglobin) within thrombus, not "flow void" (compare to Case 617). MR angiography can distinguish between patent and thrombosed portions of an aneurysm when the nature of a low intensity zone is ambiguous on routine scans (see Case 601).

Parasellar aneurysms usually arise from the cavernous segment of the internal carotid artery. They commonly cause diplopia, as in Case 635. Both patent and thrombosed parasellar aneurysms can mimic other cavernous masses on CT scans. MR characterizes such lesions by demonstrating flow and/or blood products.

The cavernous angioma in Case 636 was extraaxial, located between the cavernous sinus and the displaced medial margin of the temporal lobe. Dural-based cavernous angiomas are often more homogeneous than this lesion, lacking the characteristic reticulation and hemosiderin ring of parynchymal hemangiomas. Such masses may enhance uniformly and be indistinguishable from mengingiomas.

Distension of the cavernous sinus by a carotid-cavernous fistula can resemble the above pathologies. Low signal intensity due to arterialized "flow void" within the widened sinus may mimic a parasellar aneurysm or present a multinodular appearance similar to a cavernous angioma (see discussion of Case 796).

DIFFERENTIAL DIAGNOSIS:
BRAINSTEM MASS IN AN ADULT

Case 637

45-year-old woman with a ten-year history
of "brainstem glioma."
(sagittal, noncontrast scan; SE 700/16)

Case 638

52-year-old woman presenting with ataxia.
(sagittal, postcontrast scan; SE 600/20)

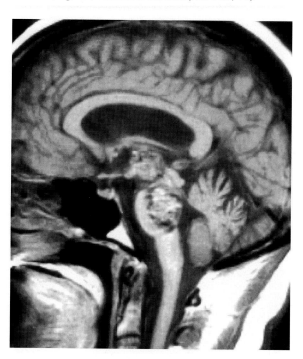

Cavernous Angioma
(same patient as Case 628)

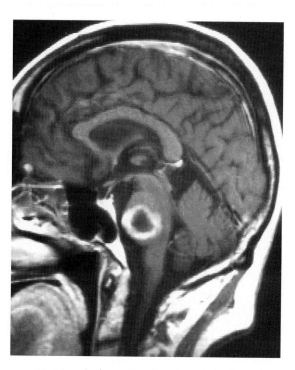

Metastasis from Carcinoma of the Lung

Cavernous angiomas commonly occur in the brainstem, where they may mimic primary or metastatic tumors. The gradual enlargement of an angioma can cause progressive symptoms suggesting an infiltrating neoplasm, as had been true in Case 637. Alternatively, the repeated occurrence and organization of small hemorrhages within or adjacent to an angioma of the brainstem may lead to a relapsing/remitting course that resembles demyelinating disease.

MR scans have now demonstrated that many patients previously assumed to have stable brainstem "tumors" have in fact harbored cavernous malformations. The characteristics of the lesion in Case 637 are highly suggestive of this diagnosis. Furthermore, the patient demonstrated accompanying cerebral lesions (see Case 628) and had a sister whose subsequent MR evaluation for seizures disclosed multiple cavernous angiomas.

Other varieties of vascular malformations may also involve the brainstem. Venous angiomas are occasionally found in this location. The pathologically common capillary telangiectasia is rarely evident on noncontrast MR scans but may cause pontine hemorrhage. True AVMs of the brainstem occur, often bordering the fourth ventricle. Bulky components of an AVM may fill the ventricle and simulate an intraventricular tumor.

Case 638 serves as a reminder that metastases should be considered whenever a posterior fossa mass is encountered in an adult (see also Cases 20-23). MR has demonstrated that the occurrence of brainstem metastases is nearly as common as the well-known incidence of cerebellar lesions. Like cavernous angiomas, brainstem metastases may be associated with additional lesions at other sites.

Case 639A

77-year-old man presenting with brain stem TIA's.
(coronal, noncontrast scan; SE 700/25)

Case 639B

Same patient (more posterior scan).
(coronal, noncontrast scan; SE 700/25)

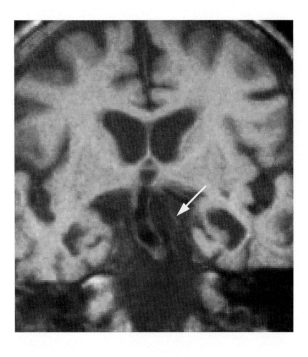

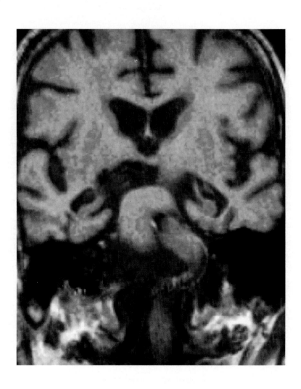

An atherosclerotic basilar artery may undergo striking elongation and fusiform ectasia in elderly patients. This so-called "dolichoectasia" may cause the tip of the artery to rise as far superiorly as the foramen of Monro.

Case 639A demonstrates the rostral basilar artery to be mildly widened and substantially elongated. The tip of the artery elevates the floor of the third ventricle. Atherosclerotic thickening of the vessel wall is apparent.

The thin tissue band angling steeply downward from the basilar tip on the left side *(arrow)* likely represents the third cranial nerve. The cisternal portion of this nerve passes between the proximal posterior cerebral and superior cerebellar arteries. Elongation of the basilar artery has carried the nerve far superiorly, so that it must descend steeply to enter the cavernous sinus. (The superior cerebellar arteries must follow a similar downward course in such cases to reach the infratentorial compartment.)

Mechanical distortion of cranial nerves is one mechanism by which dolichoectatic basilar arteries produce symptoms. Brainstem ischemia due to atherosclerotic disease affecting the origin of perforating vessels is a more common presentation. Hemorrhage is uncommon.

The scan in Case 639B demonstrates a more ectatic segment of the basilar artery. This portion of the vessel is filled with intraluminal signal intensity rather than "flow void," suggesting slow flow and/or thrombus. The ectatic artery acts as a cerebellopontine mass, deforming the adjacent brainstem. In such cases axial CT scans can be misinterpreted as demonstrating an enhancing extraaxial neoplasm.

Dolichoectasia of the supraclinoid internal carotid arteries or proximal middle cerebral arteries may also occur but is less common than basilar artery involvement.

An aneurysmal arteriopathy resembling adult dolichoectasia has been noted in children with AIDS. This ectasia of basal arteries correlates pathologically with destruction of the internal elastic lamina and thinning of the media.

VASCULAR TORTUOSITY CAUSING CRANIAL NEUROPATHY

Case 640

49-year-old woman with a history of long-standing
right hemifacial spasm.
(axial partition from a three-dimensional,
time-of-flight GRE sequence)

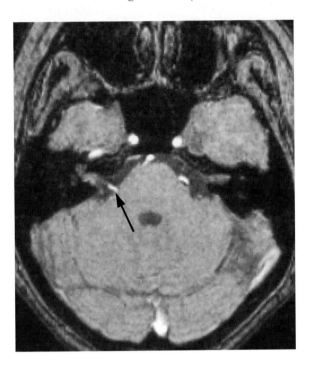

Case 641

6-year-old boy with "seizures" since infancy
manifested by facial twitching.
("chin-up" AP projection from a three-dimensional,
time-of-flight GRE sequence)

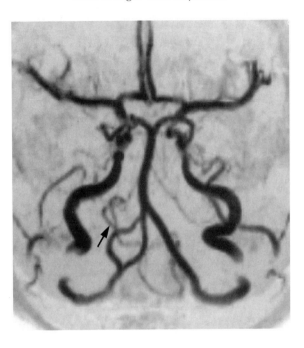

Some patients experience recurrent symptoms due to distortion of cranial nerves by adjacent vessels. Both tic douloureux (trigeminal nerve) and hemifacial spasm (facial nerve) may be caused by contact of an artery or vein with the nerve near its junction with the brainstem ("entry zone"). Although CT and MR scans rarely image the microvascular anatomy responsible for most cases of nerve irritation, occasional symptomatic arterial loops can be identified.

In Case 640, flow is demonstrated within a loop of the right AICA, which appears to be in direct contact with the facial nerve *(arrow)*. Surgery confirmed this finding. Facial spasm ceased after the artery was separated from the nerve.

Case 641 illustrates fenestration of the distal right vertebral artery. The right PICA *(arrow)* originates from the superior arm of the fenestration and courses further superiorly into the cerebellopontine angle. At surgery, this vessel was found to distort the cisternal portion of the facial nerve,

accounting for the history of hemifacial spasm that had mimicked a seizure disorder.

Prominent arterial loops within the cerebellopontine angle are commonly seen in asymptomatic patients. The significance of such vascular tortuosity depends on correlation with symptoms and anticipated surgery. Even if a notable arterial loop is not directly responsible for distortion of the symptomatic cranial nerve, demonstration of the regional vascular anatomy is important preoperative information for a surgeon contemplating microvascular decompression.

Potentially symptomatic arterial loops are occasionally apparent on routine MR scans, particularly in the coronal plane. MR angiograms offer a much more sensitive evaluation in the setting of irritative cranial neuropathy. The above scans demonstrate that examination of both the individual partition images and the three-dimensional composite view is important for analysis of vascular detail.

Case 642

32-year-old woman presenting with a two-day history of worsening headaches and papilledema. (sagittal, noncontrast scan; SE 750/20)

Case 643

12-day-old girl presenting with seizures. (sagittal, noncontrast scan; SE 600/15)

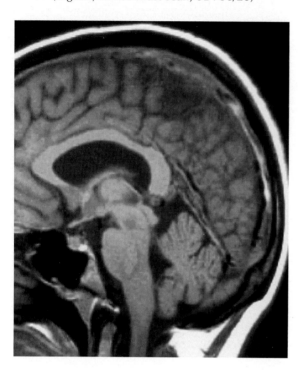

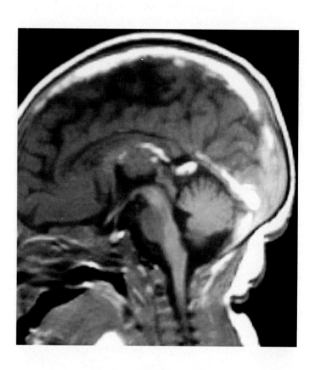

Dural sinus thrombosis can cause a confusing variety of nonspecific symptoms in patients of any age. Standard and angiographic MR images provide a highly accurate, noninvasive method to establish the diagnosis.

On routine noncontrast spin echo scans (away from the margins of the imaging volume), the dural sinuses should contain little signal. Thrombosis and stasis replace this normal "flow void" with variable intraluminal intensity.

In Case 642 the superior sagittal sinus is filled with a mixture of isointense and high intensity components. Other thrombosed dural sinuses may be completely isointense or strikingly hyperintense (as in Case 643) on T1-weighted images. Gradient echo pulse sequences (maximizing flow-related enhancement) may be used to distinguish between slow flow and thrombus within a vascular structure.

The straight sinus is also thrombosed in Case 642, as was the left transverse sinus. The patient gave a history of chronic otitis and mastoiditis, which likely precipitated thrombophlebitis of the sigmoid sinus. Other factors associated with an increased incidence of dural sinus thrombo-

sis include pregnancy, coagulopathy, dehydration, head trauma, the presence of antiphospholipid antibodies (e. g., lupus anticoagulant and anticardiolipin antibody), and some specific chemotherapeutic agents (e.g., L-asparaginase).

Case 643 demonstrates extensive dural sinus (and deep venous) thrombosis in the neonatal period. This occurrence is more frequent that has been previously recognized. The responsible mechanism may involve hemoconcentration, coagulopathy, and/or mechanical compression of the dural sinuses by calvarial molding during delivery. Affected infants typically present at age one to two weeks with irritability, seizures, or deepening lethargy. MR scans often demonstrate more extensive thrombosis than seen in adults. However, the prognosis for such infants is surprisingly good; most recover completely and develop normally.

MR venography is useful for assessing the patency of dural sinuses in equivocal cases. Either two-dimensional time-of-flight or phase-contrast techniques are capable of demonstrating the presence or absence of slow venous flow (see Case 188).

Case 644

60-year-old woman presenting with a week-long history of vague bihemispheral symptoms.
(coronal, noncontrast scan; SE 2500/30)

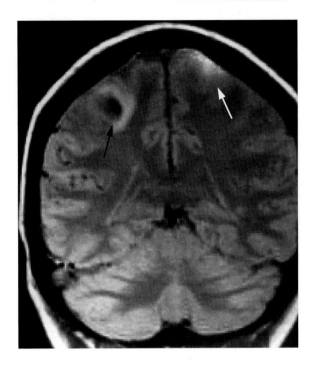

Case 645

12-day-old girl presenting with seizures.
(sagittal, noncontrast scan; SE 600/15)

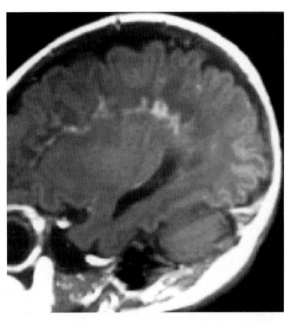

(same patient as Case 643)

The clinical course of patients with superior sagittal sinus thrombosis (SSST) usually reflects the extent to which thrombus propagates into cortical veins. In about 70% of cases there is no clinical or MR evidence of venous infarction, and a complete recovery is made.

Other patients experience cerebral edema and/or hemorrhage due to obstruction of venous drainage. Evidence of venous infarction in patients with SSST is most often found in superficial, parasagittal locations. The hemorrhagic infarct near the right hemisphere vertex *(black arrow)* and superficial edema on the left side *(white arrow)* in Case 644 are typical findings. Subcortical hemorrhage due to dural sinus thrombosis may occur at a considerable distance proximal to the occluded segment of the sinus.

Discovery of parasagittal edema or hemorrhage should raise the possibility of sagittal sinus thrombosis. Scattered areas of cerebral edema due to SSST may resemble the appearance of primary white matter disease (such as progressive multifocal leukoencephalopathy; see Cases 367-371) or cortical arterial watershed infarction (see Cases 488-490).

Since head trauma may predispose to SSST, small areas of parasagittal hemorrhage and edema should not be casually attributed to contusion or shearing injury in such cases.

The periventricular hemorrhages in Case 645 are probably secondary to thrombosis of the deep venous system. This pathophysiology of venous congestion represents another possible mechanism for hemorrhagic periventricular damage in the perinatal period—along with germinal matrix hemorrhages and periventricular leukomalacia. Deep hemispheric hemorrhages are rarely seen in adults with dural sinus thrombosis.

Other potential secondary findings on scans of patients with dural sinus thrombosis include focal or generalized cerebral swelling (which may precede any evidence of edema), tentorial congestion/hyperemia, leptomeningeal enhancement (see Case 386-2), and communicating hydrocephalus due to impaired resorption of CSF. Venous hypertension secondary to dural sinus occlusion should be considered in the differential diagnosis of "external hydrocephalus" in infants and children.

Case 646

32-year-old woman presenting with
headaches and papilledema.
(axial, noncontrast scan; SE 3000/90)

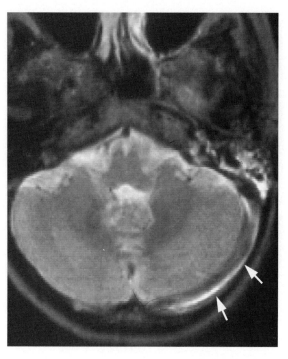

(same patient as Case 642)

Case 647

68-year-old woman presenting with headaches after
surgery for a cholesteatoma of the right ear.
(coronal, postcontrast scan; SE 600/15)

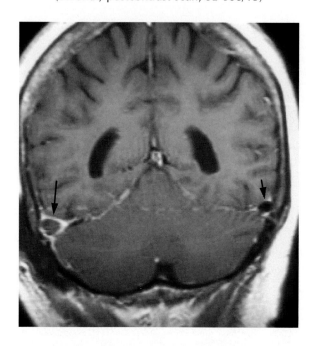

Superior sagittal sinus thrombosis is often accompanied or precipitated by thrombosis of the transverse sinus.

Propagation of infection from the petrous bone to cause thrombophlebitis of the sigmoid and transverse sinuses was a common cause of increased intracranial pressure ("otitic hydrocephalus") in children prior to the widespread availability of antibiotics. This etiology of dural sinus thrombosis is still observed on occasion, as in Case 646. The patient in this case gave a history of chronic left otitis media, and the scan confirms inflammatory thickening of mucosa in the left mastoid region. The left transverse sinus *(arrows)* demonstrates uniformly high intensity due to thrombus replacing the expected "flow void."

On postcontrast scans, the lumen of a thrombosed dural sinus usually fails to enhance. Peripheral enhancement of dura at the margins of the sinus results in a ring or "empty triangle" appearance, first observed on CT scans in cases of superior sagittal sinus thrombosis. Case 647 illustrates this pattern *(long arrow;* see Case 386-2 for another example).

The amount of central enhancement normally demonstrated within the transverse sinus, sigmoid sinus, or jugular vein is variable. In some cases, substantial intraluminal signal is present, suggesting relatively slow flow. In other cases (as in the left transverse sinus of Case 647; *short arrow)*, "flow void" is observed even on postcontrast images.

MR angiograms frequently demonstrate artifactual "filling defects" within the flow pattern of a transverse sinus that can be misinterpreted as intraluminal thrombus (see Case 188D). Inflow from large tributary veins (e.g., the vein of Labbe) and large arachnoid granulations are the most common causes of such pseudolesions.

Fluid is present within the scalp in the right retromastoid region of Case 647.

DIFFERENTIAL DIAGNOSIS:
LOCALIZED EDEMA ADJACENT TO THE TRANSVERSE SINUS

Case 648

15-year-old girl presenting with a seizure.
(coronal, noncontrast scan; SE 2500/90)

Case 649

36-year-old woman with a long history of seizures.
(coronal, noncontrast scan; SE 2800/90)

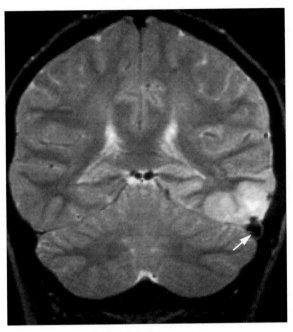

Venous Infarction
(due to transverse sinus thrombosis)

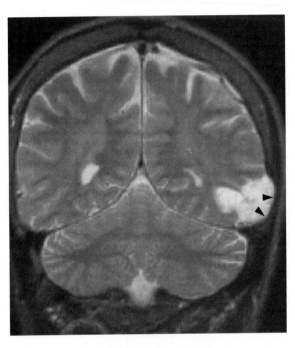

Low Grade Astrocytoma

Localized edema due to acute venous infarction may resemble a superficial mass lesion. The clinical presentation and MR appearance in Case 648 mimic the low grade glioma in Case 649.

T1-weighted scans in Case 648 demonstrated high signal intensity thrombus occluding the left transverse sinus. The low intensity within the distended sinus on the above scan *(arrow)* is due to T2-shortening from deoxyhemoglobin. It is important to realize that low signal intensity within the lumen of a dural sinus on T2-weighted scans does not necessarily represent normal "flow void."

The long-standing glioma in Case 649 is associated with localized erosion of the adjacent inner table *(arrowheads)*. This evidence of chronic mass effect may accompany superficial lesions of any kind (compare to Cases 70, 675, and 676).

REFERENCES

Anderson SC, Shah CP, Murtagh FR: Congested deep subcortical veins as a sign of dural venous thrombosis: MR and CT correlation. *J Comput Assist Tomogr* 11:1059-1061, 1987.

Aoki N: Extracerebral fluid collections in infancy: role of magnetic resonance imaging in differentiation between subdural effusion and subarachnoid space enlargement. *J Neurosurg* 81:20-23, 1994.

Atlas SW: Intracranial vascular malformations and aneurysms: current imaging applications. *Rad Clin North Am* 26:821-837, 1988.

Atlas SW: MR imaging is highly sensitive for acute subarachnoid hemorrhage . . . Not! *Radiology* 186:319-322, 1993.

Atlas SW, Grossman RI, Goldberg HI, et al: Partially thrombosed giant intracranial aneurysms: correlation of MR and pathologic findings. *Radiology* 162:111-114, 1987.

Atlas SW, Grossman RI, Gomori JM, et al: Hemorrhagic intracranial malignant neoplasms: spin-echo MR imaging. *Radiology* 164:71-77, 1987.

Atlas SW, Mark AS, Fram EK, Grossman RI: Vascular intracranial lesions: applications of gradient-echo MR imaging. *Radiology* 169:455-462, 1988.

Atlas SW, Mark AS, Grossman RI, Gomori JM: Intracranial hemorrhage: gradient-echo MR imaging at 1.5 T. Comparisons with spin echo imaging and clinical applications. *Radiology* 168:803-805, 1988.

Augustyn GT, Scott JA, Olson E, et al: Cerebral venous angiomas: MR imaging. *Radiology* 156:391-396, 1985.

Award IA, Robinson JR Jr, Mohanty S, Estes ML: Mixed vascular malformations of the brain: clinical and pathogenetic considerations. *Neurosurgery* 33:179-188, 1993.

Awasthi D, Voorhies RM, Eick J, Mitchell WT: Cerebral amyloid angiopathy presenting as multiple intracranial lesions on magnetic resonance imaging. *J Neurosurg* 75:458-469, 1991.

Ball WS Jr: Nonaccidental craniocerebral trauma (child abuse): MR imaging. *Radiology* 173:609-610, 1989.

Ballantyne ES, Page RD, Melaney JFM, et al: Coexistent trigeminal neuralgia, hemifacial spasm, and hypertension: preoperative imaging of neurovascular compression. Case report. *J Neurosurg* 80:559-563, 1994.

Barkovich AJ, Atlas SW: Magnetic resonance of intracranial hemorrhage. *Rad Clin North Am* 26:801-820, 1988.

Bernardi B, Zimmerman RA, Savino PJ, Adler C: Magnetic resonance tomographic angiography in the investigation of hemifacial spasm. *Neuroradiology* 35:606-611, 1993.

Biondi A, Scialfa G, Scotti G: Intracranial aneurysms: MR imaging. *Neuroradiology* 30:214-218, 1988.

Bourgouin PM, Tampieri D, Johnston W, et al: Multiple occult vascular malformations of the brain and spinal cord: MRI diagnosis. *Neuroradiology* 34:110-111, 1992.

Bourgouin PM, Tampieri D, Melancon D, et al: Superficial siderosis of the brain following unexplained subarachnoid hemorrhage: MRI diagnosis and clinical significance. *Neuroradiology* 34:407-410, 1992.

Bracchi M, Savoiardo M, Triulzi F, et al: Superficial siderosis of the CNS: MR diagnosis and clinical findings. *AJNR* 14:227-236, 1993.

Bradley WG Jr: MR appearance of hemorrhage in the brain. *Radiology* 189:15-26, 1993.

Bradley WG Jr, Schmidt PG: Effect of methemoglobin formation on the MR appearance of subarachnoid hemorrhage. *Radiology* 156:99-103, 1985.

Bradley WG, Waluch V: Blood flow: magnetic resonance imaging. *Radiology* 154:443-450, 1985.

Brooks RA, Di Chiro G, Patronas N: MR imaging of cerebral hematomas at different field strengths: theory and applications. *J Comput Assist Tomogr* 13:194-206, 1989.

Brown E, Prager J, Lee H-Y, Ramsey RG: CNS complications of cocaine abuse: prevalence, pathophysiology and neuroradiology. *AJR* 159:137-147, 1992.

Cammarata C, Han JS, Haaga JR, et al: Cerebral venous angiomas imaged by MR. *Radiology* 155:639-644, 1985.

Ciricillo SF, Dillon WP, Fink ME, Edwards MSB: Progression of multiple cryptic vascular malformations associated with anomalous venous drainage. *J Neurosurg* 81:477-481, 1994.

Clark RA, Watanabe AT, Bradley WG Jr, Roberts JD: Acute hematoma: effects of deoxygenation, hematocrit, and fibrin-clot formation and retraction on T2 shortening. *Radiology* 175:201-206, 1990.

Curling OP, Kelly DL, Elster AD, Craven TE: An analysis of the natural history of cavernous hemangiomas. *J Neurosurg* 75:702-708, 1991.

DeMarco JK, Dillon WP, Halback VV, Tsuruda JS: Dural arteriovenous fistulas: evaluation with MR imaging. *Radiology* 175:193-199, 1990.

Destian S, Sze G, Krol G, et al: MR imaging of hemorrhagic intracranial neoplasms. *AJNR* 9:1115-1122, 1988.

Damiano TR, Truwit CL, Dowd CF, Symonds DL: Posterior fossa venous angiomas with drainage through the brain stem. *AJNR* 15:643-652, 1994.

Dooms GC, Uske A, Brant-Zawadzki M, et al: Spin-echo MR imaging of intracranial hemorrhage. *Neuroradiology* 28:132-138, 1986.

Ebeling JD, Tranmer BI, Davis KA, et al: Thrombosed arteriovenous malformations: a type of occult vascular malformation. *Neurosurgery* 23:605-610, 1988.

Ebisu T, Naruse S, Horikawa Y, et al: Nonacute subdural hematoma: Fundamental interpretation of MR images based on biochemical and in vitro MR analysis. *Radiology* 171:449-454, 1989.

Edelman RR, Wentz KU, Mattle HP, et al: Intracerebral arteriovenous malformations: evaluation with selective MR angiography and venography. *Radiology* 173:831, 1989.

Epstein MA, Packer RJ, Rorke LB, et al: Vascular malformations with radiation vasculopathy after treatment of chiasmatic/hypothalamic glioma. *Cancer* 70:887-893, 1992.

Erdman WA, Weinreb JC, Cohen JM, et al: Venous thrombosis: clinical and experimental MR imaging. *Radiology* 161:233-238, 1986.

Fobben ES, Grossman RI, Atlas SW, et al: MR characteristics of subdural hematoma and hygromas at 1.5 T. *AJNR* 10:687-693, 1989.

Gaen AD, Pile-Spellman J, Heros RC: A pneumatized anterior clinoid mimicking an aneurysm on MR imaging. Report of two cases. *J Neurosurg* 71:128-132, 1989.

Gentry LR: Primary neuronal injuries. *Neuroimaging Clin N Amer* 1:411-432, 1991.

Gentry LR, Gordersky JC, Thompson B: MR imaging of head trauma: review of the distribution and radiopathologic features of traumatic lesions. *AJNR* 9:101-110, 1988.

Gentry LR, Gordersky JC, Thompson BH: Traumatic brain stem injury: MR imaging. *Radiology* 171:177-187, 1989.

Gentry LR, Gordersky JC, Thompson B, Dunn VD: Prospective comparative study of intermediate-field MR and CT in the evaluation of closed head trauma. *AJNR* 9:91-100, 1988.

Gentry LR, Thompson B, Gordersky JC: Trauma to the corpus callosum: MR features. *AJNR* 9:1129-1138, 1988.

Gomori JM, Grossman RI: Mechanisms responsible for the MR appearance and evolution of intracranial hemorrhage. *Radiographics* 8:427-440, 1988.

Gomori JM, Grossman RI, Bilaniuk LT, et al: High field MR imaging of superficial siderosis of the central nervous system. *J Comput Assist Tomogr* 9:972-975, 1985.

Gomori JM, Grossman RI, Goldberg HI, et al: High-field spin-echo MR imaging of superficial and subependymal siderosis secondary to neonatal intraventricular hemorrhage. *Neuroradiology* 29:339, 1987.

Gomori JM, Grossman RI, Goldberg HI, et al: Intracranial hematoma: imaging by high-field MR. *Radiology* 157:87-93, 1985.

Gomori JM, Grossman RI, Goldberg HI, et al: Occult cerebral vascular malformations: high-field MR imaging. *Radiology* 158:707-713, 1986.

Gomori JM, Grossman RI, Hackney DB, et al: Variable appearances of subacute intracranial hematomas on high-field spin-echo MR. *AJNR* 8:1019-1026, 1987.

Graves VB, Duff TA: Intracranial arteriovenous malformations: current imaging and treatment. *Invest Radiol* 25:952-960, 1990.

Grossman RI, Gomori JM, Goldberg HI, et al: MR imaging of hemorrhagic conditions of the head and neck. *Radiographics* 8:441, 1988.

Groswasser Z, Reider-Groswasser I, Soroker N, Machtey Y: Magnetic resonance imaging in head injury patients with normal late computed tomography scans. *Surg Neurol* 27:331-337, 1987.

Hackney DB, Lesnick JE, Zimmerman RA, et al: MR identification of the bleeding site in subarachnoid hemorrhage with multiple intracranial aneurysms. *J Comput Assist Tomogr* 10:878-880, 1986.

Han JS, Kaufman B, Alfidi RJ, et al: Head trauma evaluated by magnetic resonance and computed tomography: a comparison. *Radiology* 150:71-77, 1984.

Harwood-Nash DC: Abuse to the pediatric central nervous system. *AJNR* 13:569-576, 1992.

Hasegawa M, Yamashima T, Yamashita J: Traumatic subdural hygroma: pathology and meningeal enhancement on magnetic resonance imaging. *Neurosurgery* 31:580-585, 1992.

Hayman LA, Taber KH, Ford JJ, Bryan RN: Mechanisms of MR signal alteration by acute intracerebral blood: old concepts and new theories. *AJNR* 12:899-907, 1991.

Hesselink JR, Dowd CF, Healy ME, et al: MR imaging of brain contusion: a comparative study with CT. *AJNR* 9:269-278, 1988.

Holtas S, Olsson M, Romner B, et al: Comparison of MR imaging and CT in patients with intracranial aneurysm clips. *AJNR* 9:891-897, 1988.

Hosoda K, Tamaki N, Masumua M, et al: Magnetic resonance images of chronic subdural hematomas. *J Neurosurg* 67:677-683, 1987.

Hulcelle PJ, Dooms GC, Mathurin P, et al: MRI assessment of unsuspected dural sinus thrombosis. *Neuroradiology* 31:217, 1989.

Huston J III, Rufenacht DA, Ehman RL, Wiebers DO: Intracranial aneurysms and vascular malformations: comparison of time-of-flight and phase-contrast MR angiography. *Radiology* 181:721-730, 1991.

Janick PA, Hackney DB, Grossman RI, Asakura T: MR imaging of various oxidation of intracellular and extracellular hemoglobin. *AJNR* 12:891-897, 1991.

Janss AJ, Galetta SL, Freese A, et al: Superficial siderosis of the central nervous system: magnetic resonance imaging and pathologic correlation. Case report. *J Neurosurg* 79:756-760, 1993.

Jaspan T, Wilson M, O'Donnell H, et al: Magnetic resonance imaging with even-echo rephasing sequences in the assessment and management of giant intracranial aneurysms. *Br J Radiol* 61:351, 1988.

Jenkins A, Hadley D, Teasdale GM, et al: Magnetic resonance imaging of acute subarachnoid hemorrhage. *J Neurosurg* 68:731-736, 1988.

Jones KM, Mulkern RV, Mantell MT, et al: Brain hemorrhage: evaluation with fast spin-echo and conventional dural spin-echo images. *Radiology* 182:53-58, 1992.

Kashiwagi S, Van Loueren HR, Tew JM Jr, et al: Diagnosis and treatment of vascular brain stem malformations. *J Neurosurg* 72:27-34, 1990.

Katayama Y, Tsubokawa T, Miyazaki S, et al: Magnetic resonance imaging of cavernous sinus cavernous hemangioma. *Neuroradiology* 33:118-122, 1991.

Kelly AB, Zimmerman RD, Snow RB, et al: Head trauma: comparison of MR and CT-experience in 100 patients. *AJNR* 9:699-708, 1988.

Kucharczyk W, Kelly WM, Davis DO, et al: Intracranial lesions. Flow-related enhancement on MR images using time-of-flight effects. *Radiology* 161:767-772, 1986.

Kucharczyk W, Lemme-Pleghos L, Uske A, et al: Intracranial vascular malformations. MR and CT imaging. *Radiology* 156:383-389, 1985.

Landi JL, Spickler EM: Imaging of intracranial hemorrhage associated with drug abuse. *Neuroimaging Clin N Amer* 2:187-194, 1992.

Lasjaunias P, Burrows P, Planet C: Developmental venous anomalies (DVA): the so-called venous angioma. *Neurosurg Rev* 9:233-244, 1986.

Leblanc R, Levesque M, Comair Y, Ethier R: Magnetic resonance imaging of cerebral arteriovenous malformation. *Neurosurgery* 21:15-20, 1987.

Lee BCP, Herberg L, Zimmerman RD, Deck MDF: MR imaging of cerebral vascular malformations. *AJNR* 6:863-870, 1985.

Lemme-Plaghos L, Kucharczyk W, Brant-Zawadzki M, et al: MR imaging of angiographically occult vascular malformations. *AJNR* 7:217-222, 1986.

Levin HS, Amparo EG, Eisenberg HM, et al: Magnetic resonance imaging after closed head injury in children. *Neurosurgery* 24:223-227, 1989.

Levin HS, Amparo EG, Eisenberg HM, et al: Magnetic resonance imaging and computerized tomography in relation to the neurobehavioral sequelae of mild and moderate head injuries. *J Neurosurg* 66:706-713, 1987.

Macchi PJ, Grossman RI, Gomori JM, et al: High field MR imaging of cerebral venous thrombosis. *J Comput Assist Tomogr* 10:10-15, 1986.

Mann CI, Dietrick RB, Schrader MT, et al: Posttraumatic carotid artery dissection in children: evaluation with MR imaging. *AJR* 160:134-136, 1993.

Marks MP, Lane B, Steinberg GK, Chang PJ: Hemorrhage in intracerebral aneurysms and arteriovenous malformations: frequency of intracranial hemorrhage and relationship of lesions. *J Neurosurg* 73:859-863, 1990.

McArdle CB, Richardson CJ, Hayden CK, et al: Abnormalities of the neonatal brain: MR imaging. Part I. Intracranial hemorrhage. *Radiology* 163:387-394, 1987.

McArdle CB, Mirfakhraee M, Amparo EG, Kulkarni MV: MR imaging of transverse/sigmoid dural sinus and jugular vein thrombosis. *J Comput Assist Tomogr* 11:831-838, 1987.

McCluney KW, Yeakley JW, Fenstermacher MJ, et al: Subdural hygroma versus atrophy on MR brain scans: "The cortical vein sign." *AJNR* 13:1335-1339, 1992.

McMurdo SK, Brant-Zawadzki M, Bradley WG, et al: Dural sinus thrombosis: study using intermediate field strength MR imaging. *Radiology* 161:83-86, 1986.

Medlock MD, Olivero WC, Hanigan WC, et al: Children with cerebral venous thrombosis diagnosed with magnetic resonance imaging and magnetic resonance angiography. *Neurosurgery* 31:870-876, 1992.

Mendelsohn DB, Levin HS, Harward H, Bruce D: Corpus callosum lesions after closed head-injury in children: MR clinical features and outcome. *Neuroradiology* 34:384-388, 1992.

Meyer FB, Huston J III, Riederer SS: Pulsatile increases in aneurysm size determined by cine phase-contrast MR angiography. *J Neurosurg* 78:879-883, 1993.

Momoshima S, Shiga H, Yuasa Y, et al: MR findings in extracerebral cavernous angiomas or the middle cranial fossa: Report of two cases and review of the literature. *AJNR* 12:756-760, 1991.

Moon KL Jr, Brant-Zawadzki M, Pitts LH, Mills CM: Nuclear magnetic resonance imaging of CT-isodense subdural hematomas. *AJNR* 5:319-322, 1984.

Nadel L, Braun IF, Kraft K, et al: Intracranial vascular abnormalities: value of MR phase imaging to distinguish thrombus from flowing blood. *AJNR* 11:1133-1140, 1990.

Naseem M, Leehey P, Russell E, et al: MR of basilar artery dolichoectasia. *AJNR* 9:391-392, 1988.

New PFJ, Ojemann RG, Davis KR, et al: MR and CT of occult vascular malformations of the brain. *AJNR* 7:771-780, 1986.

Noorbehesht B, Fabrikant JI, Enzmann DR: Size determination of supratentorial arteriovenous malformations by MR, CT, and angio. *Neuroradiology* 29:512, 1987.

Ogawa T, Inugami A, Shimosegawa E, et al: Subarachnoid hemorrhage: evaluation with MR imaging. *Radiology* 186:345-351, 1993.

Olsen WL, Brant-Zawadzki M, Hodes J, et al: Giant intracranial aneurysms: MR imaging. *Radiology* 163:431-435, 1987.

Orrison WW, Gentry LR, Stimac GK, et al: Blinded comparison of cranial CT and MR in closed head injury evaluation. *AJNR* 15:351-356, 1994.

Ostertun B, Solymosi L: Magnetic resonance angiography of cerebral developmental venous anomalies: its role in differential diagnosis. *Neuroradiology* 35:97-104, 1993.

Padayachee TS, Bingham JB, Graves MJ, et al: Dural sinus thrombosis: diagnosis and follow-up by magnetic resonance angiography and imaging. *Neuroradiology* 33:165-167, 1991.

Pfleger MJ, Hardee EP, Contant CF Jr, Hayman LA: Sensitivity and specificity of fluid-blood levels for coagulopathy in acute intracerebral hematomas. *AJNR* 15:217-224, 1994.

Prayer L, Wimberger D, Stiglbauer R, et al: Haemorrhage in intracerebral arteriovenous malformations: detection with MRI and comparison with clinical history. *Neuroradiology* 35:424-427, 1993.

Rapacki TFX, Brantley MJ, Furlow TW, et al: Heterogeneity of cerebral cavernous hemangiomas diagnosed by MR imaging. *J Comput Assist Tomogr* 14:18-25, 1990.

Raybaud CA, Strother CM, Hald JK: Aneurysms of the vein of Galen: embryonic considerations and anatomical features relating to the pathogenesis of the malformations. *Neuroradiology* 31:109-128, 1989.

Rigamonti DE, Drayer BP, Johnson PC, et al: The MRI appearance of cavernous malformations (angiomas). *J Neurosurg* 67:518-524, 1987.

Rigamonti D, Johnson PC, Spetzler RF, et al: Cavernous malformations and capillary telangiectasia: a spectrum within a single pathological entity. *Neurosurgery* 28:60-64, 1991.

Rigamonti D, Spetzler D: The association of venous and cavernous malformations: report of four cases and discussions of the pathophysiological, diagnostic and therapeutic implications. *Acta Neurochir (Wien)* 92:100-105, 1988.

Rinkel GJE, Wijdicks EFM, Vermeulen M, et al: Nonaneurysmal perimesencephalic subarachnoid hemorrhage: CT and MR patterns that differ from aneurysmal rupture. *AJNR* 12:829-834, 1991.

Rippe DJ, Boyko OB, Spritzer CE, et al: Demonstration of dural sinus occlusion by the use of MR angiography. *AJNR* 11:199-201, 1990.

Robinson JR Jr, Awad IA, Magdinec M, Paranandi L: Factors predisposing to clinical disability in patients with cavernous malformations of the brain. *Neurosurgery* 32:730-736, 1993.

Robinson JR Jr, Awad IA, Thomas J, et al: Pathological heterogeneity of angiographically occult-vascular malformations of the brain. *Neurosurgery* 33:547-555, 1993.

Ruggieri P, Poulos N, Masaryk T, et al: Occult intracranial aneurysms in polycystic kidney disease: screening with MR angiography. *Radiology* 191:33-40, 1994.

Sato Y, Yuh WTC, Smith WL, et al: Head injury in child abuse: evaluation with MR imaging. *Radiology* 173:653-657, 1989.

Saton S, Kadoya S: Magnetic resonance imaging of subarachnoid hemorrhage. *Neuroradiology* 30:361, 1988.

Schuierer G, Huk WJ, Laub G: Magnetic resonance angiography of intracranial aneurysms: comparison with intra-arterial digital subtraction angiography. *Neuroradiology* 35:50-54, 1993.

Seidenwurm D, Berenstein A: Vein of Galen malformation: clinical relevance of angiographic classification and utility of MRI in treatment planning. *Neuroradiology* 33(suppl):153-155, 1991.

Seidenwurm D, Berenstein A, Hyman A, Kowalsla H: Vein of Galen malformation: correlation of clinical presentation, arteriography, and MR imaging. *AJNR* 12:347-345, 1991.

Seidenwurm D, Meng T-K, Kowalski H, et al: Intracranial hemorrhage lesions: evaluation with spin-echo and gradient-refocused MR imaging at 0.5 and 1.5 T. *Radiology* 172:189-194, 1989.

Sklar EML, Quencer RM, Bowen BC, et al: Magnetic resonance applications in cerebral injury. *Rad Clin North Am* 30:353-366, 1992.

Smith HJ, Strother CM, Kikuchi Y, et al: MR imaging in the management of supratentorial intracranial AVMs. *AJNR* 9:225-235, 1988.

Smith KA, Kraus GE, Johnson BA, et al: Giant posterior communicating artery aneurysm presenting as third ventricle mass with obstructive hydrocephalus. *J Neurosurg* 81:299-303, 1994.

Snow RB, Zimmerman RD, Gandy SE, Deck MDF: Comparison of magnetic resonance imaging and computed tomography in the evaluation of head injury. *Neurosurgery* 18:45-52, 1986.

Stein SC, Spettell C, Young C, Ross SE: Delayed and progressive brain injury in closed-head trauma: radiologic demonstration. *Neurosurgery* 32:25-31, 1993.

Stone JL, Crowell RM, Gandhi YN, Jafar JJ: Multiple intracranial aneurysms: magnetic resonance imaging for determination of the site of rupture. *Neurosurgery* 23:97-100, 1988.

Strother CM, Eldevik P, Kikuchi Y, et al: Thrombus formation and structure and the evolution of mass effect in intracranial aneurysms treated by balloon embolization: Emphasis on MR findings. *AJNR* 10:787-796, 1989.

Sze G, Krol G, Olson WL, et al: Hemorrhagic neoplasms: MR mimics of occult vascular malformations. *AJNR* 8:795-802, 1987.

Sze J, Simmons B, Krol G, et al: Dural sinus thrombosis: verification with spin-echo techniques. *AJNR* 9:679-686, 1988.

Tash R, DeMerritt J, Sze G, Leslie D: Hemifacial spasm: MR imaging features. *AJNR* 12:839-842, 1991.

Tash RE, Kier EL, Chyatte D: Hemifacial spasm caused by a tortuous vertebral artery: MR demonstration. *J Comput Assist Tomogr* 12:492-494, 1988.

Tien RD, Wilkins RH: MRA delineation of the vertebrovascular system in patients with hemifacial spasm and trigeminal neuralgia. *AJNR* 14:34-36, 1993.

Tomlinson FH, Houser OW, Scheithauer BW, et al: Angiographically occult vascular malformations: a corelative study of features on magnetic resonance imaging and histologic examination. *Neurosurgery* 34:792-800, 1994.

Toro VE, Gever CA, Sherman IL, et al: Cerebral venous angiomas: MR findings. *J Comput Assist Tomogr* 12:935-940, 1988.

Truwit CL: Venous angioma of the brain: history, significance and imaging findings. *AJR* 159:1299-1307, 1992.

Tsuruda JS, Shimakawa A, Pelc JN, Saloner D: Dural sinus occlusion:

evaluation with phase-sensitive gradient-echo MR imaging. *AJNR* 12:481-488, 1991.

Uchino A, Imador H, Ohno M: Magnetic resonance imaging of intracranial venous angioma. *Clinical Imaging* 14:309-314, 1990.

Vogl TJ, Bergman C, Villringer A, et al: Dural sinus thrombosis: value of venous MR angiography for diagnosis and follow-up. *AJR* 162:1191-1198, 1994.

Walenga JM, Marmon JF: Coagulopathies associated with intracranial hemorrhage. *Neuroimaging Clin N Amer* 2:137-152, 1992.

Watanabe AT, Mackey JK, Lufkin RB: Imaging diagnosis and temporal appearance of subarachnoid hemorrhage. *Neuroimaging Clin N Amer* 2:53-59, 1992.

Wilberger JE Jr, Deeb Z, Rothfus W: Magnetic resonance imaging in cases of severe head injury. *Neurosurgery* 20:571-576, 1987.

Wilms G, Bleus E, Demaerel P, et al: Simultaneous occurence of developmental venous anomalies and cavernous angiomas. *AJNR* 15:1247-1254, 1994.

Wilms G, Demaerel P, Marchal G, et al: Gadolinium-enhanced MR imaging of cerebral venous angiomas with emphasis on their drainage. *J Comput Assist Tomogr* 15:199-206, 1991.

Wilms G, Marchal G, Vas Hecke P, et al: Cerebral venous angioma: MR imaging at 1.5 Tesla. *Neuroradiology* 32:81-85, 1990.

Wilms G, Vanderschueren G, Demaerel PH, et al: CT and MR in infants with pericerebral collections and macrocephaly: benign enlargement of the subarachnoid spaces versus subdural collections. *AJNR* 14:855-860, 1993.

Wong BW, Steinberg GK, Rosen L: Magnetic resonance imaging of vascular compression in trigeminal neuralgia: case report. *J Neurosurg* 70:132-134, 1989.

Worthington BS, Kean DM, Hawkes RC, et al: Nuclear magnetic resonance imaging in recognition of giant intracranial aneurysms. *AJNR* 4:835-836, 1983.

Yoon HC, Lufkin RB, Vinuela F, et al: MR of acute subarachnoid hemorrhage. *AJNR* 9:404-405, 1988.

Yousem DM, Flamm ES, Grossman RI: Comparison of MR imaging with clinical history in the identification of hemorrhage in patients with cerebral arteriovenous malformations. *AJNR* 10:1151-1154, 1989.

Yuh WTC, Simonson TM, Wang A-M, et al: Venous sinus occlusive disease: MR findings. *AJNR* 15:309-316, 1994.

Zimmerman RA, Bilaniuk LT, Hackney DB, et al: Head injury: early results of comparing CT and high-field MR. *AJNR* 7:757-764, 1986.

Zimmerman RD, Ernst RJ: Neuroimaging of cerebrovenous thrombosis. *Neuroimaging Clin N Amer* 2:463-485, 1992.

Zimmerman RD, Heier LA, Snow RB, et al: Acute intracranial hemorrhage: intensity changes on sequential MR scans at 0.5 T. *AJNR* 9:47-58, 1988.

CHAPTER 11

Hydrocephalus and Cysts

Case 650

10-year-old girl presenting with headaches.
(axial, noncontrast scan; SE 2500/28)

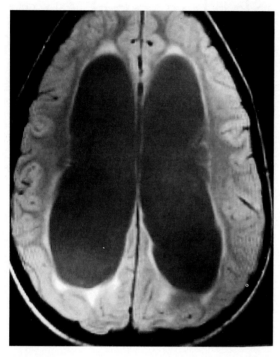

Hydrocephalus due to a Cerebellar Astrocytoma

Case 651

32-year-old woman presenting with headaches and
a large head.
(axial, noncontrast scan; SE 3000/70)

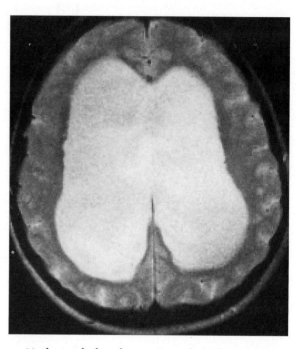

Hydrocephalus due to Aqueductal Stenosis

Although the diagnosis of hydrocephalus is easily made by CT, MR is valuable for assessing etiology. Many cases of hydrocephalus are caused by obstruction at the level of the aqueduct or fourth ventricle. Sagittal and coronal MR views free from bone artifact provide much better visualization of the midbrain and posterior fossa than CT scans.

The contrast sensitivity of MR also may demonstrate intraventricular or periventricular lesions that have low attenuation resembling CSF on CT studies. Such pathologies (e.g., pilocytic astrocytomas or parasitic cysts) can be mistaken for or camouflaged by distended ventricular chambers on CT scans (see Cases 128 and 664).

Cases 650 and 651 illustrate marked symmetrical enlargement of the lateral ventricular bodies. Hydrocephalic lateral ventricles may become hugely dilated, occupying most of the supratentorial compartment. Except in extreme cases, the thinness of the residual cortical mantle is an unreliable predictor of postshunt recovery.

The posterior bodies, atria, and occipital horns of hydro-cephalic ventricles are often larger than the frontal horns. This disparity may increase after shunting, with the greatest reduction in ventricular size occurring anteriorly.

Some children have large heads as a consequence of having large brains. Several pathological syndromes (e.g., mucopolysaccharidoses, gangliosidoses) are associated with "megalencephaly," but many children with large brains are functionally normal. Clinical clues to "benign megalencephaly" include normal head shape, head growth curves parallel to standards, the absence of increased intracranial pressure, normal neurological development, and large head size of a parent.

Children with benign megalencephaly often have moderately large ventricles. They may also demonstrate prominent subarachnoid spaces. The latter finding provides a clue to the diagnosis, since hydrocephalic expansion of ventricles usually effaces sulcal markings. Occasionally "benign" communicating hydrocephalus causes large ventricles and sulci in a child, with a stable appearance or improvement on follow-up scans.

Case 652

26-year-old woman presenting with positional headaches.
(axial, noncontrast scan; SE 2500/28)

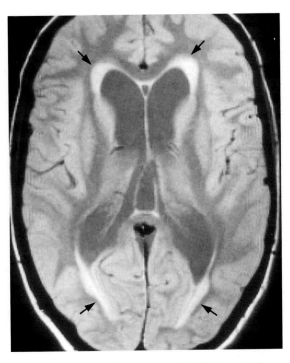

**Hydrocephalus due to a Colloid Cyst of the
Third Ventricle**

Case 653

7-year-old girl presenting with ataxia.
(axial, noncontrast scan; SE 2500/45)

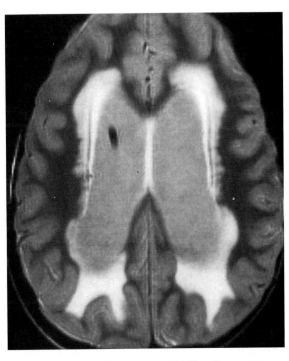

Hydrocephalus due to a Cerebellar Astrocytoma

As the lateral ventricles enlarge in hydrocephalus, the tight junctions between ependymal cells are eventually disrupted. This discontinuity may allow cerebrospinal fluid under pressure to leak into the periventricular white matter. The normal centripetal movement of interstitial fluid from the brain through the subependymal region into the ventricles is also impaired by high intraventricular pressure. These factors cause a localized or diffuse layer of increased fluid around the ventricular margins.

Periventricular edema due to hydrocephalus is well demonstrated by MR, like other causes of increased water content in cerebral white matter. Cases with an equivocal CT appearance may be obvious on MR studies.

The zone of periventricular edema bordering hydrocephalic ventricles may be smooth and uniform, as in Case 652. Other cases present a broader and more irregular band of edema, as seen in Case 653. This "shaggy" morphology occurs with acute and/or severe elevation of intraventricu-

lar pressure. Regardless of severity, the fluid accumulation within periventricular white matter is usually most prominent near the frontal horns and trigones of the lateral ventricles.

Periventricular edema is best demonstrated on MR scans with "intermediate" weighting (long TR and short TE values). On T2-weighted scans, the high signal intensity of ventricular CSF may merge with the high intensity of subependymal fluid.

On the preceding page, a small amount of periventricular edema surrounds the dilated lateral ventricles in Case 650. Although the ventricles in Case 651 are even larger, there is no convincing demonstration of increased periventricular fluid. This discrepancy reflects the more acute development of hydrocephalus in Case 650. The aqueductal stenosis in Case 651 has probably been present for decades, causing gradual and progressive ventricular enlargement without acute elevation of intraventricular pressure.

Case 654A

7-day-old girl.
(axial, noncontrast scan; SE 2800/30)

Case 654B

Same patient.
(axial, noncontrast scan; SE 2800/90)

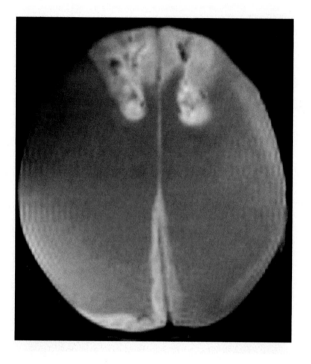

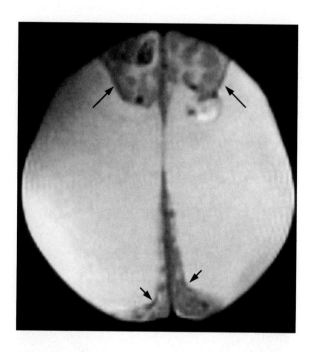

Several congenital abnormalities are associated with large supratentorial CSF spaces that may resemble hydrocephalic ventricles.

Hydranencephaly represents loss of normal brain tissue due to an embryologic insult. Major portions of the cerebral hemispheres are absent, and the supratentorial region is filled with fluid. In most cases the posterior fossa and diencephalon are preserved. This finding suggests that the hemispheric deficiency is due to agenesis, hypoplasia, and/or occlusion of the supraclinoid internal carotid arteries.

Case 654 is somewhat unusual because the absence of cerebral tissue is limited to the distribution of the middle cerebral arteries. Parasagittal parenchyma is spared both anteriorly, in the distribution of the anterior cerebral arter-

ies *(long arrows,* Case 654B), and posteriorly, in the distribution of the posterior cerebral arteries *(short arrows,* Case 654B).

Hydranencephaly may be mistaken for severe hydrocephalus. However, the scattered remnants of cortex in hydranencephaly do not form a complete rim around the hemisphere, as does the compressed cortical mantle of hydrocephalus.

A diffuse postnatal anoxic or inflammatory insult may also resemble hydranencephaly when widespread damage to cerebral tissue spares the posterior fossa and diencephalon. A ghost of once-normal hemispheric structures is usually visible in such cases.

Compare the transcerebral clefts in this case of hydranencephaly to schizencephaly, as discussed in Cases 742 to 745.

Case 655A

2-month-old girl presenting with a large head.
(coronal, noncontrast scan; SE 600/14)

Case 655B

Same patient.
(axial, noncontrast scan; SE 600/14)

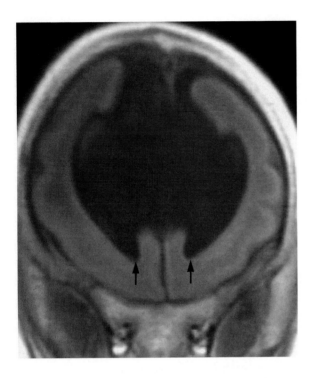

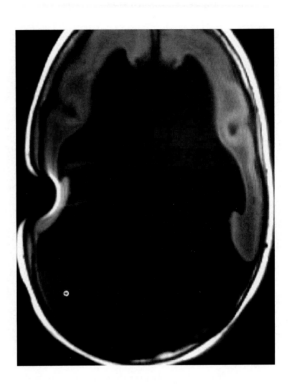

Holoprosencephaly is a developmental malformation characterized by absent or incomplete cerebral hemispherization. A horseshoe-shaped forebrain ("holoprosencephalon") surrounds a central monoventricle.

The typical batwing morphology of the single-chambered ventricle is seen anteriorly in Case 655. Inferior pointing of the frontal horns is prominent (*arrows,* Case 655A). This finding also occurs in less severe syndromes of midline dysgenesis (such as septooptic dysplasia; see Cases 728 and 729), and in some cases of Chiari II malformation.

A midline "dorsal cyst" is often found posterior and superior to cerebral tissue in cases of holoprosencephaly. The cyst may communicate broadly with the monoventricle, as seen above, or be an isolated, interhemispheric structure.

Dorsal interhemispheric cysts can also accompany other congenital malformations of the brain, notably agenesis of the corpus callosum (see Cases 720-722).

Absence of the septum pellucidum does not by itself imply holoprosencephaly (or milder forms of midline cerebral dysgenesis). The septum may become markedly thinned or frankly dehiscent in severe hydrocephalus, with resulting communication between the lateral ventricles.

Cerebral cortex in Case 655 is abnormally smooth, demonstrating a lack of gyral development (see Cases 732-735). Metallic artifact in the right parietal region in Case 655B is due to a shunt valve.

Cases 730 and 731 provide further discussion of holoprosencephaly.

Case 656A

66-year-old woman presenting with imbalance and vertigo.
(coronal, postcontrast scan; SE 650/15)

Case 656B

Same patient.
(axial, noncontrast scan: SE 2500/90)

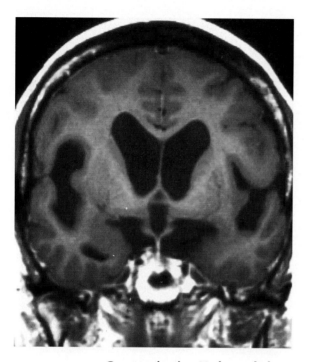

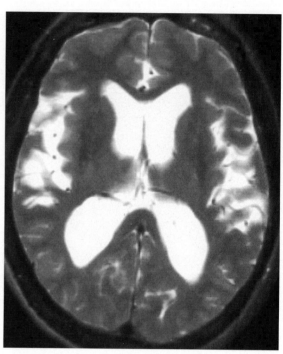

Communicating Hydrocephalus Associated with a Small Acoustic Schwannoma

Hydrocephalic expansion of all four ventricles suggests impairment of CSF flow or absorption along the surface pathways from the foramen magnum through the tentorial incisura to the parasagittal arachnoid granulations. This "communicating" pathophysiology contrasts with localized ventricular obstruction and is a common cause of infantile and adult hydrocephalus.

In infants, communicating hydrocephalus is frequently congenital and idiopathic but may also develop after meningitis or intracranial hemorrhage. Communicating hydrocephalus in adults often follows an inflammatory meningeal process, either infectious (meningitis) or hemorrhagic (trauma or aneurysm rupture). Meningeal carcinomatosis may also present in this manner. Contrast-enhanced scans and CSF analysis to exclude meningeal pathology are important whenever ventricular enlargement is noted in the absence of an obstructing lesion.

Intracranial and spinal tumors may be associated with communicating hydrocephalus due to high CSF loads of cells, hemorrhage, and/or protein. Choroid plexus papillomas, ependymomas, and acoustic schwannomas (as in Case 656) are among the masses with this tendency.

Multiplanar MR can support the diagnosis of communicating hydrocephalus by documenting widened superficial CSF pathways in addition to diffuse ventricular enlargement. In Case 656, the sylvian cisterns are prominently expanded with a tight contour that suggests active distention. The absence of atrophic sulci in other sites supports the interpretation of focal cisternal enlargement as a manifestation of communicating hydrocephalus.

Some adults develop low grade communicating hydrocephalus with no history of meningitis, subarachnoid hemorrhage, or tumor. This "normal pressure hydrocephalus" may be difficult to distinguish from atrophy in an elderly patient. Several clues are helpful in this situation: (1) the margins of hydrocephalic ventricles appear stretched, while the margins of atrophic ventricles are less distended; (2) hydrocephalic expansion of the lateral ventricles includes prominent temporal horn enlargement (*without* accompanying enlargement of the choroidal fissures), while the temporal horns are less dilated in most cases of cerebral atrophy; and (3) enlargement of the third ventricle is definite in hydrocephalus but less impressive in patients with atrophy.

Case 657

49-year-old woman complaining of headaches.
(sagittal, noncontrast scan; SE 600/14)

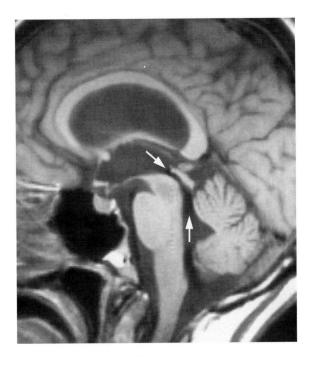

Case 658

64-year-old man presenting with dementia.
(axial, noncontrast scan; SE 2500/90)

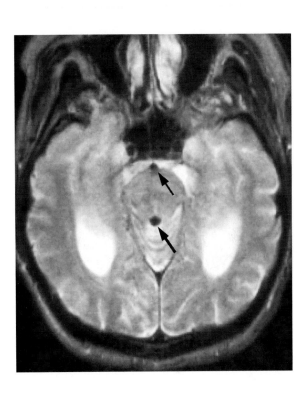

The flow of CSF through the ventricular system is pulsatile, reflecting the transmission of cardiac systole and diastole to the cerebral hemispheres. CSF flow velocity is greatest where ventricular diameters are narrowest, notably at the aqueductal level. Normal aqueductal flow is bidirectional (see Case 264), with the magnitude of the caudal systolic component exceeding the rostral diastolic component.

In the presence of communicating hydrocephalus (or hydrocephalus due to fourth ventricular obstruction), CSF flow through the aqueduct may become hyperdynamic, with greater caudal and rostral excursions. The cause of this increased pulsatility has been suggested to be the reduced elasticity or compliance of the distended lateral ventricles and cerebral hemispheres. In any event, the greater velocity and turbulence of aqueductal flow in such cases may cause increased signal loss within the aqueduct.

Prominent aqueductal signal loss can therefore be a clue to abnormal CSF hydrodynamics. Although the finding is not specific and may be seen in some cases of atrophy, its presence should lead to consideration of hydrocephalus (and its absence argues against the diagnosis.) The degree

of aqueductal signal loss depends on the pulse sequence employed, especially the amount of motion compensation.

In Case 657, abnormally "black" CSF is seen within the aqueduct. Unusually low signal intensity extends from the aqueduct into the posterior third ventricle and into the rostral fourth ventricle (arrows), suggesting increased excursion and/or turbulence of aqueductal CSF flow. A similar finding is present at the foramen of Magendie.

Case 658 demonstrates signal loss within the aqueduct (thick arrow) that is comparable to "flow void" within the basilar artery (thin arrow). Low signal intensity due to exaggerated CSF flow is often most apparent on T2-weighted scans, when more static ventricular chambers are filled with high signal intensity.

Midsagittal scans such as Case 657 can be useful in other respects to distinguish communicating hydrocephalus from atrophy. Superior bowing of the corpus callosum and inferior bulging of the third ventricular floor (causing partial effacement of the interpeduncular cistern) on such scans can help to support the diagnosis of active ventricular distention. (See Cases 130, 144, 272, 273, 275, 659, and 661.)

Case 659

38-year-old woman presenting with diplopia.
(sagittal, postcontrast scan; SE 600/20)

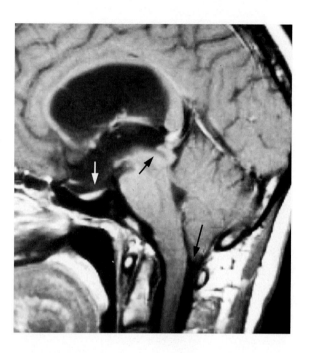

Case 660

32-year-old woman presenting with headaches and
a large head.
(coronal, noncontrast scan; SE 700/16)

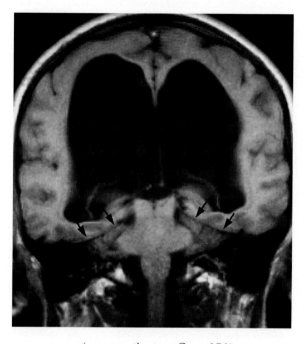

(same patient as Case 651)

Aqueductal stenosis is a major cause of infantile hydrocephalus. Most cases are due to a congenital abnormality, usually "forking" or "gliosis." Infantile aqueductal stenosis may also follow ependymitis from infection or intraventricular hemorrhage. Cases of congenital origin often present in adulthood, when the borderline capacity of a narrowed aqueduct is further compromised or exceeded by some superimposed event.

The CT diagnosis of aqueductal stenosis has been based on (1) enlargement of the lateral and third ventricles without fourth ventricular expansion and (2) the absence of other lesions mimicking obstruction at the aqueductal level (see Cases 124 and 661). MR now adds direct visualization of the aqueduct to these secondary observations. Multiplanar display and the absence of bone artifact in the posterior fossa contribute to an excellent view of midbrain anatomy on MR scans.

In Case 659, the lateral and third ventricles are distended (including inferior bowing of the third ventricular floor; *white arrow*), while the fourth ventricle is small. This disparity localizes obstruction to the aqueductal level. The proximal aqueduct is dilated *(short black arrow)* while the lumen of the distal aqueduct is not visualized, further defining the site of stenosis.

The posterior fossa in Case 659 is crowded due to longstanding expansion of the supratentorial compartment. The brainstem is closely applied to clivus, and the cerebellar tonsils extend below the plane of the foramen magnum *(long black arrow)*.

Adults presenting with hydrocephalus due to aqueductal stenosis often demonstrate evidence of chronic ventricular enlargement. In Case 660, the markedly dilated lateral ventricles are associated with a small posterior fossa. (Arrows mark the low tentorium.) This finding suggests intrauterine or infantile onset of aqueductal compromise, with developmental expansion of the supratentorial compartment at the expense of the posterior fossa.

Case 661

15-year-old girl presenting with headaches
and papilledema.
(sagittal, noncontrast scan; SE 600/14)

Case 662

19-year-old woman presenting with blurred vision.
(sagittal, noncontrast scan; SE 600/20)

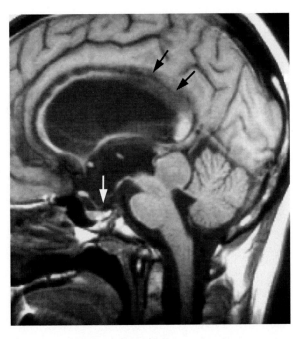

Glioma of the Midbrain Tectum

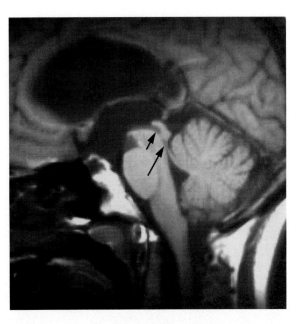

Aqueductal Stenosis

Case 661 demonstrates obstruction of the aqueduct due to the localized mass effect of a tectal glioma. (See Case 125 for an axial scan of this lesion.) The sagittal MR display clearly defines both the luminal compromise and the responsible tumor.

As discussed in Chapter 4, many midbrain gliomas are small, low grade lesions. Patients who have carried the diagnosis of "benign aqueductal stenosis" on the basis of CT scans deserve an MR exam to exclude a subtle, obstructing glioma.

In Case 662, the proximal aqueduct is distended *(short arrow)*, while the lumen of the distal aqueduct is small *(long arrow)*. The junction between the segments represents the precise level of aqueductal compromise. Benign stenosis commonly occurs between the middle and distal thirds of the aqueduct, where an anatomical narrowing called the "inferior constriction" is normally located.

Both of the above cases demonstrate hydrocephalic stretching of the corpus callosum. In addition, callosal

edema is present, particularly posteriorly in Case 661 *(black arrows)*. Edema between the transversely oriented axons of the corpus callosum often exhibits a striated appearance on sagittal or axial scans. Inferior bowing of the floor of the third ventricle is prominent in Case 661 *(white arrow)*.

In addition to small midbrain masses, another group of pathologies can mimic benign aqueductal stenosis. Cysts or tumors with fluid-like intensity values (e.g., cysticercosis, ependymal cyst, pilocytic astrocytoma, or epidermoid cyst) may obstruct the third ventricle while blending with the surrounding CSF. These masses can be easily overlooked, leading to the incorrect diagnosis of aqueductal stenosis.

Close attention to the intensity values of "CSF" within the enlarged third or fourth ventricles is warranted in all cases of hydrocephalus. "Intermediate" or "balanced" spin echo pulse sequences (long TR, short TE) are particularly useful for demonstrating subtle intraventricular lesions. In some cases, intraventricular contrast is required for diagnosis.

Case 663

8-month-old girl presenting with an enlarging head.
(axial, noncontrast scan; SE 2500/30)

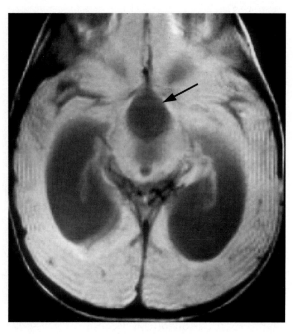

Aqueductal Stenosis

Case 664

18-year-old man shunted for presumed aqueductal stenosis.
(axial, noncontrast scan; SE 2500/90)

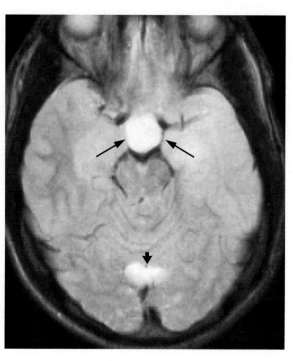

Suprasellar Arachnoid Cyst

The diagnosis of aqueductal stenosis requires careful exclusion of other lesions. As discussed on the preceding page, small midbrain masses can obstruct the aqueduct while causing minimal abnormalities of CT density or contour. Alternatively, fluid-intensity lesions may be overlooked as they occupy or compress the third ventricle. Such lesions can be hidden within CSF or mistakenly interpreted as a dilated ventricle.

A hydrocephalic third ventricle is seen in Case 663 *(arrow)*. This structure may act as a suprasellar mass, causing erosion of the dorsum sella and expansion of the sella itself.

The suprasellar arachnoid cyst in Case 664 *(long arrows)* mimicked an enlarged third ventricle on a preshunt CT study. The diagnosis of aqueductal stenosis was assumed. Subsequent evaluation demonstrated a suprasellar cyst that had compressed the third ventricle to cause obstructive hydrocephalus. An ependymal cyst or a cysticercosis cyst arising within the third ventricle could present identical images.

Other midline lesions that may mimic third ventricular distention include hypothalamic gliomas (see Case 242), craniopharyngiomas (see Cases 229 and 232), and rare cysts of the septum pellucidum.

A second small arachnoid cyst is present beneath the tentorial apex in Case 664 *(short arrow)*.

Shunted ventricles sometimes collapse to tiny residual slits, as was true in Case 664. Chronic ventricular collapse may be associated with low compliance. Subsequent shunt malfunction can cause a rapid increase in pressure with little expansion of ventricular volume. Small ventricular size does not exclude shunt malfunction in such cases.

Case 665

23-month-old boy with a history of posterior fossa surgery for resection of ependymoma.
(sagittal, noncontrast scan; SE 1000/16)

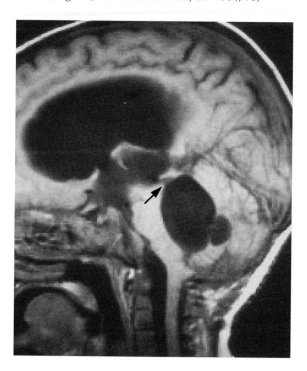

Case 666

3-year-old girl with a history of communicating hydrocephalus and recurrent shunt infection.
(sagittal, noncontrast scan; SE 600/20)

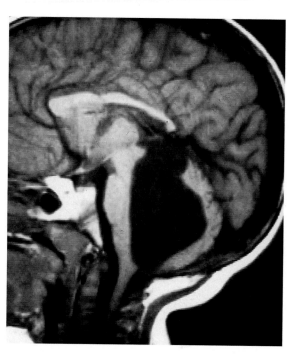

Occasional cases of hydrocephalus are complicated by "trapping" or isolation of a portion of the ventricular system. The fourth ventricle in particular may become obstructed both rostrally and caudally.

"Trapping" of the fourth ventricle is a potential complication of shunting in cases with obstruction of the fourth ventricular foramina. Reduction in the caliber of a previously distended aqueduct and/or reactive aqueductal gliosis may lead to functional disconnection of the fourth ventricle from the supratentorial ventricles. The fourth ventricle is then isolated both superiorly and inferiorly. Continued production of CSF within a "trapped" fourth ventricle leads to an expanding mass, which can cause life-threatening compression of the brainstem.

In Case 665, the entire ventricular system is hydroce-

phalic. Postoperative adhesions and/or residual or recurrent tumor have obstructed the outlets of the fourth ventricle. At the same time, there is impaired communication between the rostral fourth ventricle and the aqueduct *(arrow)*, causing the fourth ventricle to enlarge as a cystic mass.

By contrast, the lateral and third ventricles in Case 666 are well decompressed by a supratentorial shunt. The fourth ventricle is strikingly dilated, implying both functional inadequacy of the aqueduct (so that the fourth ventricle is isolated from drainage by the shunt) and obstruction of fourth ventricular outlet foramina. The degree of compression of the brainstem and cerebellum is comparable to that of a large fourth ventricular tumor (compare to Cases 148 and 149).

Case 667

1-year-old boy presenting with a large head.
(sagittal, noncontrast scan; SE 500/20)

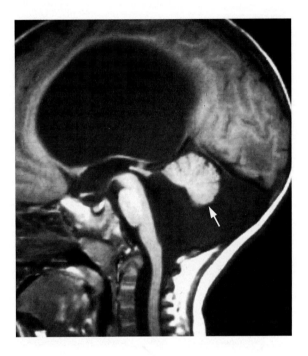

Case 668

8-month-old girl.
(axial, noncontrast scan; SE 2500/90)

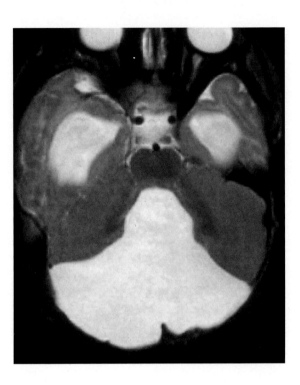

The Dandy-Walker malformation is an uncommon cause of congenital hydrocephalus. Hallmarks of this syndrome include (1) hypoplasia and malrotation of the cerebellar vermis and (2) a "roofless" fourth ventricle, which opens dorsally into a large posterior fossa cyst.

The sagittal MR plane has improved understanding of the Dandy-Walker malformation. As seen in Case 667, "absence" of the vermis on low axial scans through the posterior fossa is due more to superior rotation of this tissue than to true aplasia. The broad communication between the fourth ventricle and the posterior fossa cyst lifts and rotates the vermis *(arrow)* superiorly against the tentorial apex. Although associated vermian hypoplasia is common, the amount of residual tissue demon-

strated by MR is greater than previously appreciated on CT studies.

The cerebellar hemispheres are variably hypoplastic in patients with Dandy-Walker malformations. In Case 668, a broad communication is present between the fourth ventricle and a slightly asymmetrical posterior fossa cyst. The cyst surrounds mildly compressed and hypoplastic hemispheres. Associated hydrocephalus is indicated by expansion of the temporal horns.

Posterior fossa arachnoid cysts (see Cases 685-688) and enlarged cisternae magnae may mimic the Dandy-Walker malformation. The integrity and position of the cerebellar vermis are keys to the differential diagnosis in such cases (see Cases 689 and 690).

DIFFERENTIAL DIAGNOSIS:
EXPANSION OF THE FOURTH VENTRICLE

Case 669

3-year-old girl with a history of shunted
hydrocephalus.
(axial, noncontrast scan; SE 3000/90)

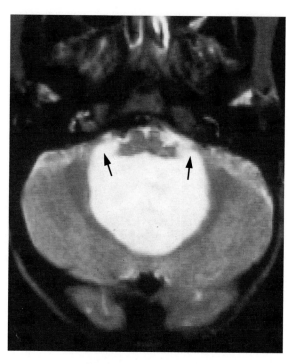

"Trapped" Fourth Ventricle
(same patient as Case 666)

Case 670

4-year-old boy presenting with headaches and
vomiting.
(axial, noncontrast scan; SE 2500/90)

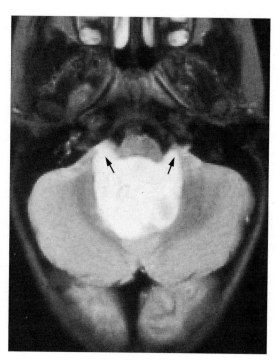

Medulloblastoma

A number of pathologies can cause or mimic distention of the fourth ventricle.

The above cases superficially resemble the Dandy-Walker malformations illustrated on the preceding page. However, vermian tissue is clearly present (albeit compressed), enclosing the posterior portion of the fourth ventricle and distinguishing these cases from the Dandy-Walker morphology.

Expansion of the fourth ventricle may reflect distention by CSF (as in Case 669) or enlargement due to an intraventricular mass (as in Case 670). The above scans both demonstrate marked compression of the brainstem and striking dilatation of the anterolateral recesses of the fourth ventricle (*arrows*).

In Case 670, the tumor demonstrates prominent prolongation of T2, which appears quite homogenous. Compare the symmetrical anterior growth of this medulloblastoma to the typically eccentric extension of fourth ventricular ependymomas into the lateral recess and cerebellopontine angle, illustrated in Cases 156 and 157.

DIFFERENTIAL DIAGNOSIS:
UNILATERAL VENTRICULAR ENLARGEMENT

Case 671

53-year-old man presenting with headaches.
(axial, noncontrast scan; SE 2500/28)

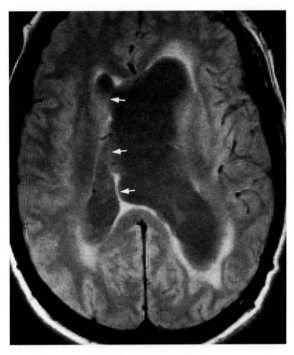

Unilateral Hydrocephalus

Case 672

16-year-old girl presenting with seizures and mild right hemiparesis.
(axial, noncontrast scan; SE 3000/30)

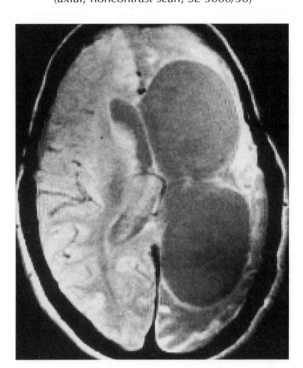

Old Hemispheric Infarction

Asymmetrical enlargement of one lateral ventricle may represent unilateral hydrocephalus. Obstruction at the foramen of Monro can be caused by a definable mass or by inapparent septation or adhesions (see Cases 673 and 674).

In Case 671, there was no evidence of an intraventricular or periventricular cyst or tumor on preshunt or postshunt studies. Asymmetrical expansion of the left lateral ventricle causes contralateral bowing of the septum pellucidum. Mass effect from the left ventricular "cyst" has obstructed the right foramen of Monro, with secondary expansion of the right lateral ventricle. Periventricular edema is present bilaterally.

Unilateral ventricular enlargement in Case 672 is attributable to volume loss throughout the left cerebral hemi-sphere. The extensive loss of tissue with relatively little residual gliosis and the patient's mild neurological deficit suggest an intrauterine event, most likely a CVA. There is less evidence of compensatory calvarial changes in Case 672 than in Case 541, which presents a similarly shrunken hemisphere. Secondary ventricular expansion caused by focal or diffuse parenchymal damage is often (inappropriately) referred to as "ex vacuo hydrocephalus."

Note that the septum pellucidum is shifted away from the large ventricle in Case 671 and toward the large ventricle in Case 672. Periventricular edema in Case 671 and widened ipsilateral subarachnoid spaces in Case 672 confirm the divergent etiologies of unilateral ventricular expansion in these cases.

DIFFERENTIAL DIAGNOSIS:
UNILATERAL HYDROCEPHALUS

Case 673

42-year-old woman presenting with headaches.
(coronal, postcontrast scan; SE 600/15).

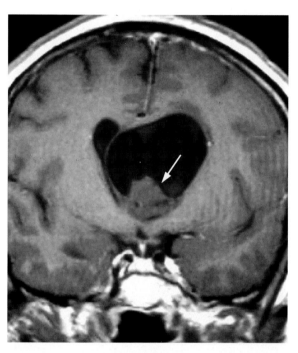

Subependymoma
(same patient as Case 118)

Case 674

2-year-old girl presenting with worsening
left hemiparesis.
(coronal, noncontrast scan; SE 600/15).

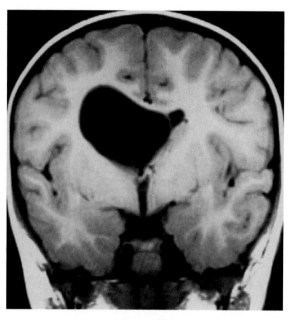

Stenotic Foramen of Monro

Occasional intraventricular or periventricular masses obstruct one lateral ventricle without compromising the contralateral foramen of Monro. The subependymoma in Case 673 is a typical example. Markedly asymmetrical hydrocephalus is apparent, with rightward bowing of the septum pellucidum and left-sided periventricular edema. Note the lack of contrast enhancement in this low grade lesion (see discussion of Case 118).

Other masses that could cause unilateral hydrocephalus include intraventricular meningiomas (see Case 267), subependymal giant cell astrocytomas in tuberous sclerosis (see Cases 266, 756, and 757), ependymomas (see Cases 115 and 309), septal or intraventricular gliomas (see Cases 113, 262, and 759), oligodendrogliomas (see Case 114), and central neurocytomas (see Case 308).

Unilateral hydrocephalus may also result from benign strictures or adhesions at the foramen of Monro, as in Case 674. Such septations are usually not definable on scans without intraventricular contrast material. The diagnosis is otherwise based on exclusion of an obstructing mass or cyst by careful examination of multiplanar, multisequence, precontrast and postcontrast MR images.

Fungal or bacterial ventriculitis is an additional rare cause of unilateral hydrocephalus.

Case 675

21-year-old woman presenting with seizures.
(sagittal, noncontrast scan; SE 600/17)

Case 676

16-year-old boy presenting with headaches.
(axial, noncontrast scan; SE 2800/90)

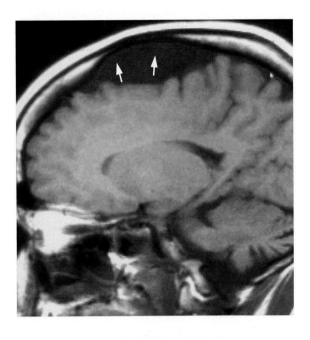

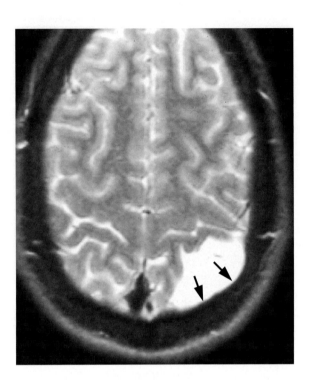

Arachnoid cysts account for about 1% of intracranial masses. They are often discovered incidentally, presenting as fluid-intensity lesions in a number of characteristic locations. The cerebral convexity is a common site, as illustrated in these cases.

Convexity arachnoid cysts usually depress the underlying cerebral cortex (but see Case 677 on the next page). The interface between the cyst and the brain is often quite angular or linear. This characteristic feature may help to distinguish extensive arachnoid cysts from subdural hygromas or chronic hematomas on CT and MR studies.

Long-term pressure from arachnoid cysts frequently causes expansion or erosion of bone. This finding is well illustrated in the above cases, with scalloping of the inner table *(arrows)*. Bone remodelling establishes the chronicity of these low grade lesions, distinguishing them from subdural collections. (Compare to erosions of the inner table by superficial low grade gliomas, as in Cases 70 and 649.)

Cortical deformity due to the arachnoid cyst in Case 675 is of questionable relevance to the patient's seizures. The cyst in Case 676 is probably incidental. Case 675 demonstrates cerebellar atrophy (possibly associated with dilantin therapy).

Case 677A

51-year-old woman presenting with mild
left hemiparesis.
(sagittal, noncontrast scan; SE 600/14)

Case 677B

Same patient.
(axial, noncontrast scan; SE 2500/90)

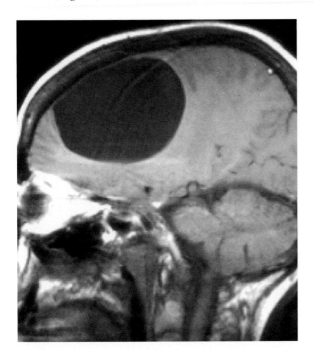

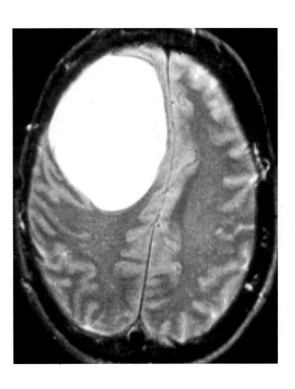

Occasional arachnoid cysts invaginate into adjacent parenchyma, as in this case. (See Case 691 for an infratentorial example.) Such extension is relatively common with other long-standing extraaxial masses (e.g., meningiomas or schwannomas; see Cases 39 and 168) but is unusual for arachnoid cysts. As a result, an appearance such as Case 677 may be misinterpreted as a cystic intraaxial lesion (e.g., ependymal cyst, neuroepithelial cyst, parasitic cyst, or cystic neoplasm).

Clues to the correct diagnosis in the above images include the meningeal base of the cyst, the simple character of the fluid, the absence of tissue nodules or irregularity along the margin, the lack of surrounding edema, and the morphology of compressed gyri and "buckled" white matter displaced by the lesion. (Compare this appearance to the similar ripples of compressed parenchyma adjacent to the meningioma in Case 49.)

Low attenuation CT lesions can be confirmed as CSF-containing cysts by magnetic resonance imaging. The signal intensity of such masses should match that of cisternal or ventricular fluid on all pulse sequences.

Case 678

38-year-old man presenting with right orbital pain.
(coronal, noncontrast scan; SE 700/16)

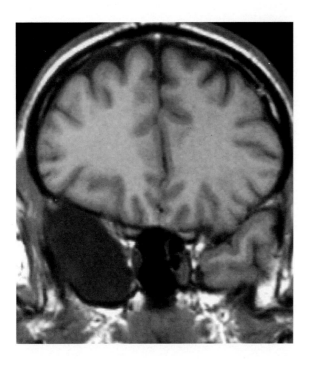

Case 679

19-year-old man complaining of headaches.
(axial, noncontrast scan; SE 2500/90)

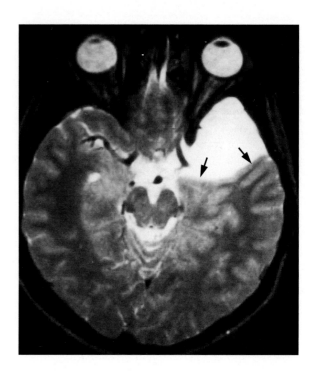

Arachnoid cysts are most common near the skull base. The anterior portion of the middle cranial fossa is a particularly frequent location for these lesions, which are usually incidental findings.

In Case 678, an arachnoid cyst has caused expansion of the middle cranial fossa on the right (compare to the volume of the middle fossa on the left side). There is little midline shift because the slow growth of the cyst has been accommodated by calvarial expansion and parenchymal hypoplasia (see discussion of Case 680).

Case 679 presents a typical T2-weighted axial scan of another patient. Note the posterior flattening and compression of the hypoplastic left temporal lobe and the straight, some-what angular margin between the cyst and the brain.

There is usually no reactive edema surrounding arachnoid cysts. The walls of the cyst do not demonstrate abnormal contrast enhancement.

Arachnoid cysts of the middle cranial fossa are occasionally complicated by subdural and/or intracystic hemorrhage. Bleeding may be spontaneous or posttraumatic and probably originates from cortical veins near the perimeter of the cyst.

An appearance similar to Case 678 is occasionally seen in children with chronic subdural hematomas of the middle cranial fossa. In adults, the major differential diagnosis is an epidermoid cyst (see Cases 292-296).

Case 680

11-year-old boy scanned after head trauma.
(coronal, postcontrast scan; SE 600/15)

Case 681

20-year-old man presenting with dizziness.
(coronal, noncontrast scan; SE 600/14)

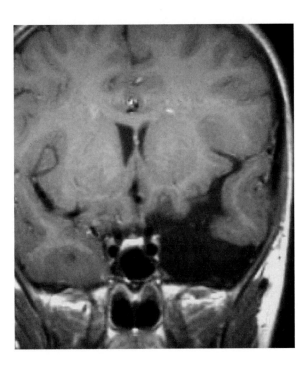

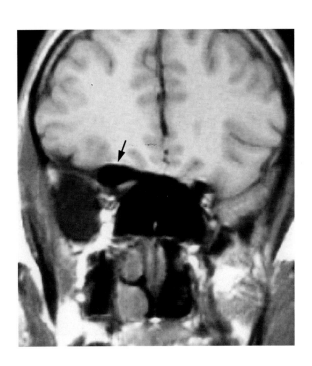

As discussed on the preceding pages, arachnoid cysts are commonly accompanied by calvarial erosion, linear or angular interfaces with underlying parenchyma, and accordion-like compression of adjacent brain tissue.

Arachnoid cysts of the middle cranial fossa may demonstrate other characteristic findings. Hypoplasia of the ipsilateral temporal lobe is common, illustrated in Case 680 (and Case 679). Debate about whether this incomplete development is primary or secondary with respect to formation of the cyst does not reduce the diagnostic significance of the association.

A less frequent finding accompanying arachnoid cysts of the middle cranial fossa is hypertrophy and prominent pneumatization of the lesser wing of the sphenoid bone. Case 681 demonstrates expansion and elevation of the anterior clinoid process on the side of the lesion *(arrow)*. This appearance adjacent to a "mass" is somewhat paradoxical, resembling "blistering" expansion of the sphenoid sinus beneath a meningioma of the planum sphenoidale (see Cases 46 and 47).

The mechanism causing this hypertrophy of bone/sinus has not been established. Speculation includes the possibilities of local meningeal traction by the cystic mass or primary parenchymal hypoplasia with secondary bone overgrowth and cyst formation.

Case 682A

25-year-old man with a four year history
of headaches.
(sagittal, noncontrast scan; SE 700/16)

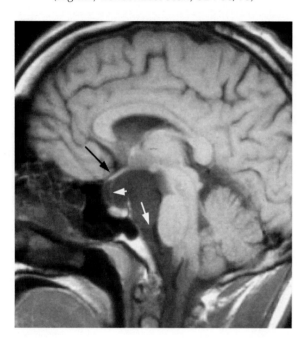

Case 682B

Same patient.
(coronal, noncontrast scan; SE 600/16)

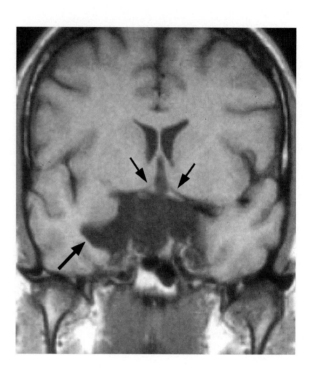

Arachnoid cysts may occur in the suprasellar region, mimicking other masses or a distended third ventricle (see Case 664). Case 682 demonstrates the characteristic morphology of these lesions.

Suprasellar arachnoid cysts are usually associated with a prominent prepontine component. The interface between the cyst and the prepontine cistern is faintly visible in Case 682A *(long white arrow)* due to the slightly higher intensity of the cyst. This feature may reflect relatively less fluid movement within the enclosed cyst as compared to subarachnoid cisterns and/or slight elevation of protein content within the lesion.

Case 682A also documents superior displacement of the optic chiasm *(black arrow)* and anterior bowing of the pituitary infundibulum *(short white arrow)*. The floor of the third ventricle is elevated, and the basilar artery and pons are posteriorly displaced. (Compare the suprasellar anatomy in this case to Case 683 on the next page.) Such evidence of mass effect distinguishes an arachnoid cyst from incidental widening of basal cisterns, which is common in children.

The coronal view in Case 682B again suggests that fluid within the suprasellar cyst is slightly higher in signal intensity than ventricular CSF. Elevation of the optic chiasm *(upper arrows)* is confirmed. The arachnoid cyst has extended into the choroidal fissure in the medial right temporal region *(lower arrow)*.

Epidermoid cysts should be included in the differential diagnosis of suprasellar masses with fluid-like intensity values (see discussion of Cases 695 and 696). Compare the lateral extension of the lesion in Case 682B to Case 293.

ARACHNOID CYSTS OF THE QUADRIGEMINAL CISTERN

Case 683

50-year-old woman presenting with TIAs.
(sagittal, postcontrast scan; SE 600/15)

Case 684

1-year-old girl presenting with hydrocephalus.
(sagittal, noncontrast scan; SE 600/14)

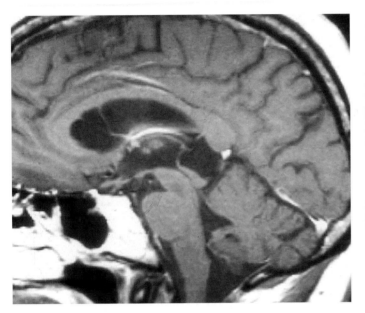

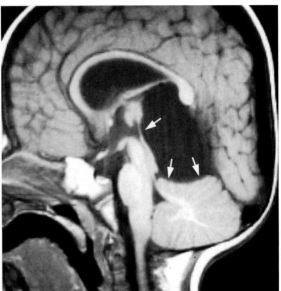

Arachnoid cysts are among the masses that may be encountered in the quadrigeminal region. They are often small and incidental (as in Case 683), but occasional large lesions are symptomatic (as in Case 684).

A pineal cyst (see Cases 268 and 269) would be considered in the differential diagnosis of Case 683.

The cyst in Case 684 causes marked inferior displacement of the cerebellum, anterior flattening of the midbrain and third ventricle, and elevation of the splenium of the corpus callosum. The combination of supratentorial and infratentorial mass effect is unique to lesions spanning the tentorial hiatus (or traversing the tentorium itself; e.g., meningiomas).

In Case 684, a scan at two months of age had demonstrated a cyst measuring one centimeter in diameter. The marked enlargement of an arachnoid cyst on follow-up studies is highly unusual but occasionally observed. Similarly, spontaneous decompression of arachnoid cysts has been noted (see Case 686).

Compression of the aqueduct in Case 684 has caused obstructive hydrocephalus. In the presence of ventricular en-

largement, the differential diagnosis of a transtentorial cyst includes a ventricular diverticulum. Such expansion of hydrocephalic ventricles may arise from the medial wall of the lateral ventricular trigone or from the posterior portion of the third ventricle. Either type of diverticulum may expand to occupy the quadrigeminal cistern and/or extend infratentorially to deform the cerebellum in a manner similar to Case 684.

A ventricular diverticulum may then be misinterpreted as a cystic mass causing obstructive hydrocephalus. Careful attention to ventricular margins in areas of potential diverticula and follow-up studies after ventriculostomy or shunting will establish the correct diagnosis in such cases. The thinned walls of distended ventricles may alternatively perforate, relieving symptoms by means of "spontaneous ventriculostomy."

The quadrigeminal cistern is a common location for both epidermoid cysts and arachnoid cysts. The differential diagnosis of these two pathologies on MR scans is discussed in Cases 695 and 696.

423

Case 685

14-month-old boy.
(sagittal, noncontrast scan; SE 600/20)

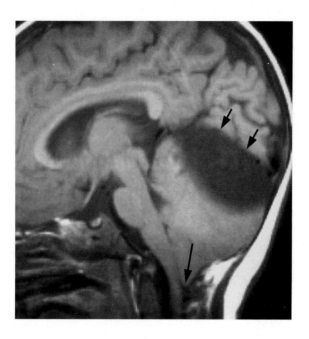

Case 686

1-year-old girl.
(sagittal noncontrast scan; SE 600/14)

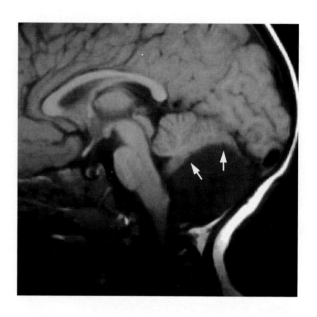

Infratentorial arachnoid cysts occur in both retrocerebellar and anterolateral locations. The former cysts may be encountered superior or inferior to the cerebellar vermis and/or hemispheres, as seen in the above cases.

The cyst in Case 685 is marginated superiorly by the tentorium *(short arrows)*. Mass effect from the lesion has crowded the posterior fossa, with ventral displacement of the fourth ventricle and caudal herniation of the cerebellar tonsils *(long arrow)*.

A supracerebellar arachnoid cyst may extend through the tentorial hiatus, compressing the brain stem and posterior third ventricle. The resultant combination of transtentorial cyst and hydrocephalus may resemble the appearance of a third ventricular diverticulum, as discussed in Case 684.

Case 686 demonstrates a midline cyst located inferior to the cerebellum. Signal intensity within the cyst is slightly higher than cisternal or ventricular CSF (see discussion of Case 682). The morphology of displaced inferior cerebellar folia and the absence of enhancement on a postcontrast

scan help to exclude the alternative diagnosis of a cystic cerebellar astrocytoma (compare to Cases 128 and 130).

Posterior fossa arachnoid cysts should not be confused with the Dandy-Walker malformation, since they are not associated with defects or malrotation of the vermis. Compare the fourth ventricular morphology in the above cases to Case 667.

The child in Case 686 returned for a follow-up study three months later. The cyst was found to have spontaneously decompressed in the interval, leaving mild hypoplasia of the inferior cerebellum as the only apparent abnormality. Although most arachnoid cysts are stable lesions, occasional cysts may be observed to enlarge or shrink (see also Case 684).

The low signal intensity within the basisphenoid in these cases suggests persistent hematopoietic marrow. This finding is common in infants and contrasts with the short T1 values of fatty marrow within the skull base in older children and adults. Fatty replacement of marrow within the clivus usually occurs by age 6 or 7.

Case 687

25-year-old woman presenting with numbness of
the arms and shoulders.
(axial, noncontrast scan; SE 3000/90)

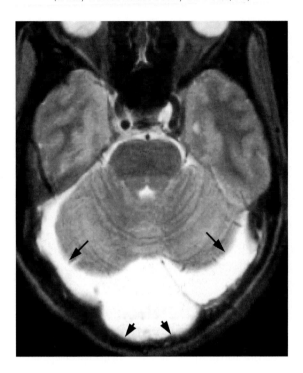

Case 688

14-month-old boy.
(axial, noncontrast scan; SE 3000/90)

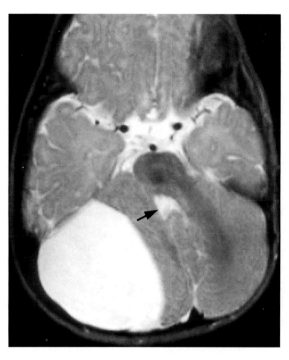

(same patient as Case 685)

The morphology and symmetry of retrocerebellar arachnoid cysts are variable. Case 687 demonstrates a midline lesion with symmetrical lateral extensions, while the cyst in Case 688 is more spherical and eccentric.

Arachnoid cysts near the occipital bone may be confused with large and/or asymmetric cisternae magnae. Evidence of mass effect favors the diagnosis of a true cyst.

In Case 687, the surface of the cerebellar hemispheres is abnormally smooth *(long arrows)* due to displacement by the lateral arms of the cyst. The midline component has caused erosion of the inner table *(short arrows)*, comparable to the supratentorial lesions in Cases 675 and 676.

The cyst is Case 688 clearly compresses underlying cerebellar tissue. The fourth ventricle *(arrow)* is displaced anteriorly and laterally.

Low signal intensity within the pons and middle cerebellar peduncles in Case 688 reflects the normal myelination of these structures in an infant. By contrast, the as yet unmyelinated white matter of the frontal and temporal lobes demonstrates high signal intensity reflecting higher water content. (Compare the relative intensity of gray and white matter within the temporal lobes in Case 688 to Case 687.)

Case 689

25-year-old woman presenting with numbness of
the shoulders and arms.
(sagittal, noncontrast scan; SE 600/20)

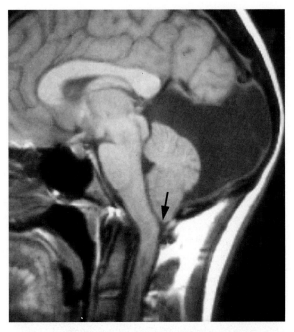

Arachnoid Cyst (and Hydromyelia)
(same patient as Case 687)

Case 690

20-year-old woman with a history of shunted
hydrocephalus.
(sagittal, noncontrast scan; SE 600/14)

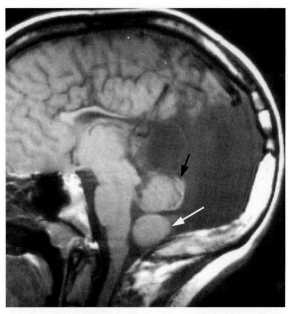

Dandy-Walker Malformation
(with tonsillar tissue as a "pseudovermis")

The large arachnoid cyst in Case 689 surrounds the cerebellum posteriorly and superiorly, representing a combination of the locations in Cases 685 and 686. This cyst is clearly not an expansion of the fourth ventricle (compare to Case 667).

Mass effect is present with enlargement of the posterior fossa and erosion of the occipital bone. More importantly, the cerebellum has been displaced anteriorly and inferiorly into the foramen magnum *(arrow)*. The resulting crowding of cerebellar tissue dorsal to the cervicomedullary junction resembles a Chiari I malformation (see Cases 712 and 713) and is similarly associated with hydromyelia (faintly seen at the caudal margin of the scan).

In Case 690 the diagnosis of a Dandy-Walker malformation is confused by the presence of tissue in the expected location of vermian hypoplasia *(white arrow)*. Coronal scans demonstrated that this tissue represents medial extension of the cerebellar tonsils secondary to hypoplasia of

the inferior vermis. True vermian tissue in this case is limited to the more superior nodule of cerebellar parenchyma *(black arrow)*.

Both cases demonstrate abnormally high position of the tentorium reflecting congenital enlargement of the posterior fossa. The tentorium normally moves posteriorly and inferiorly as the cerebral hemispheres develop. Intrauterine presence of a cyst or mass within the posterior fossa prevents normal tentorial descent. (Compare to the appearance of exaggerated tentorial descent as in Cases 660, 714, and 715.)

The corpus callosum is markedly hypoplastic in Case 690. Agenesis or dysgenesis of the corpus callosum is present in about 20% of patients with the Dandy-Walker malformation. Less common associated congenital abnormalities include gray matter heterotopias, polymicrogyria, and occipital encephaloceles.

DIFFERENTIAL DIAGNOSIS:
CYSTIC CEREBELLAR MASS

Case 691

87-year-old woman presenting with headaches.
(coronal, noncontrast scan; SE 600/17)

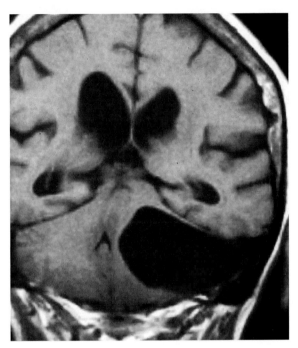

Invaginating Arachnoid Cyst

Case 692

48-year-old woman presenting with ataxia.
(coronal, noncontrast scan; SE 700/16)

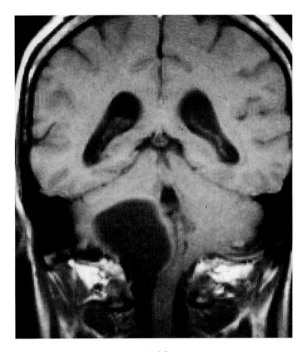

Hemangioblastoma

As discussed in Case 677, occasional arachnoid cysts burrow into underlying brain tissue rather than displacing it. The reasons for this unusual occurrence have not been established. Possible factors include early extension of the cyst into a sulcus (see Case 682B) or meningeal adhesions limiting convexity spread of the lesion.

The mass in Case 691 resembles a cystic cerebellar neoplasm. Clues to the correct diagnosis include the CSF-like content of the cyst, its base against the petrous bone, and the absence of a mural nodule. The relatively small shift of the fourth ventricle also favors a long-standing lesion. A postcontrast scan demonstrated no peripheral enhance-

ment, supporting the diagnosis of a benign cyst. At surgery the lesion was documented to be extraaxial, originating from the meninges.

Case 692 is an example of a largely cystic hemangioblastoma (compare to Case 140). The signal intensity of the fluid is mildly but definitely higher than that of ventricular CSF. A small tissue nodule at the caudal pole of the cyst enhanced intensely after contrast injection, establishing the diagnosis of a cystic neoplasm. The differential diagnosis includes a cystic astrocytoma, which is rarer in adults (see Case 141).

Case 693

31-year-old man presenting with a left sixth
nerve palsy.
(axial, postcontrast scan; SE 600/20)

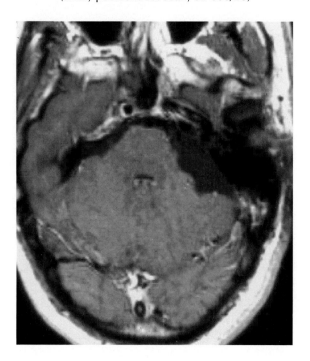

Case 694

15-year-old girl presenting with right-sided
facial pain.
(axial, noncontrast scan; SE 2500/90)

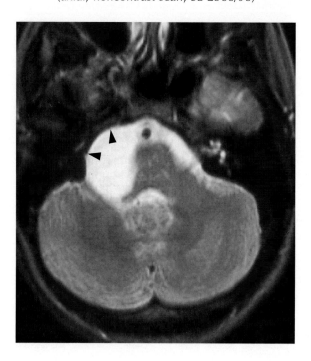

The cerebellopontine angle is a common location for in-fratentorial arachnoid cysts. The lesions in Cases 693 and 694 are typical examples.

Signal intensity within the cysts is very close to cisternal or ventricular CSF on all pulse sequences. Margins are well defined. A smooth border (either linear or rounded) as in Case 694 is more characteristic than the mild irregularity of Case 693, which resembles the morphology of an epidermoid cyst (compare to Cases 292, 294, and 295).

The cyst in Case 694 has caused erosion of the adjacent petrous bone *(arrowheads)*. This characteristic feature of arachnoid cysts helps to distinguish them from epidermoid tumors.

Masses within the cerebellopontine angle can account for a variety of cranial neuropathies. Syndromes caused by intermittent aberrant firing of sensory or motor neurons (e.g., trigeminal neuralgia and hemifacial spasm) and steadily progressive palsies (e.g., sixth nerve) may both be caused by cisternal tumors or cysts. Distortion of cranial nerves by adjacent vascular structures is another potential extraaxial etiology of cranial neuropathies (see Cases 640 and 641).

Case 695

31-year-old man presenting with a left sixth
nerve palsy.
(axial, postcontrast scan; SE 600/14)

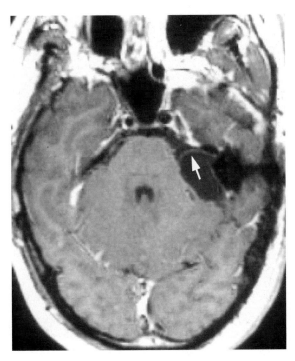

Arachnoid Cyst
(same patient as Case 693)

Case 696

51-year-old man presenting with right
facial numbness.
(axial, postcontrast scan; SE 700/20)

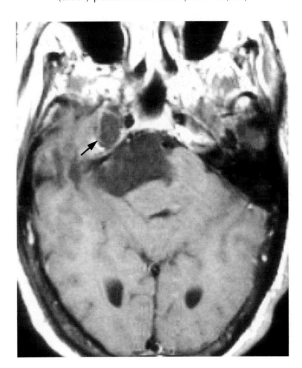

Epidermoid Cyst
(same patient as Case 292)

Magnetic resonance imaging can help to distinguish between arachnoid cysts and epidermoid cysts of the cerebellopontine angle. (Other locations in which the same differential diagnosis is important are the suprasellar region and the quadrigeminal cistern.) The signal intensity of these lesions is usually similar: long T1 and T2 values, with no contrast enhancement. However, their morphologies are typically characteristic.

Epidermoid cysts are soft, lobulated, infiltrating masses that tend to surround vessels and cranial nerves (see Case 292). By contrast, arachnoid cysts are usually unilocular and smoothly margined, stretching and displacing adjacent neurovascular structures. Bone erosion is commonly associated with arachnoid cysts and rarely seen with epidermoid cysts.

Scalloped erosion of the petrous apex is suggested adjacent to the lesion in Case 695. The neurovascular bundle (seventh and eighth cranial nerves) crossing to the internal auditory canal is anteriorly displaced and bowed *(arrow)*.

By contrast, neural structures can be seen within (i.e., surrounded by) the epidermoid mass in Case 696. The mass has extended ventrally into Meckel's cave *(arrow)*. The presenting symptom of facial numbness may reflect this component of the lesion or be due to distortion of the fifth nerve more proximally, where it is surrounded by the cisternal portion of the mass. Arachnoid cysts rarely extend across the petrous apex in this manner.

Occasional schwannomas within the cerebellopontine angle are cystic masses, as seen in Cases 167 and 171. Infrequently a cystic meningioma is encountered at this site. Coronal and sagittal MR scans help to establish the correct diagnosis in such cases by demonstrating the solid components of complex tumors.

"Racemose cysts" of cysticercosis may involve the cerebellopontine angle (or the suprasellar, sylvian, or prepontine cisterns). Another rare pathology in this differential diagnosis is a neurenteric cyst, which more commonly occurs in the spinal canal (see Cases 1091 and 1092).

Case 697

9-year-old girl with seizures and a history
of a stroke in infancy.
(coronal, noncontrast scan; SE 600/14)

Case 698

27-year-old man presenting with seizures and stable
right hemiplegia.
(coronal, noncontrast scan; SE 3000/80)

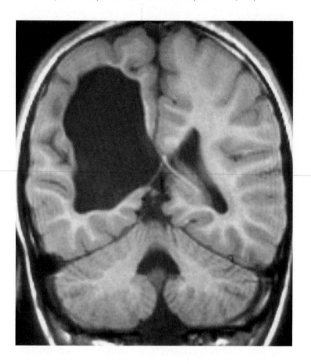

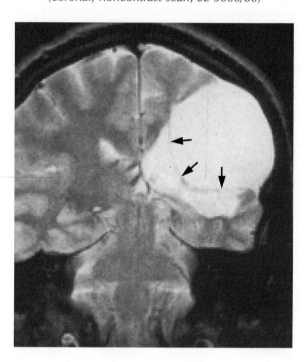

The term "porencephalic cyst" is variously applied to cystic lesions that form in regions of cerebral encephalomalacia. The strict use of the phrase refers to localized expansion of the ventricular system into an area of parenchymal damage.

Case 697 is an example of this occurrence. Porencephalic expansion of the right ventricular trigone indicates the site of the childhood CVA.

Porencephalic cysts may grow and exert pressure, probably due to incomplete communication with the parent ventricle or subarachnoid pathways. Such lesions present a paradoxical appearance of mass effect in the midst of atrophy.

In Case 698, a large cyst of CSF-like intensity extends from the ventricular margin to the cortical surface of the left hemisphere. The overlying inner table is mildly eroded. A thin layer of tissue *(arrows)* separates the cyst from the ventricular chamber. Although the cyst itself is clearly "tight" and associated with mass effect, ipsilateral ventricular enlargement suggests a porencephalic origin. The left hemicranium is slightly smaller than the right, supporting a history of parenchymal damage.

Compare the lack of tissue separating the intraaxial cyst from the adjacent ventricle in Case 698 to the appearance of an invaginating extraaxial arachnoid cyst in Case 691.

DIFFERENTIAL DIAGNOSIS:
CYST AT THE CEREBRAL SURFACE

Case 699

48-year-old man presenting with headaches.
(coronal, noncontrast scan; SE 600/14)

Case 700

22-year-old man with a history of seizures and
"cerebral palsy."
(coronal, noncontrast scan; SE 2500/28)

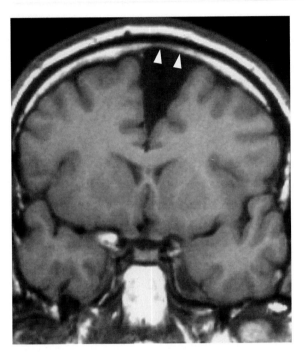

Arachnoid Cyst

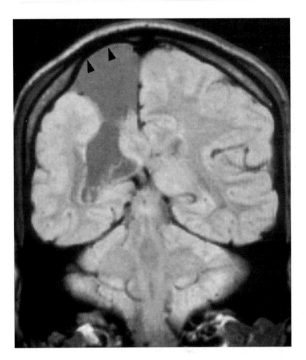

Porencephalic Cyst

Convexity arachnoid cysts occasionally involve the interhemispheric region, as in Case 699. The lateral margin of the lesion is quite linear. Mild erosion of the adjacent inner table is present superiorly *(arrowheads)*. The underlying cerebral cortex is intact although displaced. These features combine to indicate the correct diagnosis of a long-standing, extraaxial lesion.

In Case 700, a superficial cyst with CSF-like intensity values is seen at the right hemisphere vertex. The location and content of the lesion and the associated erosion of the overlying calvarium *(arrowheads)* might suggest an arachnoid cyst.

The key to the correct diagnosis in Case 700 is the status of the underlying cerebral parenchyma. The right hemisphere is small, with expansion of the right lateral ventricle. These features imply old volume loss and suggest that the superficial cyst has arisen in a region of encephalomalacia. Unlike Case 699, there is a gap between medial and lateral hemispheric cortex. Adjacent gliosis is not well seen on this scan but supports the MR diagnosis of porencephaly in other cases.

Fatty marrow within large anterior clinoid processes is present bilaterally in Case 699. This normal variant may be asymmetrical and can mimic a partially thrombosed aneurysm of the paraclinoid internal carotid artery.

Case 701

25-year-old woman with mild hemiparesis and a history of CVA in infancy.
(sagittal, noncontrast scan; SE 600/17)

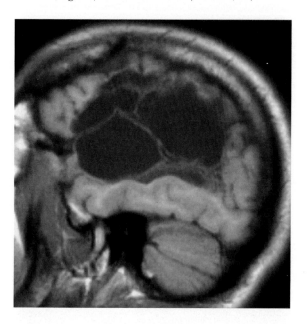

Case 702

18-month-old boy with a history of herpes encephalitis at two months of age.
(sagittal, noncontrast scan; SE 600/20)

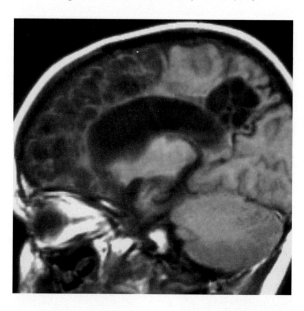

Areas of cystic encephalomalacia may occur as the result of ischemia, infection, or developmental insults. These regions may be small and numerous ("multicystic encephalomalacia") or large and unilocular, as in "porencephaly" (see Cases 697 and 698). The gliotic reaction that surrounds and contains zones of cystic encephalomalacia is a more mature response to cerebral injury than the generalized dissolution of tissue often seen in cases of intrauterine or premature perinatal damage.

In Case 701, a group of relatively large cysts occupies the sylvian region. The location of the lesion suggests old infarction involving the distribution of the middle cerebral artery. The size of the cysts is intermediate between the larger lesions of Cases 697 and 698 and the appearance of Case 702.

Neonatal herpes encephalitis is often diffuse and devastating (see Case 403). Infection in older infants may demonstrate a more multifocal pattern, illustrated by Case 702. Encephalomalacia extends from the cerebral surface to the ventricular margin in the frontal region. A multicystic morphology of fluid spaces loculated by bands of scar tissue is seen throughout this area. A smaller zone with similar characteristics is present in the deep parietal lobe.

The multicystic nature of encephalomalacia is better demonstrated on MR scans than by CT studies, which may fail to define septations traversing and partitioning zones of low attenuation.

Case 703

9-year-old boy with "cerebral palsy."
(sagittal, noncontrast scan; SE 600/14)

Case 704

2-month-old boy born at 32-weeks' gestation.
(sagittal, noncontrast scan; SE 600/14)

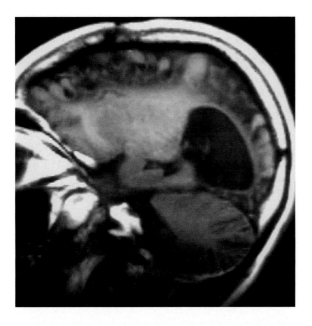

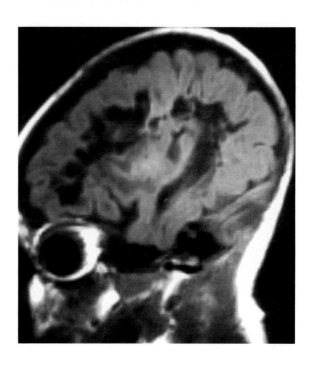

Hypoxic/ischemic damage to cerebral tissue occurring near the end of gestation or in the perinatal period can result in a pattern of multicystic encephalomalacia. The morphology of alternating cavitation and gliosis is a nonspecific response of maturing brain, with a similar appearance seen after infectious insults (see Case 702). However, the location or distribution of parenchymal damage may suggest the timing of hypoxic/ischemic injury.

In Case 703, the multiple cysts are concentrated within subcortical white matter along parasagittal bands that approximate the arterial watersheds (see Cases 488 and 492). As discussed in Chapter 9, diffuse ischemia or hypoxia late in gestation typically causes greatest damage to tissues at the intersection of the cortical watershed and intrahemispheric watershed zones. The location of multicystic en-

cephalomalacia in Case 703 is compatible with such a hypoxic/ischemic insult.

Prominent dilatation of the ventricular trigone in Case 703 indicates severe volume loss in the parietal region. This finding probably reflects "end of the line" watershed injury, as discussed in Cases 492 and 493.

The multiple cysts in Case 704 are predominantly periventricular. This distribution suggests a diffuse hypoxic/ischemic insult at an earlier stage of cerebral development. The appearance may be considered to be a multicystic expression of periventricular leukomalacia, illustrating the variable spectrum of this disorder. (Compare to Cases 500 and 501 where dissolution of white matter is more prominent than cavitation.)

Case 705A

58-year-old woman complaining of dizziness.
(coronal, postcontrast scan; SE 600/15)

Case 705B

Same patient.
(axial, noncontrast scan; SE 3000/80)

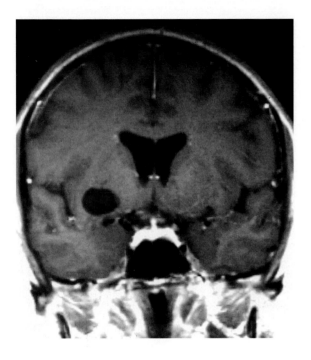

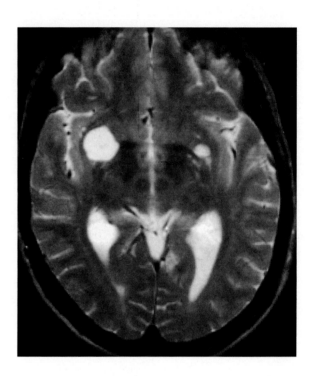

Small developmental cysts occur in several characteristic locations within the cerebral hemispheres. A particularly common site is the sublenticular region, as illustrated above.

One or more cysts ranging in diameter from a few millimeters to several centimeters may be found unilaterally or bilaterally near the inferior margin of the putamen. The occurrence of cysts in this location has been suggested to represent localized exaggeration of prominent perivascular spaces accompanying lenticulostriate arteries into the basal ganglia.

Prominent perivascular spaces or "sublenticular cysts" are incidental and asymptomatic. They are distinguished from mass lesions by their characteristic location, sharply defined margins, round shape, lack of contrast enhancement, and absence of associated edema. The typical location of sublenticular cysts is inferior to the site of most ganglionic infarctions. The common presence of bilateral (albeit asymmetrical) cysts helps to establish the diagnosis of a developmental variant in ambiguous cases.

Gelatinous pseudocysts within the basal ganglia due to cryptococcus could cause an appearance similar to Case 705. Such lesions are typically round and nonenhancing, measuring five to ten millimeters in diameter. They are caused by fungal disease ascending from basal cisterns along perivascular spaces accompanying the lenticulostriate arteries into the brain. The clinical setting of basal meningitis usually distinguishes cryptococcal pseudocysts from the normal variant illustrated above.

Compare the sublenticular location of the cysts in this case to the appearance of pallidal necrosis from carbon monoxide poisoning in Case 554A.

Another example of an incidental sublenticular cyst is seen in Case 625.

Case 706

67-year-old woman presenting with confusion.
(axial, postcontrast scan; SE 700/15)

Case 707

21-year-old man with a history of seizures.
(coronal, noncontrast scan; SE 2800/90)

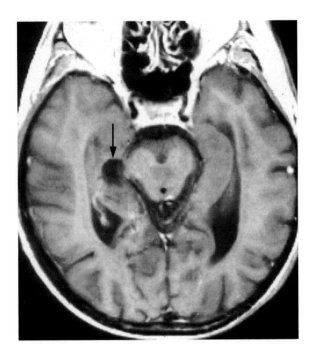

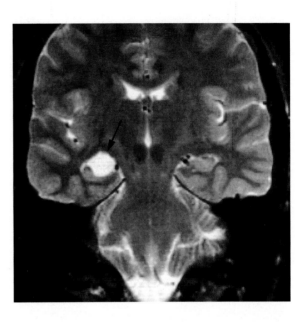

Another common location of developmental cysts is in the choroid fissure. Such cysts may be either neuroepithelial or arachnoidal in origin.

Cases 706 and 707 present typical examples of this entity. The cysts are usually quite round on axial and coronal scans, with a characteristic spindle shape paralleling the long axis of the temporal lobe (and choroid fissure) on sagittal images. They are often about one centimeter in diameter. Intensity values within choroid fissure cysts are close to those of CSF, and there is no associated contrast enhancement or reactive parenchymal edema.

As with the sublenticular cysts discussed on the preceding page, recognition of choroid fissure cysts as a developmental variant is important to avoid mistaking them for other lesions. It is possible that a parasitic cyst (e.g., cysticercosis) could present a similar appearance in this location,

but an incidental cyst would be much more common. Low grade gliomas can involve the medial temporal lobe; cysts of the choroid fissure should be considered in the differential diagnosis of such lesions. (Compare Case 707 to Cases 78, 452, and 453.)

Despite the proximity of choroid fissure cysts to the hippocampal formation, most patients with this finding do not experience seizures (or other referrable symptoms). EEG studies did support right temporal origin of seizures in Case 707.

Cysts measuring a few millimeters in diameter may be demonstrated within the hippocampal formation on high resolution scans. The small size and usual multiplicity of these incidental structures distinguish them from more medial cysts of the choroid fissure.

Case 708

2-year-old boy with a "brain tumor" reported on an outside CT scan.
(sagittal, noncontrast scan; SE 600/20)

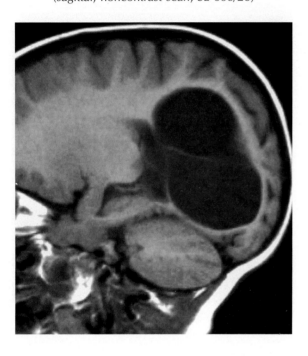

Case 709

2-year-old boy being evaluated for hypothyroidism.
(axial, postcontrast scan; SE 600/15)

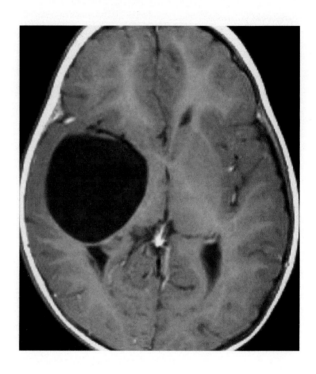

When a cyst is encountered within the brain, diagnostic considerations include cystic neoplasm, abscess, parasitic cysts, cystic encephalomalacia or porencephaly, and dermoid or epidermoid cysts. The diagnosis of a benign developmental or "neuroepithelial" cyst is entertained when alternative etiologies have been excluded.

Sporadic cysts may occur anywhere within cerebral parenchyma and may be unrelated to fissures or ventricles. They likely arise from neuroepithelial or ependymal cell rests enclosed during embryogenesis. Although the above patients are children, neuroepithelial cysts may be incidentally discovered or present in adulthood.

The large cyst in Case 708 demonstrates at least one fold or septation. Location of the cyst adjacent to the ventricular margin suggests possible origin from aberrant ependy-

mal development. Mass effect from the lesion causes anterior displacement of the lateral ventricle, but there is no evidence of surrounding edema. Ependymal cysts may also arise within ventricular chambers, causing obstructive hydrocephalus while blending with surrounding CSF in a manner analogous to parasitic intraventricular lesions.

The cyst in Case 709 had been observed to triple in size within one year. Despite this rapid growth, the cyst appears benign. Margins are smoothly rounded and well-demarcated, demonstrating no abnormal contrast enhancement. Surgery disclosed a simple unilocular neuroepithelial cyst, with no communication to the subarachnoid space or ventricular system. The mechanism by which such cysts may enlarge has not been established. (Compare to the occasional dramatic growth of arachnoid cysts, as in Case 684.)

DIFFERENTIAL DIAGNOSIS:
TEMPORAL LOBE CYSTS

Case 710

47-year-old man presenting with seizures.
(coronal, postcontrast scan; partition from
three-dimensional GRE sequence)

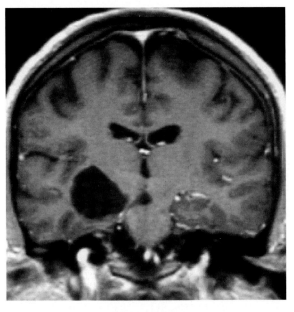

Epidermoid Cyst
(same patient as Case 293)

Case 711

64-year-old woman presenting with
left hemiparesis.
(coronal, post-contrast scan; SE 600/14)

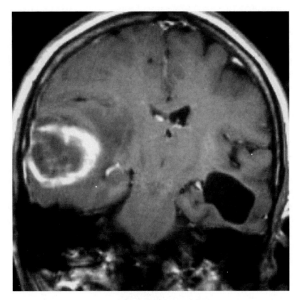

Neuroepithelial Cyst
(and contralateral glioblastoma multiforme)

As discussed on the preceding page, the diagnosis of a developmental or "neuroepithelial" cyst should be entertained only after alternative etiologies have been considered.

Case 710 demonstrates that epidermoid cysts can invaginate into cerebral parenchyma to mimic an intraaxial lesion. (Compare to the dermoid cyst in Case 288.) The epidermoid mass in this case has apparently developed within and widened the choroid fissure. The well-defined, homogeneous, nonenhancing appearance of the lesion closely resembles a simple fluid-containing cyst.

The left temporal cyst in Case 711 is sharply defined, with no associated contrast enhancement. It is centered within white matter of the temporal lobe, lateral to the temporal horn. (Compare to the medial location of the choroid fissure cysts in Cases 706 and 707.) Possible "ball-valve" communication with the temporal horn cannot be excluded, but the cyst could also have arisen from ependymal duplication or compartmentalization.

REFERENCES

Altman NR, Naidich TP, Braffman BH: Posterior fossa malformations. *AJNR* 13:691-724, 1992.

Atlas W, Mark AS, Fram EK: Aqueductal stenosis: evaluation with gradient echo imaging. *Radiology* 169:449-453, 1988.

Baker LL, Barkovich AJ: The large temporal horn: MR analysis in developmental brain anomalies versus hydrocephalus.

Barkovich AJ, Kjos BO, Norman D, Edwards MS: Revised classification of posterior fossa cysts and cystlike malformations based on the results of multiplanar MR imaging. *AJNR* 10:977-988, 1989.

Barkovich AJ, Newton TH: MR of aqueductal stenosis. Evidence of a broad spectrum of tectal distortion. *AJNR* 10:471-476, 1989.

Bourekas EC, Raji MR, Dastur KJ, et al: Retroclival arachnoid cyst. *AJNR* 13:353-354, 1992.

Bradley WG, Kortman KE, Burgoyne B: Flowing cerebrospinal fluid in normal and hydrocephalic states: appearance on MR image. *Radiology* 159:611-616, 1986.

Bradley WG Jr, Whittemore AR, Watanabe AS, et al: Association of deep white matter infarction with chronic communicating hydrocephalus: implications regarding the possible origin of normal-pressure hydrocephalus. *AJNR* 12:31-39, 1991.

Britton J, Marsh H, Kendall B, et al: MRI and hydrocephalus in childhood. *Neuroradiology* 30:310-314, 1988.

Choi SK, Starshak RJ, Meyer GA, et al: Arachnoid cyst of the quadrigeminal plate cistern: report of two cases. *AJNR* 7:725-728, 1986.

Czervionke LF, Daniels DL, Meyer GA, et al: Neuroepithelial cyst of the lateral ventricles: MR appearance. *AJNR* 8:609-613, 1987.

Dross PE, Lally JF, Bonier B: Pneumosinus dilatans and arachnoid cyst: a unique association. *AJNR* 13:209-211, 1992.

El Gammal T, Allen MB Jr, Brooks BS, Mark EK: MR evaluation of hydrocephalus. *AJNR* 8:591-597, 1987.

Fitz CR: Disorders of ventricles and CSF spaces. *Semin US CT MR* 9:216-230, 1988.

Gammal T, Allen M, Brooks B, et al: MR evaluation of hydrocephalus. *AJR* 149:807, 1987.

Gandy SE, Heier LA: Clinical and magnetic resonance features of primary intracranial arachnoid cysts. *Ann Neurol* 21:342-348, 1987.

Garcia Santos JM, Martinez-Lage J, Ubeda AG, et al: Arachnoid cysts of the middle fossa: a consideration of their origins based on imaging. *Neuroradiology* 39:395-358, 1993.

Gideon P, Stahlberg F, Thomsen C, et al: Cerebrospinal fluid flow and production in patients with normal pressure hydrocephalus studied by MRI. *Neuroradiology* 36:210-215, 1994.

Hanigan WC, Wright R, Wright S: Magnetic resonance imaging of the Dandy-Walker malformations. *Pediatr Neurosci* 12:151-156, 1985-1986.

Jack CR, Mokri B, Laws ER Jr, et al: MR findings in normal pressure hydrocephalus: significance and comparison to other forms of dementia. *J Comput Assist Tomogr* 11:923-931, 1987.

Jinkins JR: Clinical manifestations of hydrocephalus caused by impingement of the corpus callosum on the falx: an MR study in 40 patients. *AJNR* 12:331-340, 1991.

Jungreis CA, Kanal E, Hirsch WL, et al: Normal perivascular spaces mimicking lacunar infarction: MR imaging. *Radiology* 169:101-104, 1988.

Kemp SS, Zimmerman RA, Bilaniuk LT, et al: Magnetic resonance imaging of the cerebral aqueduct. *Neuroradiology* 29:430-436, 1987.

Kimura M, Tanaka A, Yoshinaga S: Significance of periventricular hemodynamics in normal pressure hydrocephalus. *Neurosurgery* 30:701-705, 1992.

Kjos BO, Brant-Zawadzki M, Kucharczyk W, et al: Cystic intracranial lesions: magnetic resonance imaging. *Radiology* 155:363-370, 1985.

Kollias SS, Ball WS Jr, Prenger EC: Cystic malformations of the posterior fossa: differential diagnosis clarified through embryologic analysis. *Radiographics* 13:1211-1232, 1993.

Kollias SS, Prenger EC, Becket WW Jr, et al: Posterior fossa cystic malformations: possible pitfalls in radiographic diagnosis. *Radiology* 185(suppl):403, 1992.

Malcolm GP, Symon L, Kendall B, Pires M: Intracranial neurenteric cysts. *J Neurosurg* 75:115-120, 1991.

Nakase H, Ishida Y, Tada T, et al: Neuroepithelial cysts of the lateral ventricle. *Surg Neurol* 37:94-100, 1992.

Novetsky GJ, Berlin L: Aqueductal stenosis. Demonstration by MR imaging. *J Comput Assist Tomogr* 6:1170-1171, 1984.

Quencer RM: Intracranial CSF flow in pediatric hydrocephalus: evaluation with Cine-MR imaging. *AJNR* 13:601-608, 1992.

Quint DJ: Retroclival arachnoid cysts. *AJNR* 13:1503-1504, 1992.

Robertson SJ, Wolpert SM, Runge VM: MR imaging of middle cranial fossa arachnoid cysts: temporal lobe agenesis syndrome revisited. *AJNR* 10:1007-1010, 1989.

Sakamoto H, Fujitani K, Kitano S, et al: Cerebrospinal fluid edema associated with shunt obstruction. *J Neurosurg* 81:179-183, 1994.

Schumacher DJ, Tien RD, Friedman H: Gadolinium enhancement of the leptomeninges caused by hydrocephalus: a potential mimic of leptomeningeal metastasis. *AJNR* 15:639-641, 1994.

Sherman JL, Componovo E, Citrin CM: MR imaging of CSF-like choroidal fissure and parenchymal cysts of the brain. *AJNR* 11:939-945, 1990.

Tsuruda JS, Chew WM, Moseley ME, Norman D: Diffusion-weighted MR imaging of the brain: value of differentiating between extraaxial cysts and epidermoid tumors. *AJNR* 11:925-931, 1990.

Weiner SN, Pearlstein AE, Eiber A: MR imaging of intracranial arachnoid cysts. *J Comput Assist Tomogr* 11:236-241, 1987.

Wester K: Gender distribution and sidedness of middle fossa arachnoid cysts: a review of cases diagnosed with computed imaging. *Neurosurgery* 31:940-944, 1992.

Wilms G, Venderschueren G, Demaerel PH, et al: CT and MR in infants with pericerebral collections and macrocephaly: benign enlargement of the subarachnoid spaces versus subdural collections. *AJNR* 14:855-860, 1993.

CHAPTER 12

Developmental Abnormalities

Case 712

34-year-old man presenting with bilateral
arm numbness.
(sagittal, noncontrast scan; SE 600/20)

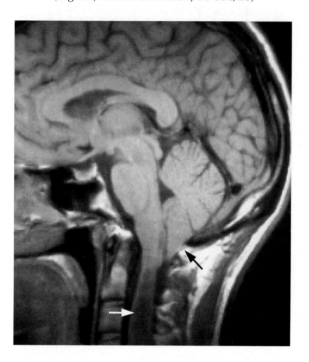

Case 713

5-year-old boy presenting with occipital headaches.
(sagittal, noncontrast scan; SE 600/20)

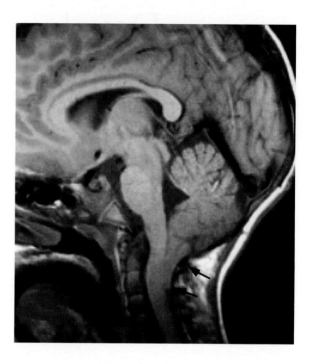

The Chiari I hindbrain malformation consists of abnormal inferior extension of the cerebellar tonsils through the plane of the foramen magnum. Caudal elongation and/or displacement of inferior vermian tissue may accompany the tonsils into the cervical spinal canal.

There is considerable variability in the position of normal cerebellar tonsils with respect to the foramen magnum. The caudal margin of the tonsils may normally reside up to two or three millimeters below a line from the basion to the opisthion. Greater degrees of tonsillar ectopia suggest congenital malformation (or acquired herniation) and may correlate with clinical symptomatology.

The morphology of low-lying cerebellar tonsils can help to distinguish normal variation from Chiari I malformation. Tonsils in the latter condition tend to be peg-shaped or inferiorly pointed, as seen in the above cases *(black arrows)*. The caudal margin of normal tonsils has a more rounded or bulbous contour.

Chiari I malformations may be incidentally encountered in patients who have no related symptoms. Alternatively, the malformation may present a variety of clinical syndromes. Crowding of tissue within the foramen magnum may compress the cervicomedullary junction, causing headaches (as in Case 713), neck pain, and/or lower cranial neuropathies.

Symptoms in other patients are due to hydromyelia, which develops in association with the Chiari I malformation in about 20% of cases. This frequent occurrence warrants careful examination of the cervical spinal cord when a Chiari I hindbrain malformation is discovered. In Case 712, a cyst within the spinal cord is faintly seen at the inferior margin of the scan *(white arrow)*.

The morphological and symptomatic equivalent of primary Chiari I malformation of the cerebellum can be produced by osseous deformity at the craniocervical junction (e.g., basilar invagination and/or platybasia; see Case 1047) or by tonsillar herniation (e.g., due to intrauterine hydrocephalus or a posterior fossa mass; see Case 689).

Case 714

3-year-old girl with a history of myelomeningocele repair at birth.
(sagittal, noncontrast scan; 600/17)

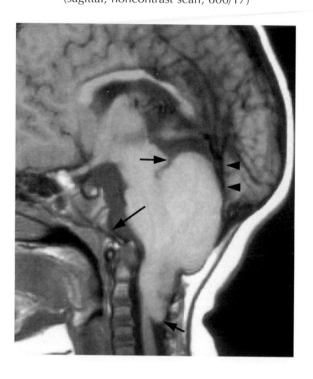

Case 715

2-year-old girl with spina bifida.
(sagittal, noncontrast scan; SE 600/17)

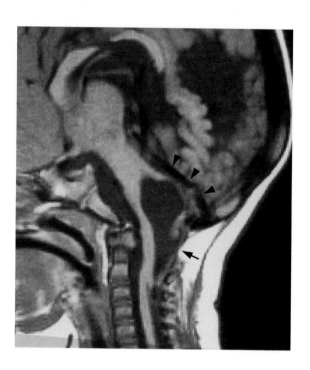

The Chiari II ("Arnold Chiari") hindbrain malformation is much more severe and complex than the Chiari I deformity. More extensive caudal herniation of the hindbrain into the cervical spinal canal is present, almost invariably associated with a lumbosacral myelomeningocele.

Case 714 illustrates a typical "cascade" of herniating tissue extending inferiorly from the small posterior fossa through the wide foramen magnum. Buckling of the caudally displaced medulla often forms a tissue layer between the herniated cerebellum and the spinal cord *(lowest arrow,* Case 714).

The fourth ventricle in Chiari II malformations is usually caudally elongated and slit-like due to tissue crowding. When a "normal"-sized or enlarged fourth ventricle is seen (as in Case 715), distention or "trapping" should be suspected (see discussion of Cases 665 and 666).

The combination of herniating posterior fossa tissue and commonly associated supratentorial hydrocephalus results in a small posterior fossa. Associated cerebellar hypoplasia is variable. Very little cerebellar tissue is present in the tiny posterior fossa of Case 715, while Case 714 demon-strates a much larger cerebellum and infratentorial compartment.

Crowding of tissue within the small posterior fossa causes characteristic patterns of bone erosion. Ventrally concave scalloping of the clivus *(long arrow,* Case 714) is typical and most apparent on sagittal MR scans after shunting has reduced intracranial pressure. A similar concave remodelling is often seen along the posterior margin of the petrous bones on axial scans.

The above cases illustrate additional abnormalities associated with the Chiari II hindbrain malformation. Hypoplasia of the corpus callosum (particularly posteriorly) is usually present, as is an abnormal gyral pattern most prominent in the medial occipital regions. "Beaking" of the midbrain tectum *(upper arrow,* Case 714) is characteristic, often reflecting both primary malformation (with fusion of colliculi into a single peak) and secondary deformity (due to long-standing lateral compression from hydrocephalic hemispheres). The straight sinus is abnormally low and vertical in both of these patients *(arrowheads).*

Case 716

18-year-old man with a history of
myelomeningocele repair at birth.
(axial, noncontrast scan; SE 3000/80)

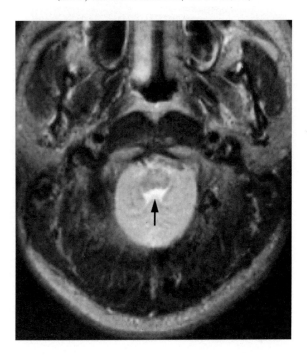

Case 717

4-year-old girl, post repair of myelomeningocele
and shunting for hydrocephalus.
(axial, noncontrast scan; SE 3000/90)

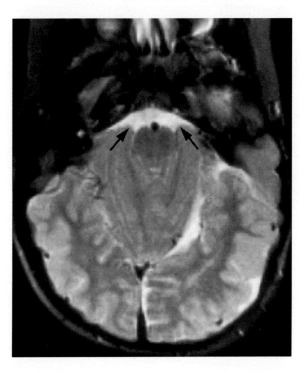

Axial scans document the crowding and deformity of infratentorial tissue in patients with Chiari II hindbrain malformations.

The abnormally large foramen magnum in Case 716 is filled by cerebellar parenchyma surrounding the lateral and posterior aspects of the medulla and low-lying fourth ventricle *(arrow)*. A similar appearance is seen in Case 717, where the cerebellar hemispheres wrap ventrally around the pons to reach the prepontine cistern *(arrows)*.

Case 717 illustrates a very narrow posterior fossa with a steeply sloping tentorium (see also Case 719). Mild concave erosion along the posterior surface of the petrous ridges is suggested medially. This remodelling of bone may be much more prominent in other cases.

The Chiari II malformation ranks with communicating hydrocephalus and aqueductal stenosis among the major causes of congenital hydrocephalus. If hydrocephalus is not present at birth, it usually develops rapidly following surgical closure of an associated myelomeningocele. Like aqueductal stenosis (see Case 660), the Chiari II malformation presents with overall cranial enlargement in the presence of a small posterior fossa.

A clue to the diagnosis of Chiari II malformation on skull films in infants is the associated calvarial dysplasia called "craniolacunae" or "Lückenschädel skull." This characteristic finding is present at birth and usually disappears by the age of one year. (Mottled skull lucency due to "convolutional impressions" from increased intracranial pressure is rarely seen before the age of two years.)

Case 718

1-year-old girl with a history of repaired
myelomeningocele and shunted hydrocephalus.
(axial, noncontrast scan; SE 3000/75)

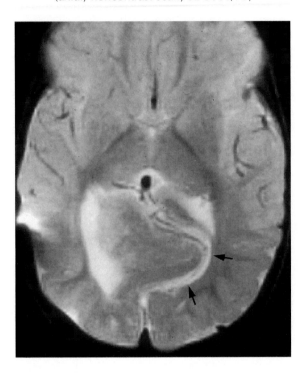

Case 719

11-month-old boy with a history of myelomeningocele repair and shunted hydrocephalus.
(coronal, noncontrast scan; SE 700/17)

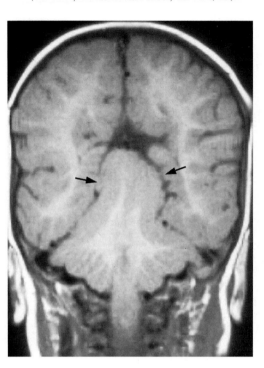

Several striking deformities of brain tissue may accompany Chiari II malformations at presentation or following treatment.

Hypoplasia and/or fenestration of the falx is common, often associated with interdigitation of gyri in the medial occipital regions. Case 718 presents a typical example of this deformity. The posterior interhemispheric fissure is bowed far to the left *(arrows)* as the right occipital lobe crosses midline.

Case 719 demonstrates the characteristically "towering" cerebellar vermis that often develops in patients with Chiari II malformations after shunting. Decompression of supra-tentorial mass effect allows the crowded cerebellum to expand superiorly, accentuated by the steeply sloping tentorium. This impressive rostral extension of bulky and dysmorphic tissue may be misinterpreted as a new midline mass, particularly on axial CT studies.

An abnormal gyral pattern on the medial surface of the cerebral hemispheres is again illustrated in Case 719.

The Chiari II malformation is occasionally accompanied by an occipital and/or cervical encephalocele containing herniated hindbrain tissue. See Cases 771 and 772 for discussion of this "Chiari III" deformity.

Case 720

37-year-old woman being evaluated for possible demyelinating disease.
(sagittal, noncontrast scan; SE 600/22)

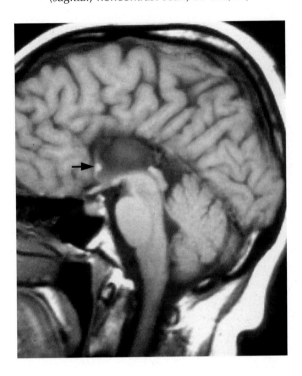

Case 721

10-month-old boy presenting with infantile spasms.
(coronal, noncontrast scan; SE 600/15)

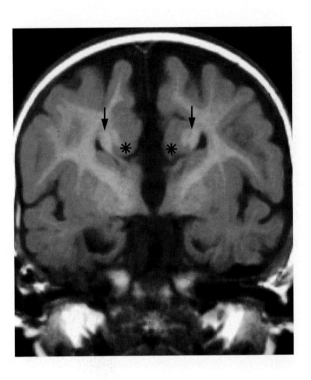

Callosal dysgenesis or agenesis is apparent on sagittal and coronal MR images. In Case 720, the expected structure of the corpus callosum is absent. Sulci on the medial surface of the hemisphere have an abnormal radial pattern, extending inferiorly to nearly reach the third ventricle and velum interpositum. The anterior commissure is hypertrophied *(arrow)*.

Case 721 demonstrates a "high-riding" third ventricle meeting the interhemispheric fissure, with no separation by crossing callosal tissue. Enlargement of the third ventricle in this position may form an "interhemispheric cyst." (A separate and larger dorsal interhemispheric cyst may be seen in some cases of callosal agenesis, as in other congenital abnormalities; see Case 655.)

The lateral ventricles in Case 721 are widely separated, resembling the head of a "longhorn steer" when viewed coronally with the third ventricle. The narrowed diameter and comma-shaped morphology of the lateral ventricles is due to indentation of their medial margin by the bundles of Probst *(arrows)*. These longitudinal fiber bands represent axons that would normally cross in the corpus callosum but have instead formed parasagittal tracts (see Case 722). Malrotated cingulate gyri are present medial to the bundles of Probst (asterisks); the gyri have not been normally "inverted" by development of a subjacent interhemispheric bridge of callosal tissue (compare to Cases 728 and 729).

Dysgenesis of the corpus callosum may be incomplete. Most common is hypoplasia of the posterior portion, indicating arrest of callosal development (which proceeds from anterior to posterior).

Agenesis or dysgenesis of the corpus callosum is frequently associated with other congenital abnormalities of the brain. Examples include the Dandy-Walker malformation, Chiari II malformation, encephaloceles, and neuronal migration abnormalities. Isolated callosal agenesis is often an incidental finding on scans obtained for unrelated complaints.

DIFFERENTIAL DIAGNOSIS:
DILATATION OF THE POSTERIOR PORTIONS OF THE LATERAL VENTRICLES

Case 722

21-year-man presenting with seizures.
(axial, noncontrast scan; SE 2500/90)

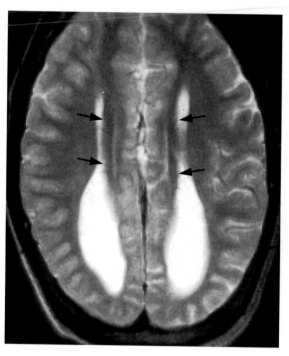

Agenesis of the Corpus Callosum

Case 723

18-month-old girl with "cerebral palsy."
(axial, noncontrast scan; SE 2800/90)

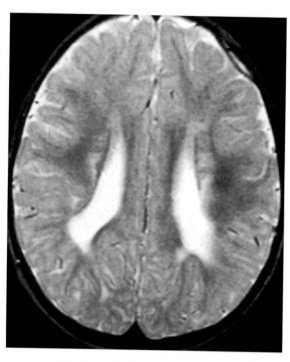

Periventricular Leukomalacia

"Colpocephaly," or dilatation of the posterior portion of the lateral ventricles, accompanies many congenital malformations. This feature may be especially prominent in agenesis of the corpus callosum, since the normal bulk and rigidity of the major forceps are missing from the posterior temporal and occipital lobes.

Case 722 presents a typical example of this finding. Also apparent is wide separation of the lateral ventricles, which are abnormally parallel. This characteristic parasagittal ventricular orientation is not present in all cases.

The posterior portions of the lateral ventricles are also enlarged in Case 723. However, the margins of the expanded ventricles are angular and irregular instead of smoothly rounded. The ventricular expansion is due to an acquired loss of periventricular white matter rather than to congenital malformation. Multiple foci of abnormal signal intensity in the periventricular regions corroborate a history of deep hemispheric insult (see discussion of Cases 498-501).

Seizures in patients with agenesis of the corpus callosum (as in Case 722) may be idiopathic or associated with recognizable accompanying abnormalities (e.g., neuronal migration disorders). Children with periventricular leukomalacia often manifest spastic diplegia and are placed in the category of "cerebral palsy," as in Case 723.

The parasagittally oriented bundles of Probst are well seen as longitudinal bands of white matter along the medial margin of the lateral ventricles in Case 722 *(arrows)*.

Case 724

36-year-old woman presenting with dizziness.
(sagittal, noncontrast scan; SE 600/15)

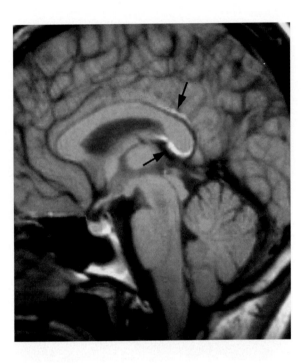

Case 725

10-year-old girl with a long history of seizures.
(sagittal, noncontrast scan; SE 600/20)

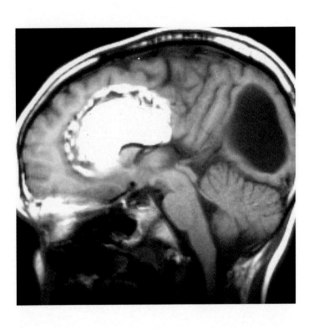

"Lipomas of the corpus callosum" are better considered to be "interhemispheric lipomas with callosal dysgenesis." The lesions are believed to result from lipomatous maldifferentiation of primitive meningeal tissue in the interhemispheric fissure. The presence of an interhemispheric lipoma may secondarily impair callosal development, resulting in hypoplasia or agenesis.

The above scans demonstrate the variable size and morphology of interhemispheric lipomas. In Case 724, a thin layer of lipomatous tissue with short T1 values outlines the normally formed splenium of the corpus callosum *(arrows)*. By contrast, the large lipoma in Case 725 is a spherical mass, associated with severe dysgenesis of the corpus callosum. (Note the characteristic associated radial pattern of medial hemispheric gyri and accompanying colpocephaly.)

Foci of low signal intensity at the perimeter of an inter

hemispheric lipoma may represent calcification, commonly demonstrated on CT scans. Such calcification usually takes the form of a thin shell within cortex adjacent to the lipoma.

"Flow voids" of major arteries are another cause for low intensity areas within a lipoma. Such vessels are engulfed when the primitive tissue ("meninx") filling fetal cisterns differentiates into fat rather than involuting normally.

In cases of callosal agenesis, the proximal anterior cerebral arteries may follow an abnormally vertical and posterior course as they ascend along the anterior margin of the third ventricle. An azygous anterior cerebral artery is often seen in this context.

Calcification or ossification within the falx may be associated with T1-shortening due to paramagnetic effects or fatty marrow elements. Such thin dural plaques should not be mistaken for interhemispheric lipomas.

Case 726

12-year-old boy with an abnormal CT scan
after head trauma.
(coronal, noncontrast scan; SE 2500/45)

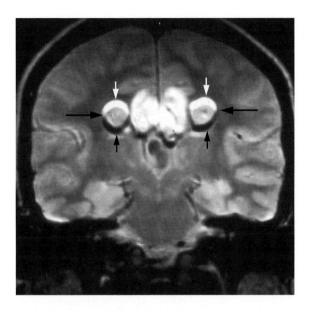

Case 727

15-year-old girl presenting with seizures.
(axial, noncontrast scan; SE 2500/90)

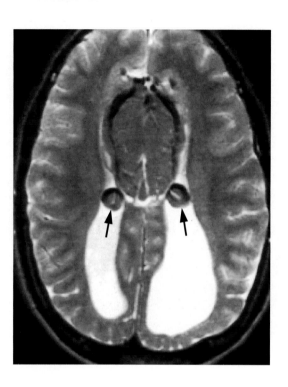

Lipomas involving the choroid plexus of the lateral ventricles commonly accompany larger interhemispheric ("callosal") lipomas. The intraventricular lesions may be unilateral or bilateral and single or multinodular. They may be continuous with the interhemispheric mass or separate from it. Choroid plexus lipomas probably develop when maldifferentiating meningeal tissue invaginates through the choroid fissure.

In both of the above cases, the satellite lipomas are bilateral and symmetrical *(long arrows)*. Associated colpocephaly is present in Case 727.

Case 726 is a good example of chemical shift artifact at the interface between aqueous and fatty tissues. The naturally lower resonance frequency of lipid protons has caused the computer to plot their signal intensity a little closer to the low end of the frequency axis than is accurate. As a result, the lipoma is misregistered against the background of aqueous tissues, being artifactually "shifted" away from the inferior tissue (leaving a "black" gap; *short black arrows*) to overlap the superior tissue (causing a "bright" superimposition of signal; *white arrows*). This finding is a useful clue to the lipid nature of a mass on MR scans.

The expected short T2 values of fatty tissue are illustrated in Case 727. All three lipomas demonstrate uniformly low signal intensity, comparable to that of subcutaneous fat in the scalp. (Chemical shift artifact is present at the anterior and posterior margins of the lipomas in Case 727.)

Low signal intensity within the third ventricle in Case 726 is due to artifact from CSF pulsation.

Case 728

1-year-old boy presenting with
developmental delay.
(coronal, noncontrast scan; SE 700/15)

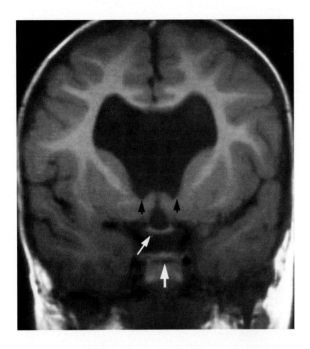

Case 729

3-year-old girl being evaluated for small stature.
(coronal, noncontrast scan; SE 600/14)

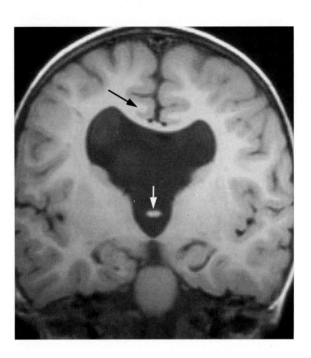

Several names have been applied to congenital malformations involving midline structures of the brain. Coexisting hypoplasia of the optic nerves and absence of the septum pellucidum has been called "septooptic dysplasia" or "de Morsier's" syndrome. The majority of such patients additionally demonstrate hypoplasia of the adenohypophysis, which may be the most important component of the complex clinically. Recently the generic nomenclature of "midline cerebral dysgenesis" has been proposed to include septooptic dysplasia and more complex malformations.

Absence of the septum pellucidum by itself has no functional significance. The finding is important only as a potential marker for associated hypoplasia of the optic nerves and/or pituitary gland. Patients with septooptic dysplasia may present with decreased visual acuity, nystagmus, or growth impairment secondary to insufficiency of the adenohypophysis.

MR scans clearly demonstrate absence of the septum pel-

lucidum. The resulting "fusion" of the lateral ventricles superficially resembles the appearance of holoprosencephaly (compare the above cases to Case 730). Inferior pointing of the frontal horns is usually prominent (*black arrows,* Case 728). This finding may also be noted in association with other congenital abnormalities, notably the Chiari II hindbrain malformation.

Because the septum pellucidum is absent, the columns of the fornix "float" characteristically within the third ventricle on coronal (or sagittal) images (*white arrow,* Case 729).

Note the small size of the optic chiasm (*thin white arrow*) and pituitary gland (*thick white arrow*) in Case 728. Case 221 presents another example of pituitary hypoplasia in septooptic dysplasia.

The corpus callosum is somewhat thin but is clearly present in the above images. As a result, the cingulate gyri have undergone normal inversion (*black arrow,* Case 729; compare to Case 721).

Case 730

32-year-old woman with a history of seizures
and "mild cerebral palsy."
(coronal, noncontrast scan; SE 600/15)

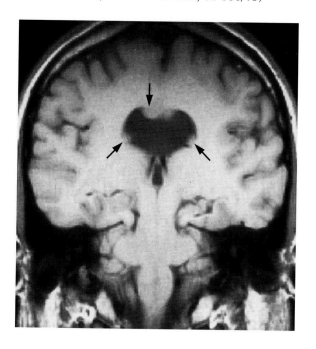

Case 731

2-month-old girl presenting with a large head.
(axial, noncontrast scan; SE 600/14)

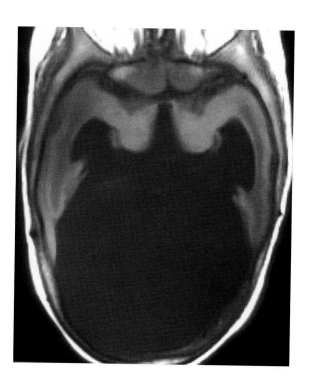

As discussed in Case 655, holoprosencephaly is a more severe midline malformation than septooptic dysplasia. Failure of normal hemisphere development results in a horseshoe-shaped forebrain ("holoprosencephalon") surrounding a central monoventricle.

Holoprosencephaly has traditionally been subdivided into lobar, semilobar, and alobar types. This somewhat artificial categorization refers to complete, partial, or absent separation of cerebral parenchyma into distinct hemispheres at the perimeter of the central ventricle. Hemispheric division (with presence of the falx) is often most complete posteriorly and least developed in the frontal region.

In Case 730, the interhemispheric fissure is bridged by tissue joining the frontal lobes (compare to the cases on the preceding pages). The single-chambered ventricle resembles the morphology of septooptic dysplasia. (See Case 655 for an example of the classic "bat wing" configuration often encountered in holoprosencephaly.) Nodules of heterotopic gray matter are present along the ventricular mar-

gins (*arrows;* see Cases 748 and 749).

Case 730 illustrates the variable severity of holoprosencephaly. The malformation demonstrated is intermediate between septooptic dysplasia and the more extensive abnormality in Case 731. Associated symptoms were correspondingly moderate.

Case 731 demonstrates partial hemispherization of the temporal lobes and thalami. However, all ventricular chambers join posteriorly to form a large cyst that occupies the posterior and superior portion of the cranium. Such a midline "dorsal cyst" is commonly found in association with cerebral malformations. The cyst may communicate with the ventricular system or be an isolated interhemispheric structure.

The hippocampal formations are severely hypoplastic in alobar and semilobar holoprosencephaly. As a result, the temporal horns in Case 731 are patulous, with a conspicuous lack of the normally complex tissue pattern along their medial margin (compare to Cases 450 and 451).

Case 732

3-month-old girl with infantile spasms.
(axial, noncontrast scan; SE 3000/30)

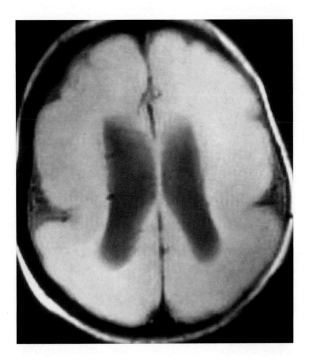

Case 733

5-year-old boy with a history of seizures.
(coronal, noncontrast scan; SE 750/20)

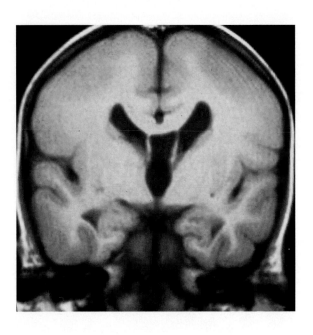

Abnormalities of neuronal migration lead to a variety of recognizable developmental malformations. Among these is lissencephaly, or "smooth brain." This disorder is characterized by thick cerebral cortex that lacks normal gyration, as seen in the above cases.

Case 732 demonstrates several associated features. Poor opercularization is present in the sylvian region, with the shallow sylvian grooves giving the brain a "figure of eight" appearance on axial images. Hypoplasia of white matter accompanies the abnormal cortical mantle. (White matter in Case 732 is represented by the thin band of relatively high signal intensity in the periventricular region.) Ventricles are typically enlarged and dysmorphic.

When smooth and thick cerebral cortex is localized rather than generalized, the condition is termed "pachygyria." Case 733 demonstrates severe pachygyria over the frontal convexity bilaterally. The temporal lobes demonstrate a more normal gyral pattern. Comparison of the cortical ribbon in the temporal regions with that of the frontal lobes helps to emphasize the gross abnormality of the latter.

Lissencephaly associated with *thin* cerebral cortex may be seen in cases of congenital CMV infection, often in association with delayed myelination and cerebellar hypoplasia.

A prominent "cavum septi pellucidi" is present in Case 733. Cysts within the septum pellucidum are a normal feature of developing brains but are usually obliterated soon after birth. Persistent cysts are most commonly found at the level of the frontal horns. Large cysts occupying most of the septum pellucidum and extending posterior to the fornix ("cavum vergae") are unusual.

Case 734

9-year-old girl presenting with seizures.
(axial, noncontrast scan; SE 3000/45)

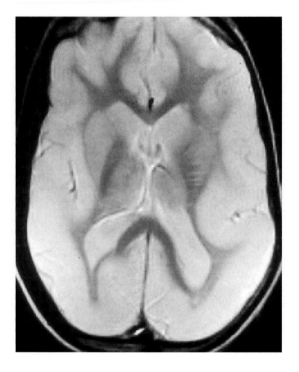

Case 735

13-year-old girl with a history of seizures.
(coronal, noncontrast scan; SE 3000/90)

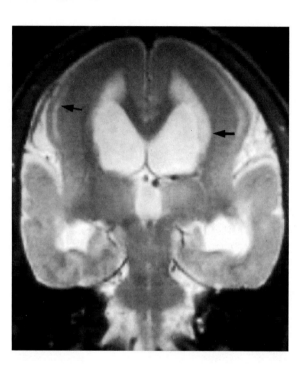

Case 734 demonstrates symmetrical pachygyria localized to the posterior portion of the cerebral hemispheres. Hypoplasia of underlying white matter and dilatation of the adjacent ventricular system accompany the marked cortical thickening. (Compare the thickness and complexity of parietal white matter to that in the frontal lobes.)

In Case 735, greatly thickened cortex occupies most of the cerebral mantle. A thin band of dysplastic underlying white matter is seen as a zone of high signal intensity in the periventricular region *(thick arrow)*. A stripe of signal abnormality near the cortical periphery *(thin arrow)* may represent the "cell sparse zone" of presumed laminar necrosis typically found in lissencephaly.

Cases 732 to 735 illustrate that pachygyria can remain strikingly symmetrical while demonstrating variable hemispheric extent. In other cases, pachygyria is entirely unilateral, with widespread or focal involvement (see Cases 738 and 739).

Focal, unilateral pachygyria can be misinterpreted as an infiltrating mass lesion (compare to Case 74). Correct interpretation in such cases is based on recognizing that the signal intensity of the questioned area matches that of gray matter on all pulse sequences.

Abnormalities of neuronal migration are commonly associated with seizures, as in the above cases.

Case 736A

7-month-old girl.
(sagittal, noncontrast scan; SE 600/14)

Case 736B

Same patient.
(axial, noncontrast scan; SE 2800/90)

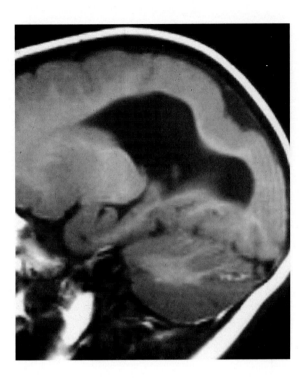

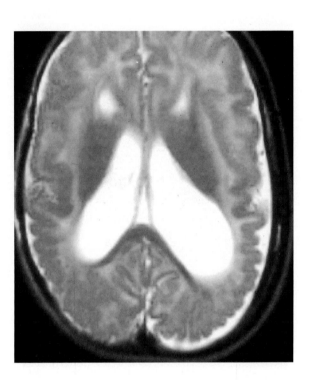

Another pattern of abnormal neuronal migration and cortical development is polymicrogyria. As the name implies, this malformation is characterized by multiple tiny "secondary" gyri on the cortical surface. These shallow irregularities are often crowded together and not clearly separated by intervening CSF spaces. As a result, the involved cortex may appear abnormally smooth, resembling pachygyria. However, polymicrogyria is usually associated with only mild cortical thickening.

In Case 736A, the cortex has a pachygyric appearance but is not as thick as in Cases 732-735. Case 736B demonstrates that the cortical contour in the parietal regions consists of multiple closely spaced ridges. This pattern contrasts with the smooth cortical surface illustrated on the preceding pages. In other cases of polymicrogyria no surface irregularity is appreciable because the secondary gyri are not individually resolved.

The T2-weighted scan in Case 736B confirms that the cortex is not prominently thickened. High signal intensity in hypoplastic subcortical white matter may represent gliosis and/or high water content due to immature myelination. White matter fronds usually do not arborize normally into areas of polymicrogyria.

Case 737

2-year-old girl presenting with developmental delay.
(axial, noncontrast scan; SE 2500/90)

Case 738

5-year-old girl presenting with a seizure.
(axial, noncontrast scan; SE 2800/90)

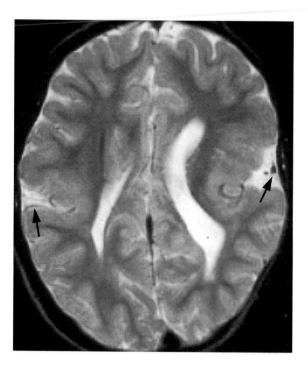

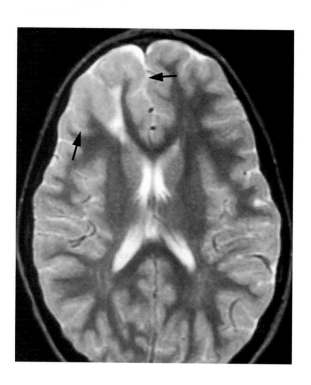

Abnormal cortical organization due to disorders of neuronal migration may be localized to small regions within one or both hemispheres. In cases of asymmetrical pachygyria or gray matter heterotopia, the prominent density and contrast enhancement of the malformed cortex may be mistaken for a mass on CT scans. Magnetic resonance imaging is valuable for demonstrating that the region in question maintains signal intensity equal to that of normal gray matter on all pulse sequences.

The sylvian and rolandic regions are commonly affected by localized cortical dysplasias, as seen bilaterally in Case 737. The mid hemispheric cortex is abnormally thick, suggesting pachygyria and/or polymicrogyria. Involved gray matter also invaginates abnormally toward the ventricular system. Such cortical infolding commonly accompanies focal pachygyria or polymicrogyria and can mimic schizencephaly (see Cases 742–744).

Prominent aberrant superficial vessels (usually veins) are often present in the distorted subarachnoid spaces overlying focal cortical dysplasia. Examples are seen bilaterally in Case 737 *(arrows)*. Such vascular channels should not be misinterpreted as a primary vascular malformation. Anomalous widening of overlying CSF spaces may help to distinguish neuronal migration disorders from mass lesions.

An area of localized cortical dysplasia is present in the right frontal region in Case 738 *(arrows)*. This unilateral lesion demonstrates cortical thickening and infolding, with focal dysplasia of underlying white matter. Compare Case 738 to the right frontal infarction in Case 502, where signal abnormality extends through the cortex.

Case 739A

5-year-old girl with seizures since birth.
(coronal, noncontrast scan; SE 800/20)

Case 739B

Same patient.
(axial, noncontrast scan; SE 2500/90)

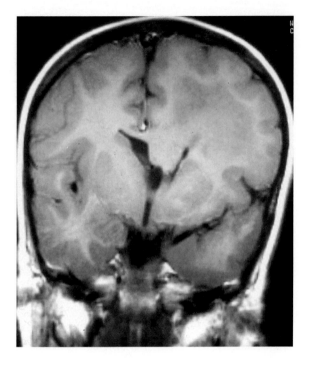

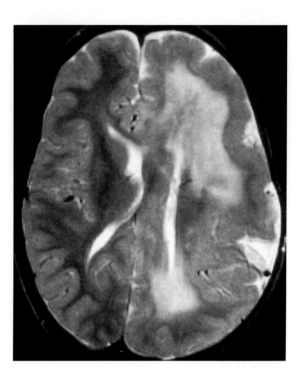

Unilateral megalencephaly is an uncommon neuronal migration abnormality extensively involving one hemisphere. The affected half of the cerebrum is enlarged, with widespread cortical thickening and hypertophied white matter. The cortical thickening may reflect pachygyria and/or polymicrogyria. White matter may be of normal signal intensity or variably dysplastic, demonstrating high intensity on T2-weighted images.

An important clue to the diagnosis in many cases is dilatation of the ipsilateral ventricle. Such ventricular enlargement is commonly associated with other neuronal migration disorders, as seen in the preceding pages. However, Case 739 demonstrates that ventricular expansion is not invariable in unilateral megalencephaly. The hemispheric enlargement and abnormal signal intensity within white matter may then suggest an infiltrating mass (see Cases 740 and 741).

The coronal scan of Case 739A documents asymmetry in the volume of the hemispheres. Bulky mass effect de-

forms the left frontal horn. Abnormal signal intensity is present in the left centrum semiovale.

The T2-weighted image in Case 739B provides key information by highlighting the abnormal thickness and contour of cortex over the left hemisphere. The pattern resembles the more common cortical dysplasias previously illustrated. Signal intensity within the dysmorphic cortical ribbon is normal. (Cortical calcification causes reduced signal intensity in occasional patients with unilateral megalencephaly.) However, the signal intensity of underlying white matter is distinctly abnormal, another common observation in cases of neuronal migration disorders (compare to Case 738).

Rare cases of tuberous sclerosis uniformly involving one cerebral hemisphere can demonstrate thick cortex, abnormal signal intensity of underlying white matter, and enlargement of the ipsilateral ventricle, resembling unilateral megalencephaly. Associated subependymal nodules usually establish the correct diagnosis in such patients.

Case 740

5-year-old girl with a history of seizures.
(axial, noncontrast scan; SE 2500/45)

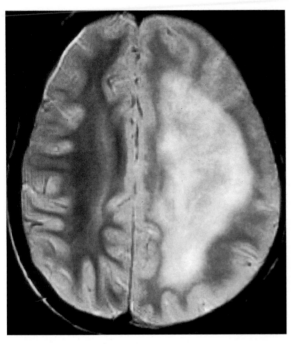

Unilateral Megalencephaly
(same patient as Case 739)

Case 741

45-year-old man presenting with worsening
hemiparesis.
(axial, noncontrast scan; SE 3000/45)

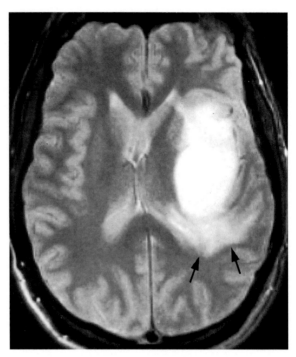

Grade III Astrocytoma

The large, confluent zone of abnormal signal intensity within the left hemisphere in Case 740 appears bulky and superficially resembles a midhemisphere mass like Case 741. As discussed on the preceding page, this presentation is within the spectrum of unilateral megalencephaly.

Clues to the diagnosis in Case 740 include (1) the increased volume of the involved hemicranium, suggesting a long-standing process; and (2) an association with dysplas-

tic cortex. The usual enlargement of the ipsilateral ventricle is not present in this case.

The glioma is Case 741 has arisen deep to the insula. Marked compression of the opercular region is present (compare the affected side to the normal right hemisphere). Edema is most extensive at the posterior pole of the mass *(arrows)*.

Case 742

8-year-old boy with a history of seizures and
"unilateral cerebral palsy."
(sagittal, noncontrast scan; SE 600/17)

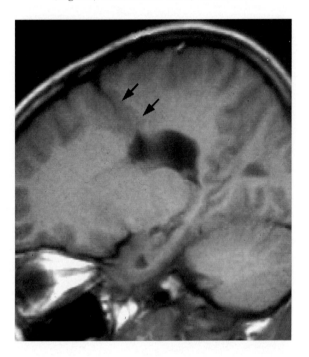

Case 743

4-year-old girl presenting with seizures
and right hemiparesis.
(axial, noncontrast scan; SE 2500/90)

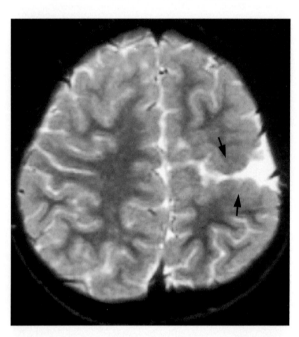

Schizencephaly is a disorder of neuronal migration characterized by a transcerebral cleft, usually extending from the lateral ventricle to the cerebral surface. Unlike encephaloclastic clefts from damage to normally formed parenchyma, schizencephalic clefts are lined by abnormal gray matter. This margin of transparenchymal cortex is clearly seen in the above cases *(arrows)*.

The clefts of schizencephaly may be unilateral or bilateral. They most frequently involve the midhemispheric region, near the central sulcus. Gray matter lining the margins of schizencephalic clefts usually demonstrates abnormal thickness and morphology. Polymicrogyria is common in these areas.

Schizencephalic clefts vary considerably in width. Many are broader than the examples above. In other cases, the margins of the clefts are closely opposed ("closed lip" schizencephaly; see Case 744).

Even narrow clefts are typically associated with small, CSF-containing diverticula at the ventricular and superficial margins of the lesion. These focal deformities of the subarachnoid space or the ventricular contour can be a clue to the presence of a largely closed cleft traversing the intervening cerebral tissue.

Case 744A

18-year-old man with a history of seizures.
(sagittal, noncontrast scan; SE 700/17)

Case 744B

Same patient.
(coronal, noncontrast scan; SE 2500/28)

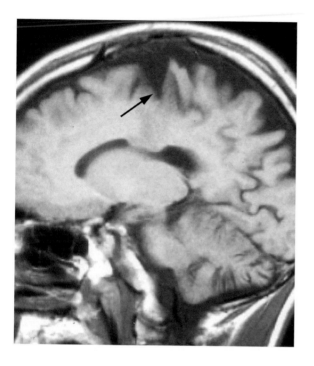

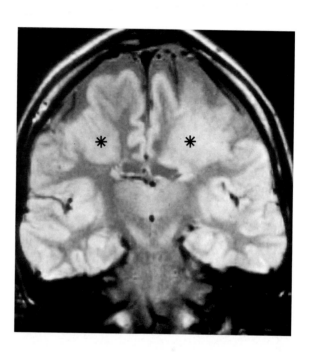

Schizencephalic clefts may be completely closed, with fusion of gray matter along the zone of disordered migration. Like localized cortical dysplasia (see Cases 737 and 738), these intraparenchymal "masses" may mimic a cerebral neoplasm. In such cases, the gray/white matter differentiation on MR scans helps to identify abnormalities of neuronal migration.

Case 744 demonstrates transcerebral columns of gray matter extending from the cerebral surface to the ventricular margin in the posterior frontal regions (asterisks, Case 744B). An associated diverticular deformity of the overlying cortical surface in Case 744A suggests a congenital lesion (arrow; compare to Case 737). Furthermore, the abnormality clearly traverses the entire thickness of the cerebral mantle, reaching and deforming the ventricular margin. Most importantly, the tissue along this band demonstrates the same signal intensity as cortical gray matter in other locations on both short and long TR pulse sequences.

A narrow schizencephalic cleft may be obscured on scans that are parallel or oblique to its plane. Multiplanar MR is more effective than CT for documenting schizencephaly by means of images that are perpendicular to the cleft. Even when a schizencephalic defect is completely closed, small diverticular deformities at the ventricular and/or cortical termination of the cleft provide a clue to the nature of the intervening abnormality.

Patients with schizencephaly often present with seizures. Focal neurological deficits may also occur, reflecting the location and size of the cleft.

Schizencephaly is accompanied by septooptic dysplasia in a large minority of cases. Evidence of one of these congenital malformations should prompt a search for the other.

Case 745

8-year-old boy presenting with seizures
and hemiparesis.
(axial, noncontrast scan; SE 3000/75)

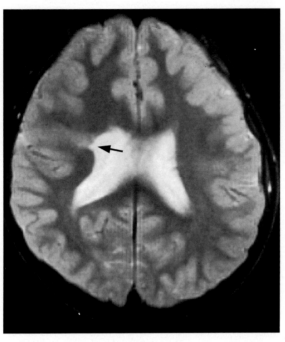

Schizencephaly
(same patient as Case 742)

Case 746

3-year-old boy presenting with
developmental delay.
(axial, noncontrast scan; SE 2800/90)

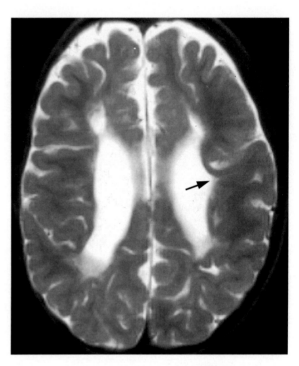

Periventricular Leukomalacia

As discussed in Cases 742-744, schizencephaly is frequently associated with a diverticular deformity at the ventricular end of the transparenchymal cleft. This focal irregularity is usually recognizable, even when the cleft itself has largely closed.

Case 745 illustrates this appearance. The localized outpouching along the lateral wall of the right lateral ventricle *(arrow)* is positioned at the base of a transhemispheric column of gray matter. (See Case 742 for better demonstration of the thin residual cleft in this patient.)

In Case 746, the focal irregularity of ventricular contours reflects localized damage to periventricular white matter. As

discussed in Cases 498-501, zones of necrosis and cavitation in periventricular leukomalacia may persist as independent cysts or coalesce with the ventricular chamber. In the latter circumstance, the lateral wall of the lateral ventricle becomes characteristically irregular and angular (see Cases 500 and 501 for other examples).

In both of the above cases, the lateral ventricles are abnormally large. Dysmorphic dilatation of ventricles commonly accompanies congenital malformations of the brain, and parenchymal loss regularly causes secondary ventricular expansion in periventricular leukomalacia. Hydrocephalus is not a consideration in either case.

BAND HETEROTOPIAS

Case 747A

15-year-old girl presenting with seizures.
(coronal, noncontrast scan; SE 2700/25)

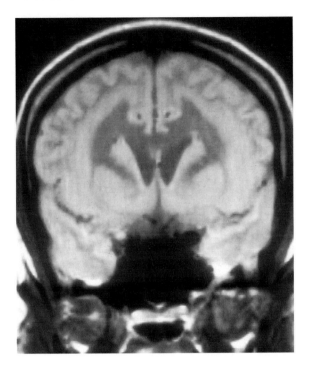

Case 747B

Same patient.
(axial, noncontrast scan; SE 2700/90)

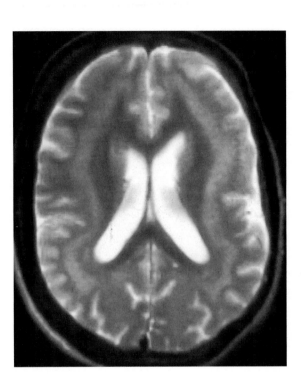

Disorders of the normal embryological migration of neurons from the germinal matrix to the cerebral cortex may take many forms. If neurons fail to leave the periventricular region, subependymal heterotopias are found (see Cases 748 and 749). If neurons fail to organize normally on reaching the surface of the brain, patterns such as pachygyria and polymicrogyria result (see Cases 732-736).

Band heterotopias represent a geographically intermediate form of neuronal migration abnormality. In these cases, waves of migrating neurons move outward from their periventricular origin but fail to reach the cerebral convexity. Instead, their migration is arrested at a location partway through the cerebral mantle. There they reside as "islands" or "bands," surrounded by midhemispheric white matter.

Like other disorders of neuronal migration, band heterotopias may be unilateral or bilateral, holohemispheric or localized. They may be centimeters thick or as thin as a millimeter.

Case 747 illustrates bilateral, symmetrically thick bands of heterotopic gray matter. These broad zones of neuronal tissue are clearly separated from the thin cerebral cortex by a narrow strip of subcortical white matter and from the lateral ventricles by a broader layer of myelinated parenchyma. Note that the midhemispheric band of abnormal tissue remains isointense to gray matter on all pulse sequences, the hallmark of heterotopic neurons.

Heterotopic gray matter within the centrum semiovale often has a more irregular and nodular morphology than the uniform bands in this case. Such islands are frequently round or amorphous in contour and markedly asymmetrical or unilateral.

Uniform and symmetrical band heterotopia like Case 747B may be misinterpreted as a leukodystrophy, since diffusely abnormal signal intensity extends throughout large regions of cerebral white matter.

Case 748

25-year-old woman with intractable seizures.
(coronal, noncontrast scan; magnetization-prepared
GRE sequence)

Case 749

4-year-old girl presenting with
developmental delay.
(axial, noncontrast scan; SE 2500/90)

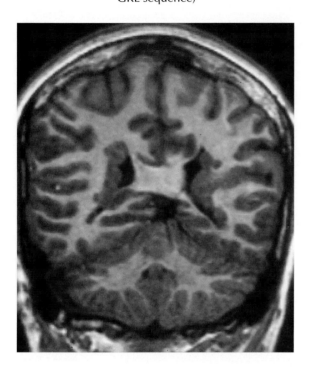

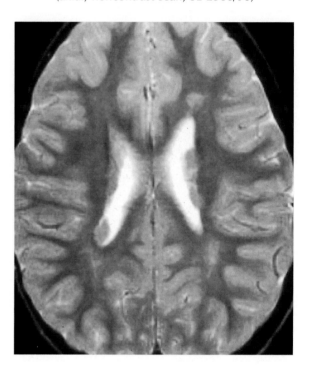

Nodules of heterotopic gray matter are commonly found along the margins of the lateral ventricles. This malformation results from an embryological failure of neurons to migrate away from the periventricular germinal matrix. The extent of involvement may vary from a few isolated nodules, as in Case 749, to a diffuse cobblestone pattern lining the ventricular wall, illustrated by Case 748. The findings may be bilaterally symmetrical or strikingly unilateral.

Isolated periventricular heterotopias are often discovered incidentally in patients with no associated symptoms. More extensive cases are usually correlated with seizures.

The key to correct identification of subependymal nodules as heterotopias is the signal intensity of the masses. They should match the intensity of normal gray matter on all pulse sequences, with no abnormal contrast enhancement. Cases 748 and 749 demonstrate this concordance.

Heavily T1-weighted gradient echo sequences with an initial inverting pulse or "magnetization preparation" accentuate the contrast between gray and white matter. Such techniques are useful for examining patients with seizures, since (1) the hippocampal formation is well defined (see discussion of mesial temporal sclerosis in Cases 450 and 451) and (2) gray matter heterotopias are sharply marginated, as in Case 748.

Case 750

5-month-old girl presenting with infantile spasms.
(coronal, noncontrast scan; SE 600/14)

Case 751

1-year-old boy with developmental delay.
(sagittal, noncontrast scan; SE 600/14)

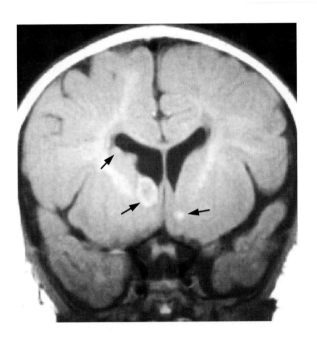

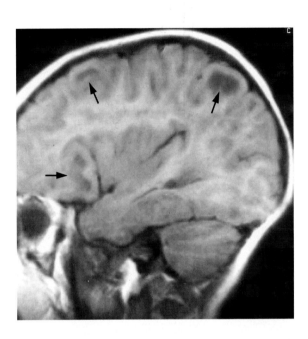

Tuberous sclerosis is one of the neurocutaneous syndromes or "neurophakomatoses," along with neurofibromatosis, Sturge-Weber syndrome, Von Hippel-Lindau disease, and ataxia telangiectasia. The disorder is inherited as an autosomal dominant trait with frequent sporadic cases. Clinical features include seizures, mental retardation, and a nodular facial rash ("adenoma sebaceum").

Hyperplastic nodules of malformed neuroglial tissue called "tubers" are commonly present along ventricular margins and within cerebral parenchyma. The characteristic subependymal nodules of tuberous sclerosis are well seen as irregularities along the ventricular margins on MR examinations. Unless there is degeneration into subependymal giant cell astrocytomas (see Cases 756 and 757), these lesions rarely exceed a few millimeters in diameter.

Subependymal nodules are often isointense on T1-weighted MR scans. In some cases, the characteristic calcification of periventricular tubers causes focal low intensity on T1-weighted images. In other instances, both subependymal and parenchymal nodules demonstrate T1-

shortening, as in Case 750 *(arrows)*. The etiology of this high intensity on T1-weighted scans is not established; fine matrix mineralization (e.g., calcium phosphate) or disordered accumulation of myelin-like lipids may play a role.

Parenchymal hamartomas in tuberous sclerosis are often larger than the subependymal nodules. The interface between cortex and subcortical white matter is a common location for such tubers. Case 751 illustrates several typical lesions *(arrows)*, demonstrating that the malformations may be clearly defined by long T1 values. More commonly, hemispheric lesions in tuberous sclerosis are relatively inapparent on T1-weighted scans (and on CT studies), with much greater conspicuity on T2-weighted images (see Cases 760-762).

Tuberous sclerosis is a common cause of infantile spasms and should be considered in this clinical context. Characteristic periventricular and parenchymal lesions on MR scans usually enable diagnosis well before specific clinical findings or CT calcifications are apparent.

DIFFERENTIAL DIAGNOSIS:
PERIVENTRICULAR NODULES

Case 752

4-year-old girl presenting with seizures.
(sagittal, noncontrast scan; SE 600/14)

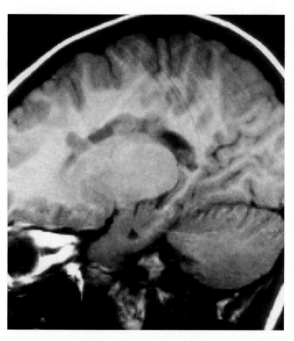

Heterotopic Gray Matter

Case 753

10-month-old girl presenting with "spasms."
(sagittal, noncontrast scan; SE 600/17)

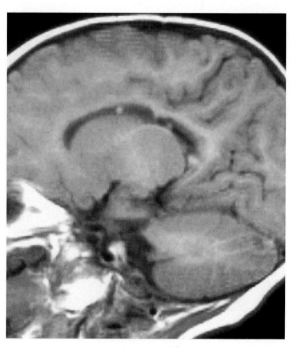

Tuberous Sclerosis

Both heterotopic gray matter and tuberous sclerosis may cause subependymal nodules in patients with seizures. Periventricular islands of heterotopic gray matter are usually larger and more amorphous than uncomplicated subependymal nodules in tuberous sclerosis, as seen above.

More importantly, the signal intensity of heterotopic gray matter matches that of cerebral cortex, while the subependymal lesions of tuberous sclerosis do not. (As discussed on the preceding page, subependymal tubers may demonstrate short, long, or intermediate T1 values.) This distinction is also apparent in the above examples.

Associated developmental anomalies (e.g., agenesis of the corpus callosum or absence of the septum pellucidum) may accompany heterotopic gray matter, confirming the diagnosis of congenital malformation.

The presence of calcification within subependymal lesions is common on CT studies of older children and adults with tuberous sclerosis. This finding is not seen in nodules of heterotopic gray matter. However, subependymal calcifications can also result from prior cerebral inflammation (e.g., congenital infection with CMV or toxoplasmosis).

Calcified tubers are usually larger and fewer than the periventricular calcifications of inflammatory disease. Congenital inflammatory disorders are also usually associated with parenchymal damage (e.g., microcephaly in CMV) and/or hydrocephalus (commonly occurring in toxoplasmosis), which would be unusual in cases of tuberous sclerosis.

DIFFERENTIAL DIAGNOSIS:
FOCAL SUPERFICIAL MASS IN A CHILD

Case 754

2-year-old girl presenting with seizures.
(sagittal, noncontrast scan; SE 600/20)

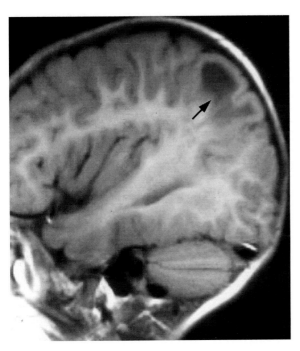

Tuberous Sclerosis

Case 755

6-year-old boy presenting with the new onset
of seizures.
(axial, postcontrast scan; SE 500/11)

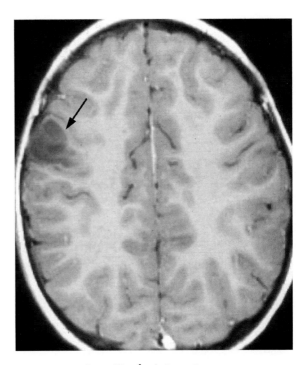

Low Grade Astrocytoma

Tuberous sclerosis can mimic a number of other pathologies, including heterotopic gray matter (see Cases 752 and 753), demyelinating disease (see Cases 762 and 763), and focal mass lesions, as illustrated above.

The cortical/subcortical "tuber" in Case 754 is similar in size, shape, location, definition, and signal intensity to the superficial glioma in Case 755. (See Cases 72 and 73 for discussion of cortical gliomas in children.) Both pathologies can involve cortex as well as subcortical white matter. Neither demonstrates abnormal contrast enhancement.

When a focal superficial lesion is encountered, a search for potential corollary findings of tuberous sclerosis is indicated. These include subependymal nodules, other hemispheric tubers, and lines or wedges of abnormal signal intensity extending radially from the ventricular wall to the cerebral surface (see Case 760). The clinical context (e.g., duration of seizures, presence or absence of associated retardation) may help to categorize cases with ambiguous scan findings.

Case 756

6-month-old boy presenting with seizures.
(axial, noncontrast scan; SE 1000/20)

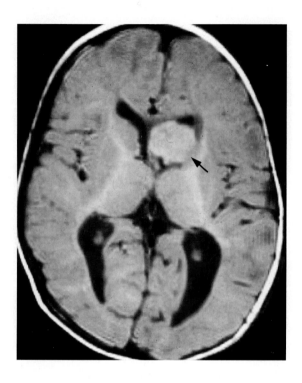

Case 757

16-year-old boy being followed with known
tuberous sclerosis.
(coronal, postcontrast scan; SE 1000/17)

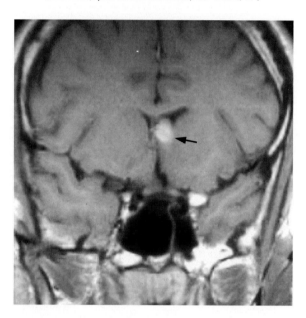

Subependymal nodules in tuberous sclerosis commonly occur near the foramina of Monro. Tubers in this location are prone to degenerate into subependymal giant cell astrocytomas, as illustrated above.

These low grade gliomas are often large, fleshy, lobulated masses. They demonstrate benign growth characteristics but may cause obstructive hydrocephalus because of their strategic location. Recurrence is rare, and prognosis is good after surgical resection.

Transformation of a benign subependymal nodule into a giant cell astrocytoma is suggested by increasing size and contrast enhancement. A lesion as large as the mass in Case 756 should be suspected of neoplastic degeneration. The differential diagnosis in such cases includes other periventricular or intraventricular tumors, as discussed on the next page.

Contrast enhancement is rarely observed in benign subependymal tubers on CT scans, so the presence of this CT finding suggests possible astrocytoma. The distinction is less clear on MR exams, which are more sensitive to small amounts of enhancement. Many static subependymal nodules do enhance on MR studies. However, prominent and/or increasing enhancement (as in Case 757) should raise the question of astrocytic transformation.

Case 758

25-year-old woman complaining
of explosive headaches.
(coronal, postcontrast scan; SE 600/14)

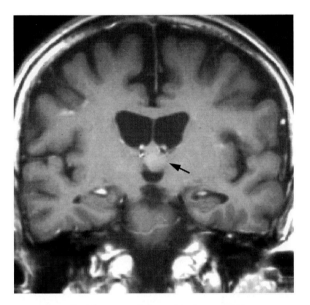

Colloid Cyst of the Third Ventricle

Case 759

3-year-old girl presenting with behavioral changes.
(axial, noncontrast scan; SE 2500/30)

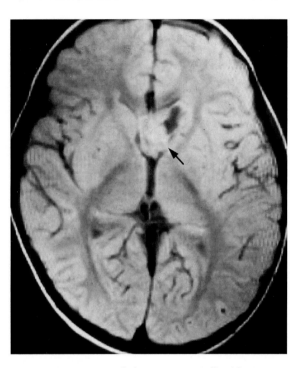

Astrocytoma of the Septum Pellucidum

Subependymal giant cell astrocytomas in tuberous sclerosis characteristically occur at the foramina of Monro, as illustrated on the preceding page. However, a number of other masses may present in this region.

Colloid cysts of the third ventricle can be identified by their origin from the third ventricular roof and their midline location. (Compare the level of the mass in Case 758 to Case 757, and note the slightly more lateral position of the giant cell astrocytoma.) The usual lack of abnormal contrast enhancement also distinguishes colloid cysts from most other neoplasms.

The glioma in Case 759 infiltrates and thickens the septum pellucidum. Like Case 758, this is a midline mass, contrasting with the typical origin of subependymal tubers and giant cell astrocytomas from the *lateral* margin of the foramen of Monro.

See Cases 103, 104, 115, 118, and 310 for other examples of gliomas involving the frontal horns of the lateral ventricles. The differential diagnosis includes intraventricular growth of a subependymal astrocytoma or oligodendroglioma, ependymoma, and subependymoma. Central neurocytomas may occur in the frontal region, as can subependymal metastases. The location is unusual but not impossible for intraventricular meningiomas (see Case 267) or choroid plexus papillomas (see Case 302). AVMs and rare inflammatory granulomas are nonneoplastic masses that can present along the ventricular margin.

Case 760

12-year-old girl presenting with seizures.
(axial, noncontrast scan; SE 2500/30)

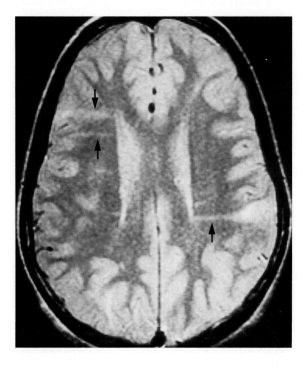

Case 761

5-month-old girl presenting with infantile spasms.
(axial, noncontrast scan; SE 2800/90)

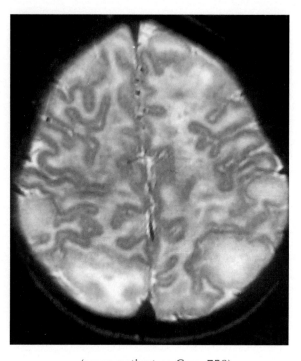

(same patient as Case 750)

Hemispheric lesions in tuberous sclerosis are more apparent on T2-weighted MR scans than on T1-weighted images or CT studies.

Case 760 illustrates multiple linear areas of high signal intensity extending from the ventricular margin to the cortical surface *(arrows)*. These striations are oriented along the direction of neuronal migration and have been termed "migration lines." Some of these rays lead to cortical/subcortical hamartomas. The finding likely reflects a combination of neuronal heterotopia, disordered myelination, and gliosis. The presence of one or more radial migration lines is highly suggestive of tuberous sclerosis.

More nodular parenchymal lesions in tuberous sclerosis are also due to heterotopic islands of abnormal neurons associated with localized demyelination and gliosis. Calcifi-

cation is occasionally seen in these foci. Abnormal contrast enhancement is rare.

Many parenchymal nodules are centered in subcortical white matter, as illustrated in Case 761 (compare to Case 754). Several of these superficial "tubers" are truly "potato-like," with expansion of gyri. Although the signal intensity of the lesions is only slightly higher than adjacent unmyelinated white matter, they are identifiable because of anatomical distortion. Subcortical tubers in older children and adults are often more sharply marginated (see Case 762).

The above cases illustrate that white matter lesions in tuberous sclerosis may have irregular, stellate morphology or rounded, mass-like contours. They are typically one or two centimeters in diameter, considerably larger than accompanying subependymal nodules.

DIFFERENTIAL DIAGNOSIS:
PATCHY LESIONS WITHIN CEREBRAL WHITE MATTER

Case 762

2-year-old boy presenting with seizures.
(coronal, noncontrast scan; SE 2500/45)

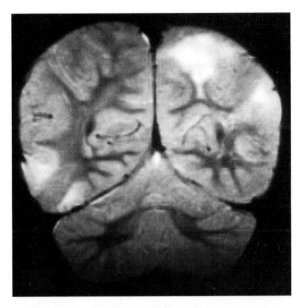

Tuberous Sclerosis

Case 763

14-year-old boy presenting with decreasing
mental status.
(axial, noncontrast scan; SE 2500/90)

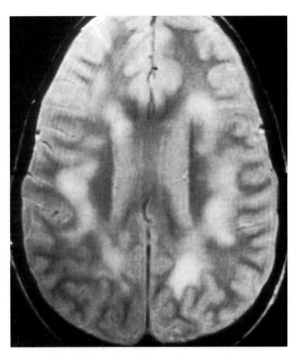

Acute Disseminated Encephalomyelitis

The patchy morphology and multiplicity of hemispheric lesions in tuberous sclerosis may resemble an inflammatory process or demyelinating disease. It is important to realize that the large, irregular subcortical white matter abnormalities in Case 762 fall within the spectrum of tuberous sclerosis. Attention to possible associated findings (e.g., subependymal nodules or migration lines) and clinical context can prevent unwarranted evaluation for leukoencephalopathy or systemic disease.

The superficial lesions of tuberous sclerosis are often more peripheral (with more cortical involvement) than demyelinating or dysmyelinating foci. In Case 763, patchy areas of signal abnormality are concentrated in central white matter, with less involvement of subarcuate fibers. Hemispheric hamartomas in tuberous sclerosis are often more mass-like than inflammatory foci, but this is not a reliable diagnostic criterion.

Cerebral vasculitis (see Case 503), mitochondrial encephalomyopathies (see Case 447), or systemic lupus erythematosus (see Cases 431 and 432) could cause multifocal lesions with combined cortical and subcortical involvement similar to Case 762. Acuity of symptoms and systemic manifestations usually distinguish these entities from tuberous sclerosis.

Case 764

4-year-old girl.
(axial, noncontrast scan; SE 2500/90)

Case 765

7 year old girl.
(axial, noncontrast scan; SE 3000/120)

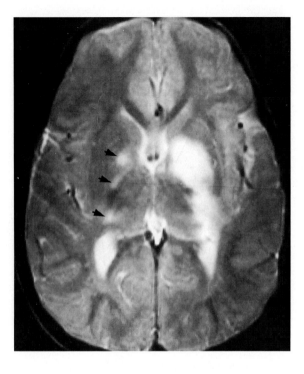

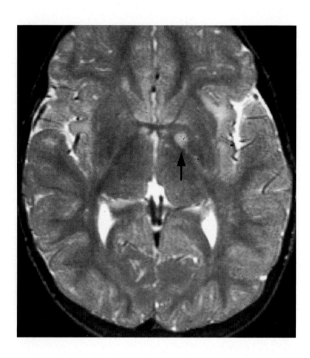

The intracranial, orbital, and spinal tumors commonly associated with neurofibromatosis are discussed in Chapters 3, 4, 13, and 15. Non-neoplastic abnormalities may also be encountered on MR scans of patients with this diagnosis.

Zones of high signal intensity on long TR images occurring deep within the cerebral hemispheres are common in children with type 1 neurofibromatosis. The basal ganglia and internal capsule are frequently involved.

These areas most often represent disordered or retarded myelination and/or hamartomatous maldevelopment, analogous to the parenchymal abnormalities of tuberous sclerosis. Most such lesions are not neoplastic and do not enlarge over time. In fact, some have been observed to disappear during years of follow-up.

However, the possibility of a developing astrocytoma warrants close observation of any patient with neurofibromatosis whose MR scan demonstrates areas of abnormal

signal intensity. Increasing size and contrast enhancement of a lesion suggest neoplasia rather than malformation (comparable to the assessment of subependymal nodules in tuberous sclerosis).

The benign deep hemispheric zones of T2-prolongation common in neurofibromatosis type 1 demonstrate variable size, multiplicity, and symmetry, as illustrated above. In Case 764, abnormality within the left basal ganglia is confluent and impressive, while smaller foci of high signal intensity are present on the right *(arrows)*. Case 765 demonstrates a small focus of abnormal intensity within the left globus pallidus *(arrow)*, which is a common site for such findings.

Neurofibromatosis should be considered among the etiologies of unilateral or bilateral ganglionic lesions (together with various anoxic, toxic, and metabolic disorders; see Cases 439, 440, 443, 444, 447, and 554).

Case 766

8-year-old girl presenting with optic gliomas.
(axial, noncontrast scan; SE 2500/100)

Case 767

7-year-old girl.
(axial, noncontrast scan; SE 3000/120)

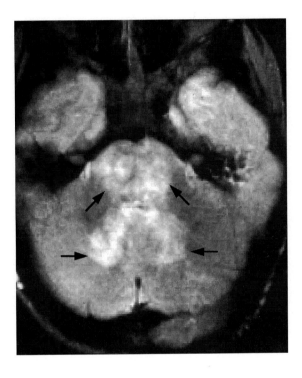

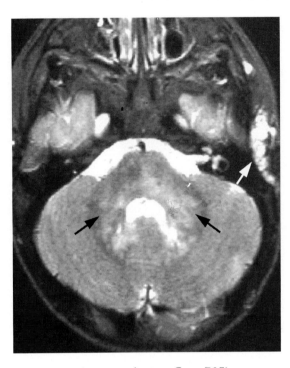

(same patient as Case 765)

The brainstem and cerebellar peduncles are other locations where non-neoplastic zones of signal abnormality commonly occur in type 1 neurofibromatosis.

The scan in Case 766 is degraded by patient motion, but extensive areas of high intensity are apparent throughout the pons and posterolateral to the fourth ventricle *(arrows)*. There was no associated mass effect or abnormal contrast enhancement. The abnormalities became progressively less conspicuous on follow-up scans over a four-year period. This course indicates that the widespread prolongation of T2 in Case 766 likely represents disordered development or immaturity of tissue that becomes more normal with age. However, the possibility of a low grade brainstem glioma must be considered when such a scan is first encountered.

Case 767 demonstrates smaller patches of signal abnormality in approximately the same distribution. In an ambiguous clinical context, this appearance could be mistaken for multifocal inflammatory disease involving the brainstem (e.g., acute disseminated encephalomyelitis or multiple sclerosis). Associated findings may help to establish the diagnosis in such cases; a subcutaneous plexiform neurofibroma is present in the left temporal region in Case 767 *(white arrow)*.

Focal or patchy areas of signal abnormality on long TR spin echo images like the lesions in Cases 764 through 767 may also be seen in the thalamus, corpus callosum, and centrum semiovale of patients with neurofibromatosis type 1.

Case 768

19-year-old man presenting with seizures.
(coronal, noncontrast scan; SE 2800/90)

Case 769

40 year old man with a history of seizures.
(coronal, noncontrast scan; SE 2600/90)

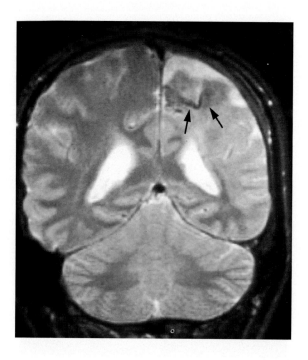

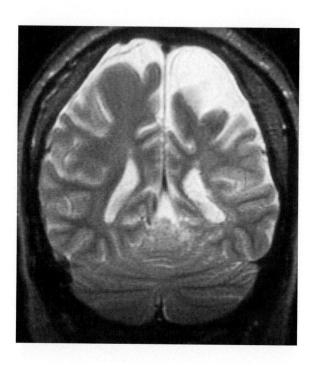

Sturge-Weber syndrome is one of the neurophakomatoses combining cutaneous and intracranial abnormalities. The external manifestation of the syndrome is a unilateral facial hemangioma or "port-wine stain" in the distribution of a division of the trigeminal nerve. This hallmark is associated with an ipsilateral venous angioma of the meninges, most common in the parietooccipital region. (An alternative name for the syndrome is "encephalotrigeminal angiomatosis.")

Cerebral cortex underlying the meningeal angioma of Sturge-Weber syndrome exhibits a characteristic "tram-track" pattern of dystrophic calcification, easily appreciated on skull films or CT scans. The calcification may be observed to develop in an infant or toddler over a period of weeks or months. (Gyriform calcification is a nonspecific response to cortical damage and can also be seen in children following encephalitis or meningitis, after treatment for CNS leukemia, and in association with disorders of neuronal migration.)

On noncontrast MR scans there may be little or no evidence of the meningeal angioma. Cortical calcification (and/or associated iron deposition) may be apparent as hazy regions of low intensity, seen in Case 768 (arrows). Vague low signal intensity may also be present within white matter in affected areas on T2-weighted scans.

Cerebral atrophy is commonly associated with Sturge-Weber syndrome and may be focal or hemispheric. Both of the above cases demonstrate reduced volume of the left parietal lobe. In Case 768, the volume of the left hemicranium is smaller than the right, with eccentric position of the falx. In Case 769, asymmetrical thickening of the calvarium on the left reflects a history of reduced volume within the left hemicranium. Sturge-Weber syndrome is one etiology for the Dyke-Davidoff-Masson syndrome, discussed in Case 541.

Case 770A

40-year-old man with a history of seizures.
(coronal, postcontrast scan; SE 600/20)

Case 770B

Same patient.
(coronal, postcontrast scan; SE 600/20)

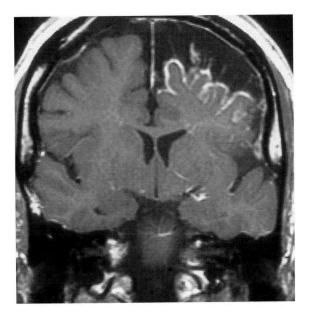

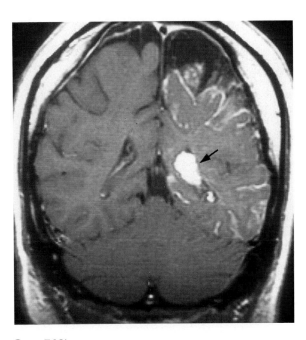

(same patient as Case 769)

A number of abnormalities may be demonstrated on postcontrast MR scans in patients with Sturge-Weber syndrome.

The meningeal angioma covering the surface of the small left hemisphere is seen as a superficial layer of enhancement in the above images. Abnormal leptomeningeal enhancement often extends beyond the area of cortical calcification and parenchymal atrophy (note the posterior temporal enhancement in Case 770B). Vascular congestion within the meninges reflecting the commonly associated abnormality of cortical venous drainage probably contributes to this diffuse involvement. In any event, Sturge-Weber syndrome should be included in the differential diagnosis of leptomeningeal enhancement (along with meningeal inflammation, neoplasm, and hyperemia).

Intense, confluent enhancement is present within choroid plexus of the left lateral ventricle in Case 770B *(arrow)*. An angioma of the ipsilateral choroid plexus is commonly associated with other findings of the Sturge-Weber syndrome. By itself, this lesion could be mistaken for a trigone meningioma (see Cases 64 and 65) or another intraventricular tumor.

Large superficial and deep veins are often seen in the region involved by Sturge-Weber syndrome. These hypertrophied and/or aberrant channels reflect associated abnormality of cortical venous drainage, with collateral flow away from the superior sagittal sinus.

Seizures are almost always a dominant feature in the clinical presentation of patients with Sturge-Weber syndrome.

Case 771

Newborn boy.
(sagittal, noncontrast scan; SE 600/14)

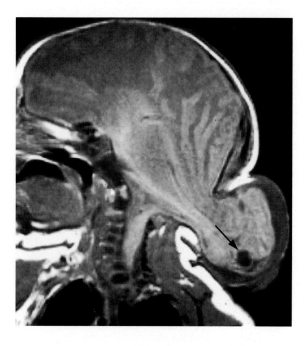

Case 772

1-day-old girl.
(sagittal, noncontrast scan; SE 600/14)

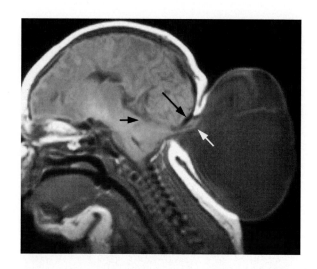

Encephaloceles are extracranial extensions of brain tissue, most commonly encountered along the skull base. Potential locations include the nose, sphenoid sinus, petrous bones, occipital region, and parietal bones. Frontonasal, parietal, and occipital meningoceles or encephaloceles are usually apparent at birth. Cephaloceles in the sphenoid or temporal region of the skull base are much more occult, often not presenting or detected until adulthood (see Cases 775 and 776).

MR is the modality of choice for noninvasive evaluation of congenital cephaloceles. Scans clearly document whether the extracranial sac is filled with brain tissue, as in Case 771, or largely contains CSF, as in Case 772.

A small amount of cerebellar parenchyma enters the superior margin of the encephalocele in Case 772 *(white arrow)*. The more amorphous zones of intermediate signal intensity in the superior portion of the encephalocele sac are artifactual.

MR scans can also demonstrate the presence of "flow void" indicating major vascular structures within cephalo-cele sacs. This is particularly relevant to the evaluation of occipital encephaloceles, which develop near major dural sinuses. In Case 771, a large vessel is imaged in cross section at the posteroinferior margin of the herniation *(arrow)*. A venous sinus is present immediately superior to the herniating cerebellar tissue in Case 772 *(long black arrow)*.

Both of the above cases demonstrate distorted morphology of intracranial parenchyma as it is pulled in the direction of the encephalocele. This traction pattern remains as evidence of the congenital malformation even after a cephalocele has been repaired.

Associated hindbrain malformations are present in the above patients. Deformed cerebellar tissue extends into the cervical spinal canal in Case 771. "Beaking" of the midbrain tectum is seen in Case 772 *(short black arrow)*. This combination of Chiari type II hindbrain deformities with an occipital and/or high cervical encephalocele is often referred to as a "Chiari III" malformation.

DIFFERENTIAL DIAGNOSIS:
EXTRACRANIAL OCCIPITAL CYST IN AN INFANT

Case 773

8-month-old girl.
(axial, noncontrast scan; SE 2500/90)

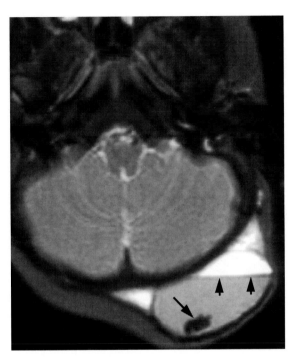

Cystic Hygroma

Case 774

1-day-old girl.
(axial, noncontrast scan; SE 1000/15)

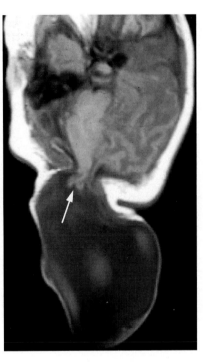

Encephalocele
(same patient as Case 772)

Not all cystic masses at the skull base are meningoceles or encephaloceles. The lesion in Case 773 *is* clearly cystic, containing a prominent sedimentation level *(arrowheads)* as well as a dependent concretion *(arrow)*. However, this mass did not communicate with the intracranial compartment at any scan level.

Cystic hygromas are loculated collections of serosanguineous fluid resulting from malformation and dilatation of cervical lymphatic channels. They usually arise in the posterior triangle of the neck but can enlarge along the skull base, as in Case 773.

Meningoceles and encephaloceles commonly involve the occipital bone. Such lesions may be associated with other congenital abnormalities, such as the Dandy-Walker malformation or Chiari hindbrain deformities.

Case 774 is an axial scan of the encephalocele illustrated in Case 772. Although substantial head tilt is present, the small tongue of cerebellar tissue entering the cephalocele sac is clearly defined *(arrow)*. (The areas of intermediate intensity within the center of the sac are artifactual.) Notice the very narrow infratentorial compartment and steeply sloping tentorium (compare to Case 717).

Case 775

71-year-old woman presenting with a one-year history of CSF rhinorrhea.
(coronal, noncontrast scan; SE 1000/22)

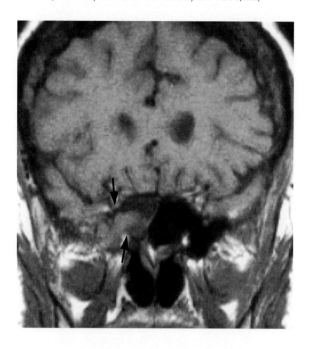

Case 776

45-year-old woman presenting with seizures.
(coronal, postcontrast scan; SE 600/14)

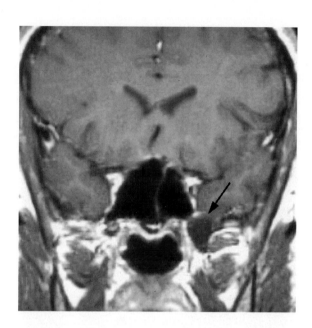

Transphenoidal meningoceles or encephaloceles are often initially occult. Midline sphenoidal encephaloceles may present in adolescence or childhood with nasopharyngeal obstruction, impaired vision, or reduced endocrine function. The latter symptoms are due to dysfunction of the optic apparatus and/or hypothalamic/pituitary axis caused by inferior displacement or traction of these structures. Parasagittal sphenoidal cephaloceles are more likely to present with meningitis, CSF rhinorrhea, or seizures, as in the above cases.

The scan in Case 775 demonstrates medial temporal gyri extending into the right side of the sphenoid sinus through a deficient lateral wall *(arrow)*. The remainder of the sinus is filled with CSF. Communication of the sphenoid sinus with the nose provides a route for CSF rhinorrhea and potential meningitis.

The cephalocele sac in Case 776 is more subtle, occurring in the left pterygoid region *(arrow)*. Meningoceles or

encephaloceles involving the medial portion of the middle cranial fossa are often associated with distortion and scarring of the adjacent temporal lobe. This parenchymal abnormality may present clinically as seizures. As a result, small lateral sphenoidal or petrous cephaloceles are among the lesions to be sought on coronal scans of epileptic patients.

The cephalocele sac in Case 776 is filled with CSF and demonstrated high signal intensity on a T2-weighted scan. This appearance had initially been interpreted as a schwannoma near the foramen ovale. Although uniform prolongation of T2 is common in schwannomas (see Case 179), the alternative possibility of a CSF-containing sac should be considered when such a lesion is encountered along the skull base. The lack of contrast enhancement within a cephalocele can distinguish it from a solid mass in otherwise ambiguous cases.

Case 777A

64-year-old man with a long history of nasal
obstruction on the right.
(axial, noncontrast scan; SE 3000/90)

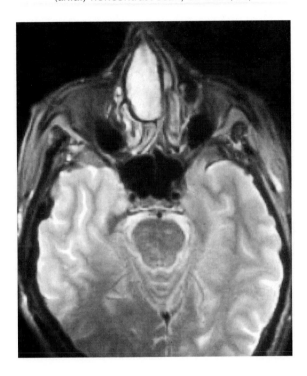

Case 777B

Same patient.
(sagittal, noncontrast scan; SE 850/20)

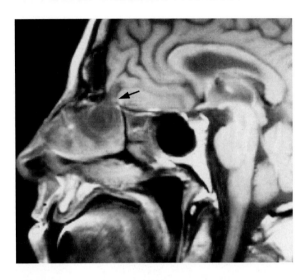

The smoothly rounded mass within the right nasal cavity in Case 777A appears to be long-standing. There is associated deviation of the nasal septum and deformity of the ipsilateral turbinates.

This appearance should raise the possibility of a nasoethmoidal encephalocele. Biopsy or removal of such masses carries the risk of CSF leak and meningitis. Important vessels or functional neural tissue may extend into the encephalocele and be susceptible to surgical injury.

Discovery of a soft tissue mass beneath the skull base warrants a careful search for bone defects or anatomical distortions linking the lesion with the intracranial compartment. In Case 777B, a defect along the floor of the anterior cranial fossa is apparent in the cribiform region *(arrow)*. The crista galli is poorly seen and presumably displaced and/or eroded. There is continuity of soft tissue between a small intracranial component and the larger intranasal mass.

Note that gyri and sulci of the frontal lobe are not pulled toward the encephalocele in this case (compare to Cases 771 and 772). Surgery confirmed an encephalocele containing dysplastic glial tissue.

Dermal sinus tracts may also span the skull base with nasal and intracranial components. However, dermal sinuses are usually not associated with significant widening of the foramen cecum and erosion or displacement of the crista galli, as is characteristic of nasoethmoidal cephaloceles.

Occasionally the stalk connecting a nasal encephalocele with its origin in the anterior cranial fossa is obliterated. The resulting island of glial tissue within the nose is often called a "nasal glioma."

Both encephaloceles and dermal sinuses involving the nasoethmoid region may predispose to isolated or recurrent meningitis.

Case 778A

6-month-old girl with a soft lump on the back
of the head.
(sagittal, noncontrast scan; SE 600/14)

Case 778B

Same patient.
(axial, noncontrast scan; SE 2800/90)

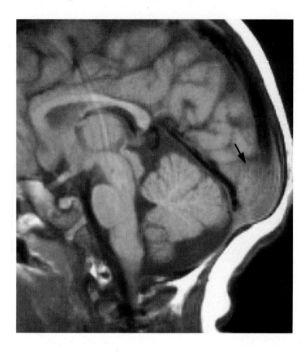

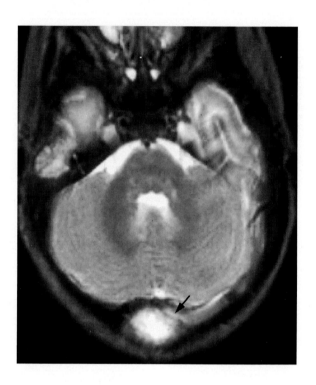

Failure of dysjunction of cutaneous and neuroectoderm leads to a dermal sinus tract from the skin surface to (or through) the dura. The spinal form of this embryological malformation is relatively common; see Cases 1089 and 1090 for discussion of the "dorsal dermal sinus syndrome."

Transcranial dermal sinuses also occur, typically in the midline. Common locations include the frontonasal region, the vertex, and the occipital area. Such sinuses may be associated with epidermoid or dermoid cysts in the epidural or intradural spaces.

Case 778 demonstrates a homogeneous midline lesion located predominantly posterior to the torcular herophili. The occipital bone overlying the mass is markedly thinned or absent. (CT would offer a better assessment of osseous deformity.)

The signal intensity of the lesion (intermediate T1 values, long T2 values) is nonspecific. Epidermoid cysts usually demonstrate lower intensity on T1-weighted scans than seen in Case 778A. However, superimposed inflammatory changes due to an associated sinus tract may modify the classic appearance. As discussed in Cases 286-289, the signal intensity of dermoid cysts is variable. Relevant factors include (1) the proportion of proteinaceous content versus lipid material, (2) the presence or absence of simple fluid (see Case 779), and (3) the presence or absence of superimposed infection.

It is important to consider dermal sinus tracts and associated dermoid or epidermoid cysts along with cephaloceles in the differential diagnosis of small, midline transcranial lesions. Both pathologies commonly involve the frontonasal and occipital regions. Traction of intracranial parenchyma toward the calvarial defect favors a cephalocele. Conversely, dermal sinuses often lead to epidural or intradural masses that displace cerebral tissue away from the skull.

Case 779A

9-month-old girl with a progressively enlarging
lump on the head.
(coronal, postcontrast scan; SE 600/14)

Case 779B

Same patient.
(axial, noncontrast scan; SE 2800/90)

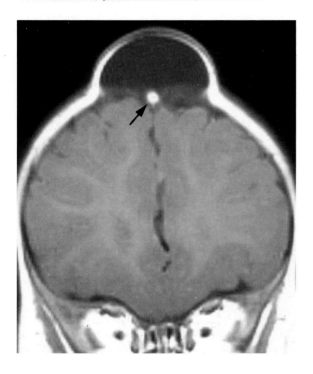

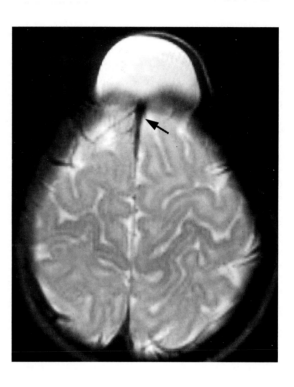

Dermoid cysts are the most common cause of a scalp mass in an infant. They are particularly frequent near the anterior fontanelle and along the course of cranial sutures. Associated dermal sinuses and intracranial extension commonly accompany lesions near the nasion and torcular (see Case 778) but rarely occur with dermoid cysts overlying the sagittal suture.

The extracranial mass in Case 779 had been observed to enlarge steadily since the newborn period. Such rapid growth would be unusual for the slow accumulation of semisolid material within a dermoid or epidermoid cyst. However, the coronal scan in Case 779A clearly indicates that the lesion is superficial to the normally formed dura and superior sagittal sinus *(arrow)*, excluding a meningocele.

At surgery, the mass proved to be a fluid-filled dermoid cyst within the scalp. A small amount of granular, greasy material was also present within the cyst.

This case demonstrates that dermoid cysts occasionally accumulate aqueous fluid. Together, Cases 778 and 779 illustrate that dermoid or epidermoid cysts may cause midline extracranial or transcranial masses clinically resembling cephaloceles.

In addition to dermoid cysts and encephaloceles, the differential diagnosis of a lump on the head of a child includes cephalohematoma, subgaleal hematoma, hemangioma, lymphangioma, neurofibroma, eosinophilic granuloma, osteoma, and sinus pericranii.

REFERENCES

Aboulezz AO, Sartor K, Geyer CA, et al: Position of cerebellar tonsils in the normal population and in patients with Chiari malformation: a quantitative approach with MR imaging. *J Comput Assist Tomogr* 1033-1036, 1985.

Altman NR, Purser RK, Post MJD: Tuberous sclerosis: characteristics at CT and MR imaging. *Radiology* 167:527-532, 1988.

Aoki S, Barkovich AJ, Nishimura K, et al: Neurofibromatosis types 1 and 2: cranial MR findings. *Radiology* 172:527-534, 1989.

Armonda RA, Citrin CM, Foley KT, Ellenbogen RG: Quantitative cine-mode magnetic resonance imaging of Chiari I malformations: an analysis of cerebrospinal fluid dynamics. *Neurosurgery* 35:214-224, 1994.

Atlas SW, Zimmerman RA, Bilaniuk LT, et al: Corpus callosum and limbic system: Neuroanatomic MR evaluation of developmental anomalies. *Radiology* 160:355-362, 1986.

Barkovich AJ: Apparent atypical callosal dysgenesis: analysis of MR findings in six cases and their relationship to holoprosencephaly. *AJNR* 11:333-339, 1990.

Barkovich AJ, Chuang SH, Norman D: MR of neuronal migration anomalies. *AJNR* 8:1009-1017, 1987.

Barkovich AJ, Fram EK, Norman D: Septo-optic dysplasia: MR imaging. *Radiology* 171:189-192, 1989.

Barkovich AJ, Gressens P, Evrard, P: Formation, maturation, and disorders of brain neocortex. *AJNR* 13:423-446, 1992.

Barkovich AJ, Jackson DE Jr, Boyer RS: Band heterotopias: a newly recognized neuronal migration anomaly. *Radiology* 171:455-458, 1989.

Barkovich AJ, Kjos BO: Nonlissencephalic cortical dysplasias: correlation of imaging findings with clinical deficits. *AJNR* 13:95-103, 1992.

Barkovich AJ, Kjos BO: Schizencephaly: correlation of clinical findings with MR characteristics. *AJNR* 13:85-94, 1992.

Barkovich AJ, Norman D: Absence of the septum pellucidum: a useful sign in the diagnosis of congenital brain malformations. *AJNR* 9:1107-1114, 1988.

Barkovich AJ, Norman D: Anomalies of the corpus callosum: correlation with further anomalies of the brain. *AJNR* 9:493-501, 1988.

Barkovich AJ, Norman D: MR imaging of schizencephaly. *AJNR* 9:297-302, 1988.

Barkovich AJ, Quint DJ: Middle interhemispheric fusion: an unusual variant of holoprosencephaly. *AJNR* 14:431-440, 1993.

Barkovich AJ, Vandermarck P, Edwards MSB, Cagen PH: Congenital nasal masses: CT and imaging features in 16 cases. *AJNR* 12:105-116, 1991.

Barkovich AJ, Wippold FJ, Sherman JL, et al: Significance of cerebellar tonsillar position on MR. *AJNR* 7:795-799, 1986.

Benedikt RA, Brown DC, Ghaed VN, et al: Sturge-Weber syndrome: cranial MR imaging with Gd-DTPA. *AJNR* 14:409-415, 1993.

Berns DH, Masaryk TJ, Weisman B, et al: Tuberous sclerosis: increased MR detection using gradient echo techniques. *J Comput Assist Tomogr* 13:896-898, 1989.

Bilaniuk L, Zimmerman R, Hochman M, et al: MR of the Sturge-Weber syndrome. *AJNR* 8:945, 1987.

Bognanno JR, Edwards MK, Lee TA, et al: Cranial MR imaging in neurofibromatosis. *AJNR* 9:461-468, 1988.

Braffman BH, Bilaniuk LT, Naidich TP, et al: MR imaging of tuberous sclerosis: pathogenesis of this phakomatosis. Use of gadopentetate dimeglumine, and literature review. *Radiology* 183:227-238, 1992.

Braffman BH, Bilaniuk LT, Zimmerman RA: The central nervous system manifestation of the phakomatoses on MR. *Radiology* 26:773-800, 1988.

Braffman BH, Bilaniuk CT, Zimmerman RA: MR of central nervous

system neoplasia of the phakomatoses. *Sem Roentgenol* 25:198-217, 1990.

Byrd SE, Bohan TP, Osborn RE, Naidich TP: The CT and MR evaluation of lissencephaly. *AJNR* 9:923-927, 1988.

Byrd SE, Naidich TP: Common congenital brain anomalies. *Rad Clin North Am* 26:755-772, 1988.

Byrd SE, Osborn RE, Bohan TP, et al: CT and MR evaluation of migrational disorders of the brain. Part I. Lissencephaly and pachygyria. *Pediatr Radiol* 19:151, 1989.

Byrd SE, Osborn RE, Bohan TP, et al: CT and MR evaluation of migrational disorders of the brain. Part II. Schizencephaly, heterotopia, and polymicrogyria. *Pediatr Radiol* 19:219, 1989.

Byrd SE, Osborn RE, Radkowski MA, et al: Disorders of midline structures: holoprosencephaly, absence of corpus callosum and Chiari malformations. *Semin US CT MR* 9:201-215, 1988.

Castillo M: Congenital abnormalities of the nose: CT and MR findings. *AJR* 162:1211-1217, 1994.

Castillo M, Bouldin TW, Scatliff JH, Suzuki K: Radiologic-pathologic correlation. Alobar holoprosencephaly. *AJNR* 14:1151-1156, 1993.

Chamberlain M, Press G, Hesselink J: MR imaging and CT in Sturge-Weber syndrome. *AJNR* 10:491, 1989.

Curnes JT, Laster DW, Koubek TD, et al: MRI of corpus callosal syndromes. *AJNR* 7:617-622, 1986.

Curnes JT, Oakes W, Boyko OB: MR imaging of hindbrain deformity in patients with and without symptoms of brain stem compression. *AJNR* 10:293-302, 1989.

Dean B, Drayer BP, Berisini DC, Bird CR: MR imaging of pericallosal lipoma. *AJNR* 9:929-931, 1988.

De La Paz RL, Brady TJ, Buonanno FS, et al: Nuclear magnetic resonance (NMR) imaging of Arnold-Chiari type I malformation with hydromyelia. *J Comput Assist Tomogr* 7:126-129, 1983.

Diebler C, Dulac O: Cephaloceles: clinical and neuroradiologic appearance. *Neuroradiology* 25:199-216.

Dietrich RB, Kocit DD, et al: Lissencephaly: MR and CT appearances with different subtypes. *Radiology* 185(suppl):123, 1992.

Dunn V, Mock T, Bell WE, et al: Detection of heterotopic gray matter in children by magnetic resonance imaging. *Magn Reson Imaging* 4:33-39, 1986.

El Gammal T, Mark EK, Brooks BS: MR imaging of Chiari II malformation. *AJNR* 8:1037-1044, 1987.

Elster AD: Radiologic screening in the neurocutaneous syndromes: strategies and controversies. *AJNR* 13:1078-1082, 1992.

Elster AD, Chen MYM: Chiari I malformations: clinical and radiologic reappraisal. *Radiology* 183:347-353, 1992.

Elster AD, Chen MYM: MR imaging of Sturge Weber syndrome: role of gadopentetate dimeglumine and gradient echo techniques. *AJNR* 11:685-689, 1990.

Gallucci M, Bozzao A, Curatolo P, et al: MR imaging of incomplete band heterotopia. *AJNR* 12:701-702, 1991.

Georgy BA, Hesselink JR, Jernigan TL: MR imaging of the corpus callosum. *AJR* 160:949-955, 1993.

Hurst R, Newman S, Cail W: Multifocal intracranial MR abnormalities in neurofibromatosis. *AJNR* 9:293, 1988.

Inoue Y, Nakajima S, Fukuda T, et al: Magnetic resonance imaging of tuberous sclerosis: further observations and clinical correlations. *Neuroradiology* 30:379, 1988.

Iwasaki S, Nakagawa H, Kichikawa K, et al: MR and CT of tuberous sclerosis: linear abnormalities in the cerebral white matter. *AJNR* 11:1029-1034, 1990.

Jinkins JR, Whittemore AR, Bradley WG: MR imaging of callosal and corticocallosal dysgenesis. *AJNR* 10:339-344, 1989.

Kingsley D, Kendall B, Fitz C: Tuberous sclerosis: a clinicoradiological evaluation of 110 cases with particular reference to atypical presentation. *Neuroradiology* 28:171-190, 1986.

Kuzniecky R, Andermann F: The congenital bilateral perisylvian syndrome: imaging findings in a multicenter study. *AJNR* 15:139-144, 1994.

Lee BCP, Engle M: MR of lissencephaly. *AJNR* 9:804, 1988.

Lipski S, Brunelle F, Aicardi J, et al: Gd-DTPA-enhanced MR imaging in two cases of Sturge-Weber syndrome. *AJNR* 11:690-692, 1990.

Martinez-Lage JF, Sola J, Casas C, et al: Atretic cephalocele: the tip of the iceberg. *J Neurosurg* 77:230-235, 1992.

McLone DG, Naidich TP: Developmental morphology of the subarachnoid space, brain vasculature, and contiguous structures, and the cause of the Chiari II malformation. *AJNR* 13:463-482, 1992.

McMurdo SK Jr, Moore SG, Brant-Zawadzki M, et al: MR imaging of intracranial tuberous sclerosis. *AJNR* 8:77-82, 1987.

Menkes JH, Curran J: Clinical and MR correlates in children with extra-pyramidal cerebral palsy. *AJNR* 15:451-458, 1994.

Menor F, Marti-Bonmati L: CT detection of basal ganglia lesions in neurofibromatosis type 1: correlation with MRI. *Neuroradiology* 34:305-307, 1992.

Menor F, Marti-Bonmati L, Mulas F, et al: Imaging considerations of central nervous system manifestations in pediatric patients with neurofibromatosis type 1. *Pediatr Radiol* 21:389-394, 1991.

Menor F, Marti-Bonmati L, Mulas F, et al: Neuroimaging in tuberous sclerosis: a clinicoradiological evaluation in pediatric patients. *Pediatr Radiol* 22:485-489, 1992.

Mirowitz SA, Sarton K, Gado M: High-intensity basal ganglia lesions on T1-weighted MR images in neurofibromatosis. *AJNR* 10:1159-1163, 1989.

Mori K: Giant interhemispheric cysts associated with agenesis of the corpus callosum. *J Neurosurg* 76:224-230, 1992.

Naidich TP, Altman NR, Braffman BH, et al: Cephaloceles and related malformations. *AJNR* 13:655-690, 1992.

Nixon JR, Houser OW, Gomez MR, Okazaki H: Cerebral tuberous sclerosis: MR imaging. *Radiology* 170:869-874, 1989.

Noorani PA, Bodensteiner JB, Barnes PD: Colpocephaly: frequency and associated findings. *J Child Neurol* 3:100, 1988.

Osborn RE, Byrd SE, Naidich TP, et al: MR imaging of neuronal migrational disorders. *AJNR* 9:1101-1106, 1988.

Payner TD, Prenger E, Berger TS, Crone KR: Acquired Chiari malformations: incidence, diagnosis, and management: *Neurosurgery* 34:429-434, 1994.

Pillay PK, Awad IA, Little JR, Hahn JF: Symptomatic Chiari malformation in adults: a new classification based on magnetic resonance imaging with clinical and prognostic significance. *Neurosurgery* 28:639-645, 1991.

Poe LB, Coleman LL, Mahmud F: Congenital central nervous system abnormalities. *Radiographics* 9:801-826, 1989.

Pont MS, Elster AD: Lesions of skin and brain. Modern imaging of the neurocutaneous syndrome. *AJR* 158:1193-1203, 1992.

Raffel C, McComb JG, Bodner S, Gilles FE: Benign brain stem lesions in pediatric patients with neurofibromatosis: case reports. *Neurosurgery* 25:959-964, 1989.

Reinarz SJ, Coffman CE, Smoker WRK, et al: MR imaging of the corpus callosum. Normal and pathologic findings and correlation with CT. *AJNR* 9:649-656, 1988.

Rice JF, Eggers DM: Basal transsphenoidal encephalocele: MR findings. *AJNR* 10:579-580, 1989.

Roach ES, Williams DP, Laster DW: Magnetic resonance imaging in tuberous sclerosis. *Arch Neurol* 44:301-303, 1987.

Rubinstein D, Youngman V, Hise JH, Damiano TR: Partial development of the corpus callosum. *AJNR* 15:869-875, 1994.

Ruge JR, Tomitashita T, Naidich TP, et al: Scalp and calvarial mass of infants and children. *Neurosurgery* 22:1037-1042, 1988.

Sato Y, Kao SCS, Smith WL: Radiographic manifestations of anomalies of the brain. *Rad Clin North Am* 29:179-194, 1991.

Sevick RJ, Barkovich AJ, Edwards MSB, et al: Evolution of white matter lesions in neurofibromatosis type 1: MR findings. *AJR* 159:171-175, 1992.

Smirniotopoulos JG, Murphy FM: The phakomatoses. *AJNR* 13:725-746, 1992.

Smith AS, Blaser SI, Ross JS, Weinstein MA: Magnetic resonance imaging of disturbances in neuronal migration: illustration of an embryologic process. *Radiographics* 9:509-523, 1989.

Smith A, Weinstein M, Quencer R, et al: Association of heterotopic gray matter with seizures: MR imaging. *Radiology* 168-195, 1988.

Stark JE, Glasier CM: MR demonstration of ectopic fourth ventricular choroid plexus in Chiari II malformation. *AJNR* 14:618-621, 1993.

Tart RP, Quisling RG: Curvilinear and tubulonodular varieties of lipoma of the corpus callosum: an MR and CT study. *J Comput Assist Tomogr* 15:805-810, 1991.

Terwey B, Doose H: Tuberous sclerosis: magnetic resonance imaging of the brain. *Neuropediatrics* 18:67-69, 1987.

Titelbaum DS, Haward JC, Zimmerman RA: Pachygyriclike changes: topographic appearance at MR imaging and CT and correlation with neurologic status. *Radiology* 173:663-668, 1989.

Truwit CL, Barkovich AJ: Pathogenesis of intracranial lipoma: an MR study in 42 patients. *AJNR* 11:665-674, 1990.

Truwit CL, Barkovich AJ, Koch TK, Ferriero DM: Cerebral palsy: MR findings in 40 patients. *AJNR* 13:67-78, 1992.

Truwit C, Williams RG, Armstrong EA, Marlin AE: MR imaging of choroid plexus lipomas. *AJNR* 11:202-204, 1990.

Uchino A, Hasuo K, Matsumoto S, Masuda K: Solitary choroid plexus lipomas: CT and MR appearance. *AJNR* 14:116-118, 1993.

Van Bogaert P, Baleriaux D, Christope C, Szliwowski HB: MRI of patients with cerebral palsy and normal CT scan. *Neuroradiology* 34:52-56, 1992.

Vogl TJ, Stemmler J, Bergman C, et al: MR and MR angiography of Sturge-Weber syndrome. *AJNR* 14:417-425, 1993.

Volpe JJ: Value of MR in definition of the neuropathology of cerebral palsy in vivo. *AJNR* 13:79-83, 1992.

Wasenko JJ, Rosenbloom SA, Duchesneau PM, et al: The Sturge-Weber syndrome: comparison of MR and CT characteristics. *AJNR* 11:131-134, 1990.

Wilms G, Van Wijck E, Dermaerel Ph, et al: Gyriform calcifications in tuberous sclerosis simulating the appearance of Sturge-Weber disease. *AJNR* 13:295-298, 1992.

Wippold FJ II, Baber WW, Gado M, et al: Pre- and post-contrast MR studies in tuberous sclerosis. *J Comput Assist Tomogr* 16:69-72, 1992.

Wolpert SM, Anderson M, Scott RM, et al: The Chiari II malformation: MR imaging evaluation. *AJNR* 8:783-792, 1987.

Wolpert SM, Scott RM, Platenberg C, Runge VM: The clinical significance of hindbrain herniation and deformity as shown on MR images of patients with Chiari II malformation. *AJNR* 9:1075-1078, 1988.

Yasumoro K, Hasuo K, Nagata S, et al: Neuronal migration anomalies causing extensive ventricular indentation. *Neurosurgery* 26:504-506, 1990.

Young JN, Oakes WJ, Hatten HP Jr: Dorsal third ventricular cyst: an entity distinct from holoprosencephaly. *J Neurosurg* 77:556-561, 1992.

Zimmerman RA, Yachnis AT, Rorke CB, et al: Pathology of findings of cerebral high signal intensity in two patients with type 1 neurofibromatosis. *Radiology* 185(suppl):123, 1992.

479

CHAPTER 13

Orbital Lesions

Case 780A

2-year-old girl with neurofibromatosis type 1,
presenting with proptosis.
(sagittal, noncontrast scan; SE 700/17)

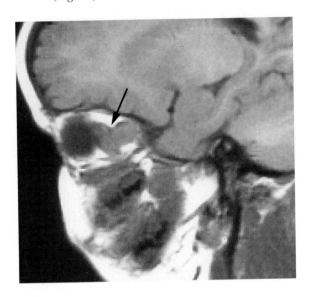

Case 780B

Same patient.
(coronal, noncontrast scan; SE 700/28)

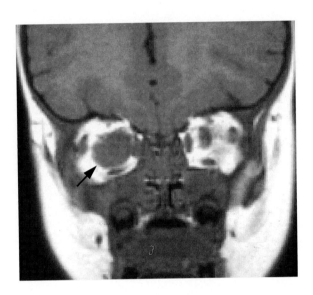

Gliomas typically cause uniform thickening of the optic nerve. Mild undulation or lobulation is common. The lesions are usually homogeneous, without calcification or prominent contrast enhancement.

Case 780A demonstrates a homogeneous, mildly lobulated mass extending from the globe to the orbital apex. Gross expansion of the right optic nerve is seen in cross section in Case 780B (compare the affected nerve to the normal optic nerve on the left).

Rotation of the head may cause coronal scans to pass through the posterior portion of one globe while demonstrating the contralateral optic nerve. This apparent asymmetry can falsely mimic an optic glioma of the posteriorly rotated side.

When a tumor of the optic nerve is discovered within the orbit, the optic chiasm should be examined to assess intracranial extension (see the next page). Similarly, the finding of a suprasellar mass should prompt careful evaluation of the intraorbital portions of the optic nerves.

Gliomas involving the optic nerve present a variety of clinical patterns. Optic nerve tumors in young patients (more frequently girls) and in patients with neurofibromatosis are often low grade lesions, behaving more like hyperplasia than neoplasm. Optic gliomas arising spontaneously in adults tend to be more aggressive tumors.

Case 781

10-year-old girl with neurofibromatosis type 1.
(sagittal, noncontrast scan; SE 600/17)

Case 782

1-year-old boy.
(coronal, noncontrast scan; SE 800/16)

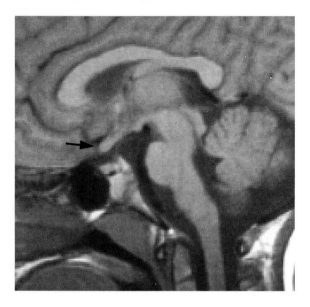

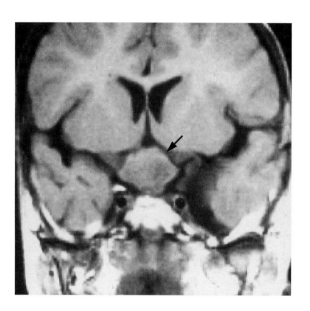

Gliomatous expansion of the optic chiasm can vary substantially in extent and morphology. Mild thickening of the chiasm is present in Case 781 *(arrow)*. Other scans demonstrated continuity of the chiasmal mass with expanded intraorbital segments of the optic nerves bilaterally. The presence of bilateral optic gliomas strongly suggests type 1 neurofibromatosis (analogous to the presumption of type 2 neurofibromatosis in patients with bilateral acoustic schwannomas).

The large, homogeneous, mildly lobulated suprasellar mass in Case 782 is centered at the location of the optic chiasm. The chiasm could not be separately identified as an independent structure displaced by the tumor. These features suggest a diagnosis of chiasmal glioma, which in this case was not associated with extension into more anterior portions of the optic pathways.

Large chiasmal gliomas may infiltrate the floor of the third ventricle and hypothalamus. It can be difficult to determine whether such a suprasellar mass is of optic or hypothalamic origin (see discussion of Cases 246 and 247).

A wide range of additional pathologies can cause chiasmal thickening or masses. An appearance similar to Case 781 may be seen secondary to optic neuritis (e.g., multiple sclerosis; see Case 795), with regression following steroid therapy. Craniopharyngiomas and cavernous angiomas are occasionally intrachiasmal, presenting morphologies similar to Case 782 (although signal intensities are usually more variable). Suprasellar meningiomas and germinomas may surround or thin the optic chiasm, so that it is no longer recognized as a discrete structure. Sarcoidosis and histiocytosis may also produce masses enveloping the chiasm.

Posterior extension of chiasmal gliomas into the optic tracts and radiations is better demonstrated on MR examinations than on CT studies. Such infiltration is usually most apparent as zones of increased signal intensity on T2-weighted images. Gliomatous involvement of the optic radiations may be symmetrical or strikingly unilateral.

Case 783

20-year-old woman with neurofibromatosis type 1,
presenting with 20/30 vision in the left eye.
(axial, noncontrast scan; SE 2800/90)

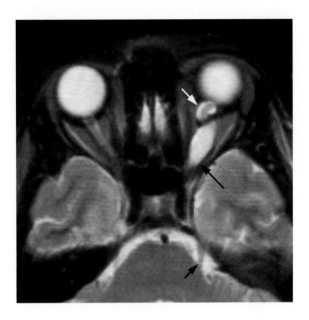

Case 784

34-year-old man presenting with decreased
vision in the left eye.
(axial, noncontrast scan; RSE 5000/100)

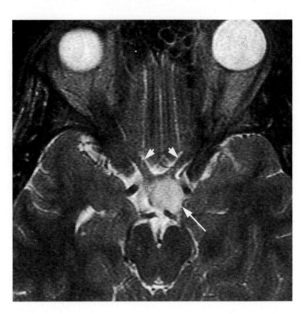

Gliomas of the optic pathway may be relatively isointense or demonstrate high signal intensity on T2-weighted scans.

Case 783 illustrates expansion and high intensity involving the intraorbital segment of the left optic nerve *(long black arrow)*. Cystic dilatation of the nerve sheath probably accounts for the very high signal surrounding the nonexpanded nerve at the junction with the globe *(white arrow)*.

Hyperplasia of astrocytes within arachnoidal tissue frequently surrounds the optic nerves in patients with neurofibromatosis type 1. This "perineural arachnoidal gliomatosis" contributes to obstruction and distention of the subarachnoid space normally encircling the nerve.

In Case 784, a chiasmal glioma is well defined as a zone of homogeneously increased signal intensity *(long arrow)*. Note the intracranial segments of the optic nerves extending from the optic canals to enter the chiasm bilaterally *(short arrows)*.

The cisternal portion of the left trigeminal nerve is imaged in Case 783 *(short black arrow)*. Case 784 demonstrates the normal anatomy of the gyrus rectus at the inferior-medial margin of the frontal lobes bilaterally.

Case 785

12-year-old boy with neurofibromatosis type 1
but no visual symptoms.
(axial, postcontrast scan; SE 600/14)

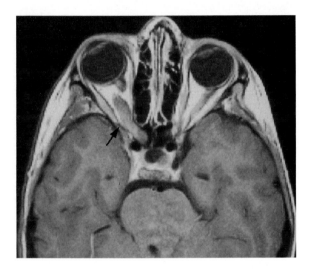

Case 786

34-year-old man presenting with decreased vision
in the left eye.
(axial, postcontrast scan; SE 550/14
with fat suppression)

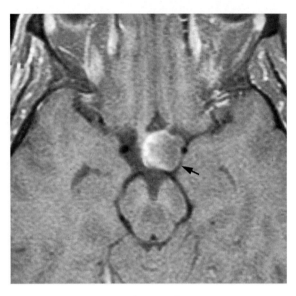

(same patient as Case 784)

Contrast enhancement within gliomas of the optic nerve or chiasm may be minimal or intense. Solid, patchy, and peripheral patterns of enhancement are encountered.

Moderate patchy enhancement is present in the posterior portion of the right optic nerve in Case 785. (This enhancement would be better distinguished from the normally short T1 of retrobulbar fat by a pulse sequence incorporating fat suppression or "saturation.") The anterior-most portion of the involved nerve is nonenhancing, resembling the sparing of this segment in Case 783.

In Case 786, an eccentric perimeter of abnormal contrast enhancement is observed. Other optic/hypothalamic gliomas enhance more uniformly (see Case 248), resembling suprasellar meningiomas or germinomas.

Posterior extension of chiasmal gliomas into the optic tracts and radiations may cause zones of T2-prolongation

that demonstrate little or no contrast enhancement. It is difficult to distinguish actual tumor invasion from disordered myelination (see Cases 764-767) or reactive edema in such cases. When present, enhancement of gliomatous infiltration of the optic radiations is usually patchy. Solid, mass-like enhancement patterns are seen in occasional aggressive and rapidly enlarging tumors.

High signal intensity on T2-weighted images and/or abnormal contrast enhancement extending from a suprasellar mass along the optic tracts is not specific for optic gliomas. Occasional craniopharyngiomas may involve the optic chiasm and follow the optic tracts posteriorly. Rarely, meningeal seeding by CNS tumors (e.g., medulloblastoma) or inflammatory disease (e.g., sarcoidosis) presents a similar appearance.

Case 787

32-year-old woman with a history of gradually diminishing visual acuity in the right eye.
(axial, noncontrast scan; SE 2500/30)

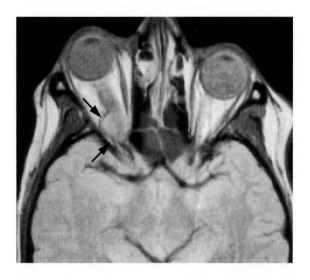

Case 788

76-year-old man presenting with a long history of worsening proptosis.
(axial, noncontrast scan; SE 2800/90)

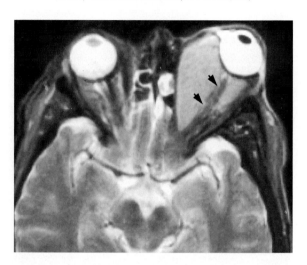

Primary orbital meningiomas most commonly arise from the optic nerve sheath. Extraconal origin from the orbital margins or presumed rests of meningeal cells is less frequent. Secondary extension of intraosseous or intracranial meningiomas into the orbit has been discussed in Chapter 2 (see Cases 45 and 54).

Like optic nerve gliomas, most nerve sheath meningiomas are nearly isointense to extraocular muscles on T1-weighted scans. The signal intensity of orbital meningiomas on long TR scans ranges from intermediate to high.

The morphology of sheath meningiomas is widely variable. Some tumors encase the nerve with a uniform, concentric layer of tumor. In other patients, an eccentric, lobulated mass extends from the nerve into the retrobulbar fat, as in Case 787 *(arrows)*. Occasionally, a nerve-sheath meningioma expands to fill the retrobulbar compartment, as demonstrated by Case 788.

Many optic sheath meningiomas develop a fusiform or elliptical shape surrounding the optic nerve. The nerve is often identifiable as a relatively uninvolved central band coursing through the mass like an axis of rotation (as in Case 788; *arrows*). This morphology is not specific but should suggest the possibility of a nerve sheath meningioma.

"Tram track" or spindle-shaped calcification surrounding the optic nerve is a common and characteristic feature on CT scans of sheath meningiomas. This finding is usually inapparent on spin echo MR images. Gradient echo sequences with more sensitivity to susceptibility-induced signal loss may provide evidence of tumor mineralization.

Patients with optic nerve sheath meningiomas are typically adults who present with progressive loss of vision or proptosis, as in the above cases.

Case 789

34-year-old man presenting with decreasing
vision in the left eye.
(coronal, postcontrast scan; SE 600/18
with fat suppression)

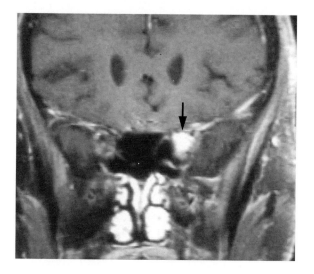

Case 790

76-year-old man presenting with proptosis.
(axial, postcontrast scan; SE 600/14)

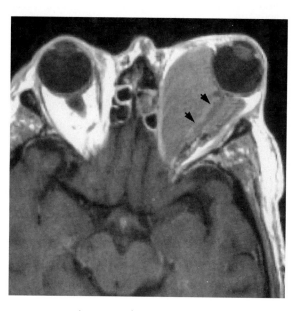

(same patient as Case 788)

Like their intracranial counterparts, most orbital meningiomas enhance intensely and uniformly. Patterns of enhancement reflect the variable morphologies of tumor growth.

Linear enhancement along the margins of the optic nerve is seen on axial or sagittal scans of meningiomas encircling the nerve as a uniform layer of thickened tissue. (Coronal scans demonstrate a ring of enhancement surrounding the nerve in such cases.) This "tram track" collar of enhancement bordering an uninvolved nerve suggests meningioma but is not diagnostic. Other pathologies that can cause perineural enhancement include orbital pseudotumor, sarcoidosis, optic neuritis (e.g., multiple sclerosis), leukemia, lymphoma, and metastases.

When orbital meningiomas are more nodular, their enhancement is more spherical. Case 789 illustrates uniform,

intense enhancement within a meningioma that is comparable in location and morphology to Case 787. This mass occupies the narrow orbital apex, crowding nerves and vessels.

Involvement of the orbital apex is seen with most nerve sheath meningiomas. However, the shape, location, and enhancement of the lesion in Case 789 are not specific; other masses (e.g., hemangioma or metastasis) could present a similar appearance.

The uniform enhancement of the tumor in Case 790 correlates with the homogeneous signal intensity in Case 788 and matches the stereotype of intracranial meningiomas. The optic nerve is also enhancing but remains outlined by surrounding tumor *(arrows)*. Proptosis and lateral displacement of the globe are apparent.

487

Case 791

38-year-old woman presenting with progressive
visual loss in the left eye.
(coronal, noncontrast scan; SE 700/17)

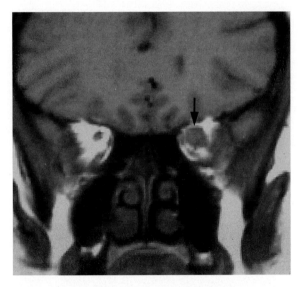

Optic Nerve Sheath Meningioma

Case 792

12-year-old boy with no visual symptoms.
(coronal, postcontrast scan; SE 600/14)

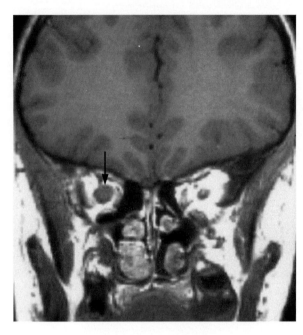

Optic Nerve Glioma
(same patient as Case 785)

A wide variety of lesions may cause thickening of the optic nerve. Non-neoplastic processes such as papilledema, optic neuritis, orbital pseudotumor, Graves' disease, and vascular malformations are included in the differential diagnosis.

Among tumors, the most important possibilities are gliomas of the nerve and meningiomas of the nerve sheath. Other neoplasms that can cause expansion of the optic nerve and/or sheath include lymphoma, leukemia, and retrobulbar metastasis.

A clinical clue to the presence of an optic nerve tumor is loss of visual acuity, which is less common with other orbital masses. This history is characteristic for adults presenting with nerve sheath meningiomas, as in Case 791. (Occasional patients report desaturation or fading of color before acuity is measurably impaired.)

Case 792 illustrates that children with neurofibromatosis may be found to have optic nerve gliomas causing little or no visual compromise. As discussed in Case 780, these tumors often behave like benign hyperplasia, with decades of stable vision.

Optic nerve sheath meningiomas are rare in children, while optic nerve gliomas are uncommon in adults. The age of the patient is therefore a clue to the likely etiology of a tumor involving the optic nerve/sheath complex.

Contrast enhancement can also help to distinguish among optic nerve lesions. As discussed on the preceding page, sheath meningiomas typically enhance intensely and with characteristic morphologies. (Convincing MR demonstration of thin enhancement along the margins of the optic nerve may require fat-suppression techniques.)

The glioma in Case 792 is moderately enhancing, compatible with low histological grade. Enhancement of optic nerve gliomas is rarely as intense as is seen with sheath meningiomas (compare Case 792 to Case 789).

DIFFERENTIAL DIAGNOSIS:
ENLARGEMENT OF THE OPTIC CHIASM

Case 793

10-year-old girl complaining of headaches.
(coronal, noncontrast scan; SE 600/17)

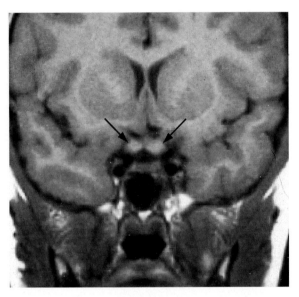

Optic Glioma
(same patient as Case 781)

Case 794

30-year-old woman presenting with visual loss.
(coronal, noncontrast scan; SE 600/15)

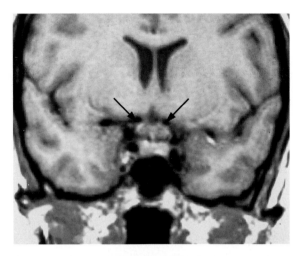

Optic Neuritis
(due to multiple sclerosis)

Both of these scans pass through the junction of the optic nerves with the optic chiasm. In each case, the normal dumbbell morphology at this location is symmetrically expanded.

The nerves/chiasm in Case 793 are normal in signal intensity, compatible with tightly packed axonal tissue. In Case 794, the signal intensity within the large nerves/chiasm is relatively lower, suggesting edema.

Comparison of the above cases demonstrates that inflammatory and neoplastic expansion of the optic nerves/chiasm can be morphologically indistinguishable. The presence and character of contrast enhancement can help with differential diagnosis (see Case 795). Associated cerebral lesions may also clarify an underlying process (e.g., plaques in multiple sclerosis or typical parenchymal signal abnormalities in neurofibromatosis; see Cases 764-767). In ambiguous cases, the clinical context (particularly acuity of symptoms) will usually distinguish between inflammatory and neoplastic involvement of the optic apparatus.

Case 795A

30-year-old woman with known multiple sclerosis presenting with rapidly progressive visual loss.
(coronal, postcontrast scan; SE 600/15)

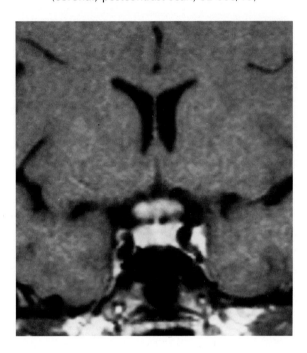

Case 795B

Same patient.
(axial, postcontrast scan; SE 600/15)

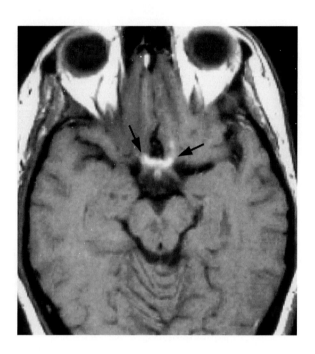

Case 795 illustrates acute optic neuritis in a patient with multiple sclerosis. The chiasm is moderately enlarged, with extensive abnormal enhancement. Compare the enhancing suprasellar mass in Case 795A with Cases 223 to 226.

The axial scan in Case 795B demonstrates abnormal enhancement at the junction of the optic nerves and chiasm *(arrows)*. Visualization of similar enhancement within the intraorbital portion of the optic nerve often requires fat saturation sequences to suppress the signal intensity of retrobulbar adipose tissue.

Contrast enhancement in cases of optic neuritis may be solid (as above), peripheral, or absent. Enhancement along the margins of the nerve may cause a "tram track" appearance that resembles nerve sheath meningiomas or other perineural tumors.

Noncontrast T2-weighted MR scans may demonstrate focal areas of high signal intensity within the optic nerve in cases of neuritis. Detection of such lesions can be increased by STIR (Short Tau Inversion Recovery) sequences and/or

large matrices (e.g., 512 × 512) providing high spatial resolution. However, noncontrast scans are often normal in the presence of clinically definite neuritis.

The most common etiology of optic neuritis is multiple sclerosis. Optic nerve involvement may precede, accompany, or follow cerebral or spinal symptoms. Inflammation may be unilateral or bilateral, affecting nerve and/or chiasm. Examination of the accompanying cerebral scan for evidence of demyelinating disease is warranted in patients with clinical optic neuritis, whether or not nerve lesions can be demonstrated.

Other potential etiologies of optic neuritis include sarcoidosis and Lyme disease. Vasculitis due to systemic lupus erythematosus, syphilis, rheumatoid arthritis, or Sjogren's syndrome can also present as optic neuritis. Rapidly progressive optic neuritis may develop after radiation of the suprasellar region (with a latency period of six months to three years). Many cases of optic neuritis are idiopathic.

Case 796A

8-year-old boy presenting with proptosis.
(axial, postcontrast scan; SE 500/14)

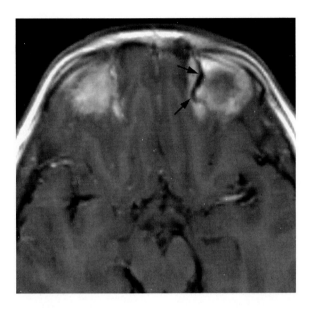

Case 796B

Same patient.
(submentovertex projection of three-dimensional,
time-of-flight GRE series)

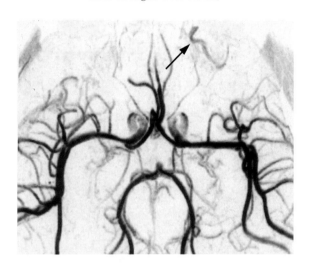

In addition to mass-like vascular lesions (hemangiomas, lymphangiomas, and varices; see Cases 797 and 798), the orbit may contain dilated vascular channels reflecting arteriovenous malformations or fistulae.

In Case 796A, a large vein in the medial portion of the left orbit *(arrows)* demonstrates prominent "flow void" on a postcontrast scan. This finding implies abnormally fast or turbulent flow. The time-of-flight MR angiogram in Case 796B visualizes the same vein *(arrow)*, confirming arterialized flow. A subsequent catheter angiogram documented a small arteriovenous fistula within the orbit.

A more common cause of enlarged orbital veins (especially in adults) is a carotid-cavernous fistula. Such arteriovenous communications may be high flow or low flow lesions. High flow fistulae are caused by a tear of the internal carotid artery as it passes through the venous compartment of the cavernous sinus. The resulting shunt of arterial blood floods the sinus and its tributaries, including the superior ophthalmic vein. These veins become enlarged, with abnormally prominent "flow voids" comparable to the above case.

Low flow carotid-cavernous fistulae are vascular malformations of the dura, often occurring spontaneously in middle-aged or elderly patients. Small dural branches of the internal and external carotid arteries supply a network of abnormal channels along the medial wall of the middle cranial fossa, shunting blood into the cavernous sinus.

In either type of carotid-cavernous fistula, stasis or reversal of flow in the superior ophthalmic vein is associated with evidence of orbital vascular congestion (e.g., proptosis and conjunctival injection) and is often accompanied by a bruit transmitted from the fistula. A corroborating MR finding is distension of the ipsilateral cavernous sinus, often containing abnormal areas of "flow void."

Case 797A

48-year-old woman presenting with inferior
displacement of the left globe.
(sagittal, noncontrast scan; SE 600/14)

Case 797B

Same patient.
(axial, noncontrast scan; SE 2800/90)

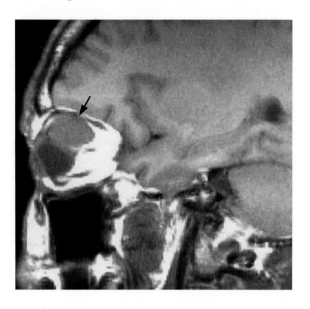

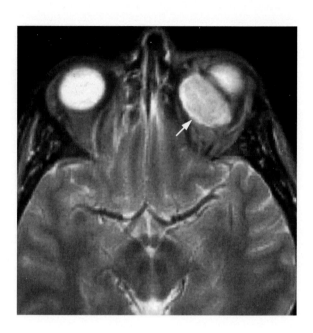

Cavernous hemangiomas are the most common masses of the adult orbit. They usually present as well-defined intraconal lesions with smooth or mildly lobulated margins. Case 797 is a typical example.

Hemangiomas are often located superior or lateral to the globe, sparing the orbital apex (unlike nerve sheath meningiomas; see Cases 787-791). The masses are nearly isointense to gray matter on T1-weighted scans. Moderately high signal intensity is usual on T2-weighted images, reflecting the fluid content of the lesion.

Other potential vascular masses within the adult orbit include varices, lymphangiomas (see Case 798), and distended vessels associated with a carotid-cavernous fistula (see Case 796). These lesions may be morphologically indistinguishable. A clinical history of positional proptosis suggests a varix; compression of the jugular vein or a valsalva maneuver during CT or MR scans may demonstrate impressive variceal enlargement.

Other benign orbital masses may resemble vascular lesions with well-defined spherical or lobulated margins and

high signal intensity on T2-weighted scans. Examples include schwannomas and plexiform neurofibromas. Orbital meningiomas have been discussed previously.

Cavernous hemangiomas often demonstrate a characteristic enhancement pattern which can help to distinguish them from other retrobulbar masses. Initial patchy enhancement occurs near the center of the hemangioma, with more uniform and extensive enhancement developing over several minutes.

Metastases from systemtic carcinomas (e.g., breast, lung) may also be considered among solid tumors of the adult orbit (although ocular metastases are more common; see Cases 804 and 805). Metastases may develop along the bony margins of the orbit, along the optic nerve, or within orbital fat. The latter presentation can be mass-like or infiltrating, resembling orbital pseudotumor or a vascular mass. Scirrhous carcinoma of the breast may incite a fibrotic reaction causing characteristic globe retraction and enophthalmus.

Case 798A

26-year-old woman presenting with mild
right proptosis.
(coronal, noncontrast scan; SE 700/17)

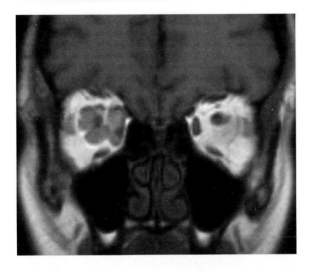

Case 798B

Same patient.
(axial, noncontrast scan; SE 3000/80)

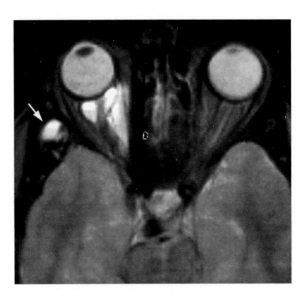

Orbital lymphangiomas can present a variety of morphologies on CT and MR images. A multilobulated and/or infiltrating appearance is typical, reflecting a lack of encapsulation (and contrasting with the more common cavernous hemangiomas). Diffuse involvement of the retrobulbar space and enhancement on postcontrast scans may mimic orbital pseudotumor or retrobulbar metastasis. Extraconal extension is common.

Case 798A demonstrates a lobulated intraconal mass surrounding the optic nerve and adjoining the medial rectus muscle. Signal intensity within the lesion is uniform and higher than that of muscle.

Like other vascular lesions, lymphangiomas are characterized by high signal intensity on T2-weighted scans. In Case 798B the optic nerve traverses a bed of bright tissue. Such T2-prolongation would be very unusual for orbital

pseudotumor and helps to distinguish between these two infiltrating lesions. (Retrobulbar metastasis may also demonstrate T2-prolongation, which is usually less marked than that of vascular masses.)

Lymphangiomas can display considerable heterogeneity. In Case 798B, small sedimentation levels are faintly seen within the orbital and extraorbital *(arrow)* components of the mass. Areas of prominent T1- and T2-shortening are often present within lymphangiomas, reflecting episodes of hemorrhage.

Lymphangiomas are highly vascular and are more prone to spontaneous bleeding than hemangiomas. Hemorrhage within a lymphangioma may cause suddenly worsening symptoms. Rapid clinical progression is otherwise unusual for vascular masses of the orbit and more compatible with inflammatory or malignant processes.

Case 799

28-year-old man presenting with fullness at the
medial margin of the right orbit.
(axial, noncontrast scan; SE 1000/23)

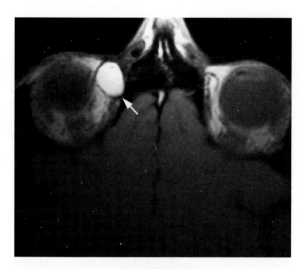

Dermoid Cyst

Case 800

83-year-old man presenting with diplopia.
(coronal, noncontrast scan; SE 500/20)

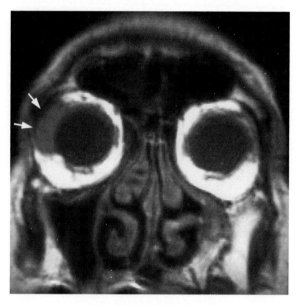

Benign Mixed Tumor of the Lacrimal Gland

A number of relatively uncommon orbital masses can be characterized by their signal intensity and/or location.

Dermoid cysts within the orbit may demonstrate T1-shortening or fat/fluid levels comparable to their intracranial counterparts (see Cases 286-289). These features are highly specific. (Scans with fat suppression eliminate potential confusion with lesions containing subacute blood products, such as an old subperiosteal hematoma.) Orbital dermoid cysts are most commonly found near the lacrimal gland (superolateral quadrant of the orbit) or at the medial orbital margin. Case 799 demonstrates a lesion in the latter location, with characteristic T1-shortening.

The differential diagnosis of a mass in the superolateral quadrant of the orbit includes tumors of the lacrimal gland (benign mixed tumors as in Case 800 or adenocarcinomas), lymphoma, metastasis, orbital dermoid cysts, sarcoidosis, and Wegener's granulomatosis. Soft tissue prominence at this site may also be seen in thyroid ophthalmopathy and in orbital pseudotumors. Remodelling or erosion of the adjacent orbital wall (present in Case 800; *arrows)* favors a long-standing, benign process.

Case 801A

2-year-old girl presenting with proptosis.
(axial, noncontrast scan; SE 2500/90)

Case 801B

Same patient.
(axial, postcontrast scan; SE 600/14)

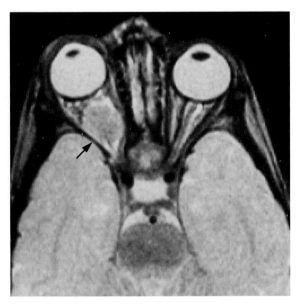

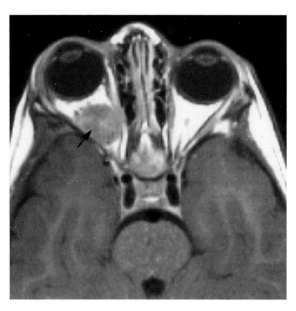

Rhabdomyosarcoma

A number of benign and malignant masses may occur within the orbit in children. Benign lesions include capillary hemangiomas (the most frequent vascular masses of the infant orbit), cavernous hemangiomas, neurofibromas, and schwannomas. Optic gliomas have been discussed in Cases 780-786.

Malignant orbital masses in children include lymphoma, leukemia, neuroblastoma, histiocytosis, and rhabdomyosarcoma. The first four of these pathologies may present as layers of thickened tissue along the orbital margins, particularly laterally. This appearance may be unilateral or bilateral, resembling thickening of rectus muscles. In other cases, lymphoma or leukemia may line the optic nerve, producing a thickened nerve/sheath complex and/or "tram track" enhancement resembling an optic sheath meningioma.

A third potential morphology for malignant orbital neoplasms is a bulky mass, as illustrated above. The tumor in

Case 801A demonstrates relatively low signal intensity on a T2-weighted scan. This appearance suggests dense cellularity and/or a fibrous stroma and argues against the diagnosis of cavernous hemangioma (compare to Case 797B).

Case 801B demonstrates moderate, patchy contrast enhancement within the mass. The tumor is intraconal, sparing the orbital apex. These features (and the pediatric presentation) would be unusual for a meningioma. The margins of the mass are well defined and smoothly rounded, unlike the lobulation commonly seen in capillary hemangiomas and lymphangiomas.

Rhabdomyosarcoma is among the malignant neoplasms of the face, pharynx, and skull base encountered in children. The mass usually arises from cell rests rather than from a particular muscle. The orbit is a frequent location for this tumor. Despite histological malignancy, the prognosis may be quite good following surgical resection and adjunctive chemotherapy.

Case 802

14-month-old boy presenting with leukokoria.
(axial, postcontrast scan; SE 600/15)

Case 803

60-year-old woman.
(sagittal, noncontrast scan; SE 800/20)

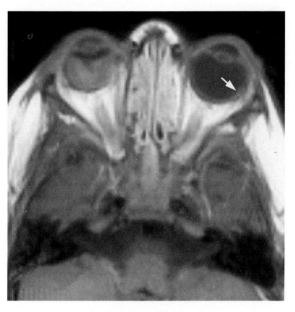

Retinoblastoma

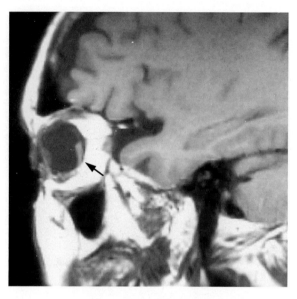

Choroidal Melanoma

The presence of an intraocular mass is usually clinically apparent. CT and MR scans are performed to characterize the lesion, detect possible contralateral tumor, and assess extraocular invasion.

Retinoblastoma is the most common ocular tumor in children. Bilateral involvement occurs in about 30% of cases. An associated pineal region tumor may occasionally be seen in such patients, often arising subsequent to the original ocular masses ("trilateral retinoblastoma"). Patients with bilateral retinoblastomas also carry a genetic predisposition to develop additional tumors (e.g., osteosarcomas within or outside of the field of initial radiation therapy).

Most children with retinoblastoma present as infants with a "white" pupil or "leukokoria." A similar appearance can be caused by a number of benign conditions including Coats' disease, persistent hyperplastic primary vitreous, and larval granulomatosis *(Toxocara canis)*.

Calcification is a hallmark of retinoblastomas. In cases of bilateral tumors, a tiny focus of calcium may be the only clue to involvement of the nonpresenting eye. CT scans are more sensitive than MR images for detecting this important finding.

In Case 802, a small left-sided retinoblastoma is seen *(arrow)*. The bulky intraocular mass on the right demonstrates only mild contrast enhancement.

Case 803 illustrates a shallow choroidal melanoma at the posterior margin of the globe *(arrow)*. Ocular melanomas may arise in the iris, ciliary body, or choroid. Choroidal melanomas are the second most common ocular malignancy in adults (after metastases; see Cases 804 and 805). These tumors sometimes demonstrate T1-shortening and T2-shortening due to the presence of paramagnetic components (melanin and/or blood products).

Other pathologies that can cause localized thickening of the ocular wall include choroidal hemangioma, inflammatory disease (e.g., sarcoidosis), and focal retinal detachment with associated hematoma or subretinal fluid.

Case 804

63-year-old woman.
(coronal, noncontrast scan; SE 600/17)

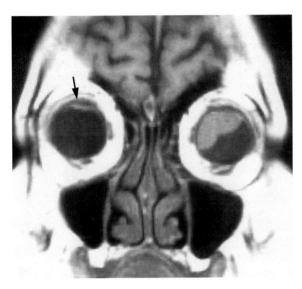

Metastatic Carcinoma of the Breast

Case 805

62-year-old woman.
(axial, noncontrast scan; SE 2000/45)

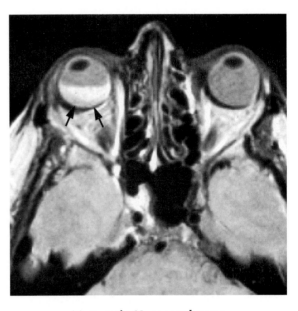

Metastatic Hypernephroma

The majority of metastases to the adult orbit are ocular. Intraocular metastases most commonly arise from carcinomas of the breast, lung, colon, and kidney. These lesions represent hematogeneous deposits in the highly vascular uveal layer (choroid, iris, ciliary body).

Metastases to the globe may demonstrate only slightly higher signal intensity than the vitreous body on T1-weighted images. More obviously increased signal often reflects accompanying retinal detachment, with subretinal fluid collections and hemorrhage.

In Case 804, a large metastatic retinal detachment is seen within the left globe. A smaller layer of abnormal tissue is present along the superior margin of the right globe *(arrow)*. Ocular metastases are bilateral in about 25% of cases.

Case 805 demonstrates the typically crescentic shape of subretinal fluid collections along the posterior margin of the right globe. The thin layer of metastatic tumor is faintly visible as a lower intensity mass *(arrows)* outlined by the surrounding detachment.

Most choroidal metastases are less intense than the vitreous body (and associated subretinal fluid collections) on heavily T2-weighted images. (Choroidal melanomas are moderately to markedly hypointense with respect to the vitreous on such sequences.)

Case 806A

47-year-old woman presenting with proptosis.
(sagittal, noncontrast scan; SE 600/20)

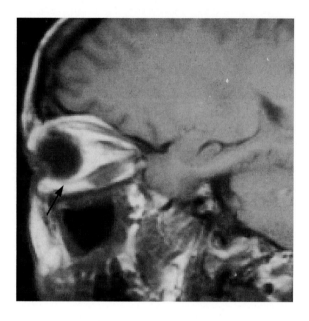

Case 806B

Same patient.
(coronal, noncontrast scan; SE 700/20)

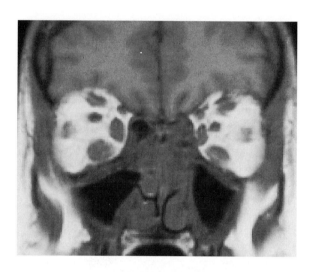

The hallmark of thyroid ophthalmopathy or "Graves' disease" is infiltration of the rectus muscles. The two eyes may be involved symmetrically or asymmetrically. Medial and inferior rectus muscles are usually affected before and to a greater extent than the lateral rectus or superior muscle group.

Case 806 illustrates these features. Thickening of rectus muscles is bilateral and approximately symmetrical. The lateral rectus muscles are least involved by the diffuse process.

Relative sparing of the tendinous insertion of affected muscles (*arrow*, Case 806A) contrasts with the appearance of orbital myositis (see discussion of Case 807).

An increased volume of orbital fat often contributes more to exophthalmos in thyroid ophthalmopathy than does enlargement of the rectus muscles. However, the muscular enlargement may cause severe compression of the optic nerve within the orbital apex.

High signal intensity may be seen within the enlarged rectus muscles on T2-weighted scans, indicating active inflammation and edema. Such cases respond better to steroid therapy than patients with thyroid ophthalmopathy whose muscular infiltration does not demonstrate T2-prolongation.

Mucosal thickening is present in the maxillary and ethmoid sinuses in Case 806.

DIFFERENTIAL DIAGNOSIS:
THICKENED RECTUS MUSCLES

Case 807

33-year-old woman with painful limitation
of upward gaze.
(coronal, noncontrast scan; SE 1000/22)

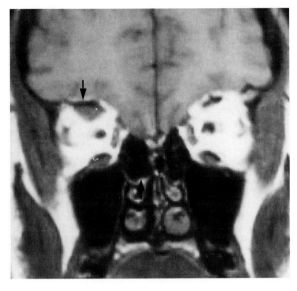

Orbital Pseudotumor

Case 808

74-year-old woman presenting with orbital
pain and diplopia.
(coronal, noncontrast scan; SE 800/17)

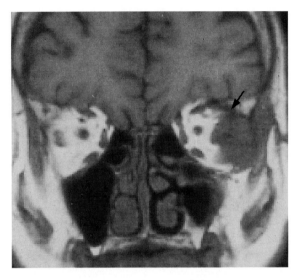

Metastatic Carcinoma of the Lung

A number of pathologies in addition to thyroid ophthalmopathy can cause thickening of one or more rectus muscles.

Case 807 demonstrates swelling of the superior muscle group (superior rectus and levator palpebrae) on the right *(arrow)*, while other rectus muscles are uninvolved. This pattern of involvement (and the presence of pain) would be unusual for thyroid ophthalmopathy, representing instead the "myositic" form of orbital pseudotumor.

The diagnosis of "orbital pseudotumor" includes a diverse group of nonspecific lymphocytic and granulomatous inflammations. Involvement may be unilateral or bilateral. In some cases, poorly defined soft tissue infiltrates the retrobulbar space, resembling orbital cellulitis, metastasis, or an amorphous vascular mass such as lymphangioma. Relatively low signal intensity within orbital pseudotumor on T2-weighted MR scans may help to distinguish this lesion from orbital metastases, which typically demonstrate higher intensity values. In other cases, orbital pseudotumor may cause swelling of rectus muscles or discrete nodules of in-

flammatory tissue that mimic primary or metastatic tumors within the orbit or lacrimal glands.

Radiographic clues distinguishing myositic pseudotumor from thyroid ophthalmopathy include (1) the tendency of pseudotumor to involve the ocular insertions of the rectus muscles, which are typically spared in thyroid ophthalmopathy, and (2) the common association of myositic pseudotumor with other evidence of orbital inflammation (e.g., scleral enhancement, preseptal edema, or hazy margins of the optic nerve). Clinical features (rapid onset, pain, and response to steroid therapy) also help to distinguish most pseudotumors from the neoplasms or endocrinopathies that they may otherwise resemble.

A variety of tumors can cause orbital masses infiltrating or surrounding rectus muscles, particularly laterally. Metastases (as in Case 808), lymphoma, and myeloma (or solitary plasmocytoma) should be considered in adults. Leukemia, lymphoma, neuroblastoma, Ewing's sarcoma, and histiocytosis can present similarly in children.

Case 809A

29-year-old woman presenting with diplopia after a blow to the right eye.
(axial, noncontrast scan; SE 690/15)

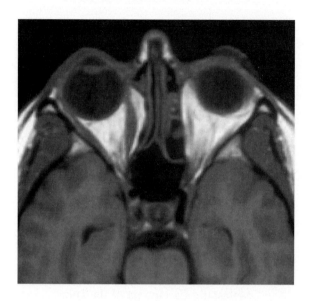

Case 809B

Same patient.
(coronal, noncontrast scan; SE 690/15)

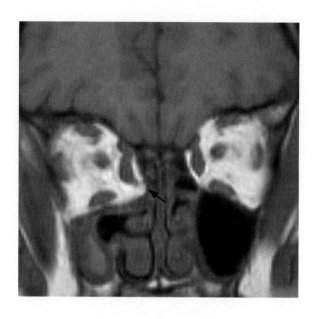

Medial "Blow-Out" Fracture

CT and MR scans display the orbital contents in cases where facial injury precludes ophthalmological evaluation. Nondisplaced fractures and radiopaque foreign bodies are better demonstrated by CT than by MR. However, retinal injury and intraocular hemorrhage may be more sensitively detected on MR studies. Hemorrhage into the vitreous body is uncommon after blunt trauma but may occur with penetrating injury.

A direct blow to the eye compresses the orbital contents into the narrowing cone of the posterior orbit. The resultant increase in intraorbital pressure may cause secondary displacement of the orbital floor or medial wall. Both CT and MR scans clearly document these so-called "blow-out" fractures, as orbital fat and muscle are seen to herniate into air-containing sinuses.

In Case 809A, orbital fat occupies a fossa formed by medial displacement of the right lamina papyracea. The medial rectus muscle is thickened and distorted as it is drawn toward the fracture.

The coronal scan in Case 809B confirms these findings. (Compare the position and morphology of the normal left medial rectus muscle to the appearance on the right.) Blow-out fractures of the orbital floor (with displacement of orbital content into the maxillary sinus) are also common and are best demonstrated in the coronal plane.

Congenital dehiscence of the lamina papyracea occurs infrequently and can resemble the appearance of a medial blow-out fracture. This possibility should be considered when orbital fat extends into the ethmoid region in patients with no history of trauma.

Case 810

44-year-old woman presenting with right-sided
proptosis and nasal obstruction.
(coronal, postcontrast scan; SE 600/14)

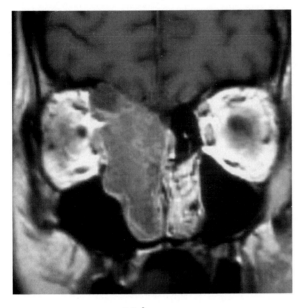

Melanoma

Case 811

36-year-old woman presenting with decreasing
visual acuity on the right.
(axial, noncontrast scan; SE 3000/75)

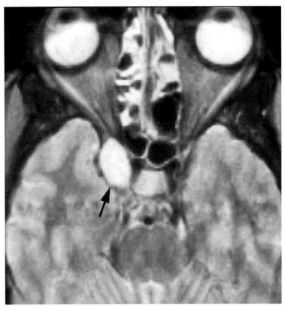

Mucocele
(within a pneumatized anterior clinoid process)

Sinus lesions are often manifested by orbital symptoms. Tumors involving the paraorbital sinuses frequently extend into the orbit and cause secondary proptosis. Among the lesions that may present in this manner are juvenile angiofibromas, esthesioneuroblastomas, and squamous cell carcinomas.

The melanoma in Case 810 fills the nose, ethmoid sinus, and the medial portion of the frontal sinus on the right. The tumor has destroyed the medial wall of the right orbit and compresses the muscle cone.

Note that the intensity of contrast enhancement within the melanoma is less than the enhancement of the contralateral nasal mucosa. This disparity is generally valid in assessing opacified sinuses on MR scans: inflammatory tissue typically enhances more intensely than neoplasm.

Case 811 demonstrates mild mucosal thickening within the ethmoid sinuses. This is a common incidental finding on cranial MR exams. Much more significant is expansion of the right anterior clinoid process *(arrow)*, which contains homogeneous high signal intensity. This small mass is strategically positioned at the margin of the optic canal, causing compression of the optic nerve.

Pneumatization of the anterior clinoid process is a common variant. The low signal intensity of air (and bone) at this location may simulate an aneurysm of the supraclinoid internal carotid artery (see Case 594). In Case 811, the pneumatized process has become obstructed, with subsequent development of an expanding mucocele.

Mucoceles are more commonly encountered in the frontal and ethmoid sinuses. They are characterized by smooth expansion of sinus walls. Mucoceles may demonstrate high or low signal intensity on either T1-weighted or T2-weighted scans, depending on the viscosity and inspissation of their proteinaceous content.

REFERENCES

Albert A, Lee BCP, Saint-Louis L, Deck MDF: MR of optic chiasm and optic pathways. *AJNR* 7:255-258, 1986.

Alvord EC, Lofton S: Gliomas of the optic nerve or chiasm. *J Neurosurg* 68:85-98, 1988.

Atlas SW: MR of the orbit: current imaging applications. *Semin US CT MR* 9:381-400, 1988.

Atlas SW, Bilaniuk LT, Zimmerman RA, et al: Orbit: initial experience with surface coil spin-echo MR imaging at 1.5T. *Radiology* 164:501-509, 1987.

Atlas SW, Grossman RI, Hackney DB, et al: STIR MR imaging of the orbit. *AJNR* 9:969-974, 1988.

Atlas SW, Grossman RI, Savino PJ, et al: Surface-coil MR of orbital pseudotumor. *AJNR* 8:141-146, 1987.

Azar-Kia B, Naheedy MH, Elias DA, et al: Optic nerve tumors: role of magnetic resonance imaging and computed tomography. *Rad Clin North Am* 25:561-582, 1987.

Barkovich AJ, Fram EK, Norman D: Septo-optic dysplasia: MR imaging. *Radiology* 171:189-192, 1989.

Beets-Tau RGH, Hendriks MJ, Ramos LMP, et al: Retinoblastoma: CT and MRI. *Neuroradiology* 36:59-62, 1994.

Bilaniuk LT, Atlas SW, Zimmerman RA: Magnetic resonance imaging of the orbit. *Rad Clin North Am* 25:509-528, 1987.

Bilaniuk LT, Farber M: Imaging of developmental anomalies of the eye and the orbit. *AJNR* 13:793-803, 1992.

Bilaniuk LT, Schenck JE, Zimmerman RA, et al: Ocular and orbital lesions. Surface coil MR imaging. *Radiology* 156:669-674, 1985.

Brown EW, Riccardi VM, Mawad M, et al: MR imaging of optic pathways in patients with neurofibromatosis. *AJNR* 8:1031-1036, 1987.

Carmody RF, Mafee MF, Goodwin JA, et al: Orbital and optic pathway sarcoidosis: MR findings. *AJNR* 15:775-783, 1994.

Char DH, Sobel D, Kelly WM, et al: Magnetic resonance scanning in orbital tumor diagnosis. *Ophthalmology* 92:1305-1310, 1985.

Daniels DL, Herfins R, Gager WE, et al: Magnetic resonance imaging of the optic nerves and chiasm. *Radiology* 152:79-83, 1984.

Daniels DL, Kneeland JB, Shimakawa A, et al: MR imaging of the optic nerve and sheath: correcting the chemical shift misregistration effect. *AJNR* 7:249-253, 1986.

Daniels DL, Yu S, Perch P, et al: Computed tomography and magnetic resonance imaging of the orbital apex. *Rad Clin North Am* 25:803, 1987.

Delfini R, Missori P, Iannetti G, et al: Mucoceles of the paranasal sinuses with intracranial and intraorbital extension: report of 28 cases. *Neurosurgery* 32:901-906, 1993.

Digre KB, Smoker WRK, Johnston P, et al: Selective MR imaging approach for evaluation of patients with Horner's syndrome. *AJNR* 13:223-227, 1992.

Engelken JD, Yuh WTC, Carter KD, Nerad JA: Optic nerve sarcoidosis: MR findings. *AJNR* 13:228-230, 1992.

Flanders AE, Espinosa GA, Markiewicz DA, Howell DD: Orbital lymphoma: role of CT and MRI. *Rad Clin North Am* 25:601-614, 1987.

Fries PD, Char DH, Norman D: MR imaging of orbital cavernous hemangioma. *J Comput Assist Tomogr* 11:418-421, 1987.

Gomori JM, Grossman RI, Shields JA, et al: Choroidal melanomas: correlation of NMR spectroscopy and MR imaging. *Radiology* 158:443-445, 1986.

Graeb DA, Rootman J, Robertson WD, et al: Orbital lymphangiomas: clinical, radiologic, and pathologic characteristics. *Radiology* 175:417-421, 1990.

Guy T, Mancuso A, Quisling RG, et al: Gadolinium DTPA-enhanced magnetic resonance imaging in optic neuropathies. *Ophthalmology* 97:592-600, 1990.

Haik BG, Saint Louis L, Smith ME, et al: Magnetic resonance imaging in the evaluation of leukokoria. *Ophthalmology* 92:1143-1152, 1985a.

Hendrix LE, Kneeland JB, Haughton VM, et al: MR imaging of optic nerve lesions: value of gadopentetate dimeglumine and fat suppression technique. *AJNR* 11:749-754, 1990.

Holman RE, Grimson BS, Drayer BP, et al: Magnetic resonance imaging of optic gliomas. *Am J Ophthalmol* 1985:100:596-601, 1985.

Hopper KD, Sherman JL, Boal DKB: Abnormalities of the orbit and its contents in children: CT and MR imaging findings. *AJR* 156:1219-1224, 1991.

Hopper KD, Sherman JL, Boal DK, Eggli KD: CT and MR imaging of the pediatric orbit. *Radiographics* 12:485-504, 1992.

Hosten N, Sander B, Cordes M, et al: Graves ophthalmology: MR imaging of the orbits. *Radiology* 172:759-762, 1989.

Hudgins PA, Newman NJ, Dillon WP, Hoffman JC: Radiation-induced optic neuropathy: characteristic appearances on gadolinium-enhanced MR. *AJNR* 13:235-238, 1992.

Imes RK, Hoyt WF: Magnetic resonance imaging signs of optic nerve gliomas in neurofibromatosis 1. *Am J Ophthalmol* 111:729-734, 1991.

Kaissar G, Kim JH, Bravo S, Sze G: Histologic basis for increased extraocular muscle enhancement in gadolinium-enhanced MR imaging. *Radiology* 179:541-542, 1991.

Komiyama M, Fu Y, Yagura H, et al: MR imaging of dural AV fistulas at the cavernous sinus. *J Comput Assist Tomogr* 14:397-401, 1990.

Langer BG, MaFee MF, Pollack S, et al: MRI of the normal orbit and optic pathways. *Rad Clin North Am* 25:429-446, 1987.

Lindblom B, Norman D, Hoyt WF: Perioptic cyst distal to optic nerve meningioma: MR demonstration. *AJNR* 13:1622-1624, 1992.

Linder B, Campos M. Schafer M: CT and MRI of orbital abnormalities in neurofibromatosis and selected craniofacial anomalies. *Rad Clin North Am* 25:787, 1987.

Mafee MF, Goldberg MF, Greenwald MJ, et al: Retinoblastoma and simulating lesions: role of CT and MR imaging. *Rad Clin North Am* 25:667-682, 1987.

Mafee MF, Linder B, Peyman GA, et al: Choroidal hematoma and effusion: evaluation with MR imaging. *Radiology* 168:781-786, 1988.

Mafee MF, Peyman GA: Retinal and choroidal detachments: role of magnetic resonance imaging and computed tomography. *Rad Clin North Am* 25:487-508, 1987.

Mafee MF, Peyman GA, Grisolano JE, et al: Malignant uveal melanoma and simulating lesions: MR imaging evaluation. *Radiology* 160:773-780, 1986.

Mafee MF, Peyman GA, Peace JH, et al: Magnetic resonance imaging in the evaluation and differentiation of uveal melanoma. *Ophthalmology* 94:341-348, 1987.

Mafee MF, Putterman A, Valvassori GE, et al: Orbital space-occupying lesions. Role of computed tomography and magnetic resonance imaging. An analysis of 145 cases. *Rad Clin North Am* 25:529-559, 1987.

Manfre L, Nicoletti G, Lombardo M, et al: Orbital "blow-in" fracture: MRI. *Neuroradiology* 35:612-613, 1993.

McArdle CB, Amparo EG, Mirfakhraee M: MR imaging of orbital blow-out fractures. *J Comput Assist Tomogr* 10:116-119, 1986.

Merandi SF, Kudryk BT: Contrast-enhanced MR imaging of optic nerve lesions in patients with acute optic neuritis. *AJNR* 12:923-926, 1991.

Mihara F, Gupta KL, Murayama S, et al: MR imaging of malignant uveal melanoma: role of pulse sequence and contrast agent. *AJNR* 12:991-999, 1991.

502

Miller DH, MacManus DG, Bartlett PA, et al: Detection of optic nerve lesions in optic neuritis using frequency-selective fat-saturation sequences. *Neuroradiology* 35:156-158, 1993.

Miller DH, Newton MR, Van der Poel JC, et al: Magnetic resonance imaging of the optic nerve in optic neuritis. *Neurology* 38:175-179, 1988.

Ohnishi T, Noguchi S, Murakami N, et al: Extraocular muscles in Graves ophthalmopathy: usefulness of T2 relaxation time measurements. *Radiology* 190:857-862, 1994.

Peyman GA, Mafee MF: Uveal melanoma and similar lesions: the role of magnetic resonance imaging. *Rad Clin North Am* 25:471-486, 1987.

Peyster RG, Augsburger JJ, Shields JA, et al: Intraocular tumor: evaluation with MR imaging. *Radiology* 168:773-780, 1988.

Peyster RG, Shapiro MO, Haik BG: Orbital metastasis: role of magnetic resonance imaging and computed tomography. *Rad Clin North Am* 25:647-662, 1987.

Pomeranz SJ, Shelton JJ, Tobias J, et al: MR of visual pathways in patients with neurofibromatosis. *AJNR* 8:831-836, 1987.

Roden DT, Savino PJ, Zimmerman RA: Magnetic resonance imaging in orbital diagnosis. *Rad Clin North Am* 26:535-544, 1988.

Rootman J, Damji KF, Dimmick JE: Malignant rhabdoid tumor of the orbit. *Ophthalmology* 96:1650, 1989.

Shen W-C, Yang D-Y, Ho WL, et al: Neurilemmoma of the oculomotor nerve presenting as an orbital mass: MR findings. *AJNR* 14:1253-1254, 1993.

Simon J, Szumowski J, Totterman S, et al: Fat suppression MR imaging of the orbit. *AJNR* 9:961-968, 1988.

Smith M, Castillo M: Imaging and differential diagnosis of the large eye, *Radiographics* 14:721-728, 1994.

Sobel DF, Kelly W, Kjos B, et al: MR imaging of orbital and ocular disease. *AJNR* 6:259-264, 1985.

Spencer G, Lufkin R, Simons K, et al: MR of a melanoma simulating ocular neoplasm. *AJNR* 8:921-922, 1987.

Sullivan JA, Harms SE: Characterization of orbital lesions by surface coil MR imaging. *Radiographics* 7:9-28, 1987.

Sullivan JA, Harms SE: Surface coil MR imaging of orbital neoplasms. *AJNR* 7:29-34, 1986.

Tien RD, Chu PK, Hesselink JR, Szumowski J: Intra- and paraorbital lesions: value of fat-suppression MR imaging with paramagnetic contrast enhancement. *AJNR* 12:245-253, 1991.

Tien R, Dillon WP: MR imaging of cavernous hemangiomas of the optic chiasm. *J Comput Assist Tomogr* 13:1087-1100, 1989.

Tien RD, Hesselink JR, Szumowski J: MR fat suppression combined with Gd-DTPA enhancement in optic neuritis and perineuritis. *J Comput Assist Tomogr* 15:223-227, 1991.

Tonami H, Nakagawa T, Ohguchi M, et al: Surface coil MR imaging of orbital blowout fractures: a comparison with reformatted CT. *AJNR* 8:445-449, 1987.

Tonami H, Tamamura H, Kimizu K, et al: Intraocular lesions in patients with systemic disease: findings on MR imaging. *AJNR* 10:1185-1190, 1989.

Tong KA, Osborn AG, Mamalis N, et al: Ocular melanoma. *AJNR* 14:1359-1366, 1993.

Walker FO, McLean WT Jr, Elster A, Stouton C: Chiasmal sarcoidosis. *AJNR* 11:1205-1207, 1990.

Wildenhain PM, Lehar SC, Dastur KJ, et al: Orbital varix. Color flow imaging correlated with CT and MR studies. *J Comput Assist Tomogr* 15:171-173, 1991.

Zimmerman RA, Bilaniuk LT: Ocular MR imaging. *Radiology* 168:875, 1988.

CHAPTER 14

Disc Disease and Spondylosis

Case 812

32-year-old woman complaining of chronic
back pain.
(axial, noncontrast scan; SE 1000/17; L4-5 level)

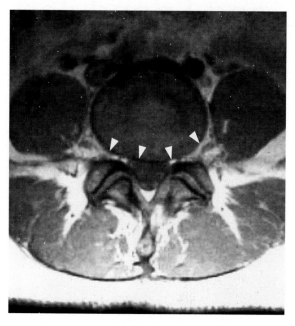

Bulging Disc

Case 813

39-year-old man presenting with left leg pain and
diminished ankle reflex.
(axial, noncontrast scan; SE 1100/19; L5-S1 level)

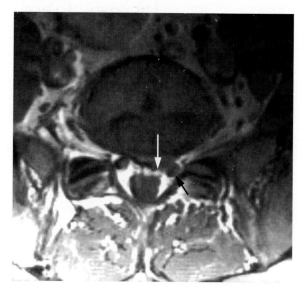

Herniated Disc

The MR demonstration of lumbar disc abnormalities is based on the differential signal intensity of bone, disc, spinal fluid, and epidural fat. In Case 812, the posterior margin of the bulging disc *(arrowheads)* is defined by the slightly lower intensity of spinal fluid within the dural sac and the higher signal intensity of epidural fat within the nerve root canals.

The posterior margin of lumbar discs is normally slightly concave at the L1 through L5 levels and nearly straight at L5-S1. Bulging discs demonstrate a uniform, symmetrical convexity. This broad curve contrasts with the focal asymmetry of disc herniation, as seen in Case 813.

The false appearance of a posterior disc bulge may be caused by oblique angulation of axial scans with respect to the disc level, most commonly seen at L5-S1. Spondylolisthesis may also cause a prominent disc "shelf" resembling a diffuse bulge (see Case 854A).

The focal protrusion of disc material in Case 813 *(white arrow)* has a small radius of curvature and a relatively abrupt angle of origin from the parent disc. This localized change in contour contrasts with the diffuse bulge in Case 812. A discontinuity in the dark line of posterior annular fibers is apparent at the base of the herniation (compare to Case 821).

Disc herniations involving the central canal are often asymmetrical. Eccentric herniations may severely distort individual nerve roots without compressing the dural sac. The disc in Case 813 displaces and compresses the proximal left S1 nerve root *(black arrow)* within the lateral recess.

Some cases present features intermediate between Cases 812 and 813, so that distinguishing between an asymmetrical disc bulge and a frank disc herniation is difficult. MR scans have demonstrated evidence of annular tears and extruded disc material in cases where the overall contour of the disc remains generally symmetrical or "bulge-like." Sagittal views are particularly useful for assessing the integrity of the annulus fibrosis (see Cases 820, 822, and 823).

Disc herniations are most common in a posterolateral direction, as in Case 813. However, midline herniations also occur (see Case 829).

Case 814

47-year-old man presenting with worsening low
back and leg pain.
(sagittal, noncontrast scan; SE 800/17)

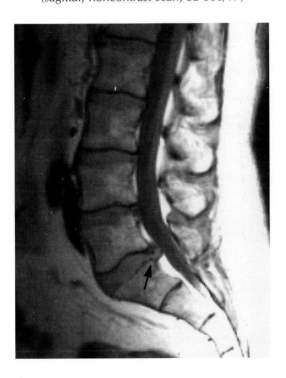

Case 815

37-year-old man presenting with back and leg pain.
(sagittal, noncontrast scan; SE 3200/90)

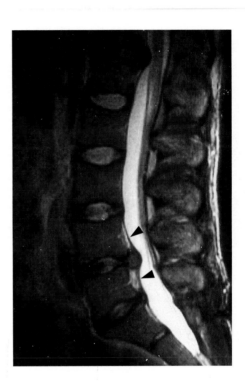

Sagittal MR scans efficiently display long segments of the spinal canal. Both extradural and intrathecal pathologies are well seen. These imaging advantages contrast with the limited coverage and poor intradural definition of standard axial CT studies.

Centrally herniated discs are outlined on T1-weighted images by the slightly lower intensity of CSF within the subarachnoid space and/or by the higher signal intensity of ventral epidural fat. In Case 814 an anterior epidural mass is centered at the L5-S1 disc level, suggesting discogenic origin. In addition to the disc herniation itself, associated edema, venous congestion, granulation tissue, and/or localized epidural hemorrhage may contribute to prominent extradural deformities (see Case 830).

The signal intensity of herniated discs is variable on long

TR spin echo images. Many herniated discs demonstrate intermediate to high intensity values on such scans (see Case 857). This apparent high water content may reflect the hydrophilic nature of herniated nuclear material and/or the presence of reactive granulation tissue. Such lesions may be best seen on "balanced" or "intermediate" spin echo images (long TR, short TE), with reduced conspicuity on more heavily T2-weighted scans.

In other cases, the signal intensity of disc herniations is relatively low, and they are well outlined by "bright" CSF on T2-weighted studies. Case 815 illustrates this appearance. The posterior longitudinal ligament and dura are tented above and below the level of the L4-5 disc herniation *(arrowheads)*. Smaller herniations are present at the L5-S1 and T12-L1 levels.

507

Case 816

21-year-old woman complaining of back pain.
(sagittal, noncontrast scan; SE 2800/45)

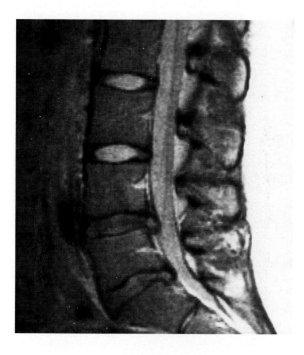

Case 817

28-year-old woman with exacerbation of back pain
after a fall.
(sagittal, noncontrast scan; SE 2500/45)

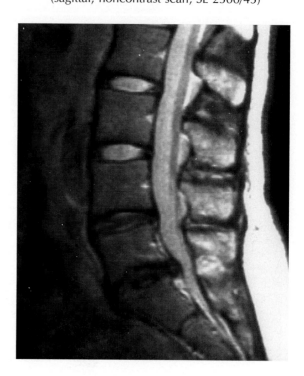

Normal intervertebral discs demonstrate generally high signal intensity on long TR spin echo images. This appearance reflects the high water content of the nucleus pulposus and the integrity of the complex polysaccharides within the nuclear matrix.

Degeneration of a disc is associated with progressive loss of long T2 values. This change probably represents both a decrease in water content and an alteration of the macromolecular matrix of the disc (with increased binding of water molecules shortening relaxation times).

Reduced "hydration signal" is apparent within the L4-5 and L5-S1 discs in each of the above cases. (Compare to the normal signal intensity at the L1 through L4 levels.) Accompanying disc herniations are present at L4-5 and L5-S1 in Case 816 and at L5-S1 in Case 817. Herniation is usually

preceded by evidence of reduced disc "hydration." However, "dehydration" of a disc is often noted in the absence of herniation (e.g., at the L4-5 level in Case 817).

Comparison of the L5-S1 level in Cases 816 and 817 demonstrates the variable signal intensity of disc herniations on long TR spin echo images. Herniated discs with low signal intensity can be difficult to distinguish from potential accompanying osteophytes.

In both of these cases the roots of the cauda equina form a dorsal band of low signal intensity within the dural sac. This normal appearance should not be mistaken for thickening of the filum terminale or an abnormally low-lying spinal cord (see Cases 1062 and 1072). Axial images will resolve confusion in most cases.

Case 818

43-year-old man presenting with a three-month
history of back pain (no prior surgery).
(axial, postcontrast scan; SE 1000/15; L4-5 level)

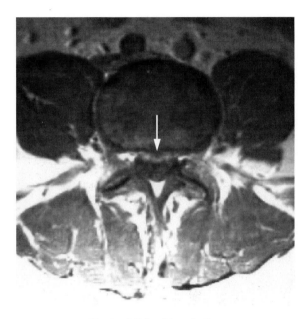

Central Disc Herniation

Case 819

38-year-old man presenting with severe right
leg pain (no prior surgery).
(axial, post-contrast scan; SE 700/17; L4 level)

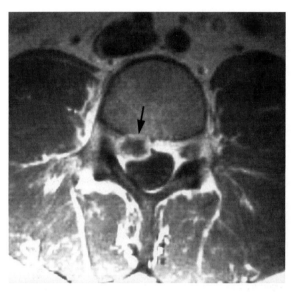

Lateral Disc Herniation
(free fragment)

The margin of herniated discs is usually outlined by a rim
of enhancement on postcontrast scans. This enhancing border has been correlated histologically with a layer of vascular granulation tissue. Marginal enhancement can help to
distinguish disc herniations from other epidural masses
(e.g., lymphoma or metastasis) or from postoperative epidural fibrosis (see Cases 839 and 840).

The above cases demonstrate that peripheral enhancement may outline disc herniations prior to surgical inter-
vention. (See Case 840 for discussion of post-operative disc
enhancement.) The small central herniation in Case 818 is
defined by the thin layer of adjacent enhancement; the herniation might otherwise be undetected on a T1-weighted
scan.

In Case 819, contrast enhancement helps to characterize
the large mass occupying the right lateral recess. This lesion is a fragment of disc material that has migrated rostrally to reside posterior to the vertebral body of L4. The
dural sac is deformed, and both the exiting right L4 nerve
root and the traversing right L5 nerve root are likely distorted.

Epidural abscesses and epidural hematomas may also
present the appearance of marginal enhancement surrounding a nonenhancing center (see Cases 981 and 1025).
These pathologies should be considered in the appropriate
clinical context.

Contrast material may diffuse from the perimeter of a herniated disc into the center on delayed scans. This gradual
accumulation of contrast over a period of minutes to hours
may obscure the initially characteristic morphology and reduce diagnostic specificity (see Case 927).

LUMBAR DISC HERNIATION: DISRUPTION OF THE ANNULUS FIBROSIS

Case 820

35-year-old woman with leg pain and a diminished
ankle reflex.
(sagittal, noncontrast scan; SE 1000/22)

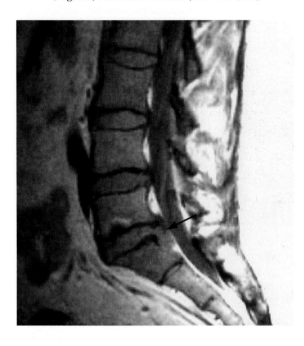

Case 821

42-year-old man presenting with left leg pain
and numbness.
(axial, noncontrast scan; SE 1000/16; L4-5 level)

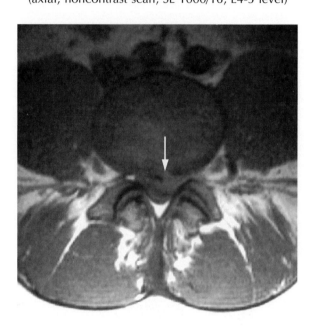

Disruption of the annulus fibrosis is necessary for herniation of nuclear material. Large annular tears may be apparent on MR scans in patients with herniated discs, as seen in the above examples. In other cases, small tears of the annulus may be imaged with no evidence of associated herniation (see Case 822).

The outer annular fibers form a dense zone at the perimeter of a normal disc. This band of collagenous tissue contains little water and is normally seen as a thick line of low signal intensity separating nuclear material from epidural fat and the thecal sac. Disruption of the outer annulus is imaged as discontinuity along the normally "dark" perimeter of a disc.

In Case 820, the posterior margin of the large disc herniation at L5-S1 interfaces directly with epidural fat. No intervening band of low intensity annulus is visible. A remnant of the disrupted annulus is seen superiorly (*arrow;* compare to the intact annular rings at the posterior margins of the L3-4 and L4-5 discs).

Case 821 demonstrates a large central to left-sided disc herniation at the L4-5 level. A focal discontinuity in the circumferential zone of annular low intensity is present at the base of the herniation (*arrow;* a similar appearance is seen in Case 813). Case 821 also illustrates that the signal intensity of herniated disc material often exceeds the intensity of the parent disc (on either T1- or T2-weighted images; see also Case 857).

A shallow Schmorl's node with reactive bone changes is present in the inferior end-plate of L5 in Case 820 (compare to Cases 831-833).

The normal plexus of epidural veins ("retrovertebral plexus") may form a prominent structure within the anterior portion of the spinal canal at midvertebral levels. This anatomical variant should not be mistaken for migration of a disc fragment. The usual proximity to the basivertebral vein at the midportion of the vertebral body helps to establish the vascular nature of the epidural "mass" in such cases.

Case 822

26-year-old man presenting with bilateral leg pain.
(sagittal, noncontrast scan; SE 2800/90)

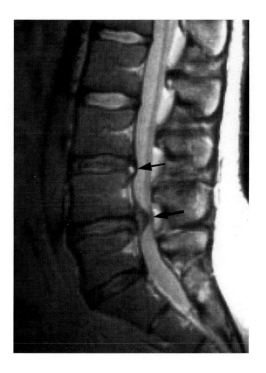

Case 823

33-year-old man complaining of chronic back pain.
(axial, noncontrast scan; SE 2000/30; L5-S1 level).

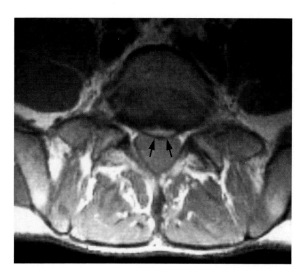

Large disruptions of the annulus fibrosis may be apparent on T1-weighted scans in association with disc herniations (see the preceding page). Smaller annular tears are best seen as focal zones of high signal intensity interrupting the normally "dark" outer annulus on long TR spin echo images.

Case 822 demonstrates reduced hydration signal at the three lowest lumbar disc levels. Herniation is present at L4-5 *(thick arrow)*. A partial thickness tear of the posterior annulus is seen inferiorly at L3-4 *(thin arrow)*. The localized high signal intensity at this site suggests an increase in water content, likely reflecting reparative granulation tissue and reactive edema.

In Case 823, a shallow zone of increased signal intensity is present along the midposterior margin of the disc *(arrows)*. This finding reflects granulation tissue and edema occupying and expanding the region of disrupted fibrous tissue. As in Case 822, a thin dark line of extreme outer annulus is present at the margin of the partial thickness tear.

An annular tear does not necessarily imply the presence of disc herniation. Reactive or reparative tissue within a disruption of the annulus may be incorrectly interpreted as herniated nuclear material.

Case 824

27-year-old man presenting with pain in the
back and right leg.
(axial, noncontrast scan; SE 1000/15; L5-S1 level).

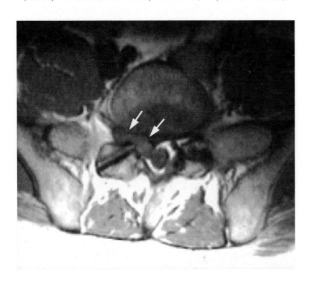

Case 825

54-year-old woman with severe left leg pain.
(axial, noncontrast scan; SE 1300/16; L4 level).

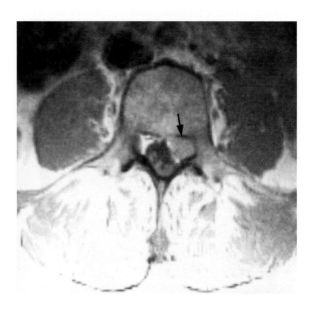

Herniated discs may compress nerve roots by distorting the dural sac, by narrowing the lateral recess, or by restricting the intervertebral foramen.

The lateral recess is formed at the anterolateral corner of the spinal canal by the junction of the vertebral body and pedicle. A lumbar nerve occupies this angle as it prepares to exit beneath the pedicle through the superior portion of the intervertebral foramen.

Posterolateral disc herniations commonly involve the region of the lateral recess, as in the above cases (see Cases 838 and 840 for additional examples). Case 824 demonstrates the amorphous, homogeneous signal intensity of herniated nuclear material replacing epidural fat within the right lateral recess and nerve root canal *(arrows)*. The proximal right S1 nerve root, which would normally reside in this location, is severely compressed.

In Case 825, a herniated nuclear fragment has ascended from the disc level to occupy the lateral recess medial to the left pedicle of L4. This homogeneous mass deforms the dural sac and compresses the proximal left L4 nerve root prior to its entry into the nerve root canal.

The appearance in Case 825 is nonspecific. Differential diagnosis would include epidural masses such as lymphoma and metastasis. A postcontrast scan in this case would likely resemble Case 819 and increase diagnostic confidence.

Adjacent lumbar nerves may share a common sleeve. A "conjoined" or "compound" sleeve is larger than an individual nerve and is located between the levels of the contributing roots. This normal variant presents as an asymmetrical structure occupying the lateral recess and may be misinterpreted as a herniated disc. However, the CSF-like signal intensity within a compound sleeve on all pulse sequences contrasts with the soft tissue values expected of disc material. In addition, the involved lateral recess is often large, favoring a congenital variation. A compound sleeve can also be identified by more caudal sections demonstrating the emergence of two separate roots.

Case 826

58-year-old woman complaining of left leg pain.
(axial, noncontrast scan; SE 1000/17; L4-5 level)

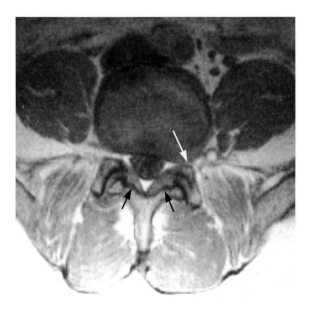

Case 827

50-year-old man presenting with right leg pain.
(sagittal, noncontrast scan; SE 800/15)

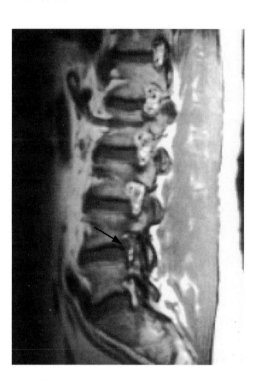

Lateral disc herniations may cause radiculopathy by compressing nerve roots as they leave the spinal canal. Disc material may extend into an intervertebral foramen and/or distort a nerve root distal to the neural canal.

In Case 826, a left lateral disc herniation *(white arrow)* occupies the inferior portion of the L4-5 nerve root canal. Compare the diameter of the right intervertebral foramen in Case 826 to the affected side.

The cephalocaudal dimension of intervertebral foramina can be difficult to judge on axial CT or MR scans. Sagittal views are helpful in this assessment. Since the orientation of lumbar nerve root canals is close to the coronal plane, sagittal MR scans provide cross-sectional views of foraminal margins and contents.

On T1-weighted images the intervertebral foramina are normally filled with high intensity fat surrounding a nerve root of intermediate intensity. (In the lumbar region the root exits close to the superior pedicle; the reverse is true in the cervical spine.) Disc material or osteophyte is well defined when encroaching into the zone of high contrast.

Case 827 demonstrates a lobulated herniation of disc material extending into the L4-5 nerve root canal *(arrow;* compare to foramina at the higher levels). The L4 root is mildly compressed between the disc margin and the overlying pedicle.

Disc herniations may occur even further laterally, distorting nerve roots as they exit from the intervertebral foramen. It is important to follow all roots through their foramina when reviewing CT and MR studies, so that foraminal or extraforaminal impingement is recognized. The surgical approach to "far lateral" root compression is a lateral exposure; traditional laminectomy will fail to identify the source of symptoms.

The symmetrical areas of tissue with intermediate signal intensity along the posterolateral margins of the spinal canal in Case 826 *(black arrows)* are the ligamenta flava. Thickening of these ligaments often accompanies degenerative disc disease and contributes to narrowing of the spinal canal or intervertebral foramina (see Cases 845 and 846).

Case 828

32-year-old man presenting with the acute onset
of severe back pain after heavy lifting.
(sagittal, noncontrast scan; SE 800/17)

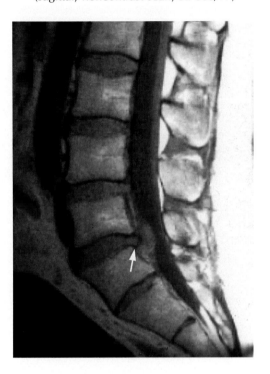

Case 829

27-year-old woman presenting with abnormal gait
and an outside CT scan interpreted as negative.
(axial, noncontrast scan; SE 1000/20; L3-4 level)

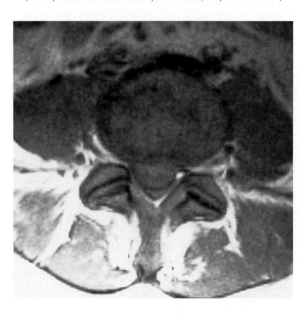

Lumbar disc herniations occasionally cause very large anterior epidural masses. Absorption of water, reactive edema, congestion of epidural veins, and epidural hemorrhage (see Case 830) may all contribute to bulky mass effect.

The diagnosis of massive herniation on MR scans is based on the lesion's location and morphology. The signal intensity of a large herniation is usually intermediate and nonspecific. However, the centering of an anterior epidural mass at the level of an intervertebral disc strongly suggests the correct diagnosis. A background of degenerative disc and/or bone changes may be supportive, along with the clinical context. Contrast enhancement (see Cases 818 and 819) can be useful in ambiguous cases.

An axial scan in Case 828 demonstrated that the large "central" herniation had in fact arisen on the left side of midline. This eccentric origin accounts for the potentially confusing appearance of an intact posterior annulus anterior to the herniation on the midsagittal image. At surgery, the entire epidural mass was found to represent edematous disc material that had emerged from a left-sided annular tear.

"Giant" disc herniations are occasionally overlooked on axial CT scans, as in Case 829. If abnormal soft tissue fills the spinal canal, there may be no recognizable interface between the herniation and the compressed dural sac.

Case 830A

59-year-old man presenting with the acute onset of
severe low back pain.
(sagittal, noncontrast scan; SE 800/15)

Case 830B

Same patient.
(sagittal, noncontrast scan; SE 2500/90)

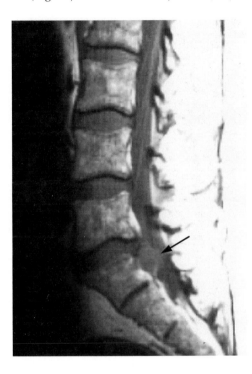

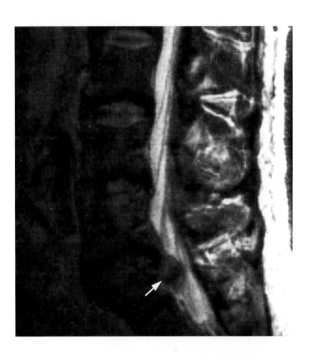

Epidural hemorrhage may contribute to the symptomatology and appearance of lumbar disc herniations. Disruption of an anterior epidural vein by a herniating disc can lead to localized bleeding that accentuates the mass effect of the herniation.

A component of epidural hemorrhage can be suspected when "giant" herniations are encountered. The signal intensity of such lesions is often intermediate and nonspecific. This is particularly true on T1-weighted scans, where T1-shortening attributable to methemoglobin is rarely observed.

In Case 830A, the large anterior epidural mass at L5-S1 is nondescript and poorly defined *(arrow)*. It is difficult to distinguish potential epidural hemorrhage from edematous inflammatory tissue or congested epidural veins, which more commonly exaggerate the bulk of a disc herniation.

On T2-weighted scans, the signal intensity within epidural hematomas is variable. Case 830B demonstrates T2-shortening within the lesion *(arrow)*, which showed even greater signal loss on subsequent axial gradient echo images. This appearance raises the question of blood products (see discussion of Cases 555-558). Simple disc fragments can appear "dark" on T2-weighted studies, but this signal loss is usually not accentuated on gradient echo scans. In other cases, the intensity of epidural hemorrhage on long TR images may be intermediate or high (see Case 866).

Epidural hematomas accompanying disc herniations usually regress spontaneously over a period of weeks to months. The resorption of such hemorrhages (together with reduction in epidural edema and venous congestion) may account for some of the spontaneously resolving disc herniations previously reported on myelographic and CT studies.

Case 831

65-year-old woman complaining of a stiff back.
(sagittal, noncontrast scan; SE 550/20)

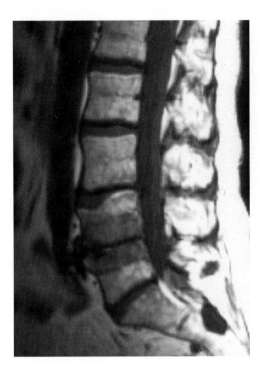

Case 832

31-year-old woman presenting with back pain.
(sagittal, noncontrast scan; SE 2500/90)

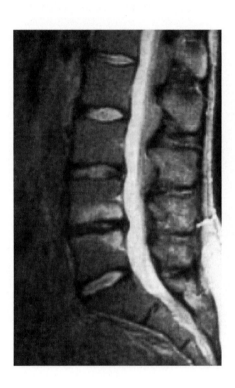

Sagittal or coronal MR scans may demonstrate reactive changes in the vertebral bodies adjacent to degenerating discs. Subchondral zones of long T1 and long T2 values are often seen, representing inflammatory edema and reactive cellular infiltration within the marrow. At a later stage, fatty atrophy of the marrow may cause the opposite pattern of signal changes: "bright" on T1-weighted images, with reduced signal intensity on T2-weighted scans (see Case 833).

The L4-5 disc space is severely narrowed in Case 831. Broad zones of low signal intensity are present in the adjacent vertebral bodies. Both reactive sclerosis and marrow edema with cellular infiltration may contribute to this appearance.

Case 832 demonstrates narrowing and reduced hydration signal at the L3-4 and L4-5 disc levels. Prominent bands of T2-prolongation are present in subchondral regions of the L4 and L5 vertebral bodies. This increase in water content suggests reactive inflammation.

Prolongation of T1 and T2 values within subchondral bone is also seen in patients with discitis and osteomyelitis (see Cases 962-965). Several features help to distinguish degenerative bone changes from osseous infection: (1) cortical end-plates are preserved in degenerative disease (except for well-defined Schmorl's nodes) and irregularly eroded by infection; (2) the adjacent disc space usually demonstrates little or no hydration signal in degenerative disease but is commonly "bright" on T2-weighted scans when inflamed by discitis; (3) associated epidural or paraspinal masses are rarely seen in degenerative disease (unless there is superimposed disc herniation) but are commonly present with discitis; and (4) contrast enhancement of affected vertebral bodies is moderate and uniform in degenerative disease, while enhancement in discitis/osteomyelitis is more irregular and intense.

The clinical context is also helpful in assessing the significance of signal abnormalities within vertebral bodies. Patients with discitis/osteomyelitis are usually in severe pain. The diagnosis is unlikely in the absence of impressive symptoms.

Case 833

71-year-old woman.
(sagittal, noncontrast scan; SE 600/15)

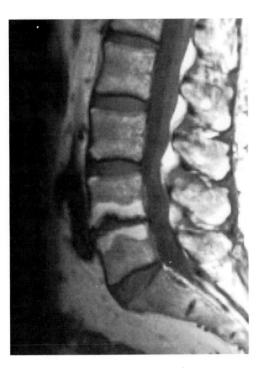

Fatty Marrow Atrophy

Case 834

49-year-old man.
(sagittal, postcontrast scan; SE 630/20)

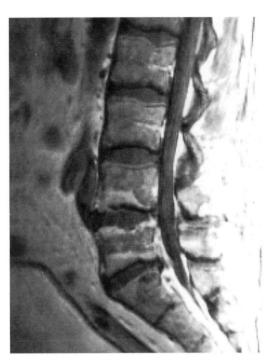

Enhancing Reactive Marrow Infiltration

Fatty marrow atrophy may cause T1-shortening within subchondral bone of lumbar vertebral bodies. This replacement of hematopoietic tissue is thought to be a late result of degenerative disc disease. In some cases, a transition from the appearance of reactive infiltration (as in Case 831) to fatty atrophy, as seen at the L4-5 level in Case 833, has been observed. (Case 853A provides another example of this finding.)

As discussed on the preceding page, reactive changes within vertebral bodies bordering degenerating discs initially include cellular infiltration and edema. Contrast enhancement is often present at this stage. Postcontrast T1-shortening may cause the involved regions to become isointense to fatty marrow. In Case 834, the subchondral zones of high signal at the L4 and L5 levels are even more intense than the adjacent normal marrow. (See the preceding page regarding distinction between enhancing degenerative changes and discitis.)

Case 835

*43-year-old woman several years after
right-sided laminectomy.
(axial, noncontrast scan; SE 1000/16; L4 level)*

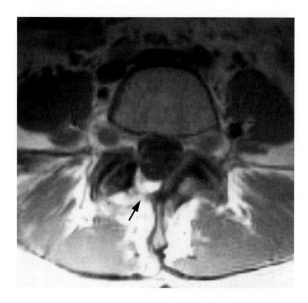

Case 836

*39-year-old man four months
after microdiscectomy.
(axial, postcontrast scan; SE 800/16; L4-5 level)*

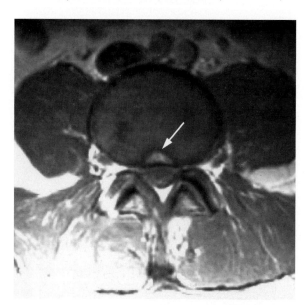

Lumbar laminectomy and discectomy lead to characteristic postoperative MR findings. A laminectomy defect is usually well defined as a gap in the the vertebral arch posterior to the facet joint. The ligamentum flavum is absent on the side of surgery.

Case 835 illustrates that both the lamina and the ligamentum flavum have been removed on the right side *(arrow)*. The dural sac bulges dorsally toward the operative defect. Epidural fibrosis is minimal in this case, and there is no evidence of recurrent disc herniation. Nerve roots are well visualized within the intervertebral foramina and within the thecal sac.

Focal contrast enhancement normally occurs along the posterior margin of intervertebral discs at the site of prior herniation and surgery. This localized finding probably reflects the presence of granulation tissue within the healing annulus. Case 836 illustrates such enhancement in the midline *(arrow)* after resection of a central herniation.

More extensive enhancement involving central portions of the disc space is unusual after uncomplicated discectomy. The possibility of infection should be considered in such cases (see Cases 974, 975 and 977).

Note that a laminectomy defect is not apparent in Case 836. "Microdiscectomy" techniques involving little or no bone removal are increasingly common. As a result, the absence of an obvious laminectomy does not preclude postoperative change as a potential etiology for abnormal findings on CT or MR scans.

Postoperative MR studies performed in the first several months after surgery often demonstrate a soft tissue "mass" at the site of the original herniation. This appearance probably reflects granulation tissue and edema filling the bed of the former herniated disc. The frequent occurrence of such pseudo-herniations limits the value of early postoperative scans.

DIFFERENTIAL DIAGNOSIS:
ABNORMAL EPIDURAL TISSUE WITHIN THE LATERAL RECESS

Case 837

42-year-old woman with persistent left leg pain six
months after laminectomy.
(axial, noncontrast scan; SE 1000/20; L4-5 level)

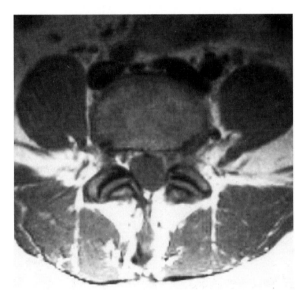

Epidural Fibrosis

Case 838

58-year-old man presenting with left leg pain.
(axial, noncontrast scan; SE 1000/70; L4-5 level)

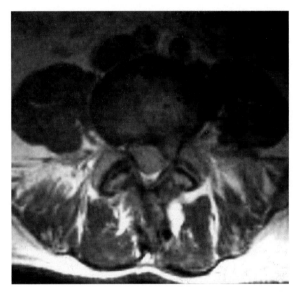

Disc Herniation

Residual or recurrent symptoms after lumbar discectomy may have many sources other than persistent or recurrent herniation at the operated level. The main purpose of scans performed in this context is to establish the presence or absence of disc herniation to help determine whether further surgery is warranted.

Following discectomy, epidural fat is often replaced or infiltrated by tissue with longer T1 values. This postoperative scarring or "epidural fibrosis" is an expected consequence of surgery and by itself is rarely significant. However, epidural fibrosis reduces or obliterates the natural contrast between a disc and epidural tissue. Amorphous, intermediate signal intensity in the region of surgery may make it difficult to diagnose or exclude disc herniation. Prominent epidural fibrosis can itself appear mass-like and simulate disc material.

In Case 837, a left-sided laminectomy defect is present. Abnormal low signal intensity surrounds the proximal left L5 nerve root within the lateral recess. (Compare to the normal L5 root on the right side.) The fact that the root can be

faintly seen in approximately normal position within the postoperative change argues against recurrent disc herniation.

The small disc herniation in Case 838 has a more mass-like contour, with better defined margins than the postoperative fibrosis of Case 837. Adjacent deformity of the dural sac is present. This finding is uncommon in cases of simple epidural fibrosis and should suggest the presence of herniated nuclear material. More importantly, the left L5 nerve root cannot be identified within the lateral recess in Case 838. This lack of visualization suggests displacement or compression of the root and contrasts with Case 837.

Long TR spin echo scans can be helpful in distinguishing between recurrent disc herniation and epidural fibrosis. Disc herniations may demonstrate either higher or lower signal intensity than surrounding postoperative changes on "intermediate" or T2-weighted images. A low intensity fibrous capsule is frequently seen at the margin of a recurrent herniation, separating it from epidural fibrosis of nearly equal intensity.

519

Case 839A

47-year-old man complaining of persistent right leg
pain nine months after L4-5 discectomy.
(axial, noncontrast scan; SE 1000/16; L4-5 level)

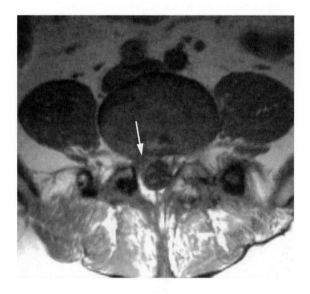

Case 839B

Same patient.
(axial, postcontrast scan; SE 1000/16; same level)

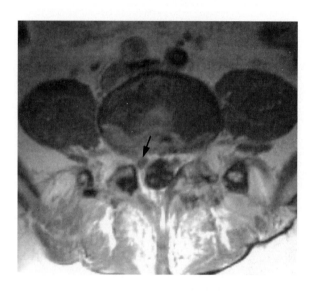

Abnormal soft tissue with a mass-like contour is present
in the right anterolateral recess of Case 839A *(arrow)*. The
ipsilateral L5 nerve root is not defined, and the overall appearance resembles the disc herniation in Case 838.

Contrast enhancement is useful for distinguishing epidural fibrosis from residual or recurrent disc herniation in
such situations. As discussed in Cases 818 and 819, scans
performed soon after the injection of contrast material usually demonstrate marginal enhancement at the perimeter of
a herniated disc. The vascular granulation and scar tissue
within zones of epidural fibrosis generally enhance more

homogeneously. That is, the early presence of contrast enhancement *within* the area of precontrast abnormality favors the diagnosis of epidural fibrosis over that of disc herniation.

In Case 839B, the majority of the "mass" within the right
lateral recess demonstrates enhancement. Enhancing scar
tissue defines the nondisplaced L5 nerve root *(arrow)*,
which was not clearly identified on the precontrast scan.
Such epidural enhancement simultaneously excludes recurrent herniation and establishes the position of symptomatic
nerve roots.

Case 840A

27-year-old woman with persistent left leg pain two
months after hemilaminectomy.
(axial, noncontrast scan; SE 800/17; L5-S1 level)

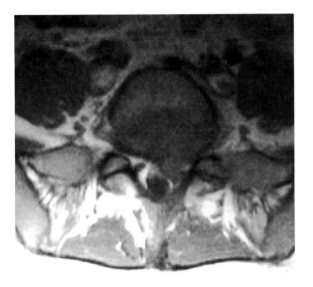

Case 840B

Same patient.
(axial, postcontrast scan; SE 800/17; same level)

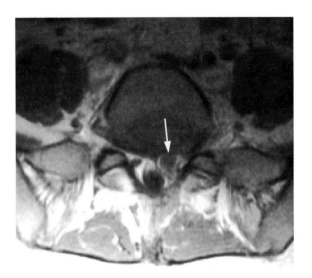

The amorphous left-sided anterior epidural mass in Case 840A is nonspecific. Both recurrent disc herniation and epidural fibrosis could present this appearance.

A postcontrast scan through the same region (Case 840B) demonstrates two components. A posterior rim of enhancing granulation tissue and fibrosis surrounds a nonenhancing disc fragment *(arrow)*. Surgery confirmed recurrent herniation.

The typical marginal enhancement of recurrent disc her-
niation in Case 840B contrasts with the usual homogeneous enhancement of epidural fibrosis in Case 839B. Scans performed immediately after contrast injection are most helpful in making this distinction. Contrast material may penetrate into the center of disc herniations on delayed scans.

It is difficult to confidently identify the proximal left S1 nerve root in either of the above images, unlike Cases 837 and 839B.

Case 841A

48-year-old man with increasing back pain one week after laminectomy and discectomy at L4-5. (sagittal, noncontrast scan; SE 700/16)

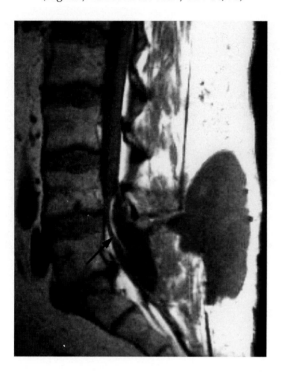

Case 841B

Same patient. (sagittal, noncontrast scan; SE 2800/90)

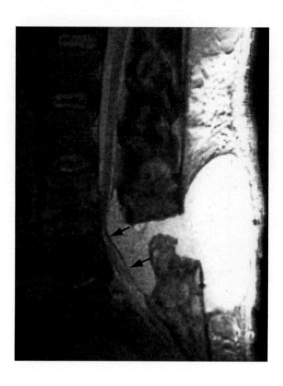

An uncommon cause of recurrent symptoms following surgery to remove a herniated disc is the development of a pseudomeningocele. These cystic collections of CSF may accumulate within epidural and paraspinal tissues when a tear of the dural sac occurs during surgery and is not completely repaired. Persistent communication with the thecal sac may cause pseudomeningoceles to enlarge, with increasing compression of adjacent nerve roots.

In Case 841A a large, fluid-filled sac is present within subcutaneous fat posterior to the lumbar spine. The appearance superficially resembles the congenital meningoceles discussed in Chapter 18. The relationship of the dorsal cyst to the dural sac is difficult to define on this T1-weighted scan. A curvilinear strand of high signal intensity within the anterior portion of the spinal canal at L4-5 *(arrow)* in fact represents a stripe of dorsal epidural fat, displaced ventrally by an epidural loculation of the cyst.

Case 841B documents the dumbbell morphology of the pseudomeningocele. A broad communication through the area of surgery connects the subcutaneous cyst with a dorsal epidural component. The epidural mass causes severe compression of the dural sac and cauda equina *(arrows)*.

Epidural or paraspinal abscesses may also cause localized fluid collections following surgery. Paraspinal abscesses are usually associated with systemic evidence of infection and severe local pain and tenderness (see Chapter 16). However, more indolent abscesses could be considered in the differential diagnosis of a pseudomeningocele, particularly if communication between the fluid collection and the dural sac is not convincingly demonstrated.

Epidural hematomas may also develop in the postoperative period to cause localized mass effect and recurrent or worsening symptoms (see Case 1020).

DURAL DIVERTICULAE

Case 842A

46-year-old man with a history of spinal trauma
and lumbar fusion twenty years earlier, now
presenting with bladder and bowel dysfunction.
(sagittal, noncontrast scan; SE 2700/90)

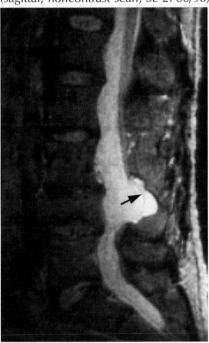

Case 842B

Same patient.
(axial, noncontrast scan; SE 1000/20; L4 level)

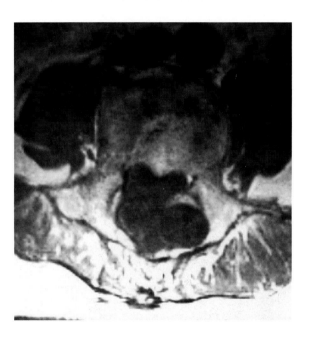

Lobulated dorsal ectasia of the dura ("dural diverticulae") may develop in patients with ankylosing spondylitis. The basis for this outpouching is not established but may include a component of chronic meningeal inflammation.

The patient in Case 842 did not have true ankylosing spondylitis. However, the lumbar fusion performed two decades earlier has apparently simulated the pathophysiology of the spondylitic disorder. The impressive lobulated dural ectasia seen here is very comparable to the pattern observed in patients with a long history of ankylosing disease.

Case 842 is distinct from Case 841 in several respects. The CSF-containing sac seen here reflects localized enlargement of the intradural compartment rather than the accumulation of extradural fluid. The ectasia in this case has developed gradually over many years, while a pseudomeningocele typically manifests within days or weeks of surgery or trauma. Finally, the morphology of the cystic CSF collection in Case 842 is characteristically lobulated, while pseudomeningoceles tend to be unilocular or dumbbell-shaped, as in Case 841.

The appearance in this case should not be confused with the dural ectasia seen in some patients with neurofibromatosis or connective tissue disorders (e.g., Marfan's syndrome or Ehlers-Danlos syndrome). In the latter conditions, dural expansion is more generalized, with smooth, concave erosion along the posterior margins of vertebral bodies. Such morphology contrasts with more focal scalloping, dorsal predominance, and limited extent of dural diverticulae in spondylitic syndromes.

The cause of the cauda equina syndrome in patients with ankylosing spondylitis and dorsal dural ectasia is probably an associated arachnoiditis. Nerve roots may become adherent or tethered to the inflamed meninges, with consequent distortion and traction. In Case 842A, the roots of the cauda equina are positioned along the posterior margin of the spinal canal at the L2-3 level. At least one root *(arrow)* follows an aberrant course into the dural diverticulae. The axial scan in Case 842B documents both the lobulated dural expansion (and bone erosion) and the distorted morphology of intrathecal nerve roots.

Case 843

77-year-old woman presenting with
pseudoclaudication.
(sagittal, noncontrast scan; SE 550/20)

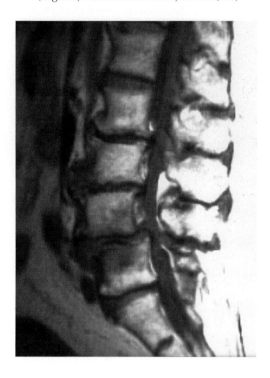

Case 844

80-year-old woman complaining of bilateral
knee pain.
(sagittal, noncontrast scan; SE 2800/90)

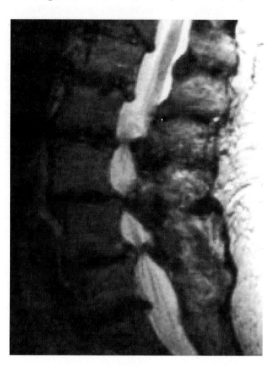

A variety of congenital and acquired factors may cause narrowing of the spinal canal at any level. Central stenosis due to degenerative changes is most common in the lumbar region. Disc bulges and osteophytes cause spondylotic ridges indenting the anterior aspect of the spinal canal. Accompanying hypertrophy of the facet joints and thickening of the ligamenta flava encroach on the posterolateral portions of the canal. The combination of these features produces a circumferential or "napkin-ring" narrowing, which encircles and constricts the dural sac. Superimposed static or dynamic subluxations exacerbate the crowding and compression of nerve roots of the cauda equina.

Sagittal MR scans effectively demonstrate narrowing of the spinal canal. In Case 843, severe disc space narrowing is present at all levels from L2 to S1. Spondylotic ridges indent the anterior aspect of the spinal canal at L2-3 and L3-4.

Ventral subluxation of L4 on L5 causes further canal compromise at this level. The normal low intensity of CSF within the thecal sac is replaced by amorphous intermediate signal intensity of compressed tissue in the region from L2 to L5. Large anterior vertebral osteophytes and reactive marrow changes within the L5 vertebral body (see Case 831) are incidentally noted.

T2-weighted sagittal scans such as Case 844 often define the posterior components of degenerative spinal stenosis more clearly than T1-weighted scans. In this case, large dorsal extradural deformities due to posterior element hypertrophy combine with a "washboard" of ventral spondylotic ridges to cause a series of napkin-ring constrictions. The nerve roots of the cauda equina are stretched centrally between these stenoses. All disc spaces in this case demonstrate severe narrowing and loss of hydration signal.

Case 845

76-year-old man with severe bilateral leg pain
on ambulation.
(axial, noncontrast scan; SE 1000/22; L4-5 level)

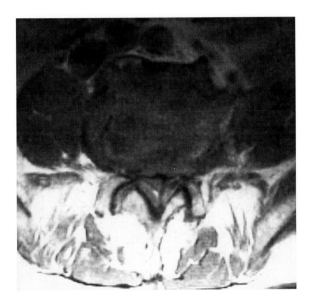

Case 846

69-year-old man presenting with back and leg pain.
(axial, noncontrast scan; SE 800/17; L3-4 level)

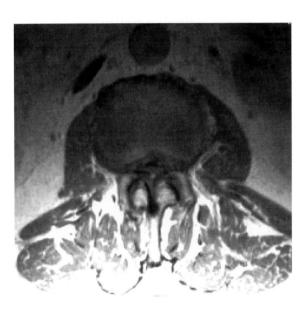

Axial scans define the cross-sectional morphology and severity of spinal stenosis. Central canal compromise is often caused by the superimposition of acquired pathology on congenitally narrow dimensions. The acquired factors may be specific processes (e.g., Paget's disease or ossification of the posterior longitudinal ligament) or simple degenerative changes.

The above cases are typical examples of the latter circumstance. The combination of disc bulge, facet hypertrophy, and thickening of the ligamentum flavum causes circumferential constriction of the lumbar canal. (Compare the size of the dural sac in these images to the more normal dimensions in Cases 835 and 837.) A complete myelographic block was demonstrated in each case.

Case 847A

18-year-old man presenting with leg spasticity.
(sagittal, noncontrast scan; SE 2500/60)

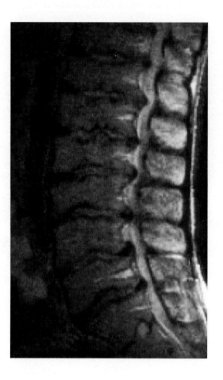

Case 847B

Same patient.
(axial, noncontrast scan; SE 1000/20; L3-4 level)

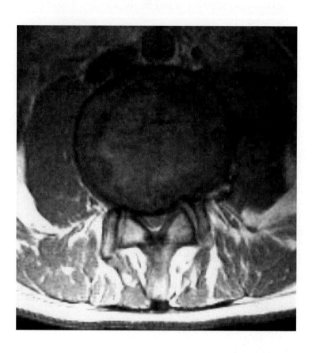

Achondroplasia is among the congenital causes of spinal stenosis. This autosomal dominant disorder results in dwarfism, with abnormal formation of enchondral bone. The head and spine are prominently affected.

Calvarial involvement characteristically results in a hypoplastic skull base. The foramen magnum is typically very small, with constriction of the cervicomedullary junction. Shelf-like hypertrophy of the posterior lip of the foramen magnum often contributes to the narrow bony dimensions.

Spinal manifestations of achondroplasia include abnormally formed vertebral bodies and high grade central canal stenosis. Case 847A demonstrates a congenitally narrow AP diameter of the lumbar canal, which is due predominantly to short pedicles. Superimposed disc bulges at all levels further constrict the canal. The axial scan of Case 847B confirms that the combination of a small bony canal and prominent disc bulging results in severe compression of the thecal sac.

Axial scans of congenitally stenotic canals often demonstrate a triangular or "trefoil" morphology, with short pedicles and medially bowing laminae. Such congenital deformity is frequently most prominent in the lumbar region.

Other systemic bone disorders that may cause multi-level spinal stenosis include Paget's disease, rickets, and diffuse idiopathic skeletal hyperostosis.

Case 848A

62-year-old man presenting with back and leg pain.
The patient was otherwise well and taking
no medications.
(sagittal, noncontrast scan; SE 550/20)

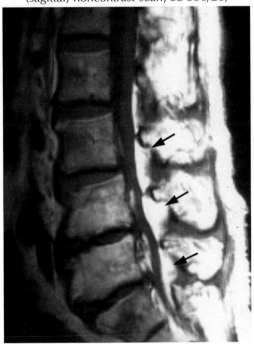

Case 848B

Same patient.
(axial, noncontrast scan; SE 1000/20; L4 level)

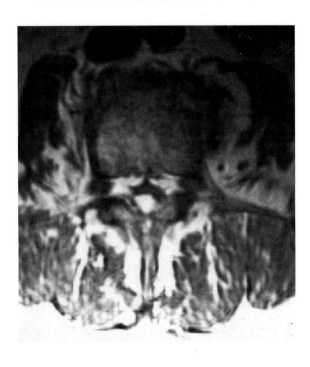

Abnormal accumulation of epidural fat is a rare cause of central canal stenosis. Symptomatic "epidural lipomatosis" is most common in the thoracic region (see Case 1022) but may also involve the lumbar canal, as in this case. Excessive exogenous or endogenous glucocorticoids (i.e., steroid therapy or Cushing's disease) is the usual clinical setting for this disorder. Uncomplicated obesity may occasionally be associated with symptomatic thickening of epidural fat.

In Case 848A, a prominent layer of epidural fat occupies the dorsal portion of the lumbar canal from L2 to S1 *(arrows)*. Ventral deposits of epidural fat are seen posterior to several vertebral bodies. The dural sac is reduced to a ribbon-like band passing between these accumulations of lipid material. The axial plane (Case 848B) confirms com-

pression and deformity of the thecal sac due to dorsal and ventral layers of epidural fat.

When the dural sac is deformed by epidural tissue demonstrating short T1 values, the possibility of hematoma should be considered along with lipomatosis. Subacute blood products (i.e., methemoglobin) may cause a subdural or epidural hemorrhage to appear "bright" on T1-weighted scans (see Cases 1019-1021). A scan performed with fat suppression techniques will establish the etiology of epidural T1-shortening in questionable cases.

Occasional angiolipomas and hemangiomas occur in the spinal epidural space, particularly in the thoracic region (see Case 889). Such tumors should also be considered in the differential diagnosis of epidural lipomatosis.

Case 849

80-year-old woman presenting with bilateral leg pain.
(axial, noncontrast scan; SE 1000/17; L4 level)

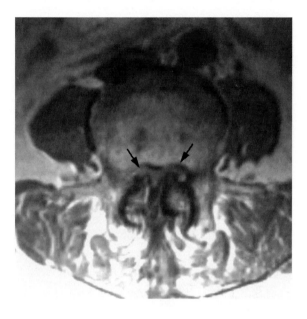

Case 850

77-year-old man with severe back pain.
(axial, noncontrast scan; SE 650/17; L4-5 level)

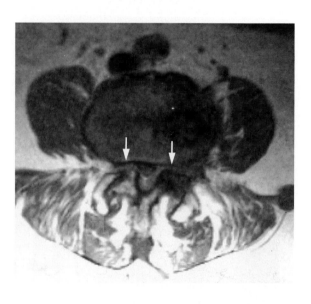

The lateral recess of the lumbar spinal canal is formed by the junction of the vertebral body and pedicle. A nerve root occupies this angle as it prepares to pass beneath the pedicle through the superior portion of the intervertebral foramen. The root may be compressed in this location by a posterolateral disc herniation, as discussed in Cases 824 and 825. Alternatively, bony narrowing of the lateral recess can severely distort the contained nerve.

The base of the superior articular facet of a lumbar vertebra forms the posterolateral margin of the lateral recess. Hypertrophy of the facet (and/or related osteophytes) may significantly narrow the recess, either alone or in combination with disc pathology.

In Case 849, hypertrophy and spurring of the facet joints encroach on the posterior portion of the lateral recesses bilaterally. The proximal L4 nerve roots are flattened antero-posteriorly *(arrows)*. High grade central canal stenosis commonly accompanies bony narrowing of the lateral recesses, as in this case.

The axial scan of Case 850 is at a slightly lower level than Case 849, passing through the junction of the lateral recesses and the intervertebral foramina. Bone overgrowth and associated spondylitic thickening of soft tissue obliterate normal epidural fat in this region. Exiting nerve roots are distorted as they traverse the constricted lateral recess and enter the nerve root canals. Moderate central canal stenosis is also present in Case 850 due to the combination of facet hypertrophy and thickening of the ligamenta flava.

Case 851

50-year-old woman presenting with back and
leg pain.
(sagittal, noncontrast scan; SE 800/17)

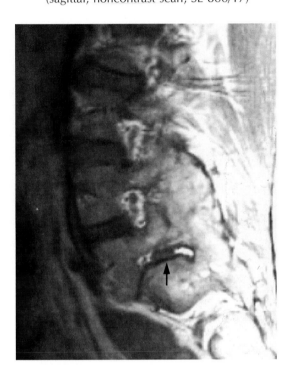

Case 852

60-year-old woman presenting with leg pain
and numbness.
(sagittal, noncontrast scan; SE 600/15)

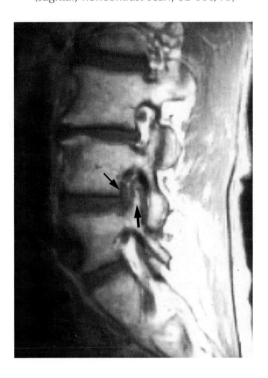

Lateral disc herniation causing foraminal compression of lumbar nerve roots has been illustrated in Cases 826 and 827. An equally important cause of foraminal compromise is bony stenosis.

Bony narrowing of a nerve root canal may develop as a consequence of disc space narrowing. Case 851 presents a typical example. Severe narrowing of the disc space (and mild spondylolisthesis) were noted at the L5-S1 level on more medial images. Associated cephalocaudal narrowing of the nerve root canal flattens the exiting L5 root *(arrow)*.

Case 852 illustrates another form of bony foraminal compromise. No significant disc space narrowing or subluxation is present. Instead, the L4-5 intervertebral foramen is constricted by hypertrophy of the superior articular facet of L5 *(thick arrow)*. A superimposed disc bulge *(thin arrow)* adds to the crowding that compresses the L4 nerve root against the overlying pedicle.

Parasagittal scans are very useful for demonstrating the relative contributions of disc and bone to compromise of an intervertebral foramen (compare Case 852 to Case 827).

Case 853A

71-year-old man presenting with L4 radiculopathy.
(sagittal, noncontrast scan; SE 700/15)

Case 853B

Same patient.
(axial, noncontrast scan; SE 1000/20; L4 level)

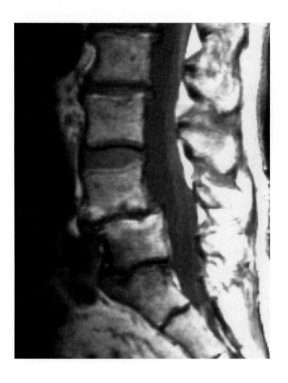

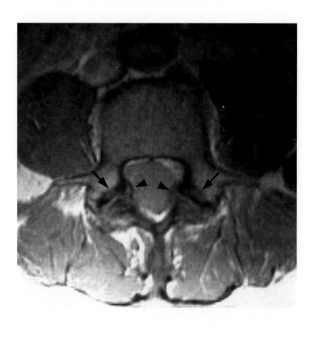

Ventral subluxation of one vertebral body on another may occur in the presence of intact vertebral arches when degenerative changes cause disc space narrowing and ligamentous laxity. (See Case 843 for an example.) Spondylolisthesis may alternatively reflect defects in the pars interarticularis of the forward-slipping vertebra. Such discontinuity of the posterior arch allows the body and superior articular facet to slide anteriorly, unrestrained by linkage to the inferior articular facet (which maintains its articulation to the next inferior vertebra).

Often spondylolysis and degenerative changes are both present at the level of subluxation, as in Case 853. The sagittal scan demonstrates severe narrowing of the disc space and reactive marrow changes (compare to Case 833), while the axial view documents narrow bilateral defects of spondylolysis *(arrows)*. Reactive sclerosis and/or callus frequently accompany a thin tissue line traversing the pars interarticularis, as seen in this case. AP elongation of the spi-

nal canal due to the mild subluxation is well demonstrated in both projections.

When present, the bone defect of spondylolysis resembles an extra facet joint crossing anterior to the normal articulation. Spondylolysis is best seen at the midvertebral level, while the facet joint is best seen at the disc level. The plane of a spondylolitic defect is typically more coronal than that of the facet joints.

Case 853B demonstrates mild soft tissue thickening at the medial margin of the spondylolitic defects *(arrowheads)*. More prominent callus formation, bone fragmentation, and granulation tissue at the site of spondylolysis may form a composite mass that encroaches on the spinal canal. Alternatively, nerve roots may be tethered within the fibrotic reaction adjacent to a pars defect.

Spondylolysis is more common at L5 than at any other lumbar level. Cervical spondylolysis occurs but is relatively rare.

Case 854A

35-year-old woman presenting with bilateral
leg pain.
(axial, noncontrast scan; SE 1000/20; L5-S1 level)

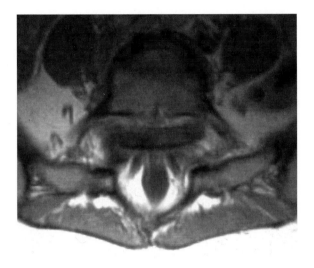

Case 854B

Same patient.
(sagittal, noncontrast scan; SE 550/20)

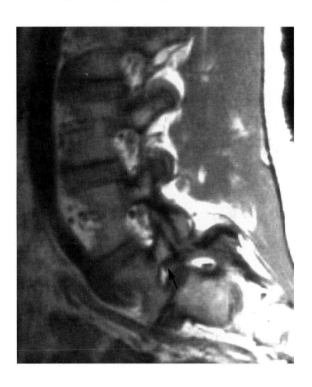

Axial CT or MR images in cases of spondylolisthesis demonstrate typical morphological features. Anterior movement of the rostral body away from its posterior arch causes the spinal canal to become elongated in anteroposterior diameter and elliptical in configuration. Since the intervertebral disc usually maintains its relationship to the caudal vertebral body, the ledge or step-off from rostral body to disc resembles a disc bulge. Case 854 illustrates these characteristic findings, which should prompt a search for associated spondylolysis.

The central canal is usually not compromised by spondylolisthesis. However, the nerve roots exiting beneath the pedicles of the forward-slipping vertebra are often distorted. Displacement of the rostral vertebra carries the lateral recesses (Case 854A) anteriorly, so that they come to lie above the nondisplaced disc. This malalignment narrows the cephalocaudal dimension of the intervertebral foramina, with consequent flattening of the exiting nerve roots.

An analysis of Case 854A presents the problem. The L5 nerve roots must pass beneath the pedicles of L5 but above the L5-S1 disc. However, both structures are imaged at the same axial level, indicating that there is little space remaining between them.

This foraminal distortion is more easily appreciated on sagittal scans such as Case 854B. The L5 nerve root is mildly flattened between the overlying pedicle and the underlying disc (*arrow;* compare to the normally rounded root morphology and abundant epidural fat in higher foramina).

Case 855

56-year-old woman presenting with back pain.
(sagittal, noncontrast scan; SE 2500/90)

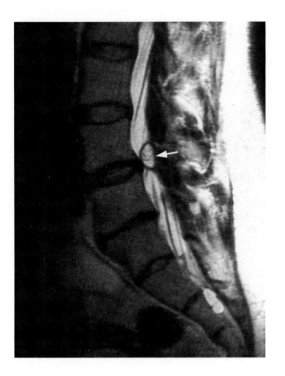

Case 856

63-year-old woman presenting with right leg pain.
(axial, postcontrast scan; SE 700/17; L4-5 level)

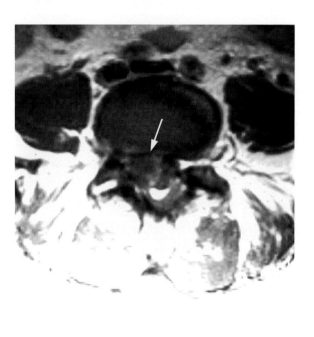

Degenerative changes of the lumbar facet joints may be associated with the development of a synovial cyst. These structures represent expansion or herniation of synovial membranes beneath or through the facet capsule/ligamentum flavum.

Synovial cysts are characteristically found at the medial aspect of the facet joint. The resultant extradural deformity along the posterolateral aspect of the spinal canal can usually be distinguished from more anteriorly based disc herniations.

Case 855 illustrates the typical appearance of synovial cysts on sagittal studies. A round mass measuring approximately one centimeter in diameter is present within the spinal canal at the L4-5 level. The lesion is defined by a thin, uniform rim of low signal intensity on a long TR spin echo image. This rim correlates with the dense perimeter of synovial cysts usually seen on CT scans and reflects calcification and/or old blood products. The center of the cyst may be heterogeneous or homogeneously "bright" on T2-weighted images.

In Case 856, the cyst is seen to reside at the medial margin of the right facet joint. The dural sac is compressed and displaced contralaterally. Enhancement is present along the margins of the cyst, most apparent medially. (See Case 924 for a sagittal view of this lesion.) Some synovial cysts demonstrate central high signal intensity on precontrast T1-weighted scans, reflecting subacute blood produces within the lesion.

The great majority of synovial cysts are found at L4-5, possibly relating to the relatively large amount of motion and facet stress occurring at this level. (As discussed in Case 853, spondylolysis is also most common at L5.)

Synovial cysts may fluctuate in size on follow-up studies, suggesting variable distention by joint effusion or fluid. Occasional cysts cause persistent compression of nerve roots and require aspiration or surgery.

DIFFERENTIAL DIAGNOSIS:
SMALL INTRASPINAL MASS WITH CENTRAL LONG T2 VALUES AND A RIM OF LOW INTENSITY

Case 857

29-year-old woman presenting with back pain.
(sagittal, noncontrast scan; SE 2500/45)

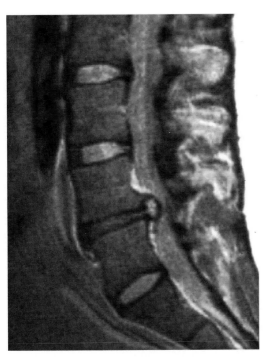

Herniated Disc

Case 858

49-year-old woman presenting with leg pain.
(sagittal, noncontrast scan; SE 2700/45)

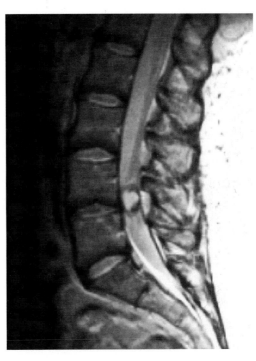

Synovial Cyst

In each of these cases a small mass with round contours is present within the spinal canal at the L4-5 level. Both of the masses demonstrate central high signal intensity surrounded by a rim of low intensity. There is reduced hydration signal within the adjacent L4-5 disc in both cases.

Case 857 is a good example of the long T2 values often seen within a herniated disc, even when the parent disc appears "dehydrated." The lesion is based against the posterior margin of the disc space. The band of low signal intensity enclosing the mass posteriorly represents intact fibers of the outer annulus and posterior longitudinal ligament partially containing the focal herniation.

The synovial cyst in Case 858 is more central with respect to the anteroposterior diameter of the spinal canal (because it arises laterally rather than ventrally). The characteristic rim of low signal intensity is somewhat more irregular in this case than in Case 855. Nevertheless, this feature combines with the size and shape of the mass, its midcanal position, and its occurrence at the L4-5 level to suggest the correct diagnosis.

Case 859

42-year-old man presenting with
bladder dysfunction.
(sagittal, noncontrast scan; SE 550/20)

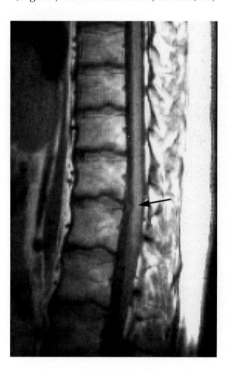

Case 860

37-year-old woman presenting with "shooting"
midthoracic pain on coughing or sneezing and
vague numbness below the waist.
(sagittal, noncontrast scan; RSE 4000/100)

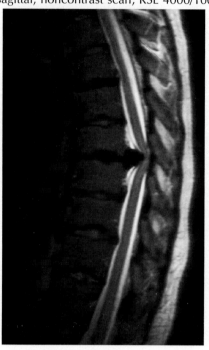

Magnetic resonance imaging has demonstrated that thoracic disc herniations are much more common than had been previously appreciated. Many such lesions are asymptomatic and clinically incidental. However, the small diameter of the thoracic spinal canal and its kyphotic curvature predispose to neurological impairment from even small anterior extradural deformities. About two thirds of patients with symptomatic thoracic disc herniations present with motor and sensory complaints, while one third experience bowel or bladder dysfunction.

In Case 859, a small disc herniation is seen at T11-12 as an indentation along the dark line of ventral subarachnoid space, dura, and posterior longitudinal ligament *(arrow)*. Slight ventral flattening of the conus medullaris confirms the presence of an extradural lesion.

Case 860 illustrates the opposite extreme in the spectrum of thoracic herniations. A very large epidural mass is based against the anterior margin of the spinal canal and centered at a disc level. The low signal intensity of the lesion correlated with dense calcification on x-ray and CT studies and matches the appearance of the adjacent disc. The spinal cord is severely displaced and compressed.

In some cases, the volume of a thoracic disc herniation seems to exceed the volume of a normal intervertebral disc. It is likely that hydration of extruded nuclear material, reactive edema, granulation tissue, focal hemorrhage, and calcification contribute to the epidural mass in such cases. (See discussion of "giant" lumbar disc herniations in Cases 828 and 829.)

Large thoracic disc herniations are often more rounded or hemispheral in morphology than in Case 860. The size and calcification of the lesion may then resemble the appearance of a spinal meningioma (see Cases 913 to 917). The relationship of such masses to a parent disc is the key feature enabling correct diagnosis.

Case 861

25-year-old man presenting with bilateral radicular
midthoracic pain.
(axial, noncontrast scan; SE 1000/17; T7-8 level)

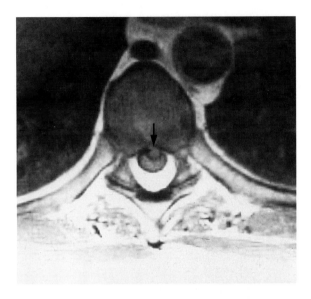

Case 862

28-year-old woman complaining of right-sided
radicular midthoracic pain.
(axial, noncontrast scan; SE 900/17; T8-9 level)

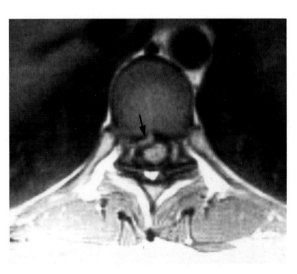

Herniated thoracic discs cause radicular pain more frequently than symptoms of cord compression. The pain may be bilateral in the presence of large or central herniations (as in Case 861) or unilateral in association with an eccentric herniation (as in Case 862). The ventral margin of the spinal cord is indented by the disc in Case 861, while the cord is not significantly deformed in Case 862.

As mentioned on the preceding page, disc herniations are a common incidental finding on MR scans of the thoracic spinal canal. However, even herniations as small as those illustrated above can cause severe local or long tract symptoms and signs. As in the lumbar and cervical regions, clinical correlation is necessary to determine the significance of small thoracic herniations.

DIFFERENTIAL DIAGNOSIS:
ANTERIOR EXTRAMEDULLARY MASS IN THE THORACIC SPINAL CANAL

Case 863

19-year-old man presenting with worsening
paraparesis.
(sagittal, noncontrast scan; SE 600/11)

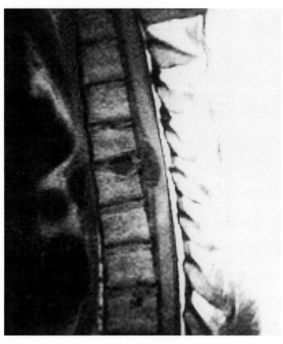

Herniated Disc

Case 864

43-year-old woman presenting with
difficulty walking.
(sagittal, noncontrast scan; SE 700/20)

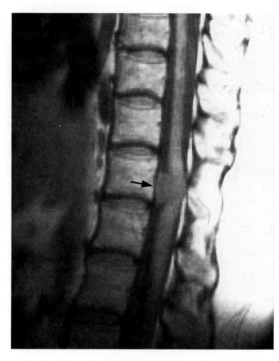

Schwannoma

As discussed in Case 860, occasional thoracic disc herniations are large lesions that can resemble intraspinal neoplasms. The herniation in Case 863 is at least as large as the tumor in Case 864 and causes substantial deformity of the spinal cord. Low signal intensity within the lesion and the parent disc space is due to calcification, which was documented on routine x-rays. The hemispheral morphology and calcification of the mass mimic a meningioma (see Cases 913-917).

Spinal schwannomas may be indistinguishable from meningiomas on precontrast or postcontrast MR studies. (Potential differentiating features are discussed in Cases 917-923.) Both types of tumors are commonly intra-

dural, causing widening of the adjacent subarachnoid space. This finding is illustrated by Case 864 and contrasts with the epidural mass effect effacing the subarachnoid space adjacent to the mass in Case 863.

A vague zone of high signal intensity within the spinal cord slightly inferior to the herniation in Case 863 may reflect subacute hemorrhage or contusion (see Case 1012). It is possible that superimposed trauma, albeit minor, exacerbated the neurological deficit caused by long-standing cord compression in this patient.

The ventral location of the tumor in Case 864 is typical of spinal schwannomas (see also Cases 918, 921, and 922).

Case 865

49-year-old man presenting with difficulty walking.
(sagittal, noncontrast scan; SE 500/15)

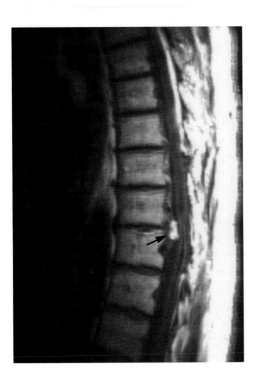

Case 866

68-year-old man with thoracic pain radiating
to the right.
(sagittal, noncontrast scan; SE 2800/45)

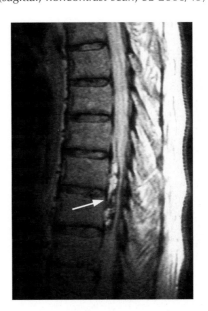

Localized epidural hemorrhage may accompany thoracic disc herniations, as is true in the lumbar region (see Case 830). The presence of blood products within the epidural space may cause heterogeneous and confusing patterns of signal abnormality.

In Case 865, a focal anterior epidural mass is centered at a disc level. This feature should raise the question of disc herniation regardless of the size, morphology, and signal intensity of an extradural lesion. At surgery, a mixture of extruded disc material, old hemorrhage, and tough fibrous tissue was found. The associated syringomyelia regressed on postoperative scans.

Case 866 demonstrates a layer of mixed high and low signal intensity along the anterior margin of the spinal canal.

The "dark" margin of the lesion on a long TR image resembles the perimeter of other masses containing small hemorrhages (e.g., the synovial cysts in Cases 855 and 858). The suspicion of hemorrhagic tissue was supported by prominent signal loss within the lesion on a subsequent gradient echo scan. At surgery, an epidural mass containing old blood products and calcification was found surrounding a degenerated central disc herniation.

Epidural abscesses often contain hemorrhage and can present a heterogeneous appearance similar to Case 866. The clinical context (acuity, degree of pain, and systemic evidence of infection) usually distinguish such cases from epidural masses representing hemorrhagic disc herniation.

Case 867

77-year-old man presenting with mild
spastic quadriparesis.
(sagittal, noncontrast scan; SE 550/15)

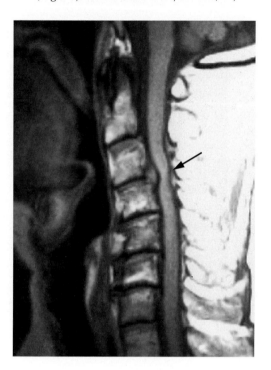

Case 868

56-year-old woman presenting with bilateral
C6 radiculopathy.
(sagittal, noncontrast scan; SE 2800/90)

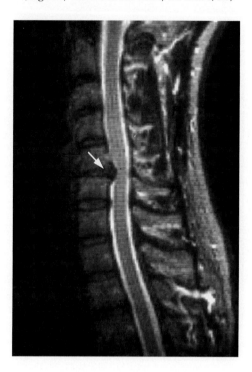

Cervical disc herniations present in a variety of clinical contexts and with a spectrum of MR appearances. The most common associated symptoms are neck and arm pain due to small or lateral herniations. Symptoms of cord compression, as in Case 867, are seen with larger herniations and/or in the setting of spinal stenosis. (Case 867 illustrates the combination of both factors.)

The signal intensity within cervical disc herniations is variable, resembling the range of appearances previously illustrated in the lumbar and thoracic regions. Most cervical herniations are relatively isointense to the parent disc and to cord parenchyma on T1-weighted scans, as seen in Case 867. On T2-weighted images, cervical herniations may demonstrate low intensity (illustrated by Case 868), intermediate values, or high intensity (see Case 870).

A small disc herniation or bulge may be difficult to appreciate on T1-weighted scans, since the low signal intensity of the annulus blends with that of the posterior longi-

tudinal ligament, dura, and ventral subarachnoid space. Techniques with "bright" CSF (i.e., spin echo sequences with long TR values or gradient echo sequences with low flip angles) demonstrate more clearly the interface between the disc margin and the dural sac. (Compare the definition of disc boundaries at the nonherniated levels in Case 867 to those in Case 868.)

Large central disc herniations may elevate or "tent" the posterior longitudinal ligament away from the adjacent vertebral bodies. Soft tissue with long T1 and T2 values then imaged between the bodies and the posteriorly displaced ligament usually represents prominent epidural veins rather than rostral or caudal migration of disc fragments.

Artifact from the thick tissue and bone of the shoulders often compromises CT scans at the lower cervical levels. Sagittal MR scans offer an alternative, artifact-free means of evaluating the cervicothoracic junction.

Case 869

26-year-old woman presenting with neck pain.
(axial, noncontrast scan; SE 800/17; C3-4 level)

Case 870

37-year-old woman presenting with right arm pain.
(axial, noncontrast scan; low flip angle GRE
sequence, C5-6 level)

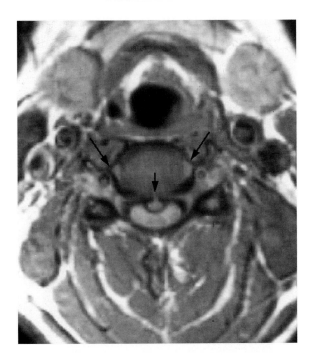

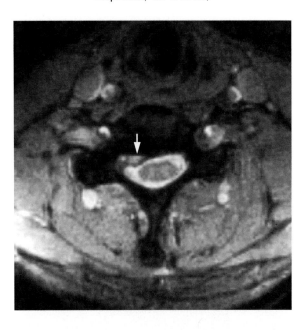

The axial perspective is as useful in the cervical spine as in the lumbar region. However, the small size of cervical vertebrae and discs requires close placement of thin sections for adequate definition of anatomical and pathological features. Even with good technique, the lack of epidural fat and the reduced contrast resolution of thin sections may make diagnosis difficult.

A small central disc herniation *(short arrow)* is well seen on the T1-weighted image in Case 869, indenting the ventral margin of the dural sac and spinal cord. A black line between the disc and the cord probably represents a combination of outer annulus, posterior longitudinal ligament, and dura. The marrow-containing uncinate processes *(long arrows)* are of higher signal intensity than the disc they enclose.

Axial scans performed with low flip angle gradient echo technique, such as Case 870, provide a myelographic effect that is useful in evaluating cervical disc herniations. Such sequences also produce high signal intensity within epidural veins of the cervical canal and neural foramina, increasing the contrast with disc material or osteophytes in both locations.

In Case 870 the spinal cord is well defined, with intramedullary discrimination of gray and white matter. A lateral disc herniation occupies the right anterolateral recess of the spinal canal near the entrance to the neural foramen.

The signal intensity of herniated discs on low flip angle gradient echo images varies from low to intermediate to bright. High intensity in the region of herniation, as in Case 870, often includes prominent epidural veins adjacent to the disc itself.

Case 871

81-year-old woman presenting with cervical myelopathy.
(sagittal, noncontrast scan; SE 2800/90)

Case 872

73-year-old man presenting with neck pain.
(sagittal, noncontrast scan; SE 2200/45)

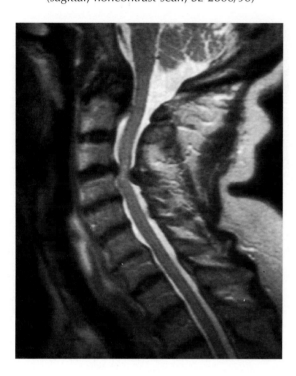

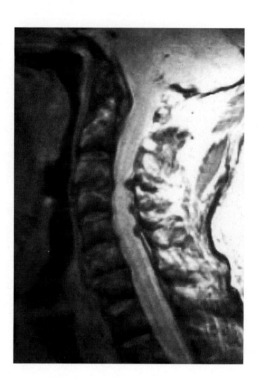

Central canal stenosis in the cervical region is often due to spondylotic ridging accompanied by thickening and buckling of dorsal ligaments. Case 871 illustrates this combination of ventral and dorsal extradural deformities. A disc bulge or herniation indents the anterior margin of the dural sac at C3-4, while thickening of posterior elements causes a dorsal impression.

The spinal cord in Case 871 is pinched between the focal extradural masses. A small area of high signal intensity is present within the mildly flattened cord, characteristic of compressive myelopathy. Both reversible edema and irreversible myelomalacia may contribute to this appearance, which may be correlated with limited postoperative improvement. Remarkable flattening of the spinal cord can be asymptomatic if epidural compression develops slowly (see Cases 876 and 1046).

Multilevel central canal stenosis in Case 872 is due predominantly to hypertrophy of dorsal ligaments. Small spondylotic ridges at several disc levels are also present. Extradural deformities are frequently best defined on "intermediate" spin echo images with long TR and short to medium TE values.

Case 873

26-year-old man presenting with right arm pain. (axial, noncontrast scan; low flip angle GRE sequence; C5-6 level)

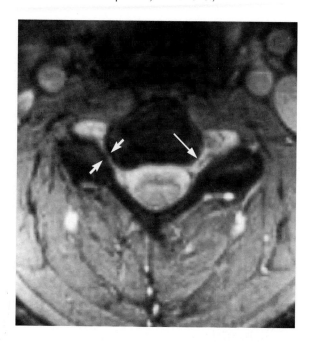

Case 874

53-year-old man presenting with neck pain. (axial, noncontrast scan; low flip angle GRE sequence; C5-6 level)

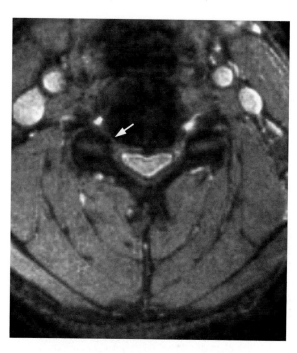

In Case 873, the left nerve root canal *(long arrow)* is seen as a band of high signal intensity reflecting its content of epidural veins and CSF-containing root sleeve. (Compare to the T1-weighted appearance of the foramina in Case 869.) By contrast, the right intervertebral foramen is severely narrowed due to hypertrophy of the uncinate process and facet joint *(short arrows)*.

A small amount of cervical scoliosis or tilt will cause asymmetrical visualization of the right and left intervertebral foramina on any one axial scan. Care should be taken to evaluate adjacent sections before foraminal asymmetry is judged to represent stenosis.

Case 874 illustrates bilateral foraminal narrowing. (The arrow points to the narrowed right nerve root canal.) Central canal stenosis is also present; compare the definition and morphology of the spinal cord in Case 874 to Case 873.

Discrimination between osteophyte and dehydrated disc material can be difficult on cervical MR scans, since both present as low intensity extradural deformities. This distinction is more easily made on CT studies.

Case 875A

38-year-old man presenting with neck
and arm pain.
(sagittal, noncontrast scan; SE 1800/60)

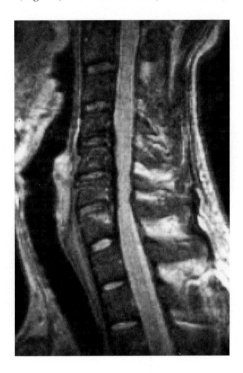

Case 875B

Same patient.
(axial, noncontrast scan; low flip angle GRE
sequence; C5-6 level)

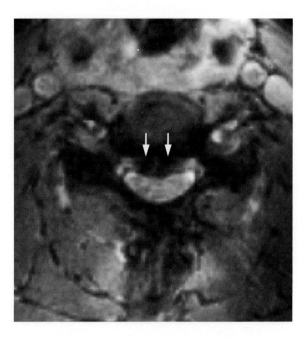

Stenosis of the cervical canal and compressive myelopathy may be caused by ossification of the posterior longitudinal ligament (OPLL). This bone formation along the posterior margin of cervical vertebral bodies may be segmental or diffuse. In either case, progressive thickening of the layer of epidural ossification causes gradual flattening of the thecal sac.

OPLL may demonstrate high or low signal intensity on T1-weighted scans, depending on the presence or absence of lipid-containing marrow elements. The latter presentation is more common. In such cases, the low intensity of

the ossified ligament may be poorly defined on T1-weighted images, due to the adjacent low intensity of the ventral subarachnoid space.

In Case 875A, a uniform layer of thickened low intensity is apparent along the posterior margin of the vertebral bodies from C4 to C7. The axial scan in Case 875B confirms that the thick layer of calcified tissue occupies the anatomical location of the posterior longitudinal ligament *(arrows)*. Both images document the associated narrowing of the spinal canal, with mild flattening of the spinal cord.

Case 876

61-year-old man presenting with abnormal posture
and quadriparesis.
(sagittal, noncontrast scan; SE 2500/90)

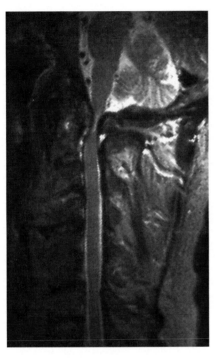

Ankylosing Hyperostosis

Case 877

2-year-old boy with spinal deformity incidentally
noted on x-rays of the pharynx.
(sagittal, noncontrast scan; SE 2500/90)

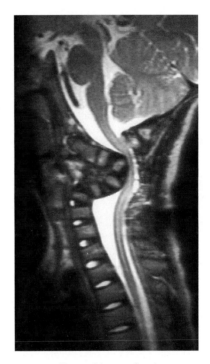

Idiopathic Kyphosis

The ability of MR scans to display long segments of the spinal canal while demonstrating the intradural consequences of vertebral abnormalities is useful for evaluation of spinal deformities. A common application of MR in this regard is the assessment of thoracic scoliosis, checking for potentially associated intradural or extradural malformations or masses and/or secondary cord compression (see Cases 937, 942, and 1081).

The above cases illustrate more unusual examples of osseous deformity involving the cervical canal. The patient in Case 876 suffers from severe constriction of the neural canal at the craniocervical junction. This stenosis is caused by subluxation and degenerative changes at the C1 level due to long-standing immobility of the remainder of the cervical spine. The thick, hyperostotic bone fusing the anterior margins of cervical vertebrae is faintly visualized, contrasting with the thin layer of denser bone along the posterior margin of vertebral bodies in Case 875.

High signal intensity within the compressed cervicomedullary junction in Case 876 may represent reversible edema and/or irreversible myelomalacia (compare to Case 871). See Cases 1044 to 1050 for additional examples of canal stenosis at the craniocervical junction.

The cause of the severe cervical kyphosis in Case 877 has not been determined. No other skeletal abnormalities have been demonstrated in this patient. The sagittal MR scan clearly documents cord deformity, with abnormal intramedullary signal. This unusual cervical gibbus was resected by an anterior approach and replaced by bone struts to reconstitute reasonable alignment of the cervical canal.

REFERENCES

Agula LA, Piraino DW, Modic MT: The intranuclear cleft of the intervertebral disk: magnetic resonance imaging. *Radiology* 155:155, 1985.

Al-Mefty O, Harkey LH, Middleton TH, et al: Myelopathic cervical spondylitic lesions demonstrated by magnetic resonance imaging. *J Neurosurg* 68:217-222, 1988.

Awwad EE, Martin DS, Smith KR Jr, Buchotz RD: MR imaging of lumbar juxtaarticular cysts. *J Comput Assist Tomogr* 14:415-417, 1990.

Barnett GH, Hardy RW Jr, Little JR, et al: Thoracic spinal canal stenosis. *J Neurosurg* 66:338-344, 1987.

Berger PE, Atkinson D, Wilson WJ, Wiltse L: High resolution surface coil magnetic resonance imaging of the spine: normal and pathologic anatomy. *Radiographics* 6:573-602, 1986.

Bergleit R, Gebarski SS, Brunberg JA, et al: Lumbar synovial cysts: correlation of myelographic MR and pathologic findings. *AJNR* 11:777-779, 1990.

Blumenkopf B: Thoracic intervertebral disc herniations: diagnostic value of magnetic resonance imaging. *Neurosurgery* 23:36-40, 1988.

Boden SD, Davis DO, Dina TS, et al: Abnormal magnetic resonance scans of the lumbar spine in asymptomatic patients. *J Bone Joint Surg* 72:403-408, 1990.

Boden SD, Davis DO, Dina TS, et al: Contrast-enhanced MR imaging performed after successful lumbar disk surgery: prospective study. *Radiology* 182:59-64, 1992.

Boden SD, Davis DO, Dina TS, et al: Postoperative diskitis: distinguishing early MR imaging findings from normal postoperative disk space changes. *Radiology* 184:765-771, 1992.

Bozzao A, Gallucci M, Masciocchi C, et al: Lumbar disk herniation: MR imaging assessment of natural history in patients treated without surgery. *Radiology* 185:135-142, 1992.

Brown BM, Schwartz RH, Frank E, Blank NK: Preoperative evaluation of cervical radiculopathy and myelopathy by surface-coil MR imaging. *AJNR* 9:859-866, 1988.

Bundschuh CV, Modic MT, Ross JS, et al: Epidural fibrosis and recurrent disk herniation in the lumbar spine: MR imaging assessment. *AJNR* 9:169-178, 1988.

Bundschuh CV, Stein L, Slusser JH, et al: Distinguishing between scar and recurrent herniated disk in postoperative patients: value of contrast-enhanced CT and MR imaging. *AJNR* 11:949-958, 1990.

Castillo M: Neural foramen remodeling caused by a sequestered disk fragment. *AJNR* 12:566-567, 1991.

Crisi G, Carpeggiani P, Trevisan C: Gadolinium-enhanced nerve roots in lumbar disk herniation. *AJNR* 14:1379-1392, 1993.

Czervionke LF: Lumbar intervertebral disc disease. *Neuroimaging Clin N Amer* 3:465-486, 1993.

Czervionke LF, Daniels DL, Ho PSP, et al: The cervical neural foramina: a correlative anatomic and MR study. *Radiology* 1:753-759, 1988.

DeRoos A, Kressel H, Spritzer C, Dalinka M: MR imaging of marrow changes adjacent to end-plates in degenerative lumbar disk disease. *AJR* 149:531-534, 1987.

Emamian SA, Skriver EB, Henriksen L, Cortsen ME: Lumbar herniated disk mimicking neuroma. *Acta Radiol* 34,fasc.2:127-129, 1993.

Enzmann DR, Rubin JB: Cervical spine: MR imaging with a partial flip angle, gradient-refocused pulse sequence. Part I. General considerations and disk disease. *Radiology* 166:467-472, 1988.

Fletcher G, Haughton VM, Ho K-C, Yu S: Age-related changes in cervical facet joints: studies with cryomicrotomy, MR and CT. *AJNR* 11:27-30, 1990.

Fox MW, Onofrio BM, Kilgore JE: Neurological complications of ankylosing spondylitis. *J Neurosurg* 78:871-878, 1993.

Friedberg SR, Fellows T, Thomas CB, et al: Experience with symptomatic spinal epidural cysts, *Neurosurgery* 34:989-993, 1994.

Gaskill MF, Lukin R, Wiot JG: Lumbar disc disease and stenosis. *Rad Clin North Am* 29:753-764, 1991.

Georgy BA, Hesselink JR: MR imaging of the spine: recent advances in pulse sequences and special techniques. *AJR* 162:923-934, 1994.

Glickstein MF, Sussman SK: Time-dependent scar enhancement in magnetic resonance imaging of the postoperative lumbar spine. *Skeletal Radiol* 20:333-337, 1991.

Gorey MT, Hyman RA, Black KS, et al: Lumbar synovial cysts eroding bone. *AJNR* 13:161-163, 1992.

Grand CM, Bank WO, Baleriaux D, et al: Gadolinium enhancement of vertebral endplates following lumbar disc surgery. *Neuroradiology* 35:503-505, 1993.

Grenier N, Greselle JF, Douws C, et al: MR imaging of foraminal and extraforaminal lumbar disk herniations. *J Comput Assist Tomogr* 14:243-249, 1990.

Grenier N, Greselle J, Vital J, et al: Normal and disrupted lumbar longitudinal ligaments: correlative MR and anatomic study. *Radiology* 171:197-205, 1989.

Grenier N, Kressel HY, Schiebler ML, et al: Normal and degenerative posterior spinal structures: MR imaging. *Radiology* 165:517-525, 1987.

Gundry CR, Heithoff KB: Epidural hematoma of the lumbar spine: 18 surgically confirmed cases. *Radiology* 187:427-432, 1993.

Haughton VM: MR imaging of the spine. *Radiology* 166:297-301, 1988.

Hedberg MC, Drayer BP, Flom RA, et al: Gradient echo (GRASS) MR imaging in cervical radiculopathy. *AJNR* 150:683-689, 1988.

Ho PSP, Yu S, Sether LA, et al: Ligamentum flavum: appearance on sagittal and coronal MR images. *Radiology* 168:469-472, 1988.

Ho PSP, Yu S, Sether LA, et al: Progressive and regressive changes in the nucleus pulposus: part I. The neonate. *Radiology* 169:87-91, 1988.

Hueftle M, Modic MT, Ross JS, et al: Lumbar spine: postoperative MR imaging with Gd-DTPA. *Radiology* 167:817-824, 1988.

Ibrahim MA, Jesmanowicz A, Hyde JS, et al: Contrast enhancement of normal intervertebral disks: time and dose dependent. *AJNR* 15:419-424, 1994.

Jackson DE, Atlas SW, Mani JR, Norman D: Intraspinal synovial cysts: MR imaging. *Radiology* 170:527-530, 1989.

Jahnke RW, Hart BL: Cervical stenosis, spondylosis, and herniated disc disease. *Rad Clin North Am* 29:777-792, 1991.

Jinkins JR: Gd-DTPA enhanced MR of the lumbar spinal canal in patients with claudication. *J Comput Assist Tomogr* 17:555-561, 1993.

Jinkins JR: MR of enhancing nerve roots in the unoperated lumbosacral spine. *AJNR* 14:193-202, 1993.

Jinkins JR, Matthes JC, Sener RN, et al: Spondylolysis, spondylolisthesis and associated nerve root entrapment in the lumbosacral spine: MR evaluation. *AJR* 159:799-803, 1992.

Jinkins JR, Osborn AG, Garrett D, et al: Spinal nerve enhancement with Gd-DTPA: MR correlation with the postoperative lumbosacral spine. *AJNR* 14:383-394, 1993.

Johnson DW, Farnum GN, Latchaw RE, et al: MR imaging of the pars interarticularis in patients with spondylolisthesis. *AJNR* 9:1215-1220, 1988.

Kent DL, Haynor DR, Larson EB, Deyo RA: Diagnosis of lumbar spinal stenosis in adults: a metaanalysis of the accuracy of CT, MR and myelography. *AJR* 158:1135-1144, 1992.

Kostelic J, Haughton MV, Sether L: Proximal lumbar spinal nerves in axial MR imaging, CT, and anatomic sections. *Radiology* 183:239, 1992.

Lane JI, Koeller KK, Atkinson JLD: Enhanced lumbar nerve roots in the spine without prior surgery: radiculitis or radicular veins? *AJNR* 15:1317-1325, 1994.

Lee SH, Coleman PE, Hahn FJ: Magnetic resonance imaging of degenerative disk disease of the spine. *Rad Clin North Am* 26:949-964, 1988.

Liu SS, Williams KD, Drayer BP, et al: Synovial cysts of the lumbosacral spine: diagnosis by MR imaging. *AJNR* 10:1239-1242, 1989.

Luetkehans TJ, Coughlin BF, Weinstein MA: Ossification of the posterior longitudinal ligament by MR. *AJNR* 8:924-925, 1987.

Maravilla KR, Lesh P, Weinreb JC, et al: Magnetic resonance imaging of the lumbar spine with CT correlation. *AJNR* 6:237-246, 1985.

Masaryk TJ, Boumphrey F, Modic MT, et al: Effects of chemonucleolysis demonstrated by MR imaging. *J Comput Assist Tomogr* 10:917-923, 1986.

Masaryk TJ, Modic MT, Geisinger MA, et al: Cervical myelopathy: a comparison of magnetic resonance and myelography. *J Comput Assist Tomogr* 10:184-194, 1986.

Masaryk TJ, Ross TS, Modic MT, et al: High-resolution MR imaging of sequestered lumbar intervertebral disks. *AJNR* 9:351-358, 1988.

Mehalic TF, Pezzuti RT, Applebaum BI: Magnetic resonance imaging and cervical spondylitic myelography. *Neurosurgery* 26:216-227, 1990.

Mirowitz SA, Shady KL: Gadopentetate dimeglumine-enhanced MR imaging of the postoperative lumbar spine: comparison of fat-suppressed and conventional T1-weighted MR scans. *AJR* 159:385-389, 1992.

Modic MT, Herfkens RJ: Intervertebral disk: normal age-related changes in MR signal intensity. *Radiology* 166:332-334, 1990.

Modic MT, Masaryk TJ, Boumphrey F, et al: Lumbar herniated disk disease and canal stenosis: prospective evaluation by surface coil MR, CT, and myelography. *AJNR* 7:709-717, 1986.

Modic MT, Masaryk TJ, Mulopulos GP, et al: Cervical radiculopathy: prospective evaluation with surface coil MR imaging, CT with metrizamide, and metrizamide myelography. *Radiology* 161:753-760, 1986.

Modic MT, Masaryk T, Paushter D: Magnetic resonance imaging of the spine. *Rad Clin North Am* 24:229-245, 1986.

Modic MT, Masaryk TJ, Ross JS, et al: Cervical radiculopathy: value of oblique MR imaging. *Radiology* 163:227-232, 1987.

Modic MT, Masaryk RJ, Ross JS, Carter JR: Imaging of degenerative disk disease. *Radiology* 168:177-186, 1988.

Modic MT, Pavlicek W, Weinstein MA, et al: Magnetic resonance imaging of intervertebral disk disease: clinical and pulse sequence considerations. *Radiology* 152:103-111, 1984.

Modic MT, Steinberg PM, Ross JS, et al: Degenerative disk disease: assessment of changes in vertebral body marrow with MR imaging. *Radiology* 166:193-199, 1988.

Murayama S, Numaguchi Y, Robinson AE: The diagnosis of herniated intervertebral disks with MR imaging: a comparison of gradient-refocused-echo and spin-echo pulse sequences. *AJNR* 11:17-22, 1990.

Nowicki BH, Haughton VM: Neural foraminal ligaments of the lumbar spine: appearance at CT and MR imaging. *Radiology* 183:257-264, 1992.

Osborn AG, Hood RS, Sherry RG, et al: CT/MR spectrum of far lateral and anterior lumbosacral disk herniations. *AJNR* 9:775-778, 1988.

Otake S, Matsuo M, Nishizawa S, et al: Ossification of the posterior longitudinal ligament: MR evaluation. *AJNR* 13:1059-1067, 1992.

Pech P, Haughton VM: Lumbar intervertebral disk: correlative MR and anatomic study. *Radiology* 156:699-701, 1985.

Ramanauskas WL, Wilner HI, Metes JJ, et al: MR imaging of compressive myelomalacia. *J Comput Assist Tomogr* 13:399-404, 1989.

Resnick D: Degenerative diseases of the vertebral column. *Radiology* 156:3-14, 1985.

Rosenbloom SA: Thoracic disc disease and stenosis. *Rad Clin North Am* 29:765-776, 1991.

Rosenblum J, Mojtahedi S, Foust RJ: Synovial cysts in the lumbar spine: MR characteristics. *AJNR* 10:S94, 1989.

Ross JS: Magnetic resonance assessment of the postoperative spine: degenerative disc disease. *Rad Clin North Am* 29:793-809, 1991.

Ross JS, Masaryk TJ, Modic MT, et al: Lumbar spine: postoperative assessment with surface-coil MR imaging. *Radiology* 164:851-860, 1987.

Ross JS, Masaryk TJ, Modic MT: Postoperative cervical spine: MR assessment. *J Comput Assist Tomogr* 11:955-962, 1987.

Ross JS, Masaryk TJ, Schrader M, et al: MR imaging of the postoperative lumbar spine: assessment with gadopentetate dimeglumine. *AJNR* 11:771-776, 1990.

Ross JS, Modic MT, Masaryk TJ, et al: Assessment of extradural degenerative disease with Gd-DTPA-enhanced MR imaging: correlation with surgical and pathologic findings. *AJNR* 10:1243-1249, 1989.

Ross JS, Modic MT, Masaryk TJ: Tears of the anulus fibrosus: assessment with Gd-DTPA-enhanced MR imaging. *AJNR* 10:1251-1254, 1989.

Ross JS, Modic MT, Masaryk TJ, et al: The postoperative lumbar spine. *Semin Roentgenol* 23:125-136, 1988.

Ross JS, Perez-Reyes N, Masaryk TJ, et al: Thoracic disk herniation: MR imaging. *Radiology* 165:511-516, 1987.

Ross JS, Ruggieri PM, Tkach JA, et al: Gd-DTPA-enhanced 3D MR imaging of cervical degenerative disk disease: initial experience. *AJNR* 13:127-136, 1992.

Ross JS, Ruggieri P, Tkach J, et al: Lumbar degenerative disk disease: prospective comparison of conventional T2-weighted spin-echo imaging and T2-weighted rapid acquisition relaxation enhanced imaging. *AJNR* 14:1215-1224, 1993.

Rubenstein DJ, Alvarez O, Ghelman B, Marchisello P: Cauda equina syndrome complicating ankylosing spondylitis: MR features. *J Comput Assist Tomogr* 13:511-513, 1989.

Russell EG: Cervical disk disease. *Radiology* 177:313-325, 1990.

Ryken TC, Menezes AH: Cervicomedullary compression in achondroplasia, *J Neurosurg* 81:43-48, 1994.

Schellinger D, Mang HJ, Vidic B, et al: Disk fragment migration. *Radiology* 175:831-836, 1990.

Schiebler ML, Grenier N, Fallon M, et al: Normal and degenerated intervertebral disk: in vivo and in vitro MR imaging with histopathologic correlation. *AJR* 157:93-97, 1991.

Sether LA, Yu S, Haughton VM, Fischer ME: Intervertebral disk: normal age-related changes in MR signal intensity. *Radiology* 177:385-388, 1990.

Silbergleit R, Gebarski SS, Brunberg JA, et al: Lumbar synovial cysts: correlation of myelographic, CT, MR, and pathological findings. *AJNR* 11:777-779, 1990.

Smith KA, Rekate HL: Delayed postoperative tethering of the cervical spinal cord. *J Neurosurg* 81:196-201, 1994.

Sobel DF, Zyroff J, Thorne RP: Discogenic vertebral sclerosis: MR imaging. *J Comput Assist Tomogr* 11:855-858, 1987.

Sotiropoulos S, Chafetz NI, Lang P, et al: Differentiation between postoperative scar and recurrent disk herniation: prospective comparison of MR, CT, and contrast-enhanced CT. *AJNR* 10:639-643, 1989.

Stollman A, Pinto R, Benjamin V, et al: Radiologic imaging of symptomatic ligamentum flavum thickening with and without ossification. *AJNR* 8:991-994, 1987.

Sze G, Kawamura Y, Neaishi C, et al: Fast spin-echo MR imaging of the cervical spine: influence of echo train length and echo spacing on image contrast and quality. *AJNR* 14:1203-1214, 1993.

Takahashi M, Yamashita T, Sakamoto Y, Kojima R: Chronic cervical cord compression: clinical significance of increased signal intensity on MR imaging. *Radiology* 173:219-224, 1989.

Tartaglino LM, Flanders AE, Vinitski S, Fiedman DP: Metallic artifacts on MR images of the postoperative spine: reduction with fast spin echo techniques. *Radiology* 190:565-572, 1994.

Teresi LM, Lufkin RB, Reicher MA, et al: Asymptomatic degenerative disk disease and spondylosis of the cervical spine: MR imaging. *Radiology* 164:83-88, 1987.

Thornbury JR, Fryback DG, Turski PA, et al: Disk-caused nerve compression in patients with acute low back pain: diagnosis with MR, CT myelography, and plain CT. *Radiology* 186:731-738, 1993.

Toyone T, Takahashi K, Kitahara H, et al: Visualization of symptomatic nerve roots. *J Bone Joint Surg* (Br) 75-B:529-533, 1993.

Tsuruda JS, Norman D, Dillown W, et al: Three-dimensional gradient-recalled MR imaging as a screening tool for the diagnosis of cervical radiculopathy. *AJNR* 10:1263-1271, 1989.

Ulmer JL, Elster AD, Matthews VP, et al: distinction between degenerative and isthmic spondylolisthesis on sagittal MR images: importance of increased anteroposterior diameter of the spinal canal ("wide canal sign"), *AJR* 163:411-416, 1994.

VanDyke C, Ross JS, Tkach J, et al: Gradient-echo MR imaging of the cervical spine: evaluation of extradural disease. *AJNR* 10:627-632, 1989.

Wagner M, Sether LA, Yu S, et al: Age changes in the lumbar intervertebral disc studied with magnetic resonance and cryomicrotomy. *Clin Anat* 1:93-103, 1988.

Walker HS, Dietrich RB, Flannigan DB, et al: Magnetic resonance imaging of the pediatric spine. *Radiographics* 7:1129, 1987.

Wasserstrom R, Mamourian AC, Black JF, Lehman RAW: Intradural lumbar disk fragment with ring enhancement on MR. *AJNR* 14:401-404, 1993.

Widder DJ: MR imaging of ossification of the posterior longitudinal ligament. *AJNR* 153:194-195, 1989.

Williams MP, Cherryman GR, Husband JE: Significance of thoracic disc herniation demonstrated by MR imaging. *J Comput Assist Tomogr* 13:211-214, 1989.

Yousem DM, Atlas SW, Goldberg HI, Grossman RI: Degenerative narrowing of the cervical spine neural foramina: evaluation with high-resolution 3DFT gradient-echo MR imaging. *AJNR* 12:228-236, 1991.

Yu S, Haughton VM, Ho PSP, et al: Progressive and regressive changes in the nucleus pulposus: part II. The adult. *Radiology* 169:93-97, 1988.

Yu S, Haughton VM, Lynch KL, et al: Fibrous structure in the intervertebral disk: correlation of MR appearance with anatomic sections. *AJNR* 10:1105-1110, 1989.

Yu S, Haughton VM, Sether LA, et al: Criteria for classifying normal and degenerated intervertebral disks. *Radiology* 170:523-526, 1989.

Yu S, Haughton VM, Sether LA, Wagner M: Comparison of MR and diskography in detecting radial tears of the annulus: a postmortem study. *AJNR* 10:1077-1082, 1989.

Yu S, Sether LA, Ho PSP, et al: Tears of the anulus fibrosus: correlation between MR and pathologic findings in cadavers. *AJNR* 9:367-370, 1988.

Yuh WTC, Drew JM, Weinstein JN, et al: Intraspinal synovial cysts: magnetic resonance evaluation. *Spine* 16:740-745, 1991.

CHAPTER 15

Tumors of the Spinal Canal

Case 878

69-year-old man presenting with back pain.
(sagittal, noncontrast; SE 550/20)

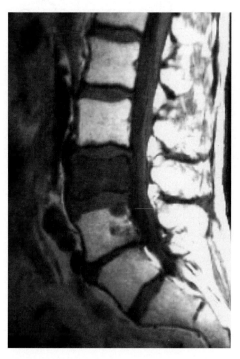

Metastatic Small Cell Carcinoma of the Lung

Case 879

70-year-old man presenting with a stumbling gait.
(sagittal, noncontrast scan; SE 800/17)

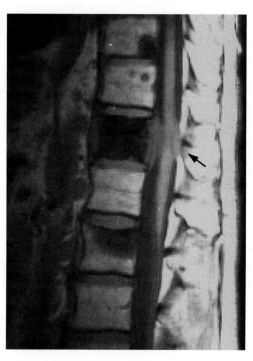

Metastatic Carcinoma of the Prostate

Vertebral and epidural metastases are usually well-defined on T1-weighted MR studies. Fat within vertebral marrow and the epidual space provides a normal background of high signal intensity. Marrow replacement by cellular infiltration (malignant or benign; see Cases 962 and 963) causes a conspicuous reduction in intensity. In Case 878, the entire vertebral body of L4 is filled with "watery" metastatic tissue. Reactive sclerosis contributes to the "dark" spots of metastatic disease within thoracic and lumbar vertebrae in Case 879.

T1-weighted images also demonstrate the contours of the spinal cord as outlined by CSF. Cord compression by epidural components of metastatic tumor can be readily assessed. In Case 879, an epidural mass at the T12 level effaces the subarachnoid space and deforms the cord *(arrow)*. The other vertebral lesions are not associated with epidural masses.

Contrast-enhanced T1-weighted scans may be less effective than noncontrast studies for detecting vertebral and epidural metastases (unless fat saturation techniques are superimposed). Metastatic lesions may enhance to a level isointense with marrow or epidural fat, masking their presence (see Case 909; also compare Cases 970 and 974).

Case 880

69-year-old man presenting with back pain.
(sagittal, noncontrast scan; SE 2800/90)

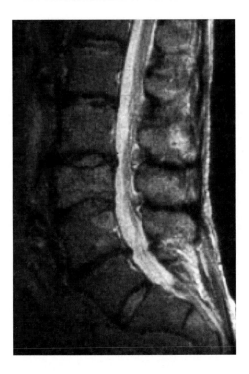

Metastatic Small Cell Carcinoma of the Lung
(same patient as Case 878)

Case 881

48-year-old man presenting with back pain.
(sagittal, noncontrast scan; low flip angle
GRE sequence)

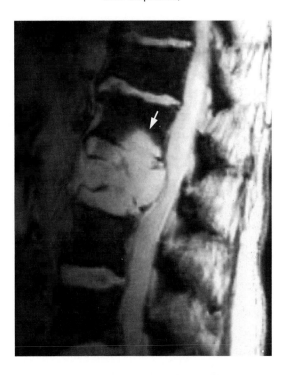

Metastatic Hypernephroma

Vertebral metastases demonstrate variable signal intensity on pulse sequences which highlight long T2 relaxation times. Some lesions are nearly isointense to surrounding marrow on T2-weighted spin echo scans, as seen in Case 880. The relative lack of T2 prolongation probably reflects a densely cellular tumor with a high nuclear to cytoplasmic ratio. (Compare to the appearance of cerebral germinomas and lymphomas, as in Cases 272 and 313.) Whatever the cause, some vertebral metastases are obvious on T1-weighted scans but inconspicuous on T2-weighted images (compare the scan in Case 878 to Case 880).

By contrast, the vertebral lesion in Case 881 demonstrates very high signal intensity on a "myelographic" gradient

echo sequence. A compression fracture of the involved body is apparent, with mild compromise of the spinal canal (see Cases 890 and 891).

Metastatic tissue has crossed the superior disc space in Case 881 to involve the adjacent vertebra *(arrow)*. This contiguous extension to an adjoining level is more characteristic of inflammatory disease but does not exclude vertebral metastasis (see Cases 970 and 971).

Rare vertebral chordomas (usually involving the C2 to C4 levels) may also extend across disc spaces. This feature can combine with characteristically long T2 values to produce an appearance very similar to Case 881.

Case 882

70-year-old man.
(sagittal, noncontrast scan; SE 500/20)

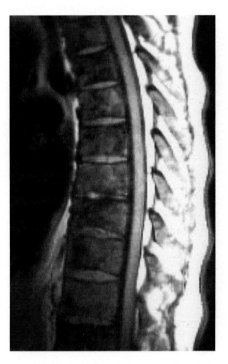

Metastatic Carcinoma of the Prostate

Case 883

25-year-old man.
(sagittal, noncontrast scan; SE 600/15)

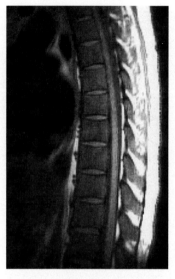

Acute Myelogenous Leukemia

Metastatic infiltration of vertebral bodies can be extensive, with uniform involvement of all visualized levels. Diffuse prolongation of T1 values throughout the spine may cause disc spaces to appear "brighter" than the adjacent vertebrae on short TR spin echo images. Cases 882 and 883 illustrate this pattern, which is the reverse of the normal relationship of signal intensities in adults (compare to Cases 878 and 879).

In addition to metastases from solid tumors, leukemia, lymphoma, myeloma, and myelofibrosis may diffusely involve the spine and cause uniform signal abnormality.

Abnormally low signal intensity may also be seen throughout the spine in hematological conditions leading to an accumulation of iron within the marrow. Among these is "anemia of chronic disease," which can be observed in patients with AIDS (see Case 959).

The spinal cord is well visualized throughout the thoracic canal in each of the above cases. There is no evidence of cord compression or epidural mass.

NORMALLY HETEROGENEOUS SIGNAL INTENSITY WITHIN THE SPINE

Case 884

74-year-old woman presenting with back pain.
(sagittal, noncontrast scan; SE 550/20)

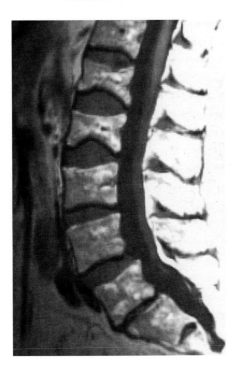

Case 885

39-year-old woman complaining of leg pain.
(sagittal, noncontrast scan; SE 550/20)

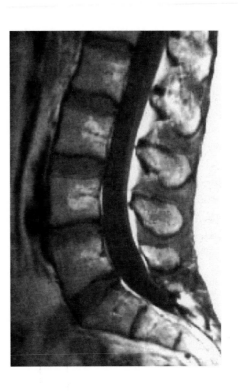

The vertebral marrow of most adults demonstrates uniformly high intensity on T1-weighted scans. However, a number of normal variations may produce a more heterogeneous appearance, which can be mistaken for multifocal metastatic disease.

Diffuse, mottled variation in the signal intensity of vertebral marrow is common in elderly patients, as illustrated in Case 884. This heterogeneity may reflect scattered fatty atrophy of the marrow alternating with zones of residual hematopoiesis. The "dark" areas within such spines on T1-weighted scans are not as well defined as focal metastases like those in Case 879 or as pervasive as the diffuse marrow infiltration in Cases 882 and 883. Clinical correlation is necessary when an appearance like Case 884 is encountered (see Case 894), but it is important to recognize this pattern as a potential normal variant.

Younger patients may have zones of signal abnormality within the midposterior portion of one or more vertebral bodies. Such areas can demonstrate T1 values that are shorter (as in Case 885) or longer (see Case 887) than adjacent marrow. They vary in size and prominence from patient to patient and from one vertebra to the next.

These normal "pseudolesions" reflect localized anatomical variation surrounding the basivertebral veins. The basivertebral vein drains the posterior half of the vertebral body, exiting through the midposterior cortex to join the anterior epidural plexus. The characteristic location of signal changes surrounding this vessel help to establish the incidental nature of the finding.

Benign compression fractures of the L1 and L2 vertebral bodies are present in Case 884.

Case 886

58-year-old woman complaining of back pain.
(sagittal, noncontrast scan; SE 550/20)

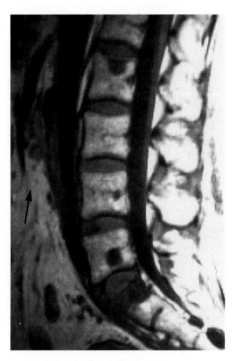

Metastatic Carcinoid Tumor

Case 887

32-year-old woman presenting with chronic
back pain.
(sagittal, noncontrast scan; SE 550/20)

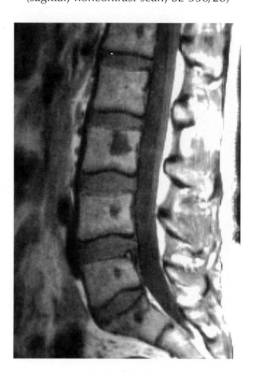

Normal Variant
(vascular spaces)

The scattered vertebral lesions in Case 886 are well defined, varying in size and location. The appearance strongly suggests metastatic disease. Associated retroperitoneal adenopathy *(arrow)* supports the diagnosis. Whenever the question of vertebral metastases is raised, a search for associated paraspinal or intraspinal masses is important (see also Case 976).

Case 887 could initially raise similar concerns. However, the "lesions" occupy the midposterior portion of each involved vertebra. This consistent location from level to level suggests an anatomical variant related to the vertebral venous system. The prolonged T1 in the region of the basi-

vertebral veins in this case may represent vascular spaces. (Compare to the appearance of focally increased marrow fat occupying similar locations in Case 885.)

Inflammatory lesions should also be considered in this differential diagnosis. Tuberculous spondylitis frequently extends beneath the anterior or posterior longitudinal ligaments to present with involvement of multiple vertebral bodies. Coccidiomycosis can also cause destruction at multiple vertebral levels due to subligamentous extension, often with sparing of the intervening disc spaces. Pyogenic vertebral osteomyelitis is usually associated with characteristic features of discitis, as discussed in Chapter 16.

Case 888

40-year-old man presenting with back pain.
(axial, noncontrast scan; SE 760/17; L4 level)

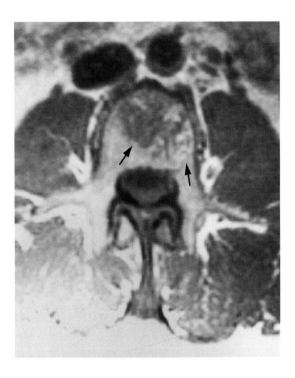

Case 889

29-year-old man presenting with back pain
and myelopathy.
(sagittal, noncontrast scan; SE 500/15)

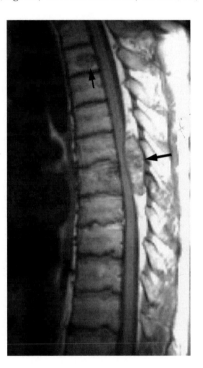

Hemangiomas are among the most common benign vertebral pathologies. These lesions consist of dilated vascular spaces replacing portions of the marrow and cancellous bone. They may occur anywhere within the vertebral body and/or posterior arch, unlike the prominent vascular spaces illustrated in Case 887. As marrow space lesions, hemangiomas must be distinguished from metastatic deposits.

The characteristic features of vertebral hemangiomas on CT scans are well recognized. A small number of vertically oriented trabeculae remain within the overall lucency caused by the hemangioma. The residual weight-bearing trabeculae are characteristically thickened, resulting in a coarse "honeycomb" or "polka-dot" pattern on axial scans and a striated texture on sagittal or coronal reconstructions.

Hemangiomas present a more variable appearance on MR studies. The lesions may have either predominantly low or predominantly high signal intensity relative to surrounding marrow on T1-weighted scans. Case 888 demonstrates a mixed pattern. High signal intensity is usually present on T2-weighted images. Margins of the hemangioma may be indistinct or sharply defined. A reticulated (axial view) or striated (sagittal or coronal view) texture may be appreciable, although less prominent than on CT studies.

Vertebral hemangiomas are often discovered incidentally (as in Case 888) and are rarely symptomatic. Occasional hemangiomas cause bone expansion or give rise to bulky paraspinal or intraspinal masses.

Case 889 illustrates epidural extension of a hemangioma involving the body and posterior arch of T7 (*large arrow*). (A smaller hemangioma is present within the body of T3; *small arrow*.) The epidural mass compresses the spinal cord and is responsible for the patient's myelopathy. The hemangiomas at T3 and T7 enhanced to become isointense with surrounding vertebral marrow and epidural fat on postcontrast scans. However, they were well defined by high signal intensity on T2-weighted images.

Aneurysmal bone cysts and osteoblastomas are other benign vertebral masses that can cause expansion of bone and secondary canal compromise.

Case 890

77-year-old woman presenting with back pain.
(sagittal, noncontrast scan; SE 550/20)

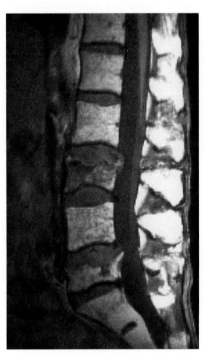

Benign Fractures

Case 891

48-year-old woman presenting with back
pain and bladder dysfunction.
(sagittal, noncontrast scan; SE 500/20)

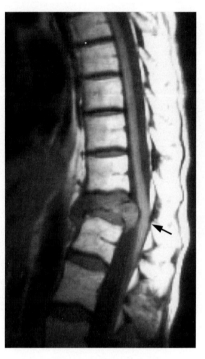

Pathological Fracture
(metastatic hypernephroma)

Compression fractures of vertebral bodies are a common feature of benign osteoporosis, with or without recognized trauma (see Cases 1009-1011). Pathological fractures of vertebral bodies are a regular manifestation of metastatic disease. Both types of fracture have an increasing incidence with patient age, and the distinction between them is a frequent clinical problem.

MR scans can be helpful in this context. Benign compression fractures that are subacute or chronic usually demonstrate residual high signal intensity due to marrow fat on T1-weighted scans. The L5 vertebral body in Case 890 is a typical example: despite the obvious loss of height, the body is normally "bright." This appearance contrasts with the replacement of marrow signal by more water-like intensity in pathological fractures, as in Case 891.

Recent benign vertebral fractures can be problematic. Hemorrhage and edema within a newly compressed verte-

bral body usually result in prolonged T1 values that may mimic metastatic infiltration. The L3 vertebra in Case 890 demonstrates this appearance, which is more prominent in other cases.

In such circumstances, secondary findings (e.g., the amount of cortical destruction or the presence of smaller lesions at other vertebral levels) may provide useful clues. STIR (Short Tau Inversion Recovery) sequences are often useful for detecting subtle vertebral metastases at other levels. Postcontrast scans with fat-suppression techniques are also valuable to define enhancing tumor, both within the compressed body and at possible additional sites. Follow-up scans are necessary to distinguish benign from malignant compression fractures in some cases.

The pathological fracture in Case 891 compresses the conus medullaris. Symptoms of conus dysfunction may also be caused by intramedullary metastases (see Case 901).

EPIDURAL MASSES ASSOCIATED WITH VERTEBRAL METASTASES

Case 892

68-year-old man.
(axial, noncontrast scan; SE 1000/20; L3 level)

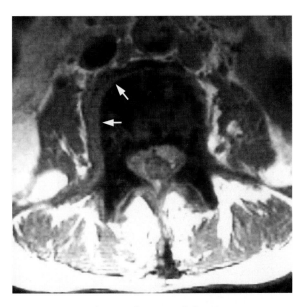

Metastatic Carcinoma of the Prostate

Case 893

59-year-old woman.
(sagittal, noncontrast scan; SE 550/20)

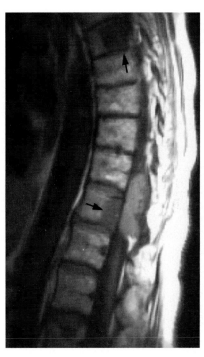

Metastatic Carcinoma of the Breast

Vertebral metastases are commonly accompanied by epidural tumor extension. Like pathological fractures, these masses may compromise the spinal canal and compress neural tissue, causing local symptoms and/or long tract findings.

The lumbar vertebral body in Case 892 is diffusely sclerotic. The epidural space is filled with soft tissue of intermediate signal intensity, replacing epidural fat and encircling the thecal sac. (Compare to the circumferential epidural lymphoma in Case 898B.) The proximal L3 nerve roots are surrounded by tumor in the lateral recesses. A layer of paraspinal tumor is present along the vertebral margins anteriorly and on the right *(arrows)*.

Case 893 demonstrates a more mass-like epidural metas-

tasis. The tumor within the spinal canal differs in signal intensity from the vertebral body of origin. By itself, the epidural mass resembles a spinal meningioma (compare to Case 913). Associated bone lesions both adjacent to and removed from the mass *(arrows)* establish the diagnosis.

The anterior epidural space is divided in the midline by a sagitally oriented band of tissue extending from the ventral surface of the dural sac to the posterior longitudinal ligament. This "ligament of Trolard" may influence the shape of slowly-growing epidural masses, causing them to initially accumulate in the lateral portions of the anterior epidural compartment (with relative sparing of the midline). Epidural metastases may demonstrate this "theater curtain" morphology.

Case 894

44-year-old man presenting with back pain.
(sagittal, noncontrast scan; SE 600/17)

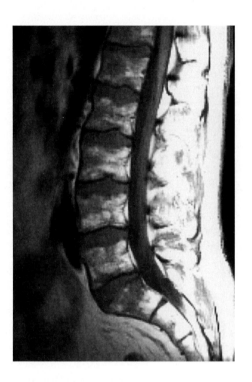

Case 895

50-year-old man presenting with back pain
and mild gait abnormality.
(sagittal, noncontrast scan; SE 550/20)

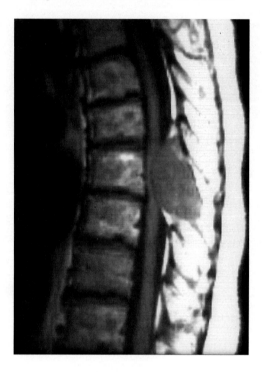

The extent and pattern of findings on MR scans of the spine in patients with myeloma are widely variable. Multifocal infiltration of spinal marrow may be encountered, as in Case 894. The heterogeneous pattern in this example resembles the potential normal variant in older patients illustrated in Case 884. More complete marrow replacement in myeloma can result in an appearance similar to Cases 882 and 883.

In other patients with myeloma, focal vertebral lesions predominate at one or several levels. Case 895 demonstrates a large mass that has expanded from the posterior arch of a midthoracic vertebra (compare to Case 893). The spinal cord is severely compressed. A background of

mottled signal intensity within all thoracic vertebral bodies is nonspecific but may reflect more generalized and subtle disease. Focal lesions within vertebral bodies (comparable to the metastases in Case 886) are also seen within the spectrum of myeloma.

Pain may be the only symptom of patients with incipient cord compression by epidural metastasis or myeloma. A high index of suspicion is warranted in cancer patients with new or worsening back pain, and prompt evaluation is indicated. Magnetic resonance imaging has replaced emergency myelography as the procedure of choice for this purpose.

DIFFERENTIAL DIAGNOSIS:
MASS EXPANDING THE POSTERIOR ARCH OF A VERTEBRA

Case 896

52-year-old man presenting with radicular
flank pain.
(axial, noncontrast scan; SE 1000/20; L3 level)

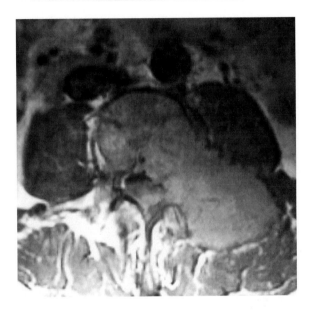

Myeloma

Case 897

62-year-old man complaining of radicular
midthoracic pain.
(axial, noncontrast scan; SE 1000/20; T6 level)

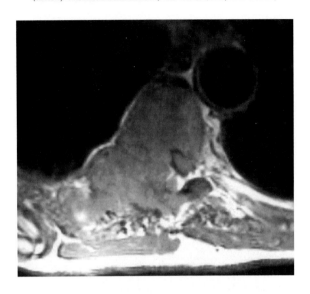

Metastatic Carcinoma of the Colon

Myeloma (or solitary plasmocytoma) is a leading consideration when an expansile tumor is discovered arising from posterior elements of the spine in adults, as illustrated in Case 896. Case 897 demonstrates that metastatic disease can also produce an expansile mass with bulky paraspinal and epidural components.

For practical purposes, metastasis and myeloma should both be considered whenever either pathology is entertained as the etiology of a spinal lesion. Both tumors can involve the vertebral body and/or the posterior arch.

In younger patients, benign bone tumors such as osteoblastomas and aneurysmal bone cysts may cause expansile lesions of the pedicle or lamina. Many aneurysmal bone cysts are multiloculated, demonstrating one or more sedimentation levels of blood products within cystic components of the mass (see Case 900-4). In other cases, aneurysmal bone cysts present as solid tissue surrounded by characteristic "egg shells" of expanded cortex (see Case 900-3).

Osteomyelitis (e.g., coccidiomycosis) is an additional rare cause of an expansile lesion arising from a vertebral body or posterior arch.

Case 898A

84-year-old man presenting with quadriparesis.
(sagittal, noncontrast scan; SE 500/20)

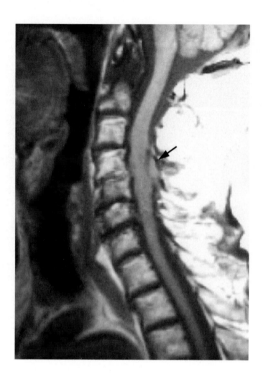

Case 898B

Same patient.
(axial, noncontrast scan; low flip angle
GRE sequence; C4-5 level)

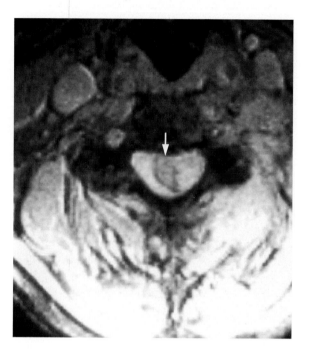

Although less common than metastasis or myeloma, lymphoma should be included in the differential diagnosis of epidural masses in adults (and in children). Like metastasis and myeloma, lymphoma may cause destructive and/or expansile lesions of vertebral bodies or posterior arches at one or more levels. However, lymphomatous epidural masses may also be present in the absence of adjacent osseous lesions. (Compare to primary epidural involvement by neuroblastoma in children; see Cases 899 and 900.)

Abnormal epidural tissue is present both ventral and dorsal to the spinal cord at the C4-5 level in Case 898A. Case 898B demonstrates that this rind encircles and deforms the thecal sac (*arrow*; compare to the epidural metastasis in

Case 892). The spinal cord is compressed, outlined by the low signal intensity of surrounding dura. (Disc space narrowing and mild subluxation at the C4-5 level are probably not related to the epidural tumor.)

Non-neoplastic epidural masses (e.g., hematoma or abscess; see Cases 980, 981, 1024, and 1025) should be considered in the differential diagnosis. These pathologies tend to have a greater longitudinal extent than epidural tumor. (However, epidural lymphoma is often more extensive than in this case and typically involves more vertebral levels than epidural metastasis.) The more rapid development of symptoms usually helps to distinguish epidural hematoma or abscess from neoplasms.

Case 899

7-year-old girl complaining of intermittent
back pain and mild gait abnormality.
(sagittal, noncontrast scan; SE 800/15)

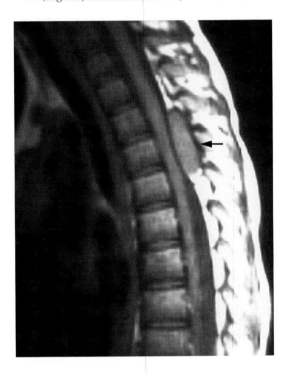

Case 900

2-month-old girl presenting with
an abdominal mass.
(coronal, noncontrast scan; SE 800/17)

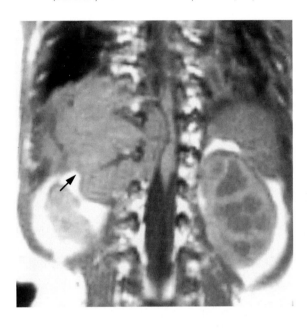

Epidural neuroblastoma is often primary, with no associated vertebral lesions. Case 899 demonstrates a smoothly marginated mass within dorsal epidural fat in the superior thoracic region *(arrow)*. The lesion extends across three vertebral levels, compressing the dural sac and spinal cord. There is no evidence of osseous infiltration or destruction.

Epidural masses in the pediatric population are frequently of paraspinal origin. In Case 900, a coronal scan establishes continuity between the paraspinal and epidural components of a large tumor. The mass extends from the right suprarenal area through two intervertebral foramina to displace the spinal cord and conus medullaris. The lesion is homogeneous in signal intensity. Calcification, which is characteristic of abdominal neuroblastoma on CT scans, is rarely appreciated on MR studies.

The differential diagnosis of an epidural and/or paraspinal mass in a child should include leukemia, lymphoma, Ewing's sarcoma, and rhabdomyosarcoma in addition to neuroblastoma. Occasional benign hemangiomas present a similar appearance.

Cases 932 and 933 illustrate examples of neuroblastoma involving the lumbosacral spinal canal.

Case 900-1A

5-year-old girl with a posterior mediastinal mass
discovered on a chest x-ray.
(coronal, noncontrast scan; SE 600/15)

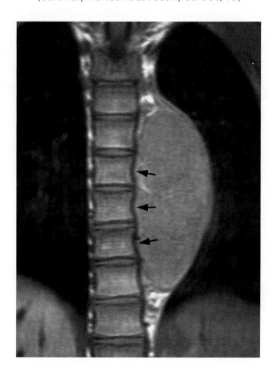

Case 900-1B

Same patient.
(sagittal, noncontrast scan; SE 2800/90)

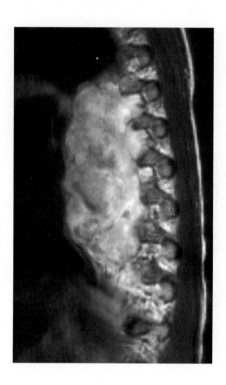

Ganglioneuromas are well-differentiated neoplasms comprised primarily of mature ganglion cells. These tumors tend to occur in older children and young adults. In some cases, they represent maturation of an earlier neuroblastoma. Ganglioneuromas frequently arise from the sympathetic chain in a paraspinal location.

The tumor in Case 900-1 is typical, presenting as a large mediastinal mass. The size of the well-defined lesion and the mild scalloping of adjacent vertebral bodies (*arrows*) suggest a slowly growing neoplasm. Note, however, that the internal architecture of the tumor appears much more complex on the T2-weighted scan in Case 900-1B than on the T1-weighted image in Case 900-1A. This heterogeneous texture cannot by itself be distinguished from more aggressive pediatric paraspinal masses.

The tumor in this case did not traverse intervertebral foramina to involve the spinal canal. Mature ganglioneuromas may do so, resembling the appearance of the neuroblastoma in Case 900.

Case 900-2A

2-year-old boy presenting with difficulty walking.
(axial, noncontrast scan; SE 700/15; T-10 level)

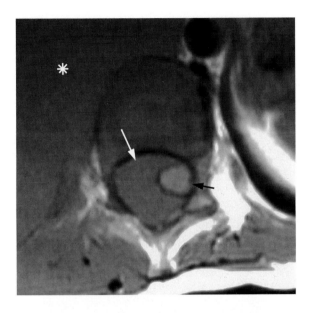

Case 900-2B

Same patient.
(sagittal, noncontrast scan; RSE 4000/96)

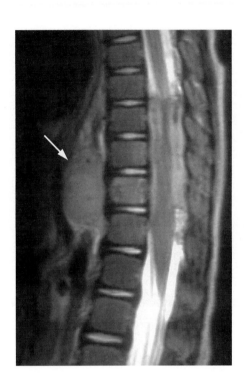

A number of childhood malignancies are characterized histologically by small round cells with little cytoplasm. The closely spaced, blue-staining nuclei in such lesions have caused them to be known as "small blue cell tumors." Included in this category are neuroblastoma, more undifferentiated primitive neuroectodermal tumors (PNET), lymphoma, rhabdomyosarcoma, and extraosseous Ewing's sarcoma. Pathological distinction among these lesions often requires special histochemical stains, electron microscopy, and/or correlation with increased levels of specific metabolites in the blood or urine. The structural and chemical characteristics of the above tumor were suggestive of a primitive neuroectodermal malignancy.

Any of the "small blue cell" neoplasms can arise in a paraspinal location with intraspinal extension. The tumor in Case 900-2A has accumulated as a large abdominal mass (*asterisk*). The lesion traversed several intervertebral foramina, with a major epidural component (*white arrow*) displacing the dural sac and spinal cord (*black arrow*). Compare this morphology to Case 900.

The scan in Case 900-2B illustrates the encircling rind of epidural tumor effacing the subarachnoid space from T-9 to T-11. A prevertebral component of the mass is demonstrated (*arrow*), as well as abnormal signal intensity within the T-11 vertebral body and the posterior portion of T-10.

Note that the epidural component of pediatric paraspinal masses as illustrated above is comparable to the adult intraspinal masses arising from vertebral metastases (compare to Cases 879 and 892).

Case 900-3

15-year-old girl presenting with back pain
and leg weakness.
(axial, noncontrast scan; SE 1000/20; T8 level)

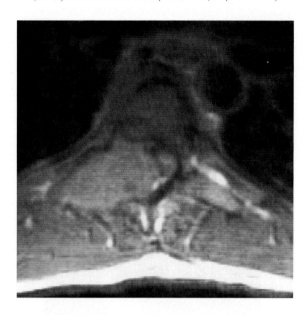

Case 900-4

10-year-old girl presenting with a stiff back
and mild difficulty walking.
(sagittal, noncontrast scan; SE 2500/80)

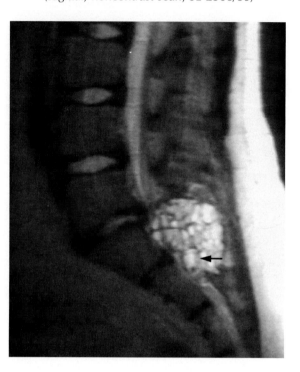

Primary vertebral tumors are an unusual cause of epidural masses and neurological symptoms. Benign lesions such as osteoblastomas and aneurysmal bone cysts may be encountered in young patients, as illustrated above.

Aneurysmal bone cysts are osteolytic masses, typically comprised of lobulated compartments containing blood. The origin of these lesions is not well established. In many cases they seem to represent a reactive process incited by a primary pathology such as fibrous dysplasia, nonossifying fibroma, osteoblastoma, or giant cell tumor. Aneurysmal bone cysts themselves are not neoplastic. About 20% of aneurysmal bone cysts occur in the spine, frequently arising from posterior elements as in these cases.

The mass in Case 900-3 has expanded from the vertebral pedicle and transverse process to involve the spinal canal. The appearance represents a pediatric analogy to the adult lesions in Cases 896 and 897. Characteristic "egg shells" of displaced cortex are often demonstrated at the periimeter of aneurysmal bone cysts on CT scans.

Case 900-3 is unusual because the mass appears homogeneous and the lesion was predominantly solid at surgery. The more typical architecture of aneurysmal bone cysts is the multicystic pattern illustrated in Case 900-4. Several of the small loculations contain sedimentation levels, suggesting the presence of blood products.

Other potential "bubbly" lesions of the sacrum in children include giant cell tumors, histiocytosis, chondrosarcoma, and hemophiliac pseudotumors. In adults, myeloma, metastases (e.g., from hypernephroma and thyroid carcinoma), and hyperparathyroidism may cause multiloculated sacral expansion. (Also see the discussion of sacral chordomas in Cases 934 and 935.)

SPINAL CHONDROSARCOMAS

Case 900-5

52-year-old man presenting with arm weakness
and difficulty walking.
(sagittal, noncontrast scan; RSE 4000/103)

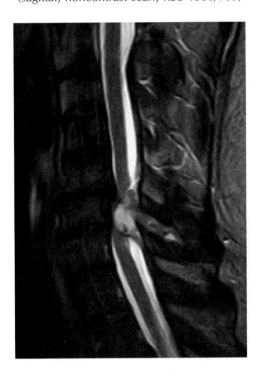

Case 900-6

34-year-old woman presenting with back pain
and paraparesis.
(axial, postcontrast scan; SE 700/17; T4 level)

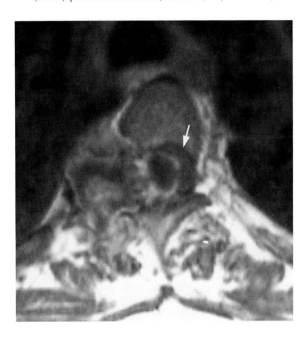

Malignant primary vertebral tumors may also cause epidural masses and spinal cord compression. Chondrosarcomas are the most common lesions to do so in adults, usually affecting patients in the 30- to 60-year-old age range. Other rare primary malignant bone tumors which occasionally involve the spinal canal include osteosarcomas (most common at ages 10 to 20), primary Ewing's sarcomas (most common at ages 15 to 25), and fibrosarcomas.

Both of the tumors illustrated above arise from the posterior arch of the involved vertebra and both demonstrate lobulated morphology. These features are typical for vertebral chondrosarcomas. The high signal intensity of the mass in Case 900-5 suggests high water content within the tumor matrix, another characteristic feature of chondroid neoplasms. Scattered areas of low signal intensity may also be seen within a chondrosarcoma on T2-weighted images due to calcification and/or hemorrhage.

The heterogeneous enhancement pattern in Case 900-6 includes both solid and peripheral components, with an overall multinodular structure. This pattern correlates with histology demonstrating a mixture of cellular tumor regions and areas that primarily contain matrix. The mass expands from its vertebral origin to produce bulky paraspinal and epidural components.

The spinal cord in Case 900-5 is well-defined and clearly compressed. The cord in Case 900-6 is less well demarcated but appears to be displaced and flattened against the left side of the spinal canal (arrow).

Case 901

55-year-old woman presenting with gait
abnormality.
(sagittal, noncontrast scan; SE 800/17)

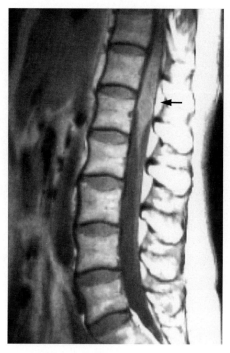

Metastasis Within the Conus Medullaris
(from carcinoma of the breast)

Case 902

57-year-old woman presenting with bilateral
leg pain and weakness.
(sagittal, noncontrast scan; SE 600/20)

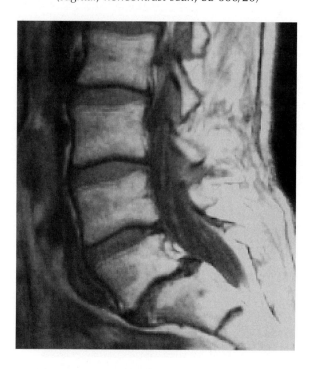

Metastases Along Roots of the Cauda Equina
(from carcinoma of the breast)

Metastases to the spinal canal most frequently involve vertebral bodies and/or the epidural space, as illustrated in the preceding pages. However, intradural metastases are more common than previously appreciated. It is important to consider this possibility when reviewing spinal MR scans of patients with cancer.

Intramedullary metastases may occur at any level of the spinal cord (see also Case 961). The conus medullaris is a particularly common site and should be carefully examined on all lumbar scans. In Case 901, the conus is expanded and demonstrates central low signal intensity. T2-weighted scans and postcontrast studies can confirm that the conus is abnormal when T1-weighted scans are equivocal.

Case 902 demonstrates distinct nodularity along the roots of the cauda equica. This studding by tumor deposits can also be appreciated on axial images (see Case 903) and is highlighted by contrast enhancement (see Cases 909 and 910).

The patient in Case 902 had undergone mastectomy and radiation for carcinoma of the breast ten years earlier. It is not uncommon to discover cerebral or spinal metastases from breast carcinoma developing a decade or more after treatment of the primary tumor.

Intradural metastases should be remembered as an occasional cause of radiculopathy, cauda equina symptoms, or conus dysfunction in patients with no preceding evidence of neoplasm. Among the primary tumors that commonly metastasize to the intrathecal compartment are carcinomas of the breast and lung and melanoma.

DIFFERENTIAL DIAGNOSIS:
THICKENED INTRADURAL NERVE ROOTS

Case 903

57-year-old woman presenting with leg pain
and weakness.
(axial, noncontrast scan; SE 1000/20; L3-4 level)

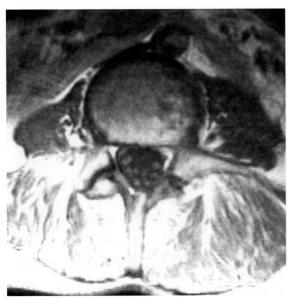

Metastatic Carcinoma of the Breast
(same patient as Case 902)

Case 904

68-year-old man presenting with progressive
leg weakness.
(axial, noncontrast scan; SE 1000/17; L4-5 level)

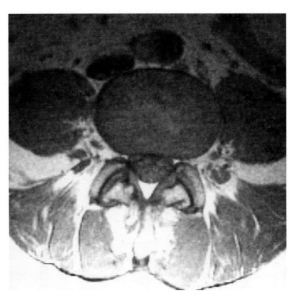

Lymphomatous Meningitis

Intrathecal nerve roots are abnormally thickened in each of the above cases. The possibility of intradural metastases should be a leading consideration when this appearance is encountered.

Case 904 illustrates that systemic lymphoma may coat the surface of intradural tissues in a manner analogous to the leptomeningeal carcinomatosis in Case 903. Thickening of nerve roots is often more uniform in lymphomatous meningitis than in cases of intradural metastases from carcinomas.

Intradural metastases may arise from CSF seeding of CNS neoplasms as well as from hematogeneous dissemination of systemic tumors. "Drop" metastases from cranial (or other

spinal) masses may cause an appearance very comparable to the above images (see Cases 907, 908, 910, and 1008).

Nerve roots of the cauda equina normally appear more prominent on postcontrast scans (particularly in the axial plane) than on precontrast studies. This mild, uniform enhancement can raise the question of carcinomatous meningitis, as discussed in Case 976.

Non-neoplastic etiologies of thickened intradural nerve roots include edema caused by mechanical compression (e.g., in cases of disc herniation or spinal stenosis), inflammation and/or adhesions secondary to arachnoiditis (see Case 1003), and rare primary hypertrophic neuropathies (e.g., Déjérine-Sottas disease).

Case 905

7-year-old boy, eleven months after resection
of a fourth ventricular ependymoma.
(sagittal, postcontrast scan; SE 600/20)

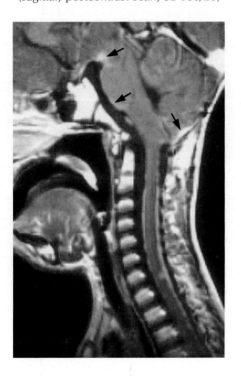

Case 906

10-year-old boy, one year after resection
of a spinal primitive neuroectodermal tumor.
(axial, postcontrast scan; SE 700/17; T12 level)

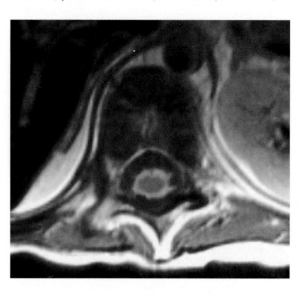

In Case 905, the surface of the cervical spinal cord is lined by abnormal contrast enhancement. Such coating or "frosting" of neural tissue is a common pattern for intradural metastases on contrast-enhanced MR studies. The appearance is particularly frequent in association with "drop" metastases from intracranial neoplasms, especially medulloblastoma and ependymoma. CSF seeding from intracranial tumors may also cause coarser intradural nodularity (see Cases 910 and 951).

Case 906 demonstrates a uniform layer of abnormal enhancement along the surface of the conus medullaris due to CSF dissemination of the patient's primitive neuroectodermal tumor. In other cases, pial-based tumor is discontinuous, asymmetrical, and/or nodular.

Superficial enhancement along cord margins as seen in Cases 905 and 906 is not specific for malignant disease. A similar appearance may be encountered in inflammatory disorders such as sarcoidosis or CMV myelitis (see Cases 995 and 998). In both disease categories, subpial spread of pathology may be associated with enhancing nodules of tissue extending into the cord from the pial surface (seen dorsally in Case 905 at the C7 level).

Case 905 also illustrates meningeal tumor spread within the posterior fossa (e.g., *arrows;* compare to Cases 160-162 and 299B).

Case 907

7-year-old boy, eleven months after resection
of a fourth ventricular ependymoma.
(sagittal, postcontrast scan; SE 600/20)

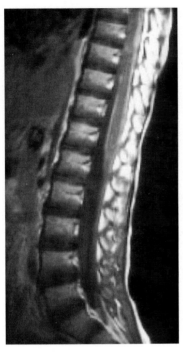

(same patient as Case 905)

Case 908

11-year-old girl with extensive intracranial
and intraspinal recurrence of a cerebral
primitive neuroectodermal tumor.
(sagittal, postcontrast scan; SE 600/15)

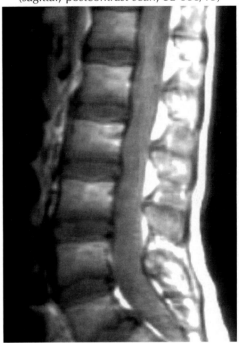

CSF-borne dissemination of intracranial tumors to the lumbar canal can present several distinct morphologies. The coating of abnormal contrast enhancement on the surface of the conus medullaris in Case 907 is comparable to the cervical involvement illustrated in Case 905.

Case 908 demonstrates pathology that is less well-defined because it is more extensive. The entire thecal sac is abnormal, with signal intensity greater than that expected for CSF. The amorphous or featureless appearance of the intradural compartment is due to the presence of cells, protein, and contrast material within the spinal fluid. This suspension surrounds the cauda equina and eliminates the normal definition of intradural anatomy. A similar appearance is occasionally seen with hematogeneous metastases of systemic origin (e.g., breast carcinoma) filling the subarachnoid space.

Primary intradural or epidural tumors may also cause a featureless lumbar canal by filling or effacing the thecal sac. Examples include intradural epidermoid masses, large intradural ependymomas (see Case 952), and epidural neuroblastomas (see Case 932).

Intradural metastatic disease within the lumbar spinal canal may alternatively present as one or more discrete masses (see Cases 910 and 951).

Case 909

90-year-old woman presenting with leg pain.
(sagittal, postcontrast scan; SE 500/15)

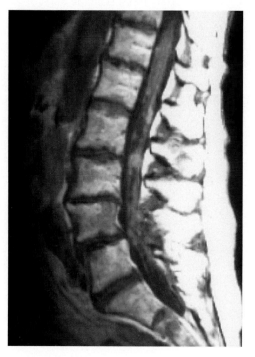

Metastatic Carcinoma of the Breast

Case 910

40-year-old man complaining of headaches
and low back pain.
(sagittal, postcontrast scan; SE 600/15)

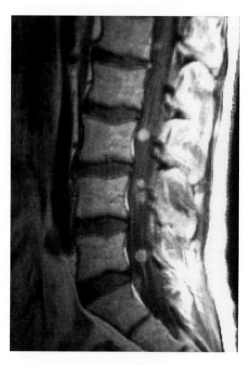

**"Drop" Metastases from a Cerebral
Glioblastoma Multiforme**

The preceding pages have demonstrated that intradural metastases can arise from hematogenous dissemination of systemic neoplasms or from CSF spread of primary CNS tumors. Cases 909 and 910 reinforce this point and illustrate the potential similarity of the two pathologies.

In Case 909, a precontrast scan showed nodularity along intradural nerve roots comparable to Case 902. The scan also demonstrated multiple, low intensity vertebral metastases. Most of the osseous lesions have enhanced to isointensity and are poorly seen on the above scan (see discussion of Cases 878 and 879).

The enhancing tumor nodules along the roots of the cauda equina in Case 910 are nonspecific and could easily represent metastases from a systemic source. Instead, they were due to CSF seeding of a malignant glioma. "Drop" metastases from gliomas are less frequent than spinal dissemination of germinomas, medulloblastomas, ependymomas, pineal cell tumors, and primitive neuroectodermal tumors.

Multiple enhancing root tumors (neurofibromas or schwannomas) in a patient with neurofibromatosis type 1 or 2 could present a pattern very similar to the above images.

Case 911

30-year-old man presenting with back pain.
(axial, postcontrast scan; SE 700/17; L2-3 level)

Case 912

17-year-old girl presenting with back pain.
(axial, postcontrast scan; SE 600/15; L3-4 level)

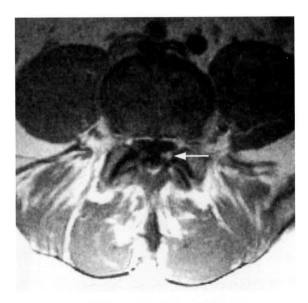

**Inflammed Root Rostral to Compression
by a Herniated Disc**

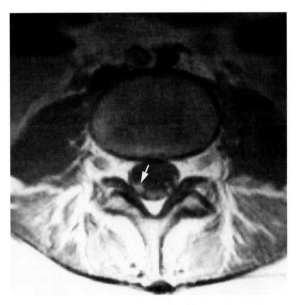

"Drop" Metastases
(from a thoracic ependymoma)

Prominent, asymmetrical contrast enhancement of an intrathecal nerve root is occasionally seen as a normal variant due to a large accompanying radicular vein. (The largest vein of the cauda equina usually courses along the filum terminale.) More often the finding is abnormal but nonspecific.

Radicular enhancement may be noted for several centimeters proximal to a site of neural compression, as in Case 911. Such enhancement is more extensive than the normal mildly increased intensity of intrathecal roots on postcontrast scans.

Inflammatory disorders (e.g., sarcoidosis, tuberculosis, herpes zoster, cytomegalovirus, arachnoiditis, and Guillain-Barré syndrome) occasionally cause focal enhancement of isolated roots. A large vessel associated with a vascular malformation could produce a similar appearance. Small nerve root tumors are characteristically intradural and intensely enhancing. Finally, intradural metastases may present in this manner, as illustrated in Case 912 and in previous cases of this chapter.

The primary tumor in Case 912 is presented as Case 953. Ependymomas of the spinal cord are frequently exophytic and may seed the cranial or spinal subarachnoid space.

Case 913

53-year-old woman with a six-month history of "rubbery" legs and diminished sacral sensation.
(sagittal, noncontrast scan; SE 800/17)

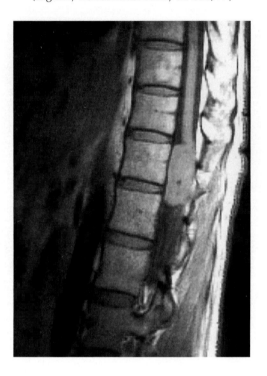

Case 914

67-year-old woman presenting with back and bilateral leg pain.
(sagittal, noncontrast scan; RSE 2300/103)

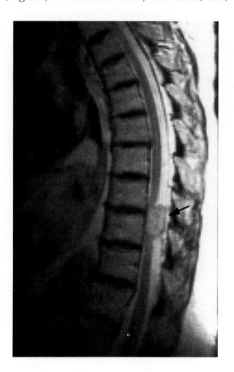

Meningiomas and schwannomas are the most common primary intradural tumors of the spinal canal. Such lesions are well outlined by surrounding CSF on T1- or T2-weighted MR scans. Although the masses may be nearly isointense to the spinal cord on noncontrast images, distortion of anatomy and capping of the tumors by spinal fluid establish their presence.

The large, homogeneous intradural meningioma in Case 913 fills the spinal canal at the level of the conus medullaris and proximal cauda equina. Cord margins are obscured and the subarachnoid space is effaced. The differential diagnosis of this intradural mass includes ependymoma and schwannoma (see Cases 923, 945, and 951).

Spinal meningiomas may demonstrate a range of signal intensities on T2-weighted scans, comparable to cerebral le-

sions (see Cases 36 to 39). Case 914 demonstrates a tumor of intermediate signal intensity and homogeneous texture. The spinal cord is anteriorly displaced and compressed. The dorsal subarachnoid space is widened at the margins of the mass, the hallmark of an intradural extramedullary process.

Spinal meningiomas are most common in the thoracic canal, often arising laterally (as in Case 913) or dorsolaterally (as in Case 914). They occur much more frequently in women than in men: the male to female ratio is about 1:4.

Ventral location within the spinal canal is common for cervical meningiomas (see Case 917). In the thoracic canal, ventral location of an intradural extramedullary mass is more typical of schwannomas (see Cases 864, 921, and 922).

Case 915

67-year-old woman presenting with back
and bilateral leg pain.
(coronal, postcontrast scan; SE 600/15)

Case 916

48-year-old woman presenting with abnormal gait.
(coronal, postcontrast scan; SE 600/15)

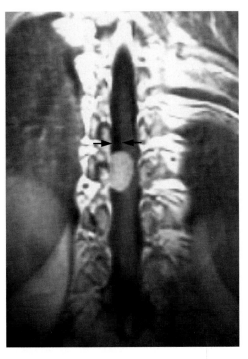

(same patient as Case 914)

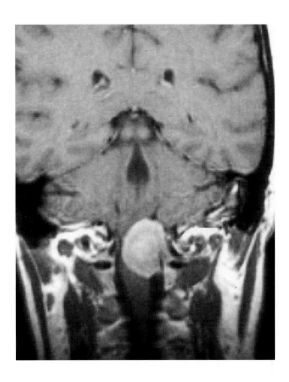

Like their intracranial counterparts, spinal meningiomas usually enhance intensely and uniformly.

In Case 915, a meningioma arises from the dorsolateral margin of the dural sac and compresses the spinal cord contralaterally and anteriorly (see Case 914). Note the widening of the subarachnoid space above and below the tumor, documenting its location as intradural but extramedullary.

The meningioma in Case 916 is centered at the C1 level. The mass occupies most of the spinal canal and distorts the cervicomedullary junction. Within the lesion a faint circular or target-like architecture can be seen. This occasional finding is highly suggestive of a meningioma.

The presence and uniformity of contrast enhancement within an intradural lesion are nonspecific. The intense, homogeneous enhancement seen above is compatible with meningioma, but schwannomas, ependymomas, and intradural metastases may have a similar appearance. On the other hand, many spinal schwannomas and ependymomas contain cystic or necrotic areas that cause an inhomogeneous pattern of enhancement (see Case 923).

The lesion in Case 915 was apparent on noncontrast scans. Contrast was given to (1) more clearly demonstrate the interface between the tumor and the spinal cord (particularly on axial images) and (2) evaluate the possibility of additional intradural masses.

DIFFERENTIAL DIAGNOSIS:
INTRADURAL EXTRAMEDULLARY MASS AT THE CRANIOCERVICAL JUNCTION

Case 917

48-year-old woman presenting with
difficulty walking.
(sagittal, noncontrast scan; SE 600/14)

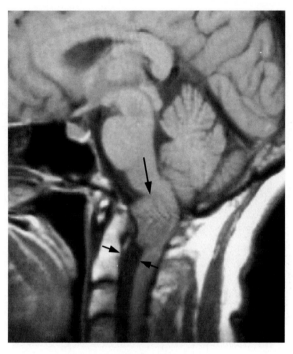

Meningioma
(same patient as Case 916)

Case 918

26-year-old woman presenting with
arm paresthesias.
(sagittal, noncontrast scan; SE 500/15)

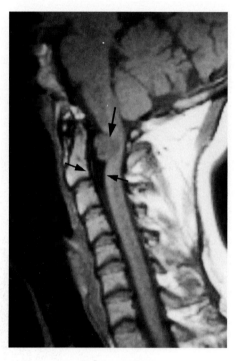

Schwannoma

Both meningiomas and schwannomas commonly occur near the foramen magnum. Both tumors may arise ventral to the spinal cord, as illustrated above. Note the widening of the anterior subarachnoid space at the margins of the mass in each case (*lower arrows*), confirming intradural location.

The two tumors are indistinguishable on these T1-weighted images. T2-weighted scans and images after contrast injection may favor one diagnosis over the other (see discussion of Cases 919, 920, and 923). However, such distinctions are usually relative rather than absolute, and the two pathologies must often be listed together in a differential diagnosis.

Fibrous "pseudotumors" may develop along the anterior margin of the foramen magnum in cases of chronic instability at C1-2 (see discussion of Cases 1044 and 1048), resembling the above lesions.

Partially or completely thrombosed aneurysms should also be considered among masses near the cervicomedullary junction (see Case 598). Peripheral or central components of T2-shortening may provide a clue to this diagnosis, even when the lesion appears isointense on T1-weighted scans (as is often the case).

Masses at the foramen magnum may present with a variety of nonspecific symptoms. Demyelinating disease was suspected in both of the above patients. Attention to the foramen magnum (and the visible segment of the cervical spinal cord) is important during review of all cranial scans, especially those obtained "for possible multiple sclerosis."

Another clinical syndrome associated with compromise of the foramen magnum is spastic diplegia, often categorized in children as "cerebral palsy." Spinal masses at the craniocervical junction or within the cervical canal should be considered in patients with such presentations.

Case 919

26-year-old woman presenting with
arm paresthesias.
(sagittal, noncontrast scan; SE 2500/80)

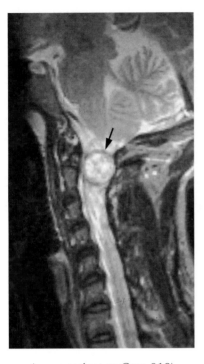

(same patient as Case 918)

Case 920

36-year-old man presenting with left arm numbness
and incoordination of the left leg.
(sagittal, noncontrast scan; SE 2300/90)

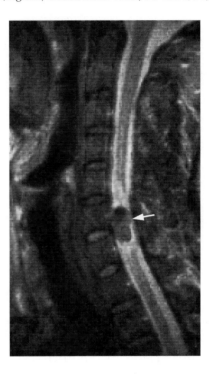

The signal intensity of spinal schwannomas on T2-weighted scans is widely variable. (Compare to the appearance of acoustic schwannomas, discussed in Cases 168 and 169.)

Some of these tumors demonstrate homogeneous or heterogeneous prolongation of T2, as illustrated in Case 919. This high signal intensity may arise from a watery tissue matrix, possibly reflecting the predominance of Antoni "B" zones with a relatively loose arrangement of cells. Alternatively, high signal intensity within schwannomas on long TR spin echo sequences may be caused by cystic or necrotic degeneration, which often occurs as these tumors enlarge. Although a faint tissue pattern of concentric circles may be suggested within some meningiomas (see Case 916), the definite ring or rim pattern of Case 919 is more commonly found in schwannomas.

Other spinal schwannomas are characterized by low signal intensity on T2-weighted scans, as in Case 920. This appearance often correlates with the presence of old blood products. Small or large areas of hemorrhage are commonly found within schwannomas at surgery or on histological examination.

The appearance in Case 920 is nonspecific. Low signal intensity may occur within meningiomas due to dense fibrous tissue or calcification. Calcified or ossified extradural lesions (e.g., osteochondromas) could also present with morphology and signal intensity resembling Case 920. Occasional cavernous angiomas of the spinal canal occur as small intradural or extradural masses with short T1 and T2 values due to the presence of subacute and chronic hemorrhage.

Case 921

34-year-old woman presenting with clumsy arms.
(sagittal, noncontrast scan; SE 800/20)

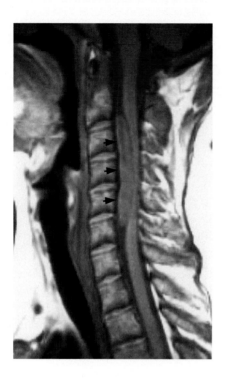

Case 922

54-year-old woman presenting with back pain
and leg weakness.
(sagittal, postcontrast scan; SE 600/15)

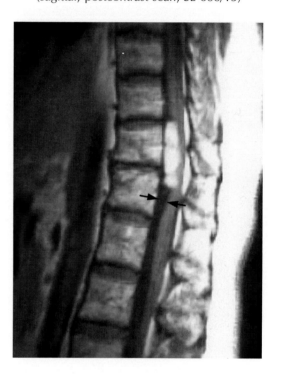

Most schwannomas of the spinal canal are round or lobulated masses, as illustrated on the preceding pages. In some cases, spinal schwannomas assume an unusually flat, plaque-like morphology. Such lesions may extend along the spine for several segments.

Case 921 demonstrates a thick layer of abnormal tissue occupying the anterior portion of the spinal canal from C2 to C6 (arrows). The length of the lesion might raise the question of an epidural process such as lymphoma or metastasis. However, the subarachnoid space is widened at the rostral and caudal margins of the tumor, indicating intradural location of the mass. At surgery, the lesion proved to be a schwannoma attached to a single cervical root.

The intensely enhancing mass in Case 922 has a similar plaque-like morphology, with mild superimposed lobulations. As in Case 921, the spinal cord is severely compressed, and caps of widened subarachnoid space are present at the poles of the mass (arrows).

A meningioma should be considered in the differential diagnosis of Case 922. "En plaque" meningiomas do occur in the spinal canal but are relatively less common than intracranial tumors with this morphology.

Examination of the remainder of the spinal canal on postcontrast images is indicated when one intradural mass is discovered. The presence of additional lesions raises the possibilities of multiple nerve root tumors (e.g., schwannomas in neurofibromatosis type 2 or neurofibromas in neurofibromatosis type 1) or intradural metastases of systemic or CNS origin (see Cases 909 and 910).

DIFFERENTIAL DIAGNOSIS:
SPINAL CANAL MASS WITH PERIPHERAL ENHANCEMENT

Case 923

44-year-old woman presenting with a three-month
history of increasing back pain
and a negative lumbar CT scan.
(sagittal, postcontrast scan; SE 550/20)

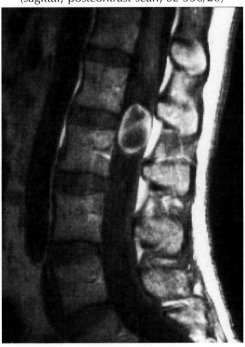

Schwannoma

Case 924

63-year-old woman presenting with leg pain.
(sagittal, postcontrast scan; SE 500/17)

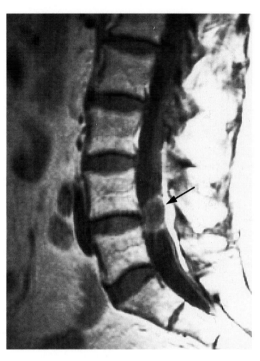

Synovial Cyst

Spinal schwannomas often contain nonenhancing areas of necrosis, hemorrhage, or cystic degeneration. As a result, schwannomas may demonstrate heterogeneous contrast enhancement, illustrated by Case 923. At surgery, this tumor was found to be both hemorrhagic and necrotic.

Peripheral contrast enhancement is also characteristic of synovial cysts, discussed in Cases 855 and 856. The typical size and shape of the lesion in Case 924 and its location at the L4-5 level are clues to the correct diagnosis. Axial scans would distinguish the epidural location of this synovial cyst from an intradural mass like Case 923.

Herniated disc fragments should be included in the differential diagnosis. They are the most common epidural masses, and they are typically outlined by enhancement on early postcontrast scans (see Cases 819 and 840).

Ependymomas of the filum terminale may be partially cystic or necrotic, resembling the above lesions. Rare cavernous angiomas within the spinal canal can also present a complex, lobulated appearance with rims of contrast enhancement.

Intrathecal masses above or within the examined region may be missed on "screening" CT examinations of the lumbar spine, as evidenced by Case 923.

Case 925A

28-year-old woman presenting with neck pain, left arm weakness, and spasticity of the left leg.
(sagittal, noncontrast scan; SE 500/15)

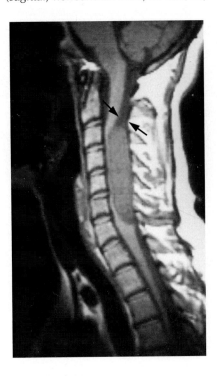

Case 925B

Same patient.
(axial, noncontrast scan; low flip angle GRE sequence; C5-6 level)

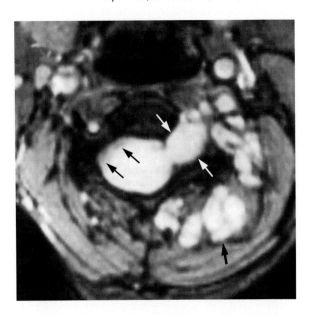

The MR characteristics of schwannomas and neurofibromas are largely indistinguishable. For this reason, they are often discussed together as "nerve sheath tumors" or "nerve root tumors." Both schwannomas and neurofibromas commonly arise from the dorsal sensory root of a spinal nerve.

Clinically and pathologically the lesions are distinct. Schwannomas occur sporadically. They originate from proliferation of schwann cells at one location on the perimeter of a nerve, leading to an eccentric mass that compresses and displaces the otherwise uninvolved axons. Neurofibromas are essentially limited to and specific for neurofibromatosis type 1. They arise from proliferation of both the internal fibroblastic and external schwann cell components of the nerve, resulting in symmetrical enlargement that surrounds individual axons. Neurofibromas are usually multiple, while schwannomas are usually solitary. (Multiple schwannomas are seen in neurofibromatosis type 2.)

The majority of nerve root tumors are entirely intradural, as illustrated by the schwannomas on the previous pages.

About 40% of nerve root tumors are extradural or demonstrate both intradural and extradural components.

Such dumbbell tumors typically involve and expand intervertebral foramina, as seen in Case 925B. The large intradural component of this tumor (which causes widening of the dorsal subarachnoid space in Case 925A) flattens the spinal cord *(thin black arrows)* contralaterally. The adjacent extradural portion of the neurofibroma extends into the left intervertebral foramen, which has been widened by chronic mass effect *(white arrows)*. A plexiform neurofibroma within dorsal soft tissues of the neck *(thick black arrow)* establishes the underlying diagnosis of type 1 neurofibromatosis.

The high signal intensity of neurofibromas on T2-weighted pulse sequences is indistinguishable from the appearance of many schwannomas (see Case 919). Central zones of low signal intensity within an otherwise "bright" tumor on T2-weighted scans is a characteristic feature seen in plexiform neurofibromas.

DIFFERENTIAL DIAGNOSIS:
MASS WITHIN AN INTERVERTEBRAL FORAMEN

Case 926

42-year-old man presenting with hearing loss
and right leg pain.
(axial, postcontrast scan; SE 900/12; L2-3 level)

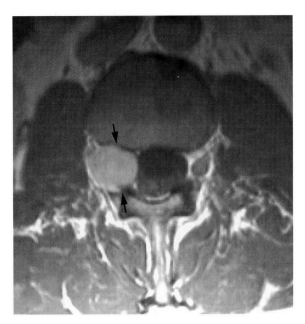

Schwannoma
(in type 2 neurofibromatosis)

Case 927

69-year-old woman presenting with left leg pain.
(axial, postcontrast scan; SE 800/17; L3 level)

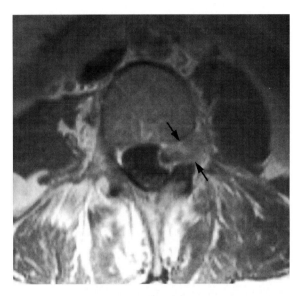

Herniated Disc

Masses within the intervertebral foramen may be neoplastic or discogenic in origin. The most common benign tumor in this location is a schwannoma, as in Case 926.

The majority of spinal schwannomas are solitary lesions. Multiple intradural and extradural schwannomas occur in patients with type 2 neurofibromatosis. Sagittal scans in Case 926 demonstrated several intensely enhancing masses within the thecal sac, resembling Cases 909 and 910.

Schwannomas often have CT attenuation values and MR intensity values resembling an enlarged root sleeve on noncontrast scans. Associated expansion of the intervertebral foramen *(arrows)* is a clue to the long-standing presence of a benign mass. Contrast enhancement confirms the solid nature of the lesion; uniform enhancement as in Case 926 is characteristic of a small and medium-sized schwannomas.

Foraminal disc herniations may resemble schwannomas on both CT and MR studies. Occasional herniated discs are accompanied by erosive changes or remodelling of adjacent bone mimicking a nerve root tumor. MR scans with contrast enhancement will usually distinguish between these entities, demonstrating peripheral enhancement at the margins of disc fragments (see Cases 819 and 840B) and more solid enhancement within neoplasms.

The enhancement pattern in Case 927 is a mixture of a peripheral component medially and a more solid and amorphous component laterally. As discussed in Chapter 14, central enhancement within disc herniations increases with time. On delayed scans, disc fragments may simulate enhancing tumors.

Lymphoma and epidural metastasis should also be included in the differential diagnosis of a foraminal mass. These pathologies are suggested when poorly defined tissue fills an intervertebral foramen without adjacent bone remodelling. Paraspinal "small blue cell" tumors and neuroblastoma can involve one or more intervertebral foramina in children (see Cases 900 and 900-2).

Finally, occasional vascular lesions can fill and expand an intervertebral foramen. Epidural cavernous angiomas may extend through a nerve root canal. A spinal dural arteriovenous fistula with predominant epidural rather than intradural drainage (see Cases 1035-1037) may also present in this manner.

DIFFERENTIAL DIAGNOSIS:
EXTRADURAL THICKENING OF A SPINAL NERVE

Case 928

40-year-old woman presenting with right leg pain.
(coronal, noncontrast scan; SE 800/22)

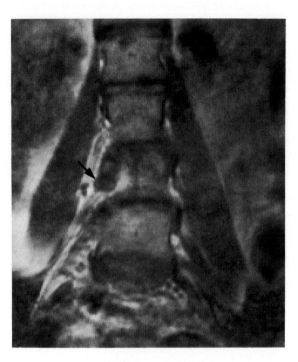

Schwannoma

Case 929

76-year-old woman presenting with severe
left neck and arm pain.
(axial, noncontrast scan; SE 1000/17)

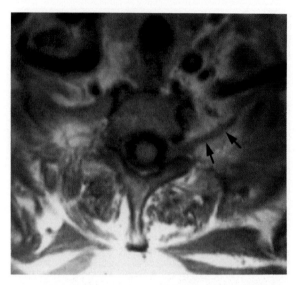

Perineural Metastatic Carcinoma of the Breast

Benign and malignant neoplasms may involve spinal nerves within or distal to the intervertebral foramen.

In Case 928, a small schwannoma is demonstrated along the course of the right L3 nerve as it passes beneath the ipsilateral pedicle to exit from the intervertebral foramen (*arrow;* compare to the normal left side). Coronal MR scans are often useful for assessing lesions involving an exiting lumbar nerve. Coronal views image a longer segment of the nerve than is visible on axial or sagittal sections, while clearly localizing pathology with respect to the overlying pedicle.

The pattern of soft tissue thickening along the left C8 nerve root in Case 929 is more linear. Paraspinal fat defines the nerve as abnormally broad and mildly irregular over a distance of several centimeters *(arrows).* This appearance is compatible with perineural spread of metastatic disease, which was established at autopsy in this patient with known carcinoma of the breast. Neuritis due to radiation therapy is usually in the clinical differential diagnosis of such cases but rarely causes impressive abnormality on MR scans. Similarly, idiopathic brachial plexitis (Parsonage Turner syndrome) usually does not result in appreciable thickening of neural structures.

Case 930

36-year-old woman presenting with left leg pain.
(coronal, postcontrast scan; SE 600/15)

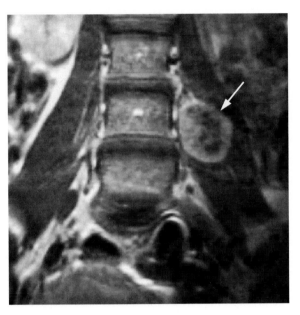

Schwannoma

Case 931

32-year-old woman presenting with sacral pain.
(axial, postcontrast scan; SE 600/15; S3 level)

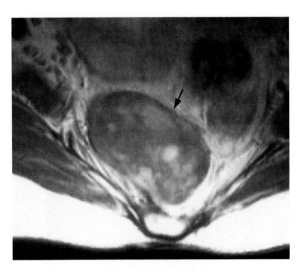

Ganglioneuroma

Schwannomas and neurofibromas are the most common primary tumors of spinal nerves and may occur at any level. As illustrated previously, many nerve root tumors have intradural and epidural components. Other schwannomas and neurofibromas are completely extraspinal, as in Case 930.

The schwannoma in this case is centered along the axis of a single root. Peripheral enhancement surrounds a nonenhancing center, which may reflect cystic or necrotic components of the tumor (compare to Case 923).

Neurofibromas also occur in the paraspinal region. When large, these tumors may present a characteristic appearance on noncontrast T2-weighted scans with a low intensity core surrounded by a perimeter of long T2 values. The central region of low intensity and little enhancement in such cases has been correlated pathologically with dense fibrous tissue.

Lateral meningoceles are an additional potential cause of a paraspinal mass in patients with neurofibromatosis type 1 (particularly in the thoracic region). These fluid-containing sacs may mimic solid paraspinal tumors on radiographic studies. MR scans can establish the diagnosis in such cases by demonstrating CSF-like signal intensity (and lack of contrast enhancement) within the lesions.

Ganglioneuromas are slowly growing tumors, containing neurons within a connective tissue matrix. Paraspinal ganglioneuromas most commonly arise from the sympathetic chain. Such tumors are often discovered incidentally. In other cases, ganglioneuromas result from maturation of neuroblastomas (see discussion of Case 900-1).

The large presacral mass in Case 931 has a somewhat whorled tissue pattern that is common within ganglioneuromas. This architecture may be apparent on precontrast or postcontrast scans.

Case 931 demonstrates that tumors of neural origin should be included in the differential diagnosis of presacral masses (along with teratomas, chordomas, and osseous lesions).

Case 932

4-year-old girl presenting with constipation.
(sagittal, noncontrast scan; SE 1000/16)

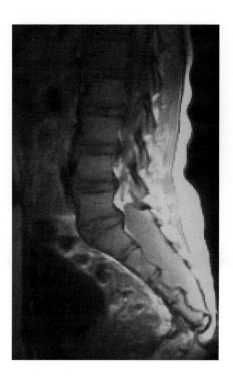

Case 933

9-year-old boy presenting with clumsiness
of the left leg.
(coronal, postcontrast scan; SE 500/15)

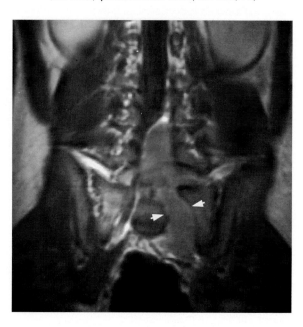

Neuroblastoma commonly involves the spinal canal in the thoracolumbar region, either as a primary epidural process or by extension from a paraspinal origin (see Cases 899 and 900).

Cases 932 and 933 illustrate a somewhat different presentation of spinal neuroblastoma within the lumbosacral region. The long-standing, slowly growing intraspinal masses in these patients have caused expansion of the spinal canal and contiguous intervertebral foramina. In Case 932, posterior scalloping of sacral vertebral bodies is apparent. In Case 933, tongues of tumor flow through widened lumbar and sacral foramina on the left side *(arrows)*. The adjacent left sacral ala is sclerotic and probably permeated by neoplasm.

Pathological examination of tumor tissue in the above cases demonstrated "mature" neuroblastoma, containing ar-

eas better classified as "ganglioneuroma." Neuroblastomas characteristically stabilize or involute after infancy, so that older children may present with low grade, long-standing versions of this tumor.

The appearance of a lobulated intraspinal mass causing scalloped bone erosion and foraminal widening may suggest the diagnosis of neurofibroma, schwannoma, or ependymoma. Neuroblastoma/ganglioneuroma should be considered among diagnostic possibilities in such cases.

Other long-standing, low grade masses (e.g., epidermoid cysts) may cause expansion of the sacral canal comparable to the scalloping in Case 932. A similar morphology may also be associated with dural ectasia (as in neurofibromatosis or Marfan's syndrome) or cysts of the sacral canal (see Cases 1030 and 1031).

SACRAL CHORDOMAS

Case 934

72-year-old man presenting with sacral pain
and difficulty with bowel movements.
(sagittal, noncontrast scan; SE 650/12)

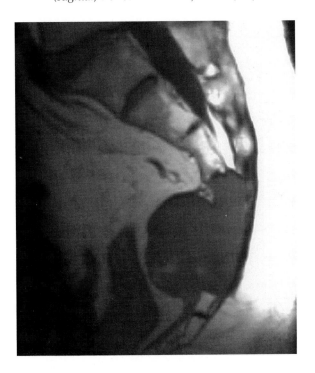

Case 935

68-year-old woman with a history of prior
sacral surgery.
(axial, noncontrast scan; SE 1500/70)

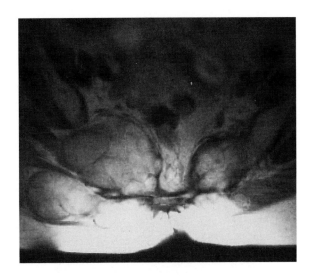

About 50% of chordomas arise from the sacrum, most commonly presenting in adults over age 60. These lobulated masses are typically expansile and should be included in the differential diagnosis of "bubbly" sacral lesions (see discussion of Case 900-4). Although sacral chordomas are slowly growing tumors, they recur and progress if incompletely resected.

The mass in Case 934 has destroyed the S4 and S5 segments, expanding ventrally into the presacral space. A thin layer of tumor extends caudally along the anterior surface of the coccyx. Many chordomas demonstrate greater heterogeneity than this lesion, including cysts and areas of hemorrhage.

The recurrent bilateral sacral tumor in Case 935 has typically long T2 values and a lobulated morphology, expanding the involved bone. This appearance correlates with the

histopathologic presence of large, vacuolated "physaliferous" cells.

Myxopapillary ependymomas (see Cases 945 and 952) occasionally arise within the sacrum or immediately dorsal to it in a "subcutaneous" location. Such tumors could cause sacral erosion resembling a chordoma.

The sacrum is intact in most cases of sacrococcygeal teratoma. These tumors usually originate near the coccyx and demonstrate more heterogeneity than chordomas on MR studies. Most sacrococcygeal teratomas occur in young children, but sporadic cases are reported in adults.

Compare the characteristics of the above masses to the clival chordoma in Case 194. Also contrast the expansion of the sacrum itself in these cases to enlargement of the sacral canal on the previous page.

Case 936

3-year-old boy with neurofibromatosis type 1.
(coronal, noncontrast scan; SE 1000/22)

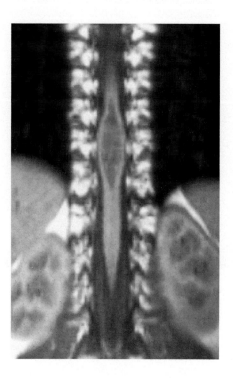

Case 937

11-year-old boy presenting with back pain,
leg weakness, and mild scoliosis.
(sagittal, noncontrast scan; SE 500/17)

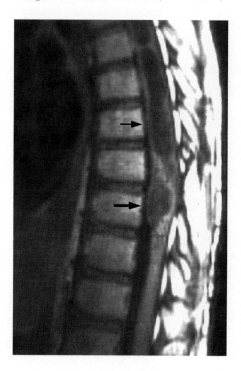

Magnetic resonance imaging far exceeds the capability of CT scanning to demonstrate intramedullary pathology. Contour abnormalities of the spinal cord are apparent on MR studies without intrathecal injection of contrast material. More importantly, MR can detect intramedullary lesions that are unaccompanied by cord expansion.

The differential diagnosis of intramedullary masses includes tumors, cysts, inflammatory processes, and vascular lesions. Within the tumor category, astrocytomas and ependymomas are the most common lesions. Of these two pathologies, astrocytomas are more frequently seen in children and in the thoracic region, as illustrated above.

On T1-weighted scans, intramedullary astrocytomas may be defined by abnormal signal intensity and/or cord expansion. The low intensity values of the tumor in Case 936 provide better than average demarcation from surrounding parenchyma. Many spinal astrocytomas are relatively isointense.

Intramedullary astrocytomas vary considerably in texture and architecture. Some tumors are homogeneously solid lesions like Case 936. Other cases demonstrate heterogenous signal intensity and/or a mixed solid/cystic morphology, as in Case 937.

The complex mass in Case 937 is located at the caudal end of a large intramedullary cyst. Contrast enhancement and surgery demonstrated an astrocytoma limited to the area of solid tissue *(large arrow)*. The extensive rostral cyst *(small arrow)* proved to represent benign syringomyelia.

Syringomyelia frequently develops secondarily when mass lesions obstruct the spinal canal, altering normal hydrodynamics. An intramedullary cyst similar to Case 937 could be observed in association with a spinal meningioma or schwannoma. (See Cases 865 and 1092 for other examples of syringomyelia secondary to spinal canal masses.)

Case 938

55-year-old man presenting with bilateral
arm numbness.
(sagittal, noncontrast scan; RSE 5000/100)

Case 939

10-year-old boy presenting with back pain.
(sagittal, noncontrast scan; SE 2500/90)

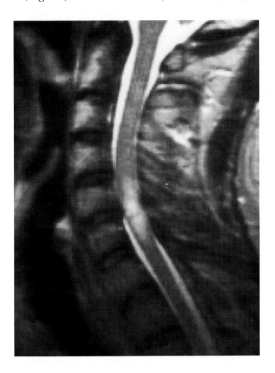

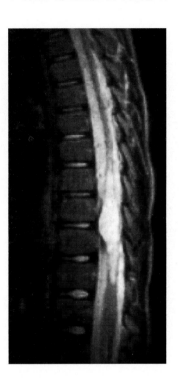

Astrocytomas usually demonstrate high signal intensity on T2-weighted scans. The region of abnormality may include components of neoplasm, adjacent gliosis, and reactive edema.

Small tumors may be limited to one or two vertebral levels, with minimal mass effect. Case 938 illustrates a very focal astrocytoma. The appearance of this lesion is nonspecific, and differential diagnosis would include myelitis (see Cases 984 and 985).

The astrocytoma in Case 939 is larger in longitudinal extent and has caused definite cord expansion. Intramedullary cysts commonly accompany spinal cord tumors (see Cases 937, 940-943, and 947) and may contribute to both mass effect and T2-prolongation. Contrast-enhanced scans help to distinguish between solid and cystic components of the tumor when an appearance like Case 939 is encountered.

Zones of T2-shortening reflecting the presence of blood products are less common within or adjacent to astrocytomas than is the case with ependymomas (see Case 946).

Back pain (especially nocturnal) is a frequent presenting complaint of children with intramedullary neoplasms. Progressive scoliosis (with or without pain) is another manifestation of intraspinal tumors in the pediatric age group.

Case 940

4-year-old boy presenting with abnormal gait.
(sagittal, noncontrast scan; SE 550/17)

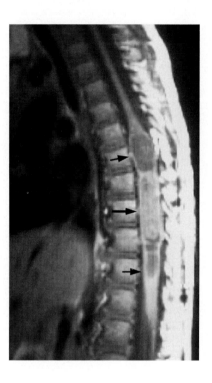

Case 941

16-year-old boy presenting with neck pain.
(sagittal, noncontrast scan; SE 2800/90)

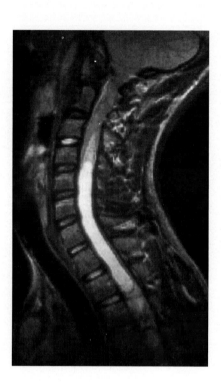

Cysts are commonly found within or adjacent to intramedullary tumors. Both astrocytomas and ependymomas (see Case 947) may contain cystic cavities lined by tumor cells and/or be bordered by benign, reactive intramedullary cysts. The distinction between primary tumor cysts and secondary syrinxes is usually best made on postcontrast scans (see Cases 942 and 948).

In Case 940, a central mass of isointense tumor tissue *(thick arrow)* is located between rostral and caudal cysts *(thin arrows)*. The solid mass enhanced uniformly, while the cyst margins did not. At surgery, neoplastic tissue was limited to the solid nodule, and the polar cysts were found to be reactive.

The majority of the intramedullary expansion in Case 941 is due to a long cyst containing uniformly high signal intensity on this T2-weighted scan. Surgery demonstrated a low grade astrocytoma at the T3 to T5 level. The cervical cyst contained simple fluid and was not lined by tumor.

Cases 942 and 943 present additional examples of spinal astrocytomas with adjacent cysts.

Case 942

13-year-old boy presenting with back pain
and scoliosis.
(coronal, postcontrast scan; SE 600/15)

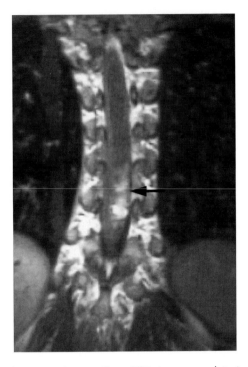

(same patient as Case 937, two years later)

Case 943

9-year-old girl presenting with a several year history
of itching on the dorsum of the feet, corroborated
by excoriation of the skin and worn shoe surfaces.
(coronal, postcontrast scan; SE 600/15)

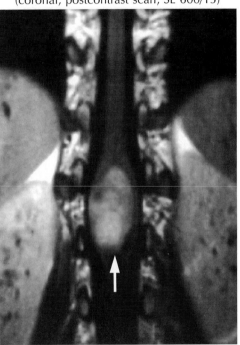

Although the majority of spinal astrocytomas are low grade lesions, these tumors characteristically enhance with contrast material. The absence of enhancement argues against neoplasm as the etiology of an intramedullary mass.

The pattern of contrast enhancement within spinal astrocytomas is highly variable. Many cases demonstrate shaggy or patchy enhancement mixed with nonenhancing portions of the tumor. Case 942 illustrates multinodular enhancement within the mass presented in Case 937. Note that there is no enhancement along the margins of the large intramedullary cyst superior to the tumor (compare to Case 948).

In Case 943, predominantly uniform enhancement is present throughout an astrocytoma within the conus medullaris. Small cysts are seen at the caudal pole of the tumor. Although the interface between the enhancing mass and adjacent parenchyma appears well-defined, astrocyto-

mas are usually poorly encapsulated. In other cases this lack of pathological demarcation is reflected by hazy or indistinct margins of contrast enhancement.

Ependymomas commonly involve the conus medullaris and cauda equina (see Cases 945, 949, and 952) and would be included in the differential diagnosis of Case 943. Occasional primitive neuroectodermal tumors and paragangliomas of the conus medullaris can present a similar appearance (see Case 960). Hemangioblastomas are rarely found in this location.

The intensely enhancing astrocytoma in Case 943 proved to be a low grade lesion. The presence and degree of contrast enhancement within spinal gliomas do not correlate with the grade of malignancy as closely as in intracranial tumors.

Case 944

21-year-old man presenting with progressive
cervical myelopathy.
(sagittal, noncontrast scan; SE 600/15)

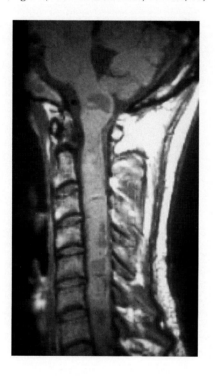

Case 945

9-year-old boy presenting with low back pain.
(sagittal, noncontrast scan; SE 600/15)

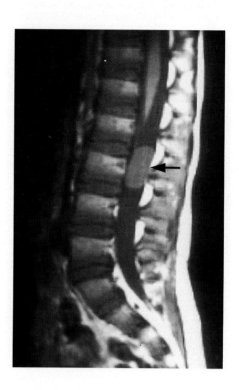

Cases 944 and 945 illustrate the variable size, complexity, and location of spinal ependymomas. The heterogeneous tumor in Case 944 expands the entire cervical spinal cord and extends into the medulla. Scattered areas of high and low signal intensity within the mass probably reflect components of hemorrhage, cystic change, and calcification. (Correlate with the T2-weighted scan of this patient in Case 946, and compare to Case 957.)

By contrast, the lumbar mass in Case 945 is homogeneous. The signal intensity and morphology of this intradural lesion suggest a meningioma, but meningiomas are rarely encountered in the lumbar region. A schwannoma would be another diagnostic possibility, although schwannomas this large are often cystic or hemorrhagic (see Cases 919 and 923). Surgery in Case 945 demonstrated a myxopapillary ependymoma arising from the filum terminale.

Ependymomas are the most common primary neoplasms of the conus medullaris and cauda equina. Myxopapillary ependymomas involving the lumbar canal are often more homogeneous than ependymomas within the cervical or thoracic region. When such tumors occur at the level of the conus medullaris, they may closely resemble a meningioma (compare Case 945 to Case 913).

The average age of patients with spinal ependymomas is about ten years older than the population presenting with astrocytomas of the cord (early forties versus early thirties). Nevertheless, the above cases indicate that young patients may develop tumors of ependymal histology. In particular, myxopapillary ependymomas of the lumbar canal *typically* occur in children and young adults, with a strong male predominance and with usually a good prognosis.

Case 946

21-year-old man presenting with cervical
myelopathy.
(sagittal, noncontrast scan; SE 2800/90)

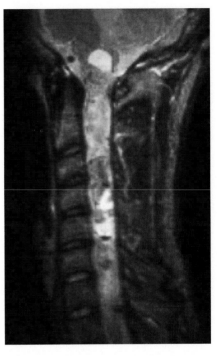

(same patient as Case 944)

Case 947

47-year-old woman presenting with neck
and back pain.
(sagittal, noncontrast scan; SE 2600/80)

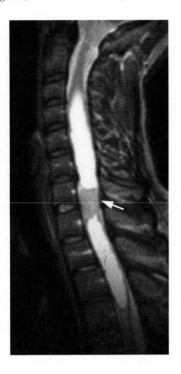

Spinal ependymomas are often strikingly complex on T2-weighted scans. Cyst formation commonly causes small or large areas of high signal intensity on long TR images, seen in Cases 946 and 947 respectively.

In addition, blood products are frequently present within or adjacent to spinal ependymomas, contributing zones of low signal intensity to their heterogeneous appearance. In Case 946, areas of T2-shortening are interspersed throughout the tumor. In other cases, caps of low signal intensity reflecting old blood products are seen at the rostral and/or caudal margins of an intramedullary ependymoma.

Case 947 presents a simpler appearance. At surgery, tumor was limited to the homogeneous solid tissue in the middle of the lesion (*arrow*). Benign rostral and caudal cysts were drained and have not recurred on follow-up studies.

Unlike astrocytomas, ependymomas are usually well encapsulated with good demarcation from surrounding parenchyma. As a result, even extensive tumors can often be completely removed with good preservation of function and excellent prognosis.

Case 948

47-year-old woman presenting with neck pain.
(sagittal, postcontrast scan; SE 500/15)

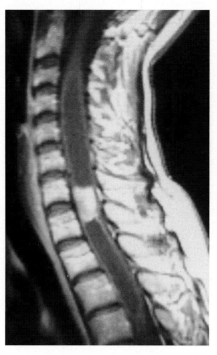

(same patient as Case 947)

Case 949

9-year-old boy presenting with low back pain.
(sagittal, postcontrast scan; SE 600/15)

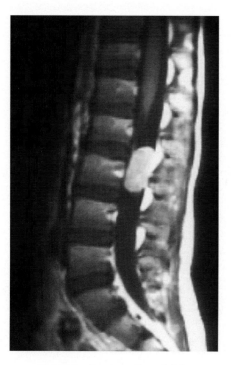

(same patient as Case 945)

Intense, homogeneous contrast enhancement is usually present within solid components of spinal ependymomas. Uniform enhancement can also be seen within astrocytomas (see Case 943), but poorly enhancing tumors are more likely to be of astrocytic origin.

The above examples provide postcontrast images for correlation with the noncontrast scans on the preceding pages. Case 948 demonstrates enhancement throughout the central mass of Case 947. No enhancement is present along the margin of the adjacent cysts, suggesting their benign nature.

Case 949 is a postcontrast view of the myxopapillary tumor in Case 945. As discussed earlier, the morphology, homogeneity, and enhancement of this lesion resemble a spinal meningioma. However, a meningioma would be extremely rare in the lumbar region of a nine-year-old boy.

Case 950

41-year-old woman with increasing
difficulty walking.
(sagittal, postcontrast scan; SE 700/20)

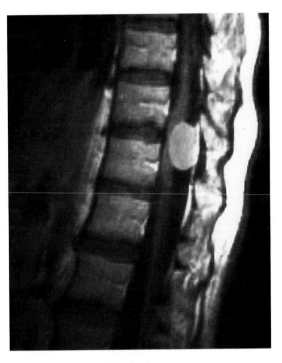

Meningioma

Case 951

38-year-old man presenting with bilateral
leg cramps and toe numbness.
(sagittal, postcontrast scan; SE 600/15)

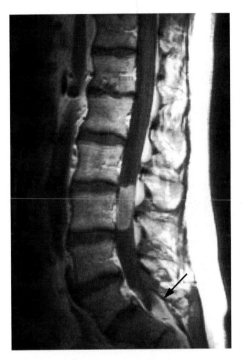

"Drop" Metastasis from a Pineal Germinoma
(treated 18 months earlier)

Myxopapillary ependymomas such as Case 949 are one of several tumors that can present as uniformly enhancing masses within the thoracolumbar canal.

Meningiomas typically demonstrate homogeneous and intense enhancement, as in Case 950. Dorsolateral location in the thoracic region of a 40- to 70-year-old woman is a characteristic setting for these lesions (see Cases 913 and 914).

Case 951 serves as a reminder that intradural metastases should be considered in the differential diagnosis of pri-mary glial or meningeal tumors within the spinal canal. A clue to the diagnosis in Case 951 is the layer of enhancing neoplasm at the caudal end of the thecal sac *(arrow)*. This gravitationally dependent cul-de-sac is commonly involved by "drop" metastases. Subtle amputation of the sac by accumulation of soft tissue may help to characterize masses at higher levels.

As discussed previously in this chapter, schwannomas as large as the above lesions usually demonstrate more heterogeneous contrast enhancement (see Case 923).

Case 952A

7-year-old girl presenting with back pain,
leg stiffness, and urinary urgency.
(sagittal, noncontrast scan; SE 2800/90)

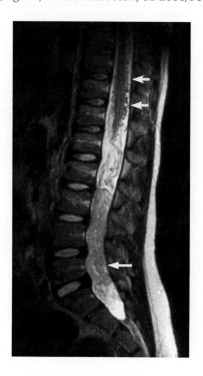

Case 952B

Same patient.
(sagittal, postcontrast scan; SE 600/15)

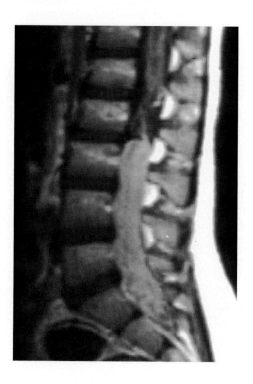

Low grade myxopapillary ependymomas of the filum terminale may enlarge to fill and expand the lumbar spinal canal. Further growth may extend through intervertebral foramina into the paraspinal region. Such bulky tumors may resemble a lobulated schwannoma or neurofibroma (or the occasional intraspinal neuroblastoma, as in Cases 932 and 933).

The signal intensity of the large intradural mass in Case 952A (*long arrow*) is intermediate and homogeneous, comparable to the intramedullary ependymoma in Case 947. The long-standing mass has caused mild scalloping of the posterior margin of the L4 and L5 vertebral bodies (compare to Case 932). Tortuous, tangled intrathecal nerve roots are seen above the tumor, reflecting a long history of traction and displacement.

Prominent vessels are present on the surface of the conus medullaris in Case 952A (*short arrows*). Distention of intrathecal veins near an ependymoma has been well-recognized myelographically and should be considered in the differential diagnosis of spinal vascular malformations. The finding may reflect congestion due to the obstructing mass effect of the tumor and/or hypervascularity of the mass itself. Spinal ependymomas are among the potential causes of intracranial superficial siderosis (see Case 591) due to recurrent small subarachnoid hemorrhages.

The postcontrast scan in Case 952B is blurred by patient motion. However, uniform enhancement throughout the tumor is apparent. Enhancement along the surface of the conus medullaris may represent the prominent vessels noted on the noncontrast scan or pial extension of tumor (compare to Case 960).

Because of their potential variation in size and morphology, ependymomas should be considered in the differential diagnosis of most masses within the lumbar canal.

Case 953

17-year-old girl presenting with cranial
nerve deficits.
(coronal, postcontrast scan; SE 550/15)

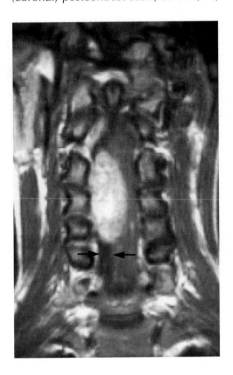

Case 954

19-year-old man presenting with back pain
after a volleyball game.
(coronal, postcontrast scan; SE 600/20)

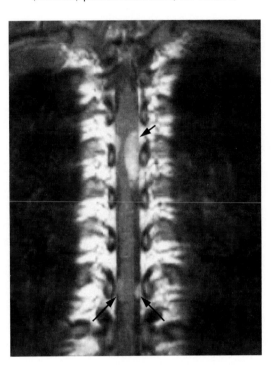

Astrocytomas and ependymomas of the spinal canal are occasionally eccentric masses. Ependymomas are particularly prone to exophytic growth, which can be associated with CSF seeding.

The patient in Case 953 was referred for a cerebral MR scan because of several cranial neuropathies. The study demonstrated leptomeningeal tumors within the posterior fossa (see Case 183), with no apparent intracranial source. The possibility of a disseminating spinal neoplasm was considered, and the cervical tumor was discovered.

Note that the exophytic ependymoma in Case 953 has displaced the spinal cord in a manner resembling an intradural, extramedullary mass (*small arrows*; compare to

Cases 915 and 950). Together with uniform contrast enhancement, this morphology mimics a meningioma or schwannoma. The rare possibility of an exophytic ependymoma should be included in the differential diagnosis of intradural, extramedullary neoplasms.

Case 954 illustrates a similar lesion. The primary ependymoma exophytically encircles the spinal cord in the superior thoracic region (*short arrow*). (Compare to the tendency of fourth ventricular ependymomas to surround the brainstem, as in Case 156.) CSF spread of the tumor has occurred, with several distant nodules enhancing along the surface of the thoracic cord more inferiorly *(long arrows)*.

Case 955

17-year-old girl.
(axial, postcontrast scan; SE 600/15; C4-5 level)

Case 956

54-year-old woman presenting with leg weakness.
(axial, postcontrast scan; SE 550/15; T10-11 level)

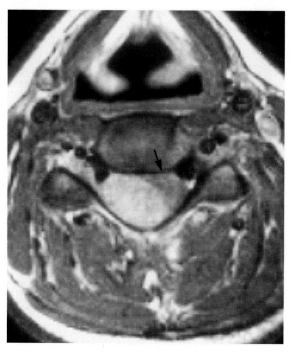

Exophytic Ependymoma
(same patient as Case 953)

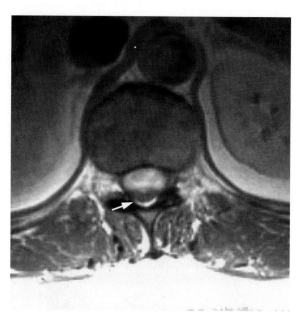

Schwannoma
(same patient as Case 922)

As discussed on the preceding page, spinal ependymomas may arise eccentrically and enlarge exophytically. The typically uniform and intense contrast enhancement within such tumors may then mimic a benign intradural, extramedullary mass.

Case 955 is an axial scan through the lesion in Case 953. The tumor is homogeneous and well demarcated from the adjacent spinal cord (*arrow*), resembling a meningioma or schwannoma.

The ventral schwannoma in Case 956 occupies most of the dural sac. The spinal cord is severely displaced and compressed dorsally (*arrow*). Uniform contrast enhancement within the lesion is typical but nonspecific. A meningioma or an intradural metastasis (of systemic or CNS origin) would be included in the differential diagnosis.

Ventral location (as in Case 956) is relatively uncommon for meningiomas below the foramen magnum. These tumors more typically arise dorsally or laterally (see Cases 914, 915, and 950).

DIFFERENTIAL DIAGNOSIS:
HETEROGENEOUS INTRAMEDULLARY MASS WITH PARTIAL ENHANCEMENT

Case 957

37-year-old man presenting with progressive
spastic quadriparesis.
(sagittal, postcontrast scan; SE 600/15)

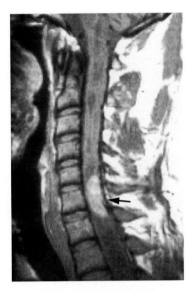

Hemangioblastoma
(surrounded by edema)

Case 958

34-year-old man presenting with neck pain
and arm weakness.
(sagittal, postcontrast scan; SE 600/15)

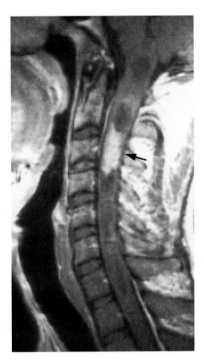

Astrocytoma

Hemangioblastomas are the third most common primary tumor of the spinal cord. They are usually small lesions, ranging in diameter from a few millimeters to a few centimeters. However, spinal hemangioblastomas often incite extensive edema and/or cyst formation within adjacent parenchyma.

Case 957 illustrates this occurrence. Noncontrast scans demonstrated mottled signal intensity throughout the cervical cord. A focal tumor mass was not defined. Intense contrast enhancement of the tumor nodule (*arrow*) in Case 957 established the appropriate site for biopsy.

At surgery, a hemangioblastoma was found to precisely conform to the margins of enhancement. The more rostral and caudal expansion of the cord was due to swampy edema, with a chain of small cysts that drained clear fluid when the tumor was removed.

Case 957 emphasizes several points regarding reactive changes within the spinal cord adjacent to an intramedullary mass: (1) parenchymal reaction may present as boggy edema or as a simple cyst (compare Case 957 to Case 948); (2) reactive cord changes may obscure the inciting tumor on noncontrast scans; and (3) contrast enhancement should guide biopsy and/or resection of intramedullary pathology.

The astrocytoma in Case 958 resembles the hemangioblastoma in Case 957: a limited area of confluent contrast enhancement is seen within the larger lesion (*arrow*). However, additional subtle areas of enhancement are present both rostral and caudal to the main nodule. These more infiltrating components of enhancement are typical of astrocytomas and are distinct from the usual solitary enhancing focus of a hemangioblastoma.

Large vascular channels may be present within or adjacent to spinal hemangioblastomas, as in the intracranial compartment (see Cases 136 to 140). A concentration of such prominent "flow voids" supports the diagnosis, although prominent superficial vessels may be associated with other intramedullary tumors (see Case 952).

Case 959

28-year-old man with AIDS.
(sagittal, postcontrast scan; SE 1000/26)

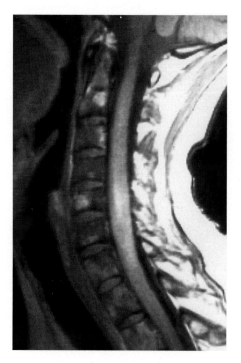

Primary CNS Lymphoma

Case 960

29-year-old woman presenting with acute
bladder dysfunction.
(sagittal, postcontrast scan; SE 550/20)

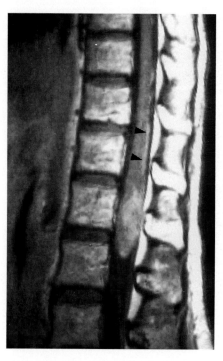

Primitive Neuroectodermal Tumor

A number of rare primary tumors may involve the spinal cord and conus medullaris. Oligodendrogliomas occasionally arise within the spinal cord, as do gangliogliomas. Primary CNS lymphoma and primitive neuroectodermal tumors may also present as intramedullary masses, as seen above.

The mildly enhancing expansion of the cervical spinal cord in Case 959 is nonspecific. (Compare to the appearance of cervical myelitis in Case 990.) The patient had a known intracerebral lymphoma. Spinal cord involvement in such cases may include CSF seeding of the central canal, which is occasionally also seen in patients with medulloblastoma.

Abnormally low signal intensity within the marrow of cervical vertebrae provides a diagnostic clue in Case 959. This finding is frequent in AIDS patients, reflecting increased iron stores due to "anemia of chronic disease."

The precontrast scan in Case 960 outlined a homogeneous, low intensity lesion within the conus medullaris, compatible with a low grade glioma. The irregular, poorly marginated contrast enhancement with subpial extension *(arrowheads)* suggests a more aggressive neoplasm. At surgery, an intramedullary primitive neuroectodermal tumor was found, with a layer of dorsal subpial extension rostral to the mass.

Case 961A

52-year-old woman presenting with cervical
myelopathy and pulmonary nodules.
(sagittal, noncontrast scan; low flip angle
GRE sequence)

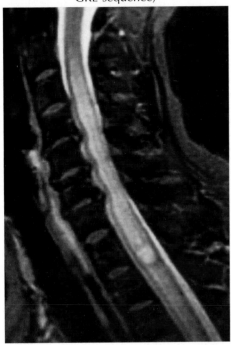

Case 961B

Same patient.
(sagittal, postcontrast scan; SE 516/19)

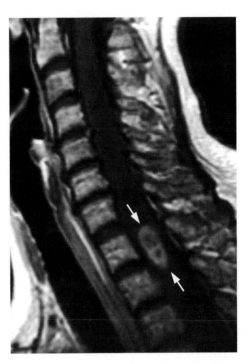

Metastatic Adenocarcinoma
(unknown primary)

Metastases to the spinal cord from systemic carcinomas are much less common than the vertebral and epidural lesions discussed at the beginning of this chapter. However, metastatic disease should be included in the differential diagnosis of myelopathy, particularly if the clinical course is rapidly progressive.

Intramedullary metastases often incite edema extending several segments beyond the tumor. Prolongation of T1 and T2 values and cord expansion are seen from C2 to T2 in the above scans. Focal contrast enhancement outlines the metastatic nodule at T1-T2 in Case 961B *(arrows)*.

Note that intramedullary edema due to inflammatory or neoplastic lesions may resemble the appearance of syringomyelia on T2-weighted scans. T1-weighted images are usually more helpful in distinguishing true intramedullary cysts from edematous parenchyma.

Carcinoma of the lung is the most common source of intramedullary metastases, and the thoracic spinal cord is the most frequent site of metastatic disease. Involvement of the conus medullaris is common (see Case 901) and warrants attention to this region on all spine scans of patients with systemic tumors.

REFERENCES

Aggarwal S, Deck JHN, Kucharczyk W: Neuroendocrine tumor (paraganglioma) of the cauda equina: MR and pathologic findings. *AJNR* 14:1003-1007, 1993.

Algra PR, Bloem JL, Tissing H, et al: Detection of vertebral metastases: comparison between MR imaging and bone scintigraphy. *Radiographics* 11:219-232, 1991.

Araki Y, Ishida T, Ootani M, et al: MRI of paraganglioma of the cauda equina. *Neuroradiology* 35:232-233, 1993.

Avrahami E, Tadmor R, Dally O, Hadar H: Earl MR demonstration of spinal metastases in patients with normal radiographs and CT and radionuclide bone scans. *J Comput Assist Tomogr* 13:598-602, 1989.

Baker LL, Goodman SB, Perkash I, et al: Benign versus pathological compression fractures of vertebral bodies: assessment with conventional spin echo, chemical-shift, and STIR MR imaging. *Radiology* 174:495-502, 1990.

Barloon TJ, Yuh WTC, Yang CJC, Schultz DH: Spinal subarachnoid tumor seeding from intracranial metastases: MR findings. *J Comput Assist Tomogr* 11:242-244, 1987.

Bazan C III: Imaging of lumbosacral spine neoplasms. *Neuroimaging Clin N Amer* 3:591-608, 1993.

Beltram J, Noto AM, Chakeres DW, Christoforidis AJ: Tumors of the osseous spine: staging with MR imaging versus CT. *Radiology* 162:565-569, 1987.

Beltram J, Simon DC, Levy M, et al: Aneurysmal bone cysts: MR imaging at 1.5 T. *Radiology* 158:689-690, 1986.

Berns DH, Blaser S, Ross JS, et al: MR imaging with Gd-DTPA in leptomeningeal spread of lymphoma. *J Comput Assist Tomogr* 12:499-500, 1988.

Brunberg JA, DiPietro MA, Venes JL, et al: Intramedullary lesions of the pediatric spinal cord: correlation of findings from MR imaging, intraoperative sonography, surgery, and histologic study. *Radiology* 181:573-579, 1991.

Burk D, Brunberg J, Kanal E, et al: Spinal and paraspinal neurofibromatosis: MR imaging. *Radiology* 162:797, 1987.

Bydder GM, Brown J, Niendorf HP, et al: Enhancement of cervical intraspinal tumors in MR imaging with intravenous gadolinium DTPA. *J Comput Assist Tomogr* 9:847-851, 1985.

Carmody RF, Yang PJ, Seeley GM, et al: Spinal cord compression due to metastatic disease: diagnosis with MR imaging versus myelography. *Radiology* 173:225-229, 1989.

Chamberlain MC, Sandy AD, Press GA: Spinal tumors: gadolinium-DTPA-enhanced MR imaging. *Neuroradiology* 33:469-474, 1991.

Cory DA, Fritsch SA, Cohen MD, et al: Aneurysmal bone cysts: imaging findings and embolotherapy. *AJR* 153:369-373, 1989.

Costigan DA, Winkelman MD: Intramedullary spinal cord metastasis. A clinicopathological study of 13 cases. *J Neurosurg* 62:227-233, 1985.

Daffner RH, Lupetin AR, Dash N, et al: MRI in the detection of malignant infiltration of bone marrow. *AJR* 146:353-358, 1986.

Davis PC, Friedman NC, Fry SM, et al: Leptomeningeal metastasis: MR imaging. *Radiology* 163:449-454, 1987.

Demachi H, Takashima T, Kadoya M, et al: MR imaging of spinal neurinomas with pathological correlation. *J Comput Assist Tomogr* 14:250-254, 1992.

De Schepper AMA, Ramon F, Van Marck E: MR imaging of eosinophilic granuloma: report of 11 cases. *Skeletal Radiol* 22:163-166, 1993.

Di Chiro G, Doppman JL, Dwyer AJ, et al: Tumors and arteriovenous malformations of the spinal cord: assessment using MR. *Radiology* 156:689-697, 1985.

Dietrich RB, Kangarloo H, Lenarsky C, Feig SA: Neuroblastoma: the role of MR imaging. *AJR* 148:937-942, 1987.

Dillon WP, Norman D, Newton TH, et al: Intradural spinal cord lesions: Gd-DTPA-enhanced MR imaging. *Radiology* 170:229-237, 1989.

Domingues RC, Mikulis D, Swearingen B, et al: Subcutaneous sacrococcygeal myxopapillary ependymoma: CT and MR findings. *AJNR* 12:171-172, 1991.

Egelhoff JC, Bates DJ, Ross JS, et al: Spinal MR findings in neurofibromatosis types 1 and 2. *AJNR* 13:1071-1077, 1990.

Epstein FJ, Farmer J-P, Freed D: Adult intramedullary astrocytomas of the spinal cord. *J Neurosurg* 77:355-359, 1992.

Fox MW, Onofrio BM: The natural history of management of symptomatic and asymptomatic vertebral hemangiomas. *J Neurosurg* 78:36-45, 1993.

Friedman DP, Flanders AE, Tartaglino LM: Vascular neoplasms and malformations, ischemia, and hemorrhage affecting the spinal cord: MR imaging findings. *AJR* 162:685-692, 1994.

Friedman DP, Tartaglino LM, Flanders AE: Intradural schwannomas of the spine: MR findings with emphasis on contrast-enhancement characteristics. *AJR* 158:1347-1350, 1992.

Ginsberg LE, Williams DW, Stanton C: Intrasacral myxopapillary ependymoma. *Neuroradiology* 36:56-58, 1994.

Godersky JC, Smoker WRK, Knutzon R: Use of magnetic resonance imaging in the evaluation of metastatic spine disease. *Neurosurg* 21:676-680, 1987.

Goy AMC, Pinto RS, Raghavendra BN, et al: Intramedullary spinal-cord tumors: MR imaging with emphasis on associated cysts. *Radiology* 161:381-386, 1986.

Hajek PC, Baker LL, Goobar JE, et al: Focal fat deposition in axial bone marrow: MR characteristics. *Radiology* 162:245, 1987.

Halliday AL, Sobel RA, Martuza RL: Benign spinal nerve sheath tumors: their occurrence sporadically and in neurofibromatosis type 1 and 2. *J Neurosurg* 74:248-253, 1991.

Hayes CW, Jensen ME, Conway WF: Non-neoplastic lesions of vertebral bodies. Findings in magnetic resonance imaging. *Radiographics* 9:883-904, 1989.

Hu HP, Huang QL: Signal intensity correlation of MRI with pathological findings in spinal neurinomas. *Neuroradiology* 34:98-102, 1992.

Ishii N, Matsuzawa H, Houkin K, et al: An evaluation of 70 spinal schwannomas using conventional computed tomography and magnetic resonance imaging. *Neuroradiology* 33:542, 1991.

Jones KM, Schwartz RB, Mantello MT, et al: Fast spin-echo MR in the detection of vertebral metastases: comparison of three sequences. *AJNR* 15:401-408, 1994.

Kaffenberger DA, Shah CP, Murtagh FR, et al: MR imaging of spinal cord hemangioblastoma associated with syringomyelia. *J Comput Assist Tomogr* 12:495-498, 1988.

Kamholtz R, Sze G: Current imaging in spinal metastatic disease. *Semin Oncol* 18:158-169, 1991.

Keslar PJ, Buck JL, Suarez ES: Germ cell tumors of the sacrococcygeal region: radiologic-pathologic correlation. *Radiographics* 14:607-620, 1994.

Klein SL, Sanford RA, Muhlbauer MS: Pediatric spinal epidural metastases. *J Neurosurg* 74:70-75, 1991.

Krol G, Sze G, Malkin M, Walker R: MR of cranial and spinal meningeal carcinomatosis, comparison with CT and myelography. *AJNR* 9:709-714, 1988.

Lanir A, Aghai E, Simon JR, et al: MR imaging in myelofibrosis. *J Comput Assist Tomogr* 10:634, 1986.

Laredo JD, Assouline E, Gelbert F, et al: Vertebral hemangiomas: Fat content as a sign of aggressiveness. *Radiology* 177:467, 1990.

Levy RA: Paraganglioma of the filum terminale: MR findings. *AJR* 160:851-852, 1993.

Li MH, Holtas S: MR imaging of spinal neurofibromatosis. *Acta Radiol* 32, fasc 4:279-285, 1991.

Li MH, Holtas S, Larsson E-M: MR imaging of intradural extramedullary tumors. *Acta Radiol* 33:207-212, 1992.

Libshitz HI, Malthouse SR, Cunningham D, et al: Multiple myeloma: appearance at MR imaging. *Radiology* 182:833-837, 1992.

Lim V, Sobel DF, Zyroff J: Spinal cord pial metastases: MR imaging with gadopentetate dimeglumine. *AJNR* 11:975-982, 1990.

Lyons MK, O'Neill BP, March WR, Kurtin DJ: Primary spinal epidural non-Hodgkin's lymphoma: report of eight patients and review of the literature. *Neurosurgery* 30:675-680, 1992.

Masaryk TJ: Neoplastic disease of the spine. *Rad Clin North Am* 29:829-846, 1991.

Mascalchi M, Arnetoli G, Pozzo G, et al: Spinal epidural angiolipoma: MR findings. *AJNR* 12:744-745, 1991.

Masuda N, Hayashi H, Tanebe H: Nerve root and sciatic trunk enlargement in Déjérine-Sottas disease: MRI appearances. *Neuroradiology* 35:36-37, 1992.

Matsumoto S, Hasu K, Uchino A, et al: MRI of intradural-extramedullary spinal neurinomas and meningiomas. *Clinical Imaging* 17:46-52, 1993.

McCormick PC, Torres R, Post KD, Stein BM: Intramedullary ependymoma of the spinal cord. *J Neurosurg* 62:523-532, 1990.

Moore SG, Gooding CA, Brasch RC, et al: Bone marrow in children with acute lymphocytic leukemia: MR relaxation times. *Radiology* 160:237-240, 1986.

Moulopoulos LA, Varma DGK, Dimopoulos MA, et al: Multiple myeloma: spinal MR imaging in patients with untreated newly diagnosed disease. *Radiology* 185:833-840, 1992.

Munk PL, Helms CA, Holt RG, et al: MR imaging of aneurysmal bone cysts. *AJR* 153:99-101, 1989.

Murota T, Symon L: Surgical management of hemangioblastoma of the spinal cord: a report of 18 cases. *Neurosurgery* 25:699-708, 1989.

Nakasu Y, Minouchi K, Hatsuda N, et al: Thoracic meningiocele vs neurofibromatosis: CT and MR findings. *J Comput Assist Tomogr* 15:1062-1064, 1991.

Nemoto Y, Inoue Y, Tashiro T, et al: Intramedullary spinal cord tumors: significance of associated hemorrhage at MR imaging. *Radiology* 182:793-796, 1992.

Nokes SR, Murtagh FR, Jones JD, et al: Childhood scoliosis: MR imaging. *Radiology* 164:791, 1987.

Olson DO, Shields AF, Sheunch CJ, et al: Magnetic resonance imaging of the bone marrow in patients with leukemia, aplastic anemia, and lymphoma. *Invest Radiol* 21:540, 1986.

Packer RJ, Zimmerman RA, Sutton LN, et al: Magnetic resonance imaging of spinal cord disease in childhood. *Pediatrics* 78:251, 1986.

Parizel PM, Baleriaux D, Rodesch G, et al: Gd-DTPA-enhanced MR imaging of spinal tumors. *AJNR* 10:249-258, 1989.

Perry JR, Deodhare SS, Bilbao JM, et al: The significance of spinal cord compression as the initial manifestation of lymphoma. *Neurosurgery* 32:157-162, 1993.

Post MJD, Quencer RM, Green BA, et al: Intramedullary spinal cord metastases, mainly of nonneurogenic origin. *AJNR* 8:339-346, 1987.

Preul MC, Leblanc R, Tampieri D: Spinal angiolipomas: report of three cases. *J Neurosurg* 78:280-286, 1993.

Rahmouni A, Divine M, Mathieu D, et al: Detection of multiple myeloma involving the spine: efficiency of fat-suppression and contrast-enhanced MR imaging. *AJR* 160:1049-1052, 1993.

Rebner M, Gebarski SS: Magnetic resonance imaging of spinal cord hemangioblastoma. *AJNR* 6:287, 1985.

Rosenthal DI, Scott JA, Mankin HJ, et al: Sacrococcygeal chordoma: magnetic resonance imaging and computed tomography. *AJR* 145-143, 1985.

Ross JS, Masaryk TJ, Modic MT, et al: Vertebral hemangiomas: MR imaging. *Radiology* 165:165-169, 1987.

Rubin JM, Aisen AM, DiPietro MA: Ambiguities in MR imaging of tumoral cysts in the spinal cord. *J Comput Assist Tomogr* 10:395-398, 1986.

Schroth G, Thron A, Guhl L, et al: Magnetic resonance imaging of spinal meningiomas and neurinomas: improvement of imaging by paramagnetic contrast enhancement. *J Neurosurg* 66:695-700, 1987.

Schuknecht B, Huber P, Buller B, Nadjimi M: Spinal leptomeningeal neoplastic disease. *Eur Neurol* 32:11-16, 1992.

Schweitzer JS, Batzdorf U: Ependymomas of the cauda equina region: diagnosis, treatment, and outcome in 15 patients. *Neurosurgery* 30:202-207, 1992.

Scotti G, Scialfa G, Colombo N, et al: Magnetic resonance diagnosis of intramedullary tumors of the spinal cord. *Neuroradiology* 29:130-135, 1987.

Scotti G, Scialfa G, Colombo N, Landoni L: MR imaging of intradural extramedullary tumors of the cervical spine. *J Comput Assist Tomogr* 9:1037-1041, 1985.

Shen W, Ho Y, Lee S, Lee K: Ependymoma of the cauda equina presenting with subarachnoid hemorrhage. *AJNR* 14:399-400, 1993.

Shen WC, Lee SK, Chang CY, Ho WL: Cystic spinal neurilemmoma on magnetic resonance imaging. *Neuroradiology* 34:447-448, 1992.

Siegel MJ, Jamroz GA, Glazer HS, Abramson CL: MR imaging of intraspinal extension of neuroblastoma. *J Comput Assist Tomogr* 10:593-595, 1986.

Silbergeld J, Cohen WA, Maravilla KR, et al: Supratentorial and spinal cord hemangioblastomas: gadolinium-enhanced MR appearance with pathologic correlation. *J Comput Assist Tomogr* 13:1048-1051, 1989.

Syklawer R, Osborn RE, Kerber CW, Glass RF: Magnetic resonance imaging of vertebral osteoblastoma: a report of two cases. *Surg Neurol* 34:421-426, 1990.

Slasky BS, Bydder GM, Niendorf HP, Young IR: MR imaging with gadolinium-DTPA in the differentiation of tumor, syrinx, and cyst of the spinal cord. *J Comput Assist Tomogr* 11:845-850, 1987.

Smoker WRK, Godersky JC, Knutzon RK, et al: The role of MR imaging in evaluation of metastatic spinal disease. *AJNR* 8:901-908, 1987.

Solero CL, Fornari M, Giombini S, et al: Spinal meningiomas: review of 174 operated cases. *Neurosurgery* 25:153-160, 1989.

Stimac GK, Porter BA, Olson DO, et al: Gadolinium-DTPA-enhanced MR imaging of spinal neoplasms: preliminary investigation and comparison with unenhanced spin echo and STIR sequences. *AJNR* 9:839-846, 1988.

Sze G: Magnetic resonance imaging in the evaluation of spinal tumors. *Cancer* 67:1229-1241, 1991.

Sze G, Abramson A, Krol G, et al: Gadolinium-DTPA/dimeglumine in the MR evaluation of intradural extramedullary spinal disease. *AJNR* 9:153-163, 1988.

Sze G, Krol G, Zimmerman RD, Deck DMF: Intramedullary disease of the spine: diagnosis of using gadolinium-DTPA-enhanced MR imaging. *AJNR* 9:847-858, 1988.

Sze G, Krol G, Zimmerman RD, Deck MDF: Malignant extradural spinal tumors: MR imaging with Gd-DTPA. *Radiology* 167:217-223, 1988.

Sze G, Merriam M, Oshio K, Jolesz FA: Fast spin-echo imaging in the evaluation of intradural disease of the spine. *AJNR* 13:1383-1393, 1992.

Sze G, Stimac GK, Bartlett C, et al: Multicenter study or gadopentetate dimeglumine as an MR contrast agent: evaluation in patients with spinal cord tumors. *AJNR* 11:967-974, 1990.

Weaver GR, Sandler MP: Increased sensitivity of magnetic resonance imaging compared to radionuclide bone scintigraphy in the detection of lymphoma of the spine. *Clin Nucl Med* 12:333-334, 1987.

Williams AL, Haughton VM, Pojunas KW, et al: Differentiation of intramedullary neoplasms and cysts by MR. *AJNR* 8:527-532, 1987.

Yochum TR, Lile RL, Schultz GD, et al: Acquired spinal stenosis secondary to an expanding thoracic vertebral hemangioma. *Spine* 18:299-305, 1993.

Yuh WTC, Zachar CK, Barloon TJ, et al: Vertebral compression fractures: distinction between benign and malignant causes with MR imaging. *Radiology* 172:215-218, 1989.

Zimmerman RA, Bilaniuk LT: Imaging of tumors of the spinal canal and cord. *Rad Clin North Am* 26:965-1007, 1988.

CHAPTER 16

Inflammatory Disorders of the Spinal Canal

Case 962

47-year-old woman presenting with fever
and back pain.
(sagittal, noncontrast scan; SE 600/20)

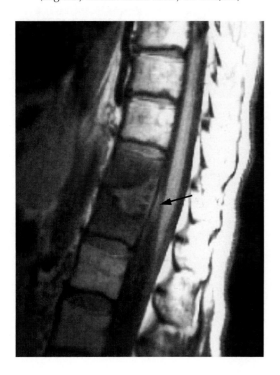

Case 963

67-year-old man presenting with severe back pain.
(sagittal, noncontrast scan; SE 600/15)

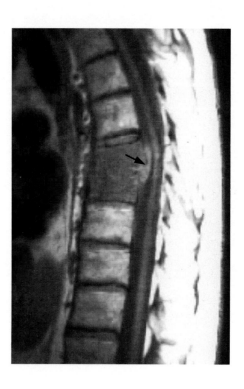

Infection of an intervertebral disc and adjacent vertebrae may occur in adults or children at any level of the spinal column. The majority of such infections are hematogenous, originating in the subchondral portion of a vertebral body and spreading to involve the adjacent disc. In young children the reverse sequence may occur: hematogenous infection may initially seed the disc before spreading to subchondral bone. Direct infection of the disc space may follow surgery or instrumentation at any age.

The radiographic hallmark of discitis is involvement of the subchondral regions of adjacent vertebral bodies. This finding is well displayed on sagittal or coronal MR studies. Infiltration of marrow by edema and inflammatory cells causes a water-like signal pattern with reduced intensity on T1-weighted images.

In Case 962, the normally "bright" signal intensity of marrow fat has been replaced throughout most of the T12 and L1 vertebral bodies. The large erosion extending from the disc space into both vertebrae is unusually prominent; often a ragged appearance of multiple smaller irregularities is found (see Case 964). A shallow area of thickened epidural tissue is present along the anterior margin of the spinal canal *(arrow)*.

Case 963 demonstrates low signal intensity occupying most of the T7 and T8 vertebral bodies. The intervening disc space is barely discernible, since cortical bone along its margins has been eroded. (Compare to cortical definition at uninvolved disc levels.) An anterior epidural mass is present *(arrow)*, displacing and compressing the spinal cord.

It is important to note that vertebral changes may be late to develop (and to resolve) during the course of discitis in some patients (see Case 978 for an example). Abnormalities of the disc space (and possible adjacent soft tissue masses) may be the only manifestation of discitis in occasional cases.

Case 964

35-year-old woman complaining of worsening back pain.
(sagittal, noncontrast scan; SE 2200/45)

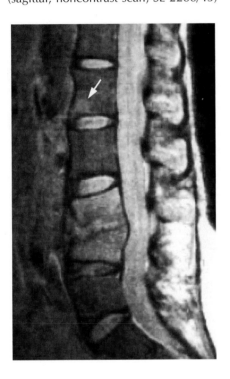

Case 965

67-year-old man presenting with severe back pain.
(sagittal, noncontrast scan; SE 2000/70)

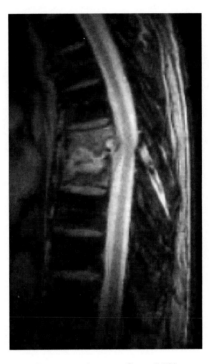

(same patient as Case 963)

The cellular infiltration and edema accompanying discitis and osteomyelitis usually cause increased signal intensity on long TR spin echo images.

In Case 964, abnormally high intensity is seen throughout the L3 and L4 vertebral bodies. Adjacent portions of the bodies have been destroyed. The intervening disc space is narrow and irregular. Signal intensity within the disc is comparable to that of the infected vertebrae. (Low intensity would be expected in a degenerated disc that has caused sterile reactive changes of neighboring bodies; see Cases 831-834.)

The T2-weighted scan in Case 965 demonstrates more pathological detail within the infected region than the accompanying T1-weighted image (see Case 963). Large, irregular erosions extend into the vertebral bodies from the disc space, resembling Case 962. Although this destruction is clearly centered at the disc level, the involved vertebral bodies are filled with inflammatory edema.

Compare the sharp definition of uninvolved vertebral margins in Cases 964 and 965 to the poor visualization of cortex bordering the infected discs. Erosion and fragmentation of adjacent vertebral end-plates are hallmarks of discitis. Inflammatory erosions are usually more numerous and irregular than the depressions caused by intravertebral disc herniations ("Schmorl's nodes"; see Case 971).

The smaller lesion within the anterior-inferior corner of the L1 vertebral body in Case 964 (arrow) illustrates that hematogenous disc space infection usually originates from seeding of subchondral bone. The term "spondylitis" may be better than "discitis" to accurately represent the vertebral component of these combined infections.

Case 966

34-year-old woman presenting with hand numbness and mildly spastic gait six months after admission for pneumonia and a mediastinal abscess.
(sagittal, noncontrast scan; SE 800/17)

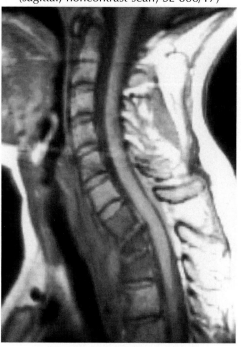

Case 967

83-year-old woman presenting with back pain and acute paraplegia.
(sagittal, noncontrast scan; SE 550/20)

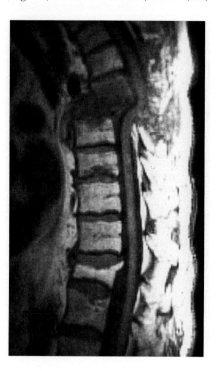

As seen on the preceding pages, discitis and osteomyelitis may cause extensive bone destruction. Cases 966 and 967 demonstrate that this loss of vertebral body height and stability may in turn lead to spinal deformity and cord compression.

In Case 966, osteomyelitis involves the C7 through T2 levels, spanning two disc spaces. Anterior wedging of the T1 vertebral body is associated with kyphotic angulation and subluxation that is beginning to compromise the spinal canal. (Note that the subarachnoid space is effaced at the cervicothoracic junction.)

The subluxation in Case 967 is more extreme, with a bayonet-like deformity of the thoracic spinal canal. Cord compression in cases of discitis/osteomyelitis may be caused by such abnormalities of alignment and/or by associated epidural inflammatory masses (as in Case 963). (The posterior arches in the involved region of Case 967 had

been resected in an attempt to decompress the spinal canal.)

Tuberculous spondylitis typically demonstrates larger paraspinal masses and less end-plate destruction than pyogenic infection. Extension beneath the anterior or posterior longitudinal ligaments is often associated with involvement of multiple vertebral bodies, mimicking metastatic disease.

A spondyloarthropathy resembling discitis/osteomyelitis may develop in patients with renal failure undergoing dialysis. The cervical spine is commonly affected by this disorder, which is believed to be caused by the accumulation and deposition of a low molecular weight protein ("beta-2-microglobulin") that is not removed by dialysis. Imaging findings include narrowing of disc spaces and erosions of adjacent vertebrae, mimicking infectious spondylitis (which must also be considered in dialysis patients).

Case 968

2-year-old boy with apparent back pain.
(sagittal, noncontrast scan; SE 2000/90)

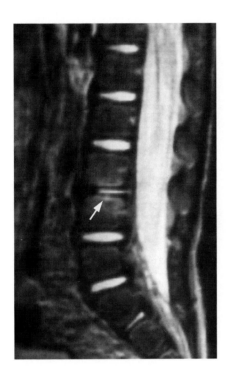

Case 969

8-month-old boy presenting with fever
and irritability.
(sagittal, noncontrast scan; SE 3000/90)

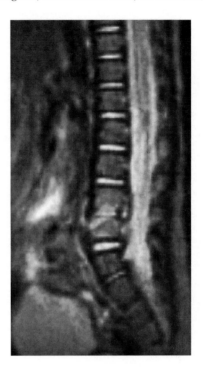

Pediatric discitis may be a low grade and self-limited inflammation, typically involving a single lumbar level. In many cases, no causative organism is established. The clinical presentation is often nonspecific and may initially suggest hip pathology or appendicitis.

Case 968 demonstrates narrowing of the L3-4 disc, with mild reduction of signal intensity. A faint haze of inflammatory edema is present within the adjacent vertebral bodies, but cortical end-plates are intact. The appearance is compatible with idiopathic nonsuppurative primary discitis.

More bone destruction is apparent at the L4-5 level in Case 969. Adjacent cortices have been eroded, and there is more prominent signal abnormality within the involved vertebral bodies. These findings suggest pyogenic infection and would support early antibiotic therapy.

DIFFERENTIAL DIAGNOSIS:
INFILTRATION/EDEMA OF ADJACENT VERTEBRAE

Case 970

45-year-old man with severe back pain.
(sagittal, noncontrast scan; SE 550/20)

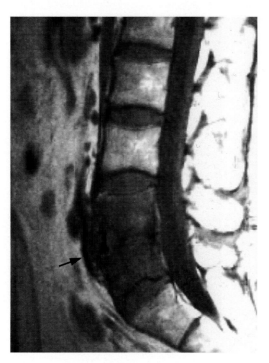

Discitis and Osteomyelitis

Case 971

61-year-old woman presenting with back pain.
(sagittal, noncontrast scan; SE 900/17)

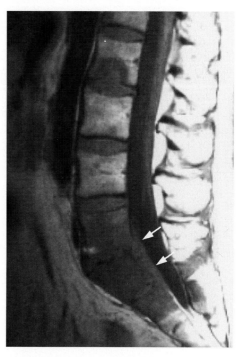

Metastatic Carcinoma of the Breast

The preceding cases in this chapter have demonstrated that discitis/osteomyelitis should be considered when abnormal signal intensity is encountered within adjacent vertebral bodies. Case 970 is another example of this pathology. The prolongation of T1 throughout the L4 and L5 vertebrae probably represents a combination of pyogenic infiltration and reactive edema. An associated prevertebral mass is present *(arrow)*. (See Case 974 for a postcontrast scan of this patient.)

Metastatic disease may also involve adjacent vertebrae, either by simultaneous hematogenous seeding or by extension across the intervening disc. In Case 971, contiguous tumor infiltrates the L5, S1, and S2 vertebral bodies. An associated anterior epidural mass is present *(arrows)*. The overall appearance simulates an inflammatory lesion. (See Case 881 for another example of metastatic disease crossing an intervertebral disc.)

Clinical context helps to distinguish between these pathologies. Evidence of systemic infection is usual in patients

with discitis. In addition, discitis/osteomyelitis is typically associated with severe back pain, which is often a more impressive component of the initial presentation than in patients with vertebral metastases.

Tuberculous spondylitis should also be considered in the differential diagnosis of pathology involving adjacent vertebral bodies. Tuberculous infection often extends beneath the anterior and/or posterior longitudinal ligament, involving several contiguous vertebrae.

A large Schmorl's node is incidentally noted within the inferior end-plate of L2 in Case 971. Disc material extends into the vertebral body, surrounded by a zone of reactive edema and/or sclerosis causing low signal intensity. Contrast this laminar architecture based at the disc space with the appearance of small vertebral metastases (as in Case 886) or localized osteomyelitis (as in Case 964).

DIFFERENTIAL DIAGNOSIS:
ANTERIOR EPIDURAL MASS CENTERED AT A DISC LEVEL

Case 972

32-year-old man presenting with back pain.
(sagittal, noncontrast scan; SE 800/17)

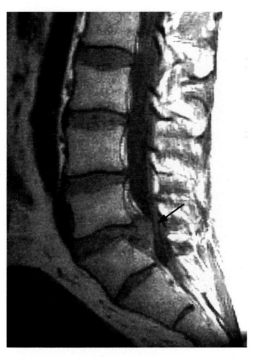

Herniated Disc

Case 973

44-year-old man presenting with rapidly increasing
back pain two weeks after lumbar discectomy.
(sagittal, noncontrast scan; SE 900/17)

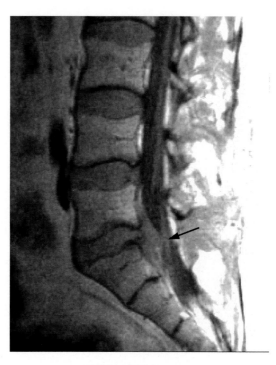

Epidural Phlegmon

An anterior epidural mass at the level of an intervertebral disc is a common manifestation of disc herniation, as in Case 972. Associated edema, granulation tissue, venous congestion, and epidural hemorrhage may contribute to the bulk of such masses (see Cases 828-830).

Case 973 illustrates that epidural infection should also be considered in this differential diagnosis. In some patients the disc space changes of infection are less impressive (or later to develop) than the epidural or paraspinal soft tissue components. The resulting appearance may simulate a herniated disc.

An epidural mass at the level of an infected disc may represent either a true abscess (see Cases 978-981) or a mound of edematous tissue referred to as a "phlegmon." An epidural phlegmon often contains small purulent pockets or "micro-abscesses."

It is very difficult to distinguish between a drainable abscess cavity and a boggy, semisolid phlegmon on MR scans. Both processes typically demonstrate intermediate to low signal intensity on T1-weighted scans and high intensity on T2-weighted studies. Contrast enhancement may be more clearly peripheral in frank abscesses, but even this appearance is not a reliable distinguishing criterion.

Case 974

45-year-old man presenting with severe back pain.
(sagittal, postcontrast scan; SE 550/20)

Case 975

52-year-old woman presenting with back pain.
(sagittal, postcontrast scan; SE 600/15)

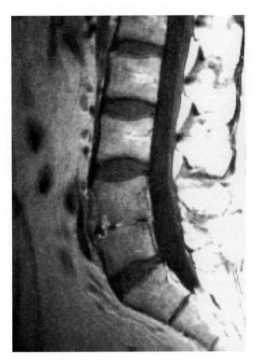

(same patient as Case 970)

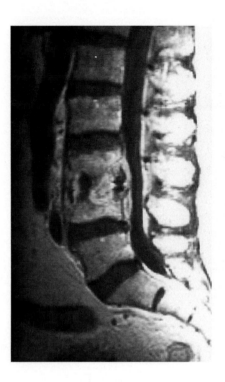

Uniform contrast enhancement throughout the involved vertebral bodies in Case 974 has caused them to become nearly isointense to normal marrow. Comparison with the precontrast scan in Case 970 illustrates that enhancement may obscure the definition of vertebral (or epidural) pathology on T1-weighted scans. This possibility is frequently of concern in the evaluation of metastatic disease to the spinal canal. Scans in such cases should not be limited to postcontrast T1-weighted images without fat suppression.

The marked disc space narrowing, erosions of cortical end-plates, and small pockets of intense enhancement within the disc in Case 974 all suggest discitis as the source of the adjacent vertebral infiltration.

Case 975 presents a different pattern of contrast enhancement in discitis. A central area of intense enhancement straddles the disc space and extends into the center of the involved vertebrae. This zone represents the core of the infection, with aggressive bone destruction comparable to Cases 962 and 965. Surrounding reactive inflammation enhances with a more uniform pattern, resembling Case 974 and appearing isointense to adjacent normal vertebrae. An associated anterior epidural mass enhances intensely, representing the postcontrast equivalent of the epidural phlegmon in Case 973.

DIFFERENTIAL DIAGNOSIS:
IRREGULAR CONTRAST ENHANCEMENT WITHIN A VERTEBRAL BODY

Case 976

66-year-old woman presenting with back pain.
(axial, postcontrast scan; SE 600/15; L2 level)

Case 977

52-year-old woman presenting with back pain.
(axial, postcontrast scan; SE 600/15; L4 level)

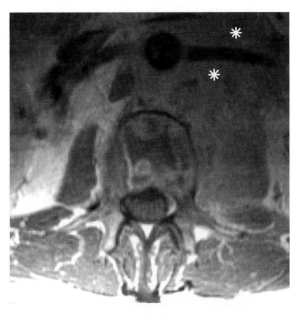

Metastatic Carcinoma of the Breast

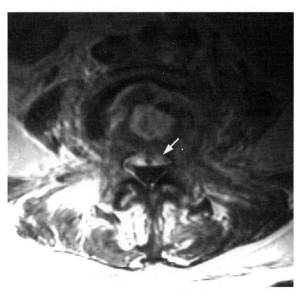

Discitis/Osteomyelitis
(same patient as Case 975)

Metastatic disease and discitis/osteomyelitis must often be considered together in the differential diagnosis of vertebral lesions (see Cases 970 and 971). Both pathologies can cause irregular enhancement within involved bodies, as illustrated above. The clinical context and pattern of spinal disease (i.e., multiplicity and continuity of affected levels) will usually differentiate between these lesions.

Both infection and metastatic disease of the spine may cause associated paraspinal and epidural masses. A large left-sided paraspinal mass in Case 976 involves the psoas region. An anterior epidural mass enhances intensely in Case 977 (*arrow*; compare to the sagittal scan in Case 975).

Retroperitoneal adenopathy, as seen in Case 976 (*asterisks*), strongly suggests the context of systemic metastases. (See Case 886 for another example.)

Intrathecal nerve roots of the cauda equina are somewhat prominent in Case 976. This can be a normal postcontrast appearance due to mild diffuse enhancement. Pathologically enlarged or inflamed roots usually demonstrate more striking and asymmetrical enhancement, often in association with unequivocal precontrast abnormality of size and/or morphology.

Case 978

84-year-old woman presenting with a two-week
history of neck pain and progressive quadriparesis.
(sagittal, noncontrast scan; SE 2500/80)

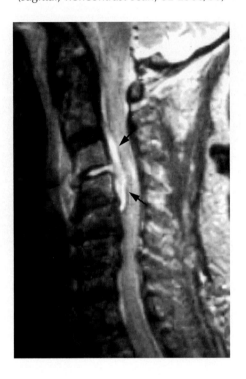

Case 979

15-year-old boy presenting with back pain,
leg numbness and leg weakness.
(sagittal, noncontrast scan; SE 600/15)

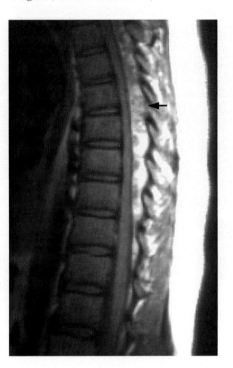

Abscesses may develop in the epidural space by direct extension of spinal infections or by hematogenous seeding from distant sources. Once established, epidural abscesses typically involve long segments of the spinal canal (e.g., 10 or 20 vertebral levels). Initial symptoms may be mild or nondescript. Rapid loss of neurological function occurs with the onset of septic thrombophlebitis extending to the spinal cord.

Anterior epidural inflammatory masses are commonly associated with discitis, as in Case 978. Abnormally high signal intensity is present within the C3-4 disc as well as within the anterior epidural abscess. No vertebral destruction is seen, again demonstrating that the extent of osseous erosion in discitis is variable and independent of the presence or size of epidural masses. Culture in this cause yielded *Staphylococcus aureus*.

By contrast, the dorsal epidural abscess in Case 979 represents hematogenous dissemination of infection, comparable to the occurrence of isolated epidural metastases. The dorsal portion of the thoracic spinal canal is a common lo-

cation for such hematogenous lesions, and *S. aureus* is the most frequently cultured pathogen.

High signal intensity within the epidural space in Case 979 likely has two sources. Dorsal epidural fat, although infiltrated by the inflammatory process, may still contribute zones of T1-shortening. In addition, hemorrhage is commonly found within epidural abscesses, and subacute blood products may cause T1-shortening in the involved region.

It is often difficult to distinguish between epidural and subdural localization of spinal empyemas. Involvement of either compartment causes compression of the dural sac. Subdural and epidural empyema should be considered in the differential diagnosis of a featureless spinal canal with obliteration of normal cord/CSF interfaces.

The differential diagnosis in Case 979 includes epidural hematoma (see Cases 1019-1021) and epidural metastasis. Rare epidural angiolipomas and hemangiomas (see Case 889) could cause a similar appearance.

Case 980

15-year-old boy presenting with back pain
and leg weakness.
(axial, postcontrast scan; SE 700/15; T6 level)

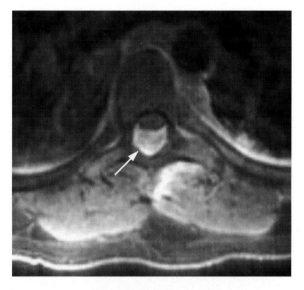

(same patient as Case 979)

Case 981

66-year-old man presenting with right-sided
radicular back pain.
(axial, postcontrast scan; SE 600/15; T8-9 level)

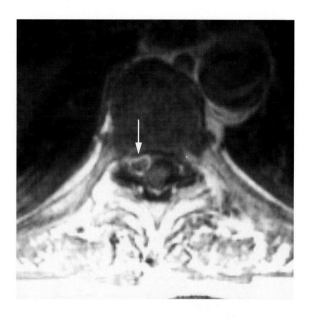

Epidural inflammatory masses may encircle the dural sac as a uniform rind of thickened tissue or be very eccentric. The former morphology resembles that of some epidural metastases, as in Cases 892 and 898. The latter appearance is illustrated by the cases above.

Contrast enhancement within the epidural abscess in Case 980 is relatively uniform. This homogeneity probably reflects leakage and accumulation of contrast material within the purulent loculations of the infected tissue.

In other cases, epidural abscesses present as nonenhancing zones surrounded by a rim of contrast material, illustrated in Case 981. Neither solid nor peripheral enhancement patterns guarantee or exclude the presence of a drainable cavity containing a macroscopic collection of pus.

In each of these cases, the dural sac is mildly deformed and compressed. Surprisingly severe and rapidly developing myelopathy in patients with small epidural abscesses often reflects septic thrombophlebitis causing impaired venous drainage and infarction within the spinal cord.

The differential diagnosis in Case 980 includes a dorsal epidural hematoma or neoplasm. An appearance resembling Case 981 may be caused by disc herniation with an associated margin of granulation tissue (compare to Case 819) or by peripheral enhancement at the margin of an epidural hematoma (see Case 1025).

A left paraspinal mass is also present in Case 980, and there is abnormally intense enhancement of inflamed muscles posterior to the spine.

Case 982

36-year-old man presenting with numbness
of the hands and feet.
(sagittal, noncontrast scan; SE 1000/20)

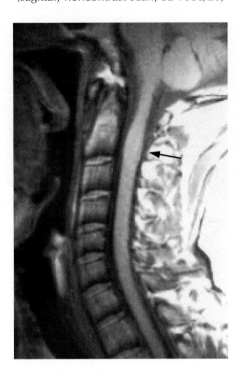

Case 983

55-year-old woman presenting with unsteady gait.
(axial, noncontrast scan; low flip angle GRE
sequence; C2-3 level)

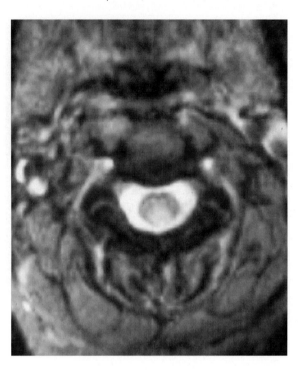

Myelitis may be caused by a variety of agents and conditions. Demyelinating disease is a leading diagnostic possibility in young and middle-aged adults. Involvement of the spinal cord in multiple sclerosis may be focal, multifocal, or diffuse.

The T1-weighted scan in Case 982 shows mild, isointense swelling of the cord at the C2-3 level. This focal expansion is nonspecific; a small primary or metastatic tumor could cause a similar appearance. However, it is important to realize that such localized swelling does occur within the spectrum of demyelinating disease. The location of this lesion (i.e., the C2-3 level) and its size (about one vertebral body in length) are both typical of multiple sclerosis within the cervical cord.

Case 983 illustrates another small demyelinating plaque within the spinal cord at the C2-3 level. The edema associated with cord lesions in multiple sclerosis usually causes prominent prolongation of T2. High signal intensity on T2-weighted scans may be very sharply defined (as in Case 983; see also Case 984) or quite hazy and indistinct (see Case 986).

The dorsal eccentricity of the lesion in Case 983 is a common feature of intramedullary demyelinating disease.

Case 984

20-year-old woman presenting with arm
and leg numbness.
(sagittal, noncontrast scan; SE 3100/90)

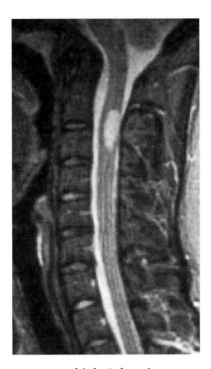

Multiple Sclerosis

Case 985

55-year-old man presenting with arm numbness
and weakness.
(sagittal, noncontrast scan; RSE 5000/100)

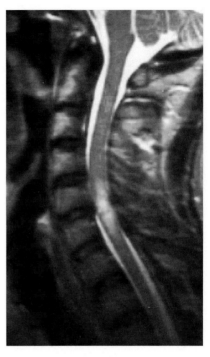

Astrocytoma

The very well-defined lesion in Case 984 is another example of focal demyelination due to multiple sclerosis. The location of the plaque within the dorsal portion of the cord at the C2-3 level and its size (approximately one vertebral body in length) are characteristic findings in this disorder.

Case 985 demonstrates that cord tumors may present a similar appearance. The astrocytoma in this case is somewhat more localized and homogeneous than usual. How-

ever, it is important to realize the potential overlap in appearance between inflammatory and neoplastic involvement of the spinal cord. (This overlap extends to contrast-enhanced images; see Cases 992 and 993.)

A cerebral scan may document intracranial demyelinating foci associated with an ambiguous cord lesion. In other cases, clinical and radiographic evidence of multiple sclerosis is limited to the spinal cord.

Case 986

39-year-old woman presenting with bilateral
arm and face numbness.
(sagittal, noncontrast scan; SE 2400/90)

Case 987

33-year-old woman presenting with diplopia
and incoordination.
(sagittal, noncontrast scan; SE 2800/90)

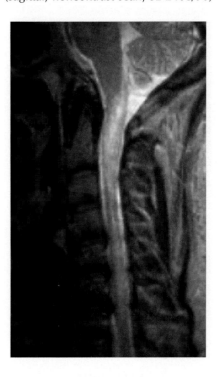

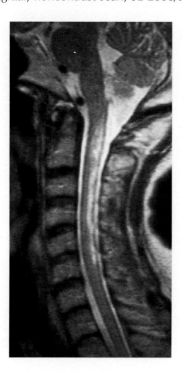

Myelitis due to multiple sclerosis may cause extensive edema involving long segments of the spinal cord. Such lesions are often patchy and poorly defined, in contrast to the focal plaques in Cases 982 and 984.

Case 986 illustrates this pattern. Hazy high signal intensity extends from the medulla to the C3 level, with additional edema at lower cervical levels. Margins of the lesion are indistinct. Cord expansion is present throughout the area of greatest involvement.

Multiple sclerosis may alternatively demonstrate a multifocal pattern, intermediate between localized disease and Case 986. The column of abnormal signal intensity paralleling the dorsal margin of the spinal cord in Case 987 represents the coalescence of multiple small areas of demyelination.

Systemic lupus erythematosus and sarcoidosis are additional potential inflammatory etiologies of diffuse cord edema and mass effect.

Case 988

2-year-old girl presenting with
progressive myelopathy.
(sagittal, noncontrast scan; SE 600/15)

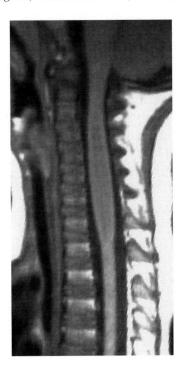

Case 989

4-year-old boy presenting with rapidly
developing quadriparesis.
(sagittal, noncontrast scan; low flip angle
GRE sequence)

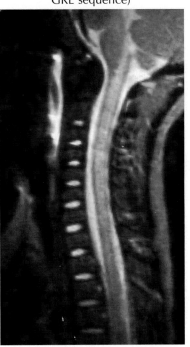

Inflammatory myelopathy with no identifiable cause is frequently called "transverse myelitis." Many such cases probably represent an autoimmune response to an antigenic challenge, analogous to acute disseminated encephalomyelitis (see Cases 361-365). Transverse myelitis ranks with multiple sclerosis as the leading causes of spinal cord inflammation in adults.

Transverse myelitis is also seen in children, as illustrated above. In both adults and children the cord swelling and dysfunction caused by transverse myelitis may mimic an intramedullary neoplasm. Expansion of the spinal cord by central edema in Case 988 resembles the astrocytoma in Case 936. Alternatively, transverse myelitis may present as extensive signal abnormality within a cord of normal size, as in Case 989.

Note that the name "transverse" myelitis is somewhat misleading. Cord involvement in the above cases is quite longitudinal, extending over many levels. In fact, transverse-myelitis typically involves longer segments of the spinal cord than multiple sclerosis.

The spectrum of intramedullary edema in transverse myelitis overlaps that of multiple sclerosis (compare Case 989 to Case 987). Clinical context (e.g., a history of optic neuritis) may help to distinguish between these inflammatory myelopathies. Alternatively, MR scans of the brain may demonstrate characteristic findings of multiple sclerosis when the pattern of spinal cord involvement is ambiguous.

Contrast enhancement usually does not separate myelitis due to multiple sclerosis from transverse myelitis. Both pathologies may demonstrate minimal or patchy enhancement. Discrete nodular enhancement favors multiple sclerosis (or another pathology) over idiopathic myelitis (see Cases 990 to 993.)

Transverse myelitis often responds dramatically to treatment with steroids. The diagnosis should be considered and a therapeutic trial entertained prior to biopsy for presumed neoplasm. A follow-up scan in Case 988 was normal after ten days of steroid administration.

Case 990

39-year-old woman presenting with numbness
of the arms and face.
(sagittal, postcontrast scan; SE 500/20)

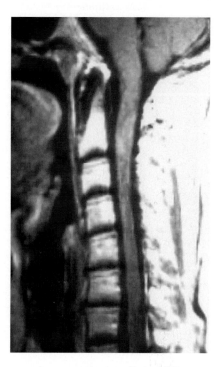

(same patient as Case 986)

Case 991

24-year-old man presenting with numbness
and paresthesias of the legs and feet.
(sagittal, postcontrast scan; SE 550/20)

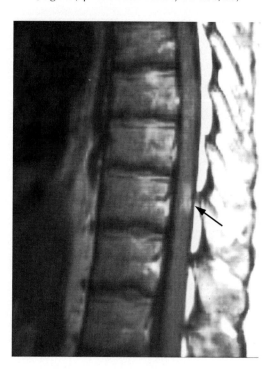

Contrast enhancement is often demonstrated at sites of active demyelination within the spinal cord. The above cases illustrate that this enhancement is typically of moderate intensity and somewhat inhomogeneous.

Case 990 is a postcontrast scan of the patient in Case 986. Comparison of the precontrast and postcontrast images suggests that much of the signal abnormality in Case 986 represents reactive edema surrounding the enhancing plaques.

The focal intramedullary enhancement in Case 991 *(arrow)* correlated with the new onset of lower extremity symptoms in a patient with known multiple sclerosis. The appearance is nonspecific. In an ambiguous clinical context the possibility of neoplasm, infection, or vascular insult (arterial or venous) would have to be considered (compare to Cases 961B, 993, and 1032B).

The absence of demonstrable cord lesions on precontrast and postcontrast MR scans does not exclude the diagnosis of myelitis due to multiple sclerosis. Some intramedullary plaques are small and/or poorly defined from surrounding parenchyma. Together with the variability introduced by slice placement and partial volume effects, these factors may limit the detection of localized pathology.

DIFFERENTIAL DIAGNOSIS:
FOCAL INTRAMEDULLARY ENHANCEMENT

Case 992

54-year-old woman presenting with gait
abnormality.
(axial, postcontrast scan; SE 800/15; C4 level)

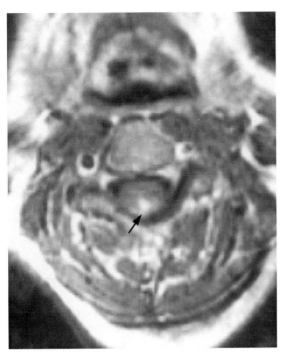

Multiple Sclerosis

Case 993

55-year-old man presenting with arm numbness
and weakness.
(sagittal, postcontrast scan; SE 600/15)

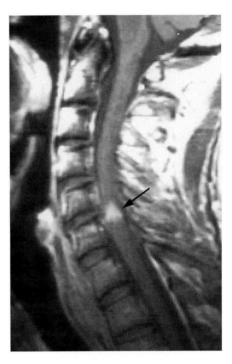

Astrocytoma
(same patient as Case 985)

Multiple sclerosis is one of several pathologies that may cause focal or multifocal enhancement within the spinal cord. The enhancing plaque in Case 992 is nonspecific. However, the dorsal location is suggestive of demyelinating disease, which typically spares central gray matter.

Primary or metastatic tumor should be included in the differential diagnosis. Astrocytomas (as in Case 993), ependymomas, and hemangioblastomas may be discovered when they are quite small. Such neoplasms may be unassociated with the characteristic cysts or hemorrhages expected of larger lesions. A pial-based hemangioblastoma in particular could closely resemble the appearance of Case 992. Metastases to the spinal cord should be considered whenever focal intramedullary lesions are found (see Case 961).

A number of vascular pathologies can also cause localized cord enhancement. Arterial and venous infarction may be extensive or limited to small regions of the spinal cord (see Case 1032B). Vascular malformations (e.g., cavernous hemangiomas) within the cord may demonstrate enhancement, often in association with surrounding blood products indicating previous hemorrhage.

Finally, a variety of additional inflammatory etiologies may produce focally enhancing cord lesions. Examples include tuberculosis and sarcoidosis (see Case 998B).

Case 994

27-year-old man presenting with arm and back pain
and cervical myelopathy.
(sagittal, noncontrast scan; SE 3000/90)

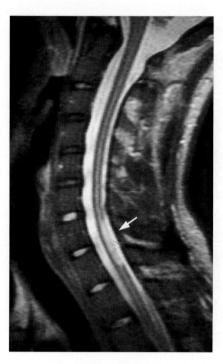

HIV Myelitis

Case 995

31-year-old man presenting with leg numbness and
paresthesias, and bowel and bladder dysfunction.
(axial, postcontrast scan; SE 800/15; T12-L1 level)

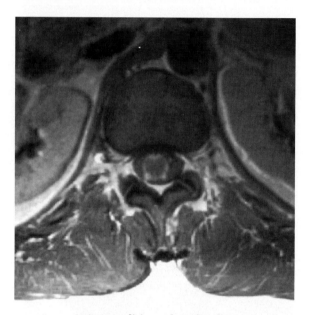

CMV Myelitis and Radiculitis

Patients with AIDS may develop meningitis, myelitis,
and/or polyradiculitis due to a variety of inflammatory
agents. Viruses (HIV, herpes simplex, varicella-zoster, and
CMV) cause the majority of such cases.

Direct infection of the spinal cord by HIV can result in
focal, multifocal, patchy, or diffuse intramedullary edema.
This range of appearances resembles the spectrum of myelitis in multiple sclerosis. The lesion in Case 994 is better
defined than in most cases of HIV myelopathy. Dorsally eccentric vacuolization and demyelination involving the posterior and lateral columns of the spinal cord have been
pathologically correlated with HIV myelitis.

CMV is recognized as a frequent cause of polyradiculitis
and myelitis involving the cauda equina and conus medullaris in AIDS patients. The pial enhancement demonstrated in Case 995 is a characteristic feature of this condition. Enhancement of individual roots within the cauda
equina may also be noted.

Myelopathy in a patient with AIDS may reflect neoplastic rather than inflammatory disease (see Case 959). Likewise, pial enhancement similar to Case 995 may be caused
by meningeal tumor coating the surface of the spinal cord
(see Cases 905-907).

Case 996

56-year-old woman previously treated with radiation therapy for esophageal carcinoma. (sagittal, noncontrast scan; SE 400/17)

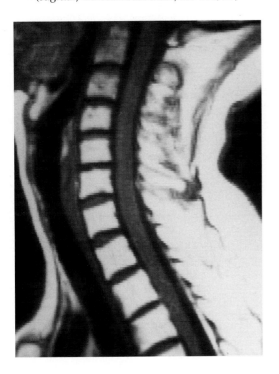

Case 997

49-year-old woman previously treated with radiation therapy for carcinoma at the skull base. (sagittal, noncontrast scan; SE 2500/120)

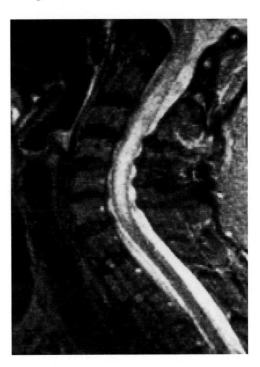

Radiation damage to the spinal cord may present subacutely or years after a course of therapy. A clinical syndrome of myelopathy in such cases is usually correlated with intramedullary edema causing long T1 and T2 values.

Such changes often extend over several vertebral levels and are associated with expansion of the spinal cord. Nodular or patchy contrast enhancement may be present. This combination of findings may mimic inflammatory myelitis or intramedullary metastasis from the originally treated tumor. (Compare the above scans to Cases 961 and 986-989.)

Case 996 demonstrates fatty atrophy within vertebral marrow, which is a clue to the history of spinal radiation.

Case 998A

42-year-old man presenting with cervical
myelopathy.
(sagittal, postcontrast scan; SE 700/11)

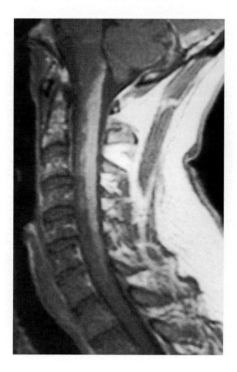

Case 998B

Same patient.
(axial, postcontrast scan; SE 600/11)

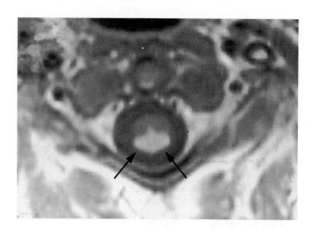

Spinal cord involvement by sarcoidosis is often pial-based, as illustrated in Case 998. A layer of abnormal contrast enhancement is present along the dorsal surface of the cord. Nodular projections of abnormal enhancement extend ventrally from this base into cord parenchyma. The affected portion of the spinal cord is widened, and T2-weighted scans demonstrated intramedullary edema.

Involvement of the cervical spinal cord is common in sarcoidosis, which occasionally causes more central intramedullary masses mimicking cord tumors. Associated intracranial disease should be sought when spinal sarcoidosis is suspected.

Compare Case 998B to Case 992.

Case 999

54-year-old woman presenting with gait
abnormality.
(sagittal, postcontrast scan; SE 600/15)

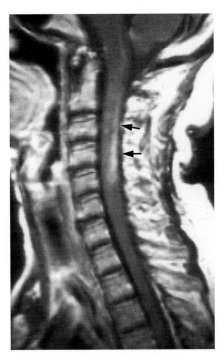

Multiple Sclerosis
(same patient as Case 992)

Case 1000

17-year-old girl presenting with cranial
neuropathies.
(sagittal, postcontrast scan; SE 600/15)

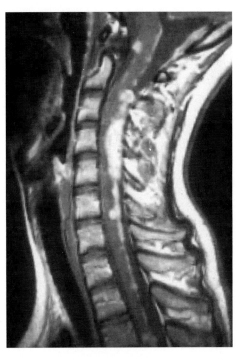

CSF Seeding from an Exophytic Ependymoma
(same patient as Case 953)

A pial-based pattern of cord enhancement is not specific for sarcoidosis. Several other inflammatory diseases can cause a similar appearance. Case 999 demonstrates that intramedullary contrast enhancement in multiple sclerosis may be eccentric (especially dorsally) and appear pial-based. Meningitis due to coccidioidomycosis may cause a thick layer of pial enhancement coating the cord. Leptomeningeal enhancement along the margins of the spinal cord has been reported in Lyme disease. Thin, superficial enhancement can be seen along the surface of the thoracic cord and conus medullaris in AIDS patients with CMV myelitis (see Case 995).

Meningeal carcinomatosis may also coat the spinal cord with a layer of tumor, which can become thick and nodular. Case 1000 illustrates this pattern; see also Cases 905-907. Several small hemangioblastomas arising at the pial surface in a patient with Von Hippel-Lindau disease could present a similar morphology.

Finally, arterial or venous infarcts of the spinal cord may demonstrate peripheral enhancement surrounding central edema.

Case 1001

40-year-old woman with a history of multiple
myelograms and lumbar operations.
(sagittal, noncontrast scan; SE 1000/22)

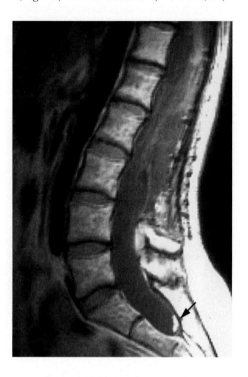

Case 1002

56-year-old woman two years after an
automobile accident.
(sagittal, noncontrast scan; SE 600/20)

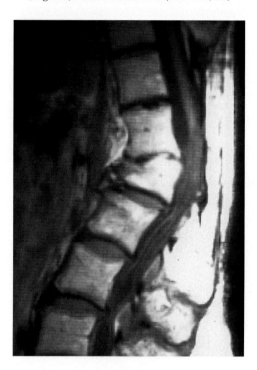

Spinal arachnoiditis may be idiopathic or secondary to inflammation caused by subarachnoid hemorrhage, meningitis, surgery, or trauma. The MR hallmark of arachnoiditis is the presence of adhesions distorting intrathecal nerve roots. The intradural course of the roots may be abnormally angled or displaced by traction from scar tissue. Alternatively, roots may be clumped together or scarred to the margins of the dural sac.

Case 1001 illustrates a wide dural sac at the thoracolumbar junction, reflecting previous laminectomies. Residual intrathecal Pantopaque is seen as small foci of T1-shortening within the caudal sac *(arrow)* and along the dorsal surface of the spinal canal in the region of surgery. The latter drop-

lets of contrast material are likely encysted or scarred in place.

Within the dural sac, the morphology of the conus medullaris and cauda equina is severely distorted. Intradural nerve roots are thick and abnormally positioned, with abrupt angulation suggesting tethering by fibrous bands.

Case 1002 demonstrates more localized arachnoiditis adjacent to a vertebral fracture. Amorphous scarring obliterates the normal contour of the conus medullaris. This fibrosis probably reflects the organization of previous hemorrhage at the level of trauma. A decompressive laminectomy is present dorsally.

DIFFERENTIAL DIAGNOSIS:
THICKENED INTRATHECAL NERVE ROOTS

Case 1003

56-year-old woman with recurrent back and leg
pain after several lumbar laminectomies.
(sagittal, noncontrast scan; SE 700/17)

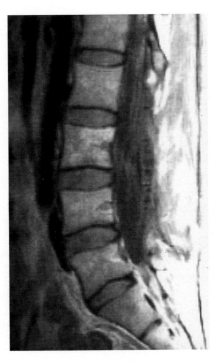

Arachnoiditis

Case 1004

68-year-old man presenting with leg pain
and weakness.
(sagittal, noncontrast scan; SE 550/25)

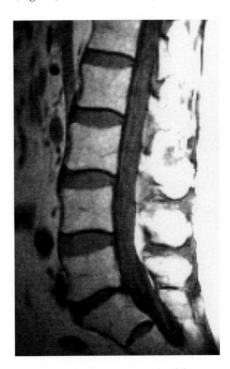

Lymphomatous Meningitis

As illustrated on the preceding page, arachnoiditis may cause extensive thickening, clumping, and distortion of intrathecal nerve roots. Case 1003 is another example of this appearance in a patient who has undergone multiple back operations. The recognition of arachnoiditis in such cases is an important factor in judging the likelihood of symptomatic improvement from additional surgery.

In Case 1004, the thickening of intradural roots is due to a coating of neoplastic cells. (Case 904 presents an axial view of this patient.) Meningeal carcinomatosis may reflect hematogenous metastases from systemic carcinomas or CSF seeding by primary intrathecal tumors. (See Cases 902, 903, 909, and 910 for additional examples.)

Neoplastic thickening of nerve roots often demonstrates contrast enhancement. Radicular enhancement is less prominent in most cases of arachnoiditis.

Arachnoiditis and meningeal carcinomatosis are among the potential etiologies of a featureless lumbar sac lacking normal definition of the conus medullaris and cauda equina. High CSF levels of cells or protein (making spinal fluid nearly isointense to neural parenchyma) may also cause this appearance. Large intradural or epidural tumors (e.g., ependymoma, as in Case 952, and neuroblastoma, as in Case 932) may fill or compress the thecal sac, obscuring intraspinal anatomy. Finally, epidural or subdural empyemas may fill the spinal canal and efface the subarachnoid space, causing an amorphous lack of intraspinal detail.

Hypertrophic neuropathies such as Déjérine-Sottas disease are a rare cause of nerve root thickening similar to the above cases.

Case 1005

48-year-old man with a history of multiple
back operations.
(sagittal, noncontrast scan; SE 2500/75)

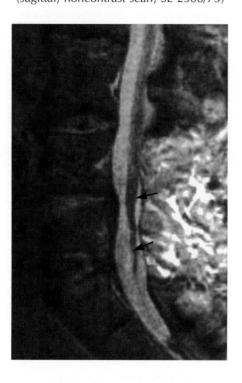

Case 1006

31-year-old man with a history of meningitis,
complaining of continuous back and leg pain.
(sagittal, noncontrast scan; SE 3300/90)

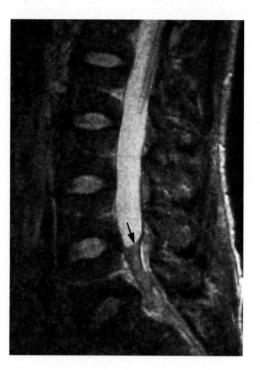

Intrathecal adhesions caused by arachnoiditis may tether nerve roots to each other or to the margins of the dural sac.

In Case 1005, an abnormally thick band of intrathecal tissue extends caudally from the conus medullaris *(arrows)*. This structure represents the aggregated nerve roots of the cauda equina, clumped together by adhesions and scarring. The resulting solitary intradural band may be misinterpreted as a tethered spinal cord or thickened filum terminale (compare to Cases 1062 and 1072).

Case 1006 illustrates the opposite pattern of arachnoiditis. The subarachnoid space appears empty because nerve roots are scarred to the perimeter of the dural sac (see Case 1007). The thecal sac terminates abnormally at the L4-5 level *(arrow)*, with the more inferior portion obliterated by scar tissue.

The differential diagnosis in Case 1006 would include an intradural mass with long T1 and T2 values causing displacement of nerve roots. Epidermoid or parasitic cysts could be considered in this category.

DIFFERENTIAL DIAGNOSIS:
CLUMPING OF INTRATHECAL NERVE ROOTS

Case 1007

31-year-old man presenting with back and leg pain.
(axial, noncontrast scan; SE 2000/80; L3 level)

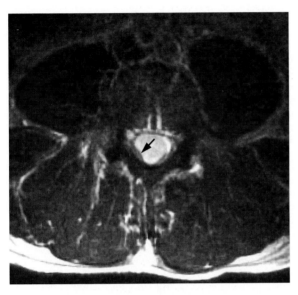

Arachnoiditis
(same patient as Case 1006)

Case 1008

17-year-old girl presenting with back pain
and cranial nerve deficits.
(axial, postcontrast scan; SE 700/15; L4-5 level)

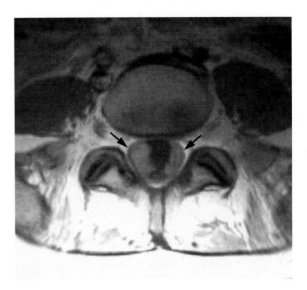

**"Drop" Metastases from a Cervical
Ependymoma**
(same patient as Case 953)

The aggregation of intrathecal nerve roots may reflect either inflammatory or neoplastic disease.

Case 1007 is an axial scan of the patient presented in Case 1006. The empty thecal sac on the sagittal view is explained on axial images by adhesion of lumbar nerve roots to the dura bilaterally (*arrow*). Note that the bulk of the roots in Case 1007 is small, contrasting with the increased mass of the roots in Case 1008.

Neoplastic coating of the cauda equina in Case 1008 is approximately symmetrical, as is often true in the inferior lumbar region. Gravitational settling of intrathecal cells makes the caudal sac a frequent location of meningeal carcinomatosis. This area should be carefully examined whenever meningeal tumor is considered clinically.

REFERENCES

Ahmadi J, Bajaj A, Destian S, et al: Spinal tuberculosis: atypical observations at MR imaging. *Radiology* 189:489-493, 1993.

Austin SG, Zee C-S, Waters C: The role of magnetic resonance imaging in acute transverse myelitis. *Can J Neurol Sci* 19:508-511, 1992.

Barakos JA, Mark AS, Dillon WP, et al: MR imaging of acute transverse myelitis and AIDS myelopathy. *J Comput Assist Tomogr* 14:45-50, 1990.

Boden SD, Davis DO, Dina TS, et al: Postoperative diskitis. Distinguishing early MR imaging findings from normal postoperative disk space changes. *Radiology* 184:765-771, 1992.

Chang KH, Han MH, Choi YW, et al: Tuberculous arachnoiditis of the spine: findings on myelography, CT, and MR findings. *AJNR* 10:1255-1262, 1989.

Chang K, Han M, Roh J, et al: Gd-DTPA-enhanced MR imaging in patients with meningitis. *AJNR* 11:69-76, 1990.

Coffe MJ, Hadley MN, Herrera GA, Morawetz RB: Dialysis-associated spondyloarthropathy. *J Neurosurg* 80:694-700, 1994.

Demaerel P, Wilms G, Van Lierde S, et al: Lyme disease in childhood presenting as primary leptomeningeal enhancement without parenchymal findings on MR. *AJNR* 15:302-304, 1994.

Edwards MK, Farlow MR, Stevens JC: Cranial MR in spinal cord MS: diagnosing patients with isolated spinal cord symptoms. *AJNR* 7:1003-1005, 1986.

Friedman DP: Herpes zoster myelitis: MR appearance. *AJNR* 13:1404-1406, 1992.

Gero B, Sze G, Sharif H: MR imaging of intradural inflammatory diseases of the spine. *AJNR* 12:1009-1019, 1991.

Heller RM, Szalay EA, Green HE, et al: Disc space infection in children: magnetic resonance imaging. *Rad Clin North Am* 26:207-210, 1988.

Holtas S, Basibuyuk N, Frederiksson K: MRI in acute transverse myelopathy. *Neuroradiology* 35:221-226, 1993.

Johnson CE, Sze G: Benign lumbar arachnoiditis: MR imaging with gadopentetate dimeglumine. *AJNR* 11:763-770, 1990.

Kelly RB, Mahoney PD, Cawley KM: MR demonstration of spinal cord sarcoidosis: report of a case. *AJNR* 9:197-199, 1988.

Kricun R, Shoemaker EL, Chovanes GI, Stephens HW: Epidural abscess of the cervical spine: MR findings in five cases. *AJR* 158:1145-1149, 1992.

Larsson E-M, Holtas S, Nilsson O: Gd-DTPA-enhanced MR of suspected spinal multiple sclerosis. *AJNR* 10:1071-1076, 1989.

Levy ML, Wieder BH, Schneider J, et al: Subdural empyema of the cervical spine: clinicopathological correlates and magnetic resonance imaging. Report of three cases. *J Neurosurg* 79:929-935, 1993.

Lexa FJ, Grossman RI: MR of sarcoidosis of the head and spine: spectrum of manifestations and radiographic response to steroid therapy. *AJNR* 15:973-982, 1994.

Malzberg MS, Rogg JM, Tate CA, et al: Poliomyelitis: hyperintensity of the anterior horn cells on MR images of the spinal cord. *AJR* 161:863-865, 1993.

Maravilla KR, Weinreb JC, Suss R, Nunnally RL: Magnetic resonance demonstration of multiple sclerosis plaques in the cervical cord. *AJNR* 5:685-689, 1984.

Merine D, Wang H, Kumar AJ, et al: CT myelography and MR imaging of acute transverse myelitis. *J Comput Assist Tomogr* 11:606-608, 1987.

Michikawa M, Wada Y, Sano M, et al: Radiation myelopathy: significance of gadolinium-DTPA enhancement in the diagnosis. *Neuroradiology* 33:286-289, 1991.

Miller GM, Baker HL Jr, et al: Spinal cord sarcoidosis: a new finding at MR imaging with Gd-DTPA enhancement. *Radiology* 173:839-843, 1989.

Modic MT, Feiglin DH, Piraino DW, et al: Vertebral osteomyelitis: assessment using MR. *Radiology* 157:157-166, 1985.

Nesbit GM, Miller GM, Baker HL Jr, et al: Spinal cord sarcoidosis: a new finding at MR imaging with Gd-DTPA enhancement. *Radiology* 173:839-843, 1989.

Numaguchi Y, Rigamonti D, Rothman MI, et al: Spinal epidural abscess: evaluation with gadolinium-enhanced MR imaging. *Radiographics* 13:545-559, 1993.

Nussbaum ES, Rigamonti D, Standiford H, et al: Spinal epidural abscess: a report of 40 cases and review. *Surg Neurol* 38:225-231, 1992.

Papadopoulos A, Gatzonis S, Gouliamos A, et al: Correlation between spinal cord MRI and clinical features in patients with demyelinating disease. *Neuroradiology* 36:130-133, 1994.

Perry JR, Fung A, Poon P, Bayer N: Magnetic resonance imaging of nerve root inflammation in the Guillain-Barré syndrome. *Neuroradiology* 36:139-140, 1994.

Post MJD, Sze G, Quencer RM, et al: Gadolinium-enhanced MR in spinal infection. *J Comput Assist Tomogr* 14:721-729, 1990.

Post MJD, Quencer RM, Montalvo BM, et al: Spinal infection: evaluation with MR imaging and intraoperative US. *Radiology* 169:765-771, 1988.

Ross JS, Masaryk TJ, Modic MT, et al: Magnetic resonance imaging of lumbar arachnoiditis. *AJNR* 8:885-892, 1987.

Sadato N, Numaguchi Y, Rigamonti D, et al: Spinal epidural abscess with gadolinium-enhanced MRI: serial follow-up studies and clinical correlation. *Neuroradiology* 36:44-48, 1994.

Sandhu FS, Dillon WP: Spinal epidural abscess: evaluation with contrast-enhanced MR imaging. *AJNR* 12:1087-1093, 1991.

Schultheiss TE, Stephens LC: Radiation myelopathy. *AJNR* 13:1056-1058, 1992.

Sharif HS: Role of MR imaging in the management of spinal infections. *AJR* 158:1333-1345, 1992.

Sharif HS, Aideyan OA, Clark DC, et al: Brucellar and tuberculosis spondylitis: comparative imaging features. *Radiology* 171:419-425, 1989.

Sklar EML, Post MJD, Lebwohl NH: Imaging of infection of the lumbo-sacral spine. *Neuroimaging* 3:577-590, 1993.

Smith AS, Blaser SI: Infections and inflammatory processes of the spine. *Rad Clin North Am* 29:809-828, 1991.

Smith AS, Weinstein MA, Mizushima A, et al: MR imaging of characteristics of tuberculosis spondylitis vs. vertebral osteomyelitis. *AJNR* 10:619-625, 1989.

Snyder RD, King JN, Keck GM, Orrison WW: MR imaging of the spinal cord in 23 subjects with ALD-AMN complex. *AJNR* 12:1095-1098, 1991.

Talpos D, Tien RD, Hesselink JR: Magnetic resonance imaging of AIDS related polyradiculopathy. *Neurology* 41:1996-1997, 1991.

Thrush A, Enzmann D: MR imaging of infectious spondylitis. *AJNR* 11:1171-1180, 1990.

Unger E, Moldofsky P, Gatenby R, et al: Diagnosis of osteomyelitis by MR imaging. *AJR* 150:605-610, 1988.

Wang P-Y, Shen W-C, Jan J-S: MR imaging in radiation myelopathy. *AJNR* 13:1049-1055, 1992.

Welk LA, Wuint DJ: Amyloidosis of the spine in a patient on long-term hemodialysis. *Neuroradiology* 32:334-336, 1990.

Yasui T, Yagura H, Komiyama M, et al: Significance of gadolinium-enhanced magnetic resonance imaging in differentiating spinal cord radiation myelopathy from tumor. Case report. *J Neurosurg* 77:628-631, 1992.

Zweig G, Russell EJ: Radiation myelopathy of the cervical spinal cord: MR findings. *AJNR* 11:1188-1190, 1990.

CHAPTER 17

Spinal Trauma, Cysts, Vascular Lesions, and Systemic Disorders

Case 1009A

53-year-old man with persistent back pain one
week after a fall from a ladder.
(sagittal, noncontrast scan; SE 550/20)

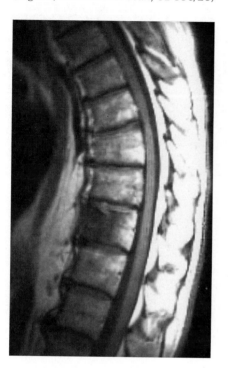

Case 1009B

Same patient.
(sagittal, noncontrast scan; low flip angle
GRE sequence)

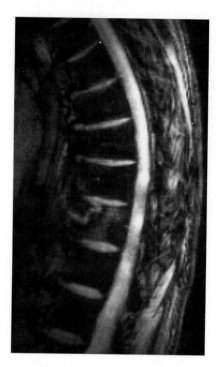

Recent compression fractures of vertebral bodies typically demonstrate altered signal intensity. The normally short T1 and T2 values of fatty marrow are replaced by water-like signal characteristics due to reactive edema and cellular infiltration.

In Case 1009 the anterior-superior corner of the T9 vertebral body has been fractured and slightly displaced. The T1-weighted scan (Case 1009A) demonstrates abnormally low signal intensity throughout the anterior portion of the involved body. The fracture line itself is best seen in Case 1009B with "myelographic" technique. Hazy areas of abnormally high intensity are present in adjacent portions of the vertebral body.

The reactive marrow edema associated with recent benign vertebral fractures may persist for weeks to months.

Eventually, the appearance of the compressed vertebra returns to the baseline of short T1 values.

During the subacute phase, posttraumatic marrow edema may mimic primary vertebral disease with secondary pathological fracture (see discussion of Cases 890 and 891). A search for additional lesions at other levels (or associated retroperitoneal or mediastinal masses) and clinical context can help to distinguish between benign and malignant vertebral fractures. Contrast-enhanced scans with fat suppression techniques may convincingly demonstrate underlying vertebral pathology at the involved level or elsewhere.

Note that the spinal canal and spinal cord are not compromised in this case, in contrast to the patients on the next page.

Case 1010

32-year-old man injured in an automobile accident
while wearing a seatbelt.
(sagittal, noncontrast scan; SE 800/17)

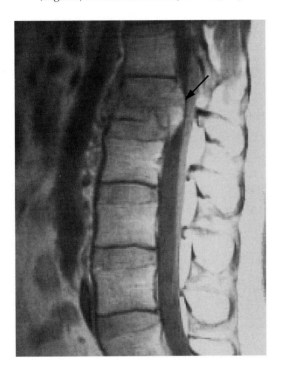

Case 1011

15-year-old boy injured in a three-wheeler
accident.
(sagittal, noncontrast scan; SE 1000/16)

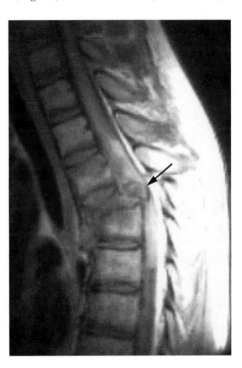

MR effectively demonstrates canal compromise and cord injury in cases of spinal trauma. Sagittal T1-weighted scans provide a rapid survey of vertebral alignment. Epidural soft tissue masses are defined, and cord compression is quantified.

Posttraumatic compromise of the spinal canal may be due to displacement of fracture fragments, associated hematomas, acute disc herniation, and/or frank dislocation. In Case 1010, a fracture of the L1 vertebral body is apparent, with posterior displacement of a bone fragment. Herniation of the T12-L1 disc and a small epidural hematoma accompany the osseous injury *(arrow)*. The conus medullaris is displaced and marginally compressed against the posterior border of the spinal canal.

Case 1011 demonstrates severe compression of the T4 vertebral body with associated dislocation. A fragment of the fractured vertebra has been displaced into the spinal canal *(arrow)*. Epidural (and possibly intradural) hemorrhage fills the canal from T2 to T6, obscuring the thecal sac and spinal cord. A localized prevertebral hematoma is present at the T5 level.

Case 1012

6-year-old girl, paraplegic after an automobile
accident, with normal spine x-rays.
(sagittal, noncontrast scan; SE 800/17)

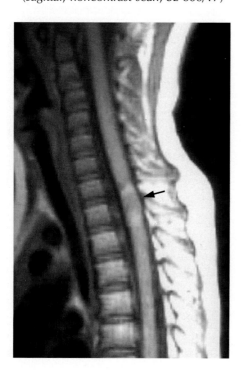

Case 1013

8-month-old girl, paraplegic after an automobile
accident, with normal spine x-rays.
(sagittal, noncontrast scan; low flip angle
GRE sequence)

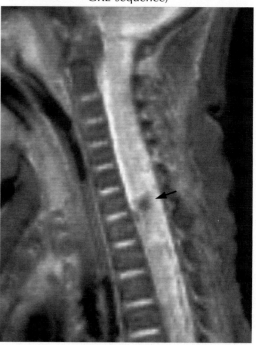

As illustrated on the preceding pages, MR scans can provide important soft tissue information in cases of spinal injury when osseous trauma is apparent on CT examinations or plain films. MR studies may also disclose neural injury when CT scans and routine radiographs are negative.

The pediatric spine is flexible and can undergo considerable subluxation without fracture. If such displacement is subsequently reduced, there may be no bony evidence of major spinal injury. The acronym "SCIWORA" (Spinal Cord Injury Without Radiographic Abnormality) has been used to describe this situation.

In Case 1012 vertebral alignment is normal. However, a zone of contusion with small areas of T1-shortening indicating subacute hemorrhage is seen within the spinal cord at the cervicothoracic junction (arrow). The child remained paraplegic, and a follow-up scan showed focal atrophy at this site (see Case 1014).

Case 1013 demonstrates a focal area of low signal intensity within the spinal cord at the C7-T1 level (arrow). This zone represents localized susceptibility effect due to a small region of acute intramedullary hemorrhage. Gradient echo sequences are more sensitive than spin echo techniques for detecting susceptibility changes caused by small amounts of blood within the brain or spinal canal (see also Case 1023B).

The demonstration of hemorrhage within an injured spinal cord has been correlated with poor prognosis. Patients whose cords contain nonhemorrhagic edema at the level of trauma have a better chance of neurological recovery.

Frank transection of the spinal cord may occur in the pediatric population and is well demonstrated by sagittal MR scans. Perinatal transection can occur during difficult breech deliveries. The most common site of transection in older children is the cervicothoracic junction, comparable to the level of cord injury in the above cases.

Case 1014

6-year-old girl, five months after
an automobile accident
(sagittal, noncontrast scan; SE 800/17)

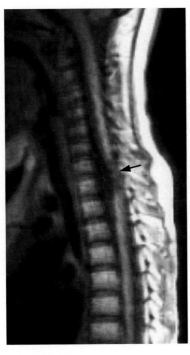

(same patient as Case 1012)

Case 1015

19-year-old woman, one year after
fracture/dislocation at C6-7.
(sagittal, noncontrast scan; SE 500/20)

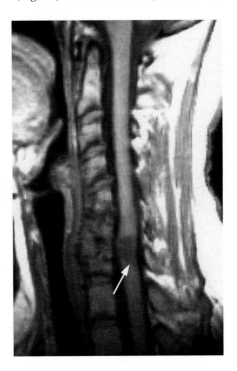

Focal injury to the spinal cord may result in localized parenchymal loss and/or cyst formation. Case 1014 is a follow-up scan of the patient presented in Case 1012. Severe atrophy is now seen at the site of the prior contusion. The spinal cord is reduced to ribbon-like thinness and appears to be tethered dorsally by adhesions.

Case 1015 illustrates cystic myelomalacia at the site of old cord injury. Rather than being atrophic as in Case 1014, the spinal cord is focally expanded by a small cyst that has formed in the damaged region. (Note that the cyst is confined to the level of prior injury, unlike the syrinxes in Cases 1017 and 1018.) A small cyst formed within a region of myelomalacia is usually not associated with further deterioration of function and rarely warrants evacuation.

However, an appearance similar to Case 1015 (localized cord "expansion") may indicate distortion of cord morphology by adhesions. Surgery to release tethering can lead to neurological improvement in such cases.

Case 1016A

3-year-old girl with persistent left arm paresis one
year after an automobile accident.
(axial, noncontrast scan; SE 800/15; C4 level)

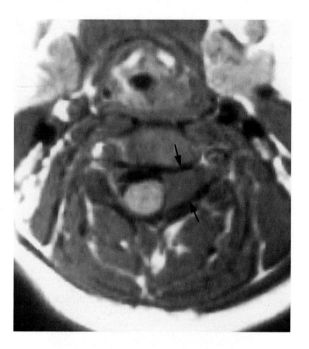

Case 1016B

Same patient.
(axial, noncontrast scan; low flip angle GRE
sequence; C4 level)

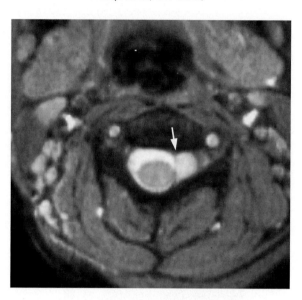

When the head and neck of a patient are turned and pulled away from a restraining or distracting force on an arm, stretch injury may occur within the brachial plexus. In severe cases, cervical nerve roots are avulsed from the spinal cord. Scans performed acutely in this setting may demonstrate a column of hemorrhage along the lateral margin of the cord at the site of the avulsed fila radicularia.

Leakage of CSF (or intrathecal contrast) from a torn cervical root sleeve is presumptive evidence of severe injury to the contained nerve. Leaking spinal fluid may form a localized or extensive pseudomeningocele, often with persistent communication to the subarachnoid space at the level of injury.

Case 1016 illustrates a posttraumatic pseudomeningocele occupying the left side of the spinal canal. The dura is faintly seen as a thin membrane separating the mildly deformed thecal sac from the epidural fluid pocket (*arrow*, Case 1016B). The pseudomeningocele in this case extended over three vertebral levels and was associated with avulsion of the C4, C5, and C6 nerve roots. (Note the lack of visualization of the left C4 dorsal root in Case 1016A, compared to the normal appearance on the right side.)

Case 1017

35-year-old man with a history of paraparesis, now presenting with increasing spasticity and arm weakness.
(sagittal, noncontrast scan; SE 550/20)

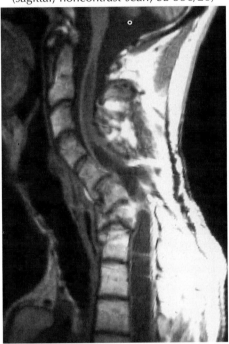

Case 1018

37-year-old man with a history of paraplegia due to fracture/dislocation at C6-7, now complaining of worsening arm numbness.
(coronal, noncontrast scan; SE 1000/20)

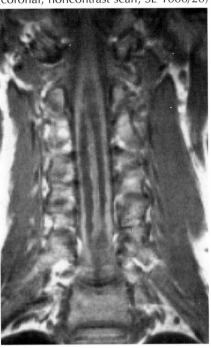

Magnetic resonance imaging has demonstrated that syringomyelia is a common delayed consequence of spinal injury. This diagnosis should be suspected when neurological function deteriorates months or years after trauma. MR is the procedure of choice for evaluating such cases. The presence of orthopedic fixation hardware usually does not contraindicate an MR scan or prevent at least partial visualization of the spinal cord.

An old fracture deformity at C7 is apparent in Case 1017. A large intramedullary cyst is present above and below the level of trauma. (Compare to the localized cystic myelomalacia in Case 1015.) The rostral extension of this cyst into the cervical spinal cord is the basis for the patient's worsening condition. Decompression of a posttraumatic syrinx is warranted and often results in a return to baseline neurological function.

Case 1018 presents an unusual double-barreled syrinx that has developed after trauma. This pattern, which has an "owl's eye" appearance on axial images, suggests symmetrical cord cavitation. In other cases, an eccentric posttraumatic syrinx is seen, resembling one of the two channels in Case 1018. Eccentric or twin-chambered morphology is rarely caused by congenital syringomyelia (see Cases 1051-1055).

Arachnoiditis occurring after spinal trauma may also be associated with the subsequent development of an intramedullary cyst. Tethering of neural elements by scar tissue is itself an important cause of late functional deterioration after spinal cord trauma, as discussed in Case 1015.

Case 1019

26-year-old man with a three-day history of increasing neck pain and leg weakness beginning after weight lifting.
(sagittal, noncontrast scan; SE 600/15)

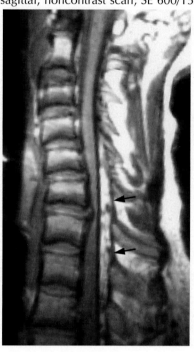

Case 1020

62-year-old man presenting with recurrent back pain one week after laminectomy.
(sagittal, noncontrast scan; SE 600/15)

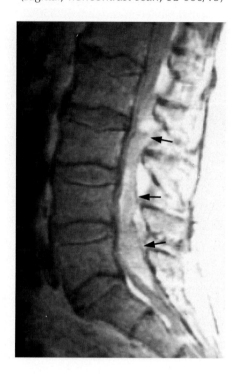

Epidural hemorrhage within the spinal canal may occur in association with disc herniation (see Case 830) or vertebral fracture (see Cases 1010 and 1011). In other patients, spinal epidural hematomas develop spontaneously or as an isolated consequence of trauma.

Spinal epidural hematomas vary widely in size and morphology. Relatively thin layers of epidural blood may cause early symptoms within small canals, as in Case 1019. The dorsal hematoma in this patient *(arrows)* combines with a disc bulge at C6-7 to compress the spinal cord.

The postoperative epidural hematoma in Case 1020 is much thicker, occupying most of the lumbar canal. The dural sac is reduced to a thin layer compressed anteriorly against the vertebral bodies. (Compare the morphology of the hematoma in Case 1020 to the postoperative pseudo-meningocele in Case 841.)

T1-shortening due to methemoglobin causes the subacute epidural hemorrhages in Cases 1019 and 1020 to be well defined. More acute epidural hematomas may be isointense on T1-weighted scans (see Case 1023), resembling other epidural pathologies. An isointense epidural (or subdural) hematoma (or empyema) is one cause of a featureless spinal canal lacking the normal definition of intrathecal nerve roots. (Imagine the appearance of Case 1020 if the hematoma did not demonstrate prominent T1-shortening.)

Both of the above hematomas extend over several vertebral levels, which is characteristic of epidural hemorrhage. Multilevel involvement is also typical of epidural abscesses and of some epidural tumors (e.g., lymphoma).

Subdural hemorrhages occur within the spinal canal and can be difficult to distinguish from epidural collections. Occasional spinal subdural hematomas develop as an extension of an intracranial hematoma or in association with spinal subarachnoid hemorrhage.

DIFFERENTIAL DIAGNOSIS:
THICK EPIDURAL TISSUE WITH SHORT T1 VALUES

Case 1021

84-year-old woman presenting with paraplegia one week after a minor fall.
(sagittal, noncontrast scan; SE 600/20)

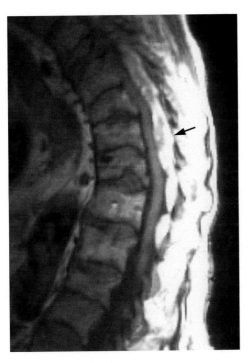

Epidural Hematoma

Case 1022

27-year-old man, moderately obese but otherwise well, presenting with mild spasticity of the legs.
(sagittal, noncontrast scan; SE 1500/30)

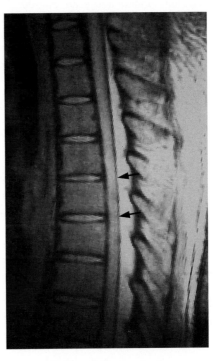

Epidural Lipomatosis

Case 1021 illustrates that spinal epidural hemorrhage may be spontaneous, occurring after trivial or unrecognized trauma. The morphology of this hematoma is distinctly lobulated, contrasting with the more linear collections on the preceding page. The superior pole of the hematoma demonstrates central areas of isointensity (see Case 1024 for an axial view of this region). In short, Case 1021 demonstrates the variable clinical context, morphology, and signal intensity of spinal epidural hemorrhage.

Lipomatosis is another potential cause of thickened epidural tissue with high signal intensity on T1-weighted scans. Abnormal accumulation of epidural fat is most often seen in the thoracic canal of patients who are obese or are exposed to high endogenous or exogenous levels of corticosteroids. The condition may cause symptomatic cord compression.

Case 1022 illustrates prominent thickening of epidural fat posterior to the thecal sac. The underlying subarachnoid space is partially effaced, and the spinal cord is mildly com-

pressed. (Compare cord definition in the midthoracic region to the appearance at the cervicothoracic junction.)

Like epidural hemorrhage, epidural lipomatosis typically extends over long segments of the spinal canal with either linear or lobulated morphology. Scans performed with fat suppression techniques can distinguish between these two pathologies in ambiguous cases. The signal intensity of lipomatous tissue will be reduced by such sequences, while the T1-shortening of aqueous protons caused by the presence of paramagnetic methemoglobin within a hematoma will be unaltered.

Epidural abscesses are often hemorrhagic (see Case 979) and should be included in the differential diagnosis of thick epidural tissue containing short T1 values. Similarly, epidural metastases containing paramagnetic substances (e.g., melanin) or subacute hemorrhage (e.g., leukemia) may present a similar appearance. Rare epidural angiolipomas and hemangiomas (see Case 889) can involve the dorsal thoracic region and resemble the more common pathologies discussed above.

Case 1023A

80-year-old woman presenting with the sudden onset of neck pain and right hemiparesis three days earlier.
(sagittal, noncontrast scan; SE 500/17)

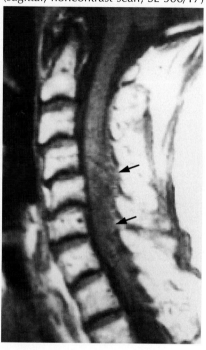

Case 1023B

Same patient.
(sagittal, noncontrast scan; low flip angle GRE sequence)

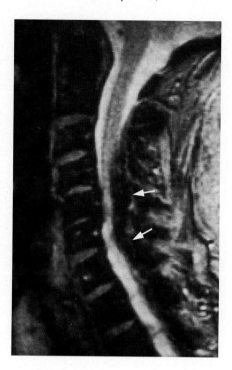

The characteristic evolution of signal intensities described for intracerebral hematomas (see Cases 555 to 558) is less rapid and less regular within extraparenchymal hemorrhages, either cranial or spinal. In particular, spinal epidural hematomas may appear isointense on T1-weighted scans for many days after the onset of bleeding. This prolonged "acute" phase may cause diagnostic confusion, mimicking other epidural processes.

In Case 1023A, a dorsal epidural mass extends from C3 to C7. The nonspecific mass is nearly isointense to cord parenchyma. However, the gradient echo sequence in Case 1023B demonstrates low signal intensity within the same region. This evidence for local magnetic susceptibility effect

correctly suggests the presence of blood products within the epidural tissue and identifies the lesion.

In some cases low signal intensity on gradient echo scans due to susceptibility effects is seen only at the margins of an epidural hematoma. The resulting dark rim around the lesion resembles the morphology of the contrast enhancement in Case 1025.

The above scans demonstrate moderate compression of the spinal cord at the C5 level due to the combination of mild subluxation and the dorsal hematoma. Susceptibility effects at interfaces on gradient echo images often exaggerate the degree of canal compromise associated with extradural deformities. The spinal canal in Case 1023B is probably not as tight as it appears.

Case 1024

84-year-old woman presenting with paraplegia.
(axial, noncontrast scan; SE 1200/20; T6-7 level)

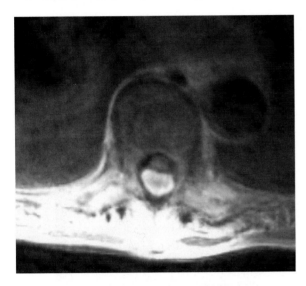

(same patient as Case 1021)

Case 1025

80-year-old woman presenting with neck pain and
right hemiparesis.
(axial, postcontrast scan; SE 700/17; C4-5 level)

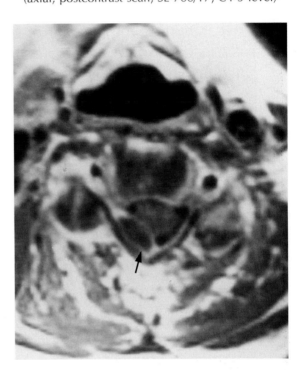

(same patient as Case 1023)

The appearance of spinal epidural hematomas on axial scans is variable, depending on the age of the collection and the presence or absence of contrast material.

In Case 1024 a midline dorsal epidural hematoma demonstrates peripheral T1-shortening surrounding a center of intermediate signal intensity. This pattern suggests subacute hemorrhage, with oxidation of methemoglobin proceeding inward from the perimeter of the clot (compare to Cases 557 and 563). Note the ventral displacement and flattening of the spinal cord, and compare this scan to the epidural abscess in Case 980.

The hematoma in Case 1025 arises posterolaterally rather than in the midline, demonstrating a more elliptical contour than Case 1024. Both of these locations and morphologies are common for spontaneous or posttraumatic epidural hemorrhages.

Peripheral high signal intensity at the margin of the lesion in Case 1025 represents contrast enhancement. The rim-enhancing morphology of an "acute" epidural hematoma resembles the appearance of some epidural abscesses (see Case 981). These two pathologies must often be considered together in the differential diagnosis of an epidural lesion.

Case 1026

59-year-old woman presenting with back pain.
(sagittal, noncontrast scan; SE 550/20)

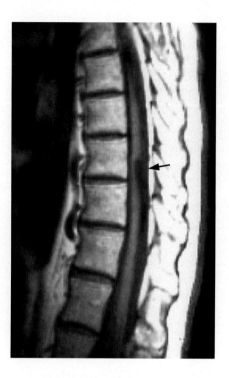

Case 1027

85-year-old woman with increasing difficulty walking, twenty years after thoracic decompression for myelopathy of unknown etiology.
(sagittal, noncontrast scan; SE 500/20)

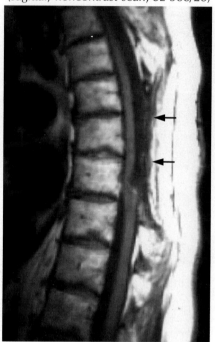

Spinal arachnoid cysts most frequently occur within the thoracic canal, particularly dorsal to the spinal cord (as in the above cases). The formation of cysts in this region likely reflects loculation of the dorsal subarachnoid space, which is normally traversed by multiple arachnoid septations. Partial obstruction of CSF circulation within a subarachnoid compartment may lead to progressive enlargement and eventual cord compression.

Arachnoiditis due to subarachnoid hemorrhage or meningitis may also cause loculation of the spinal subarachnoid space. In Case 1027 it was not clear whether an arachnoid cyst was present at the time of initial surgery or formed subsequently in the operative region.

Like arachnoid cysts overlying the cerebral convexity (see Cases 675 and 676), spinal arachnoid cysts often demonstrate linear or angular margins. In each of the above cases, the interface between the cyst and the spinal cord is quite straight. Cord compression is present in both patients.

The lesions in Cases 1026 and 1027 appear to be benign and extraaxial (but see Case 1029). A contrast-enhanced scan could be considered to exclude the rare possibility of an exophytic, cystic tumor (e.g., hemangioblastoma arising at the pial surface).

Case 1060 presents an arachnoid cyst within the cervical spinal canal.

Case 1028A

58-year-old man presenting with back pain.
(sagittal, noncontrast scan; SE 550/20)

Case 1028B

Same patient.
(axial, noncontrast scan; SE 2500/90)

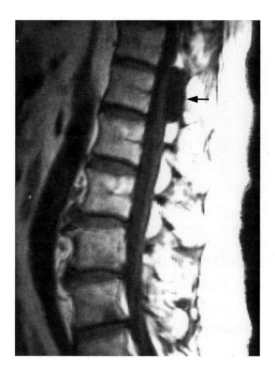

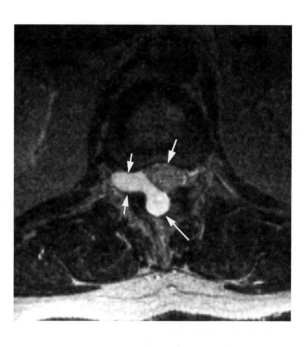

Occasional spinal arachnoid cysts are encountered in the epidural space, most commonly in the dorsal thoracic or lumbar region. This occurrence requires a congenital or acquired defect in the dura through which a loculation of the subarachnoid space can extend. Transmitted pulsation from the thecal sac and/or "ball-valve" restriction of bidirectional flow at the neck of the cyst may then lead to its enlargement. Some epidural "meningeal cysts" arise from a pedicle that originates where a dorsal nerve root penetrates the dura.

In contrast to the typically flat morphology of intradural arachnoid cysts as seen on the preceding page, extradural cysts are often round and lobulated. The spherical margins of the lesion in Case 1028A are outlined by dorsal epidural fat. Case 1028B demonstrates lobulated contours of the mass extending into the right intervertebral foramen *(short arrows)* and eroding the posterior vertebral arch in the midline *(long arrow)*. The dural sac is mildly displaced *(midsized arrow)*.

Compare the long-standing lobulated extradural cyst in this case to the similarly chronic dural diverticulae in Case 842 and to the acquired dorsal pseudomeningocele in Case 841.

Case 1029A

44-year-old man presenting with progressive myelopathy.
(sagittal, noncontrast scan; SE 600/15)

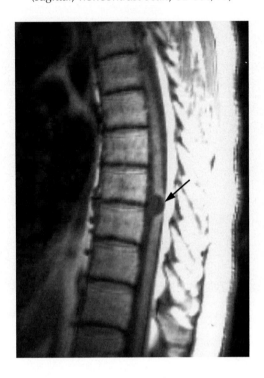

Case 1029B

Same patient.
(axial, noncontrast scan; SE 700/15; T9-10 level)

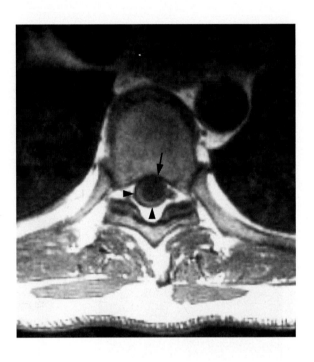

Another uncommon cystic lesion of the spinal canal is the benign intramedullary cyst. These idiopathic masses are often eccentric and exophytic, mimicking an intradural extramedullary process.

Case 1029 illustrates a round lesion of low signal intensity occupying most of the spinal canal in the midthoracic region. Spinal cord parenchyma is draped around the posterior and lateral margins of the embedded cyst (*arrowheads*, Case 1029B). A postcontrast scan demonstrated no abnormal enhancement at the perimeter of the cyst or within the cord.

The differential diagnosis in this case is broad. An intradural extramedullary tumor (such as a small schwannoma) could present a similar morphology in this location with long T1 and T2 values but would be expected to enhance with contrast material. An intradural extramedullary parasitic cyst (e.g., cysticercosis) could be considered in the appropriate clinical context. A neurenteric cyst is unlikely in the absence of adjacent vertebral deformity (see Cases 1091 and 1092). An arachnoid cyst of the thoracic canal is improbable given the ventral location and round morphology of the lesion (compare to Cases 1026 and 1027). A cystic intramedullary tumor is largely excluded by the absence of associated contrast enhancement.

At surgery, a benign "neuroepithelial" cyst was found to arise exophytically from the spinal cord. Although this lesion is relatively rare, the characteristic appearance as demonstrated above has enabled preoperative diagnosis in a number of cases.

Case 1030

61-year-old man presenting with back pain.
(sagittal, noncontrast scan; SE 500/15)

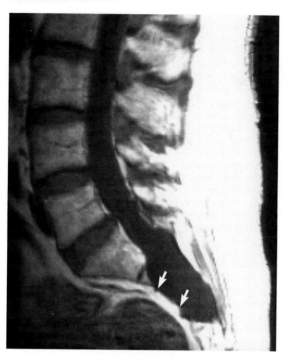

Intrasacral Meningocele

Case 1031

18-year-old man presenting with left
S1 radiculopathy.
(axial, noncontrast scan; SE 2500/45; S1 level)

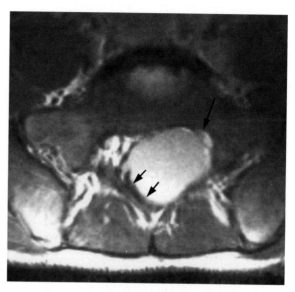

Perineural Cyst
("Tarlov" cyst)

CSF-containing masses are commonly found within the sacral canal. These may arise from the thecal sac or from sacral nerve roots. The benign and long-standing nature of the lesions is indicated by smooth erosion of adjacent bone, as seen in the above cases.

Among sacral cysts arising from the thecal sac are intrasacral or "occult" meningoceles, illustrated by Case 1030. Instead of tapering and terminating normally, the dural sac broadens within the sacral canal. Mass effect and CSF pulsation have caused erosion of the sacrum both anteriorly *(arrows)* and posteriorly. In some cases, an enlarged caudal sac balloons into the pelvis as an anterior sacral meningocele.

Another variety of sacral cyst is analogous to the extradural arachnoid cyst occasionally found at higher levels of the spinal canal (see Case 1028). A pedicle or neck communicates from the tip of the caudal sac to a sacral epidural cyst, which can fill and expand the sacral canal. Such lesions lack the broad communication with the dural sac of Case 1030. As a result, their signal intensity is usu-

ally higher than normal CSF due to elevated protein content and/or lack of pulsation-related signal loss.

"Tarlov" or perineural cysts arise from nerve root sleeves rather than from the dural sac. These cystic diverticula or ectasias may occur at any level but are particularly common in the sacral region. They are a frequent incidental finding but can enlarge to cause compressive radiculopathy.

In Case 1031 a large perineural cyst occupies much of the sacral canal. The left S1 nerve is displaced and compressed at the anterolateral margin of the cyst *(long arrow)*. The cyst displaces the dural sac and other roots posteriorly and to the right *(short arrows)*.

Sacral root sleeve cysts are often bilateral. They may accompany sacral nerves into the pelvis, mimicking the dural ectasia seen in connective tissue disorders such as Marfan's syndrome.

Epidermoid cysts should also be considered in the differential diagnosis of expansile masses within the sacral canal demonstrating long T1 and T2 values.

Case 1032A

27-year-old woman who developed paraplegia
following surgery to remove a herniated disc
at T10-11.
(sagittal, noncontrast scan; SE 2800/90)

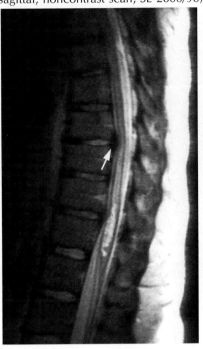

Case 1032B

Same patient.
(sagittal, postcontrast scan; SE 600/15)

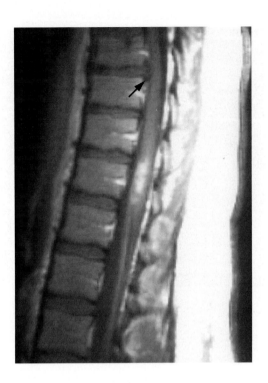

Infarction of the spinal cord may occur in a variety of clinical contexts. The most common association is an atherosclerotic aneurysm of the thoracolumbar aorta, either before or after surgery. Other possible etiologies include vasculitis (e.g., syphilis, collagen vascular disease), systemic embolization, trauma, and coagulopathy.

The thoracic spinal cord and conus medullaris are the regions most commonly affected by cord ischemia, although cervical cord infarcts also occur. Central gray matter of the cord is more severely damaged by ischemia than the peripheral white matter tracts (see Case 1033).

Case 1032 demonstrates typical findings in an atypical context. Abnormal high signal intensity involves central gray matter of the conus medullaris on a T2-weighted scan (Case 1032A). The center of the lesion is sharply defined, with an adjacent zone of less distinct signal abnormality extending rostrally into the thoracic region. Intense contrast enhancement is present within the infarct (Case 1032B).

The site of disc herniation at T10-11 *(arrows)* indents the ventral subarachnoid space and causes mild deformity of the spinal cord. It is conceivable that this epidural compression could lead to local compromise of the anterior spinal artery. A number of cases of spinal cord infarction secondary to disc herniation have been reported, including demonstration of embolic nuclear material within the anterior spinal artery. No other etiology for cord infarction was apparent in this young patient.

Equivocal swelling of the conus medullaris is seen in the above scans. Occasional cord infarcts demonstrate sufficient mass effect to resemble intramedullary tumors. In most cases the cord margins are not significantly expanded, and the differential diagnosis includes inflammatory or degenerative disorders (e.g., multiple sclerosis or amyotrophic lateral sclerosis). Compare the enhancing lesion in Case 1032B to Cases 960, 961B, 991, and 993.

DIFFERENTIAL DIAGNOSIS:
CENTRAL SIGNAL ABNORMALITY WITHIN THE CONUS MEDULLARIS

Case 1033

75-year-old man with acute paraplegia following angioplasty for renal artery stenosis.
(axial, noncontrast scan; SE 2500/45; T12-L1 level)

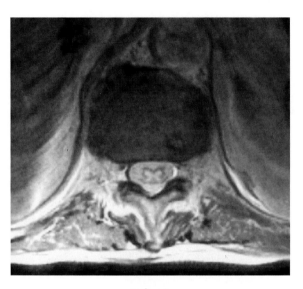

Infarct

Case 1034

68-year-old woman presenting with progressive impairment of bowel and bladder function.
(axial, noncontrast scan; low flip angle GRE sequence; T12-L1 level)

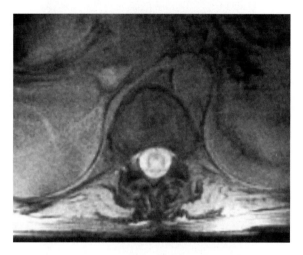

Metastatic Carcinoma of the Breast

Case 1033 illustrates abnormally high signal intensity within central gray matter of the conus medullaris. This pattern is characteristic of spinal cord infarction. The relative sparing of white matter tracts probably reflects both the greater metabolic demand of cell bodies and the collateral blood supply to the perimeter of the cord.

However, abnormal signal intensity confined to gray matter of the spinal cord is not specific for ischemia. Similar images may be obtained in patients with inflammatory or degenerative neuronal disorders (e.g., poliomyelitis). Intramedullary edema due to dural arteriovenous fistulae may also predominantly involve central gray matter.

Some cases of spinal cord ischemia affect only a portion of the gray matter anatomy demonstrated in Case 1033. For

example, involvement limited to the anterior horns of the cord may present a "snake eyes" or "owl's eyes" morphology.

Case 1033 reinforces two points made on the preceding page: (1) spinal cord infarction should be considered as the potential etiology of myelopathy in patients with atherosclerotic disease and (2) the conus medullaris is a common site of cord ischemia, so that infarction should be included in the differential diagnosis of a conus lesion.

The conus medullaris is also a frequent location for intramedullary metastases, as discussed in Chapter 15 (see Case 901). Case 1034 demonstrates edema within the conus due to a small metastatic nodule, which was defined on a postcontrast scan.

Case 1035

73-year-old man presenting with rapidly worsening
back pain and paraparesis.
(sagittal, postcontrast scan; SE 600/15)

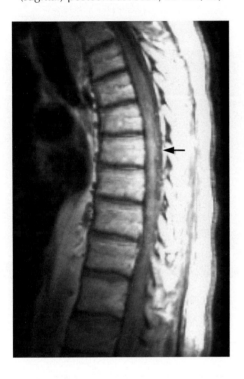

Case 1036

52-year-old woman with a several year history of
thoracic myelopathy.
(sagittal, noncontrast scan; RSE 3500/119)

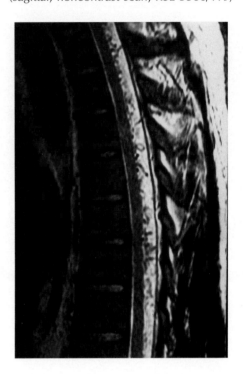

Several types of arteriovenous malformations may be found within the spinal canal. The most common is the dural arteriovenous fistula, or "radiculomedullary fistula." This lesion consists of an arteriovenous shunt occurring within the dura near the exit of a spinal nerve root. Intradural venous drainage from the fistula floods the valveless coronal venous plexus on the surface of the spinal cord. The transmitted pressure and flow distends perimedullary veins for multiple levels rostral and/or caudal to the shunt. Venous hypertension impairs drainage of spinal cord parenchyma, causing intramedullary edema and occasionally frank infarction.

A broad range of findings has been noted on MR scans of patients with spinal dural arteriovenous fistulae. In some cases the MR scan is normal, with no evidence of a fistula that is subsequently proven angiographically and/or surgically. (Myelography with water-soluble contrast material may be helpful for delineation of small, distended veins on the surface of the cord in patients with negative MR scans in the face of high clinical suspicion.)

Other patients demonstrate nonspecific cord edema and swelling, reflecting passive congestion due to venous hypertension (see Case 1037). Patchy intramedullary contrast enhancement (as in Case 1035) and/or pial enhancement may be present but is nonspecific.

Finally, distended intradural veins may be visualized with variable definition. In some cases the presence of dilated pial vessels causes a subtle irregularity or "fuzziness" along the surface of the spinal cord. In other patients, a few tortuous "flow voids" can be specifically identified at the cord margin, as seen along the dorsal surface of the cord in the midthoracic region in Case 1035 *(arrow)*. In some cases, contrast enhancement convincingly demonstrates abnormal vascular channels on the surface of the cord when noncontrast scans are equivocal. Only occasionally are distended intradural veins as well seen as in Case 1036.

The presence of dilated perimedullary vessels is not specific for spinal vascular malformations. Occasional tumors (especially ependymomas and hemangioblastomas) may cause a similar appearance (see Case 952A).

DIFFERENTIAL DIAGNOSIS:
EDEMA AND SWELLING OF THE CONUS MEDULLARIS

Case 1037

64-year-old man presenting with a two-year history
of worsening myelopathy.
(sagittal, noncontrast scan; SE 800/17)

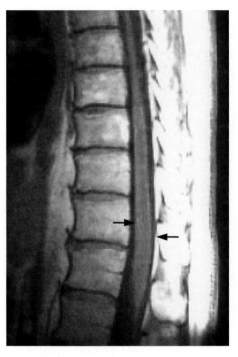

Dural Arteriovenous Fistula

Case 1038

68-year-old woman presenting with progressive
conus dysfunction.
(sagittal, noncontrast scan; SE 350/17)

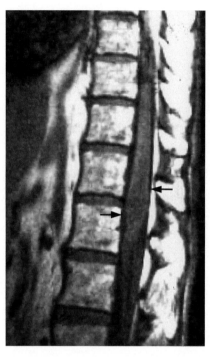

Metastatic Carcinoma of the Breast

The expansion and low signal intensity involving the thoracic cord and conus medullaris in Case 1037 were due to edema caused by a spinal dural arteriovenous fistula. Distended intradural vessels are only equivocally suggested on the MR scan but were demonstrated angiographically.

A history of long-standing progressive myelopathy is characteristic of patients with spinal dural AV fistulae. Such symptoms should suggest the diagnosis, particularly in middle-aged or elderly men. (The male to female ratio of this disorder is about 8 to 1.) Intramedullary edema is a common finding in such cases and may be diffuse (as in Case 1037) or confined to central gray matter (resembling Case 1033).

Spinal dural arteriovenous fistulae can be successfully obliterated angiographically or surgically. They represent an important treatable cause of myelopathy. The prognosis is best when the diagnosis is made prior to the onset of extensive intramedullary edema.

Case 1038 is a reminder that metastatic disease should always be suspected when a lesion is found within the conus medullaris of an adult. An enhancing intramedullary nodule was demonstrated on a postcontrast scan.

INTRADURAL ARTERIOVENOUS MALFORMATIONS

Case 1039

59-year-old woman presenting with paraparesis.
(sagittal, noncontrast scan; SE 500/20)

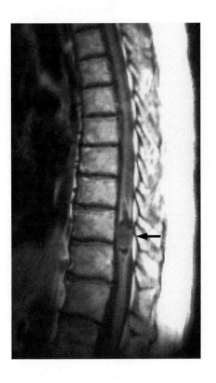

Case 1040

45-year-old man presenting with back and leg pain.
(sagittal, noncontrast scan; SE 2800/90)

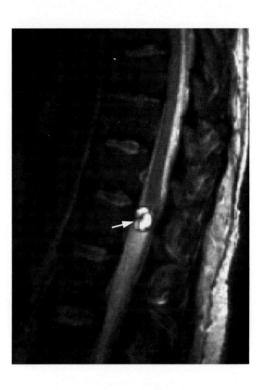

True arteriovenous malformations (AVMs) are much less common within the spinal canal than the dural arteriovenous fistulae illustrated on the preceding pages. Intradural AVMs may occur within the spinal cord (as in Case 1039) or in an extramedullary location (as in Case 1040). The lesions demonstrate variable patency. The AVMs in both of the above cases were thrombosed and angiographically "occult."

Low signal intensity capping the rostral and caudal portions of the lesion in Case 1039 may reflect calcification and/or hemosiderin from old hemorrhage. This appearance resembles the common finding of blood products at the margins of some intramedullary tumors. The potential resemblance of intramedullary AVMs and primary neoplasms is compounded by the occasional presence of dilated superficial vessels adjacent to cord tumors (due to hyperemia and/or partial venous obstruction).

The extramedullary mass at the surface of the conus medullaris in Case 1040 is nonspecific. A thrombosed vascular malformation is a rare etiology for such a lesion. Differential diagnosis would include a necrotic or hemorrhagic schwannoma (see Case 923) or an unusual ependymoma. The mass demonstrated intense enhancement on a postcontrast scan.

Case 1041

58-year-old woman scanned three days after the
acute onset of severe backache and headache.
(sagittal, noncontrast scan; SE 500/20)

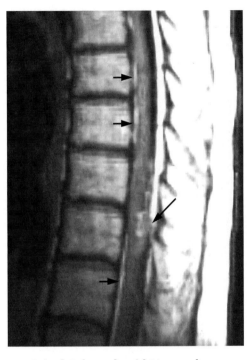

Spinal Subarachnoid Hemorrhage

Case 1042

59-year-old woman presenting with paraparesis.
(sagittal, noncontrast scan; low flip angle
GRE sequence)

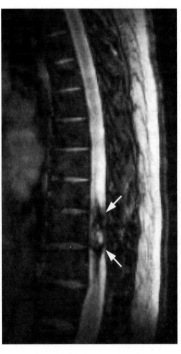

Occult Arteriovenous Malformation
(same patient as Case 1039)

Linear and nodular areas of T1-shortening are present along the margins of the spinal cord in Case 1041. Axial images confirmed the intradural, extramedullary location of the high intensity zones, which are due to subarachnoid hemorrhage. Despite a thorough work-up including spinal angiography, the source of the bleeding was not determined.

Compare Case 1041 to the examples of intracranial subarachnoid hemorrhage in Cases 589 and 590, to the subacute spinal epidural hematomas in Cases 1019 and 1021, and to enhancing subarachnoid carcinomatosis outlining the spinal cord in Cases 905-907.

As is true in the intracranial compartment, spinal subarachnoid hemorrhage may accumulate locally to form a focal hematoma. This sequestration of blood is common in the dorsal subarachnoid space of the thoracic canal, where arachnoid septations are numerous. (See the discussion of spinal arachnoid cysts in Cases 1026 and 1027.)

Such subarachnoid hematomas may mimic vascular intradural masses. The small dorsal accumulation of blood at the T10 level in Case 1041 *(long arrow)* closely resembled the appearance of Case 1042 on gradient echo images.

Case 1042 demonstrates the intramedullary mass of Case 1039 surrounded by flame-shaped zones of low signal intensity extending into adjacent parenchyma. The susceptibility-induced signal loss at the margins of this occult AVM is caused by the presence of blood products (mainly hemosiderin) and is emphasized by the gradient echo pulse sequence. Similar peripheral and/or interstitial T2-shortening may also be seen in cavernous angiomas, which occur in both intramedullary and intradural extramedullary locations.

A spinal source should be considered when no other etiology is found for intracranial subarachnoid hemorrhage. This is particularly true if (1) the hemorrhage is concentrated in the posterior fossa and/or (2) back pain is a prominent initial symptom.

Case 1043

56-year-old man presenting with headaches.
(sagittal, noncontrast scan; SE 600/15)

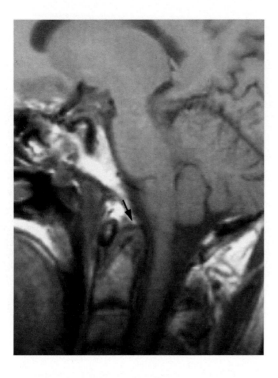

Case 1044

70-year-old woman presenting with neck pain.
(sagittal, noncontrast scan; SE 800/17)

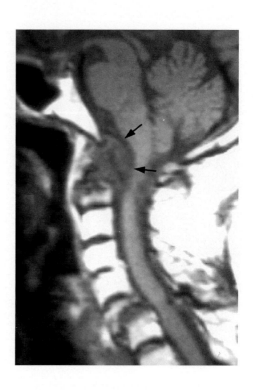

Synovial inflammation in rheumatoid arthritis may involve the articulation of the odontoid process with the anterior arch of C1 and the transverse ligament. Erosion of the odontoid often develops, with a surrounding pannus of thickened soft tissue. These findings are demonstrated in Cases 1043 and 1044.

Bone erosion and soft tissue inflammation at the C1-C2 articulation may lead to ligamentous laxity and subluxation. The head and C1 may move ventrally with respect to the odontoid process and the remainder of the cervical spine, widening the atlantodental interval and narrowing the spinal canal at C1-2.

Chronic instability at C1-C2 can also result in the development of a fibrous mass along the ventral margin of the foramen magnum. Such "pseudotumors" may themselves cause compressive myelopathy. Case 1044 illustrates a mound of inflammatory and reactive tissue occupying the anterior portion of the foramen magnum *(arrows)*. The location and effect of the lesion resemble the tumors in Cases 917 and 918.

A compression fracture of C6, subluxation at C6-7, posterior fusion of vertebral bodies at C4-5, and fatty marrow atrophy are also apparent in Case 1044.

Case 1045

53-year-old woman presenting with neck pain.
(sagittal, noncontrast scan; SE 800/17)

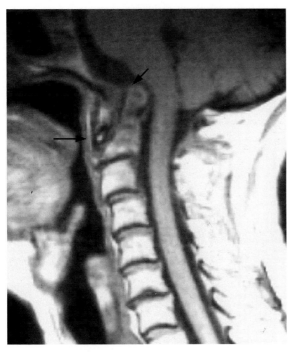

Rheumatoid Arthritis

Case 1046

10-year-old boy presenting with quadriparesis.
(sagittal, noncontrast scan; SE 600/15)

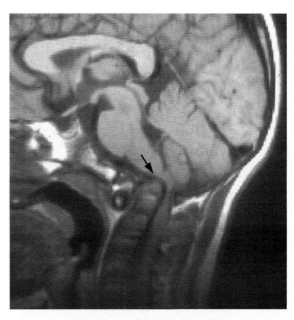

Congenital Subluxation at C1-2

A number of conditions may involve subluxation at C1-2 allowing the odontoid process to ascend into the foramen magnum. The most common cause of a "high-riding" odontoid process in adults is rheumatoid arthritis, as illustrated in Case 1045. In this patient, the dens *(short arrow)* has risen through the ring of C1 *(long arrow)* to present as a premedullary mass (compare to Case 1048).

Superior displacement of the odontoid in rheumatoid arthritis is aggravated by "cranial settling" due to erosion and reduced height of the lateral masses of C1. Resultant distortion of the medulla or cervicomedullary junction may be much more severe than demonstrated in Case 1045.

The deformity of the craniocervical junction in Case 1046 was congenital and idiopathic. Many patients with abnor-

mal flattening of the skull base ("platybasia") suffer from compromise of the foramen magnum due to associated basilar invagination with encroachment of the dens (see Cases 1047 and 1048 on the next page). The displaced odontoid process in Case 1046 has caused severe distortion and compression of the cervicomedullary junction. Transoral resection of the odontoid was performed to relieve the brainstem deformity in this case.

Compare the degree of compression of the cervicomedullary junction in Case 1046 to the adult patient in Case 876. Remarkable thinning of the medulla or spinal cord may be surprisingly well tolerated if the deformity progresses gradually. Eventual symptoms may then lead to the discovery of a ribbon-like band of flattened parenchyma.

Case 1047

34-year-old man presenting with headaches.
(sagittal, noncontrast scan; SE 600/20)

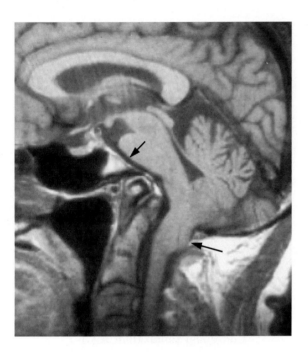

Case 1048

58-year-old woman presenting with occipital pain
(and a history of posterior decompression
of the foramen magnum).
(sagittal, noncontrast scan; SE 600/14)

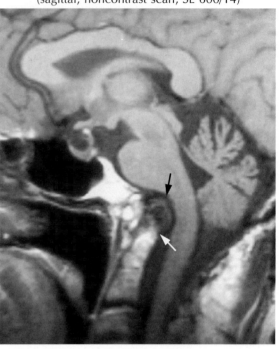

As seen in the previous pages, both congenital deformity and acquired pathology can cause abnormal alignment (and instability) at the craniocervical junction. Superimposed degenerative changes often contribute to clinical consequences in either instance.

In Case 1047, the clivus is congenitally short and flat *(short arrow)*. The elongated odontoid process represents the anterior margin of the foramen magnum. The belly of the pons is flattened, and the medulla is kinked. Cerebellar tissue extends through the foramen magnum dorsal to the spinal cord *(long arrow)*, representing a Chiari I hindbrain deformity (see Cases 712 and 713). Basilar invagination is associated with parenchymal malformation in about 30% of cases.

The clivus in Case 1048 is also somewhat flat. The odon-

toid process projects above the plane of the atlas *(white arrow)*. A degenerative pseudomass consisting of calcified fibrous tissue has developed at the top of the odontoid process *(black arrow)*, deforming the ventral medulla.

Soft tissue thickening in the region of the odontoid process may reflect old trauma and/or ligamentous laxity, with excessive motion between C1 and C2. Whatever the cause, the mound of degenerative change can act as an anterior epidural mass and cause myelopathy, requiring resection and/or decompression.

Acquired disorders such as Paget's disease and osteomalacia can soften the skull base and lead to basilar impression, resembling the anatomical distortion of the above cases.

DOWN SYNDROME INVOLVING THE CRANIOCERVICAL JUNCTION

Case 1049

31-year-old man with a six-month history of abnormal gait due to increasing leg spasticity and ataxia.
(sagittal, noncontrast scan; SE 800/17)

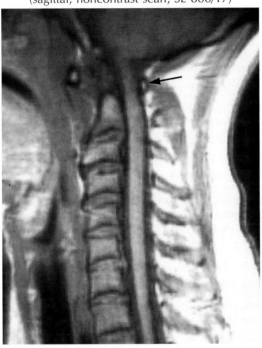

Case 1050

2-year-old boy presenting with mild spasticity.
(sagittal, noncontrast scan; SE 600/20)

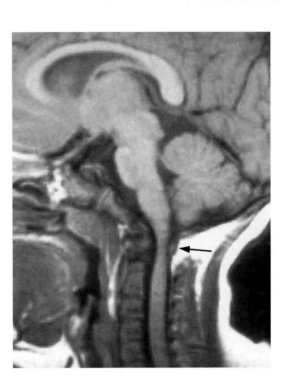

Subluxation at C1-2 due to ligamentous laxity is common in Down syndrome (trisomy 21). Case 1049 illustrates wide separation between the anterior arch of C1 and the hypoplastic odontoid process. The spinal canal is correspondingly narrowed, with reduced distance between the posterior arch of C1 *(arrow)* and the base of the dens. Compression of the spinal cord may be exacerbated by head movement or trauma in such cases.

Atlantoaxial subluxation is less prominent in Case 1050. However, constriction of the craniocervical junction is present, due predominantly to the abnormally short posterior arch of C1 *(arrow)*. This common malformation in pa-

tients with Down syndrome may combine with C1-2 subluxation to cause severe cord compression.

In addition to causing neural compression, lesions crowding or narrowing the foramen magnum may predispose to the development of syringomyelia (see Cases 689 and 712).

Other congenital syndromes often associated with compromise of the foramen magnum are achondroplasia (see discussion of Case 847), osteopetrosis, and the mucopolysaccharidoses. The latter are characterized by ligamentous laxity at C1-2, a hypoplastic odontoid process, and intraspinal soft tissue masses due to the deposition of mucopolysaccharides.

REFERENCES

Anson JA, Spetzler RF: Surgical resection of intramedullary spinal cord cavernous malformations. *J Neurosurg* 78:446-451, 1993.

Avrahami E, Tadmor R, Ram Z, et al: MR demonstration of spontaneous acute epidural hematoma of the thoracic spine. *Neuroradiology* 31:89-92, 1989.

Barkovich AJ, Sherman JL, Citrin CM, Wippold FJ II: MR of postoperative syringomyelia. *AJNR* 8:319-328, 1987.

Barnwell SL, Dowd CF, Davis RL, et al: Cryptic vascular malformations of the spinal cord: diagnosis by magnetic resonance imaging and outcome of surgery. *J Neurosurg* 72:403-407, 1990.

Bassi P, Corona C, Contri P, et al: Congenital basilar impression: correlated neurological syndromes. *Eur Neurol* 32:238-243, 1992.

Beers GJ, Raque GH, Wagner GG: MR imaging in acute cervical spine trauma. *J Comput Assist Tomogr* 12:755-761, 1988.

Bundschuh CV, Modic MT, Kearney F, et al: Rheumatoid arthritis of the cervical spine: surface-coil MR imaging. *AJNR* 9:565-571, 1988.

Casselman JW, Jolie E, Dehaene I, Meeus L: Gadolinium-enhanced MR imaging of infarction of the anterior spinal cord. *AJNR* 12:561-562, 1991.

Chakeres DW, Flickinger F, Bresnahan JC, et al: MR imaging of acute spinal cord trauma. *AJNR* 8:5-10, 1987.

Cone RO, Flournoy J, MacPherson RI: The craniocervical junction. *Radiographics* 1:1-37, 1981.

Coffe MJ, Hadley MN, Herrera GA, Morawetz RB: Dialysis-associated spondyloarthropathy. *J Neurosurg* 80:694-700, 1994.

Curati WL, Kingsley DPE, Kendall BE, Moseley IF: MRI in chronic spinal cord trauma. *Neuroradiology* 35:30-35, 1993.

Davis PC, Reisner A, Hudgins PA, et al: Spinal injuries in children: role of MR. *AJNR* 14:607-617, 1993.

Davis SW, Levy LM, LeBihan DJ, et al: Sacral meningeal cysts: evaluation with MR imaging. *Radiology* 187:445-448, 1993.

DiChiro G, Doppman JL, Dwyer AJ, et al: Tumors and arteriovenous malformations of the spinal cord: assessment using MR. *Radiology* 156:689-697, 1985.

Dietemann JH, De la Palavesa MMF, Kastler B, et al: Thoracic intradural arachnoid cyst: possible pitfalls with myelo-CT and MR. *Neuroradiology* 33:90-91, 1991.

Doppman JL: Epidural lipomatosis. *Radiology* 171:581-582, 1989.

Doppman JL, DiChiro G, Dwyer AJ, et al: Magnetic resonance imaging of spinal arteriovenous malformations. *J Neurosurg* 66:830-834, 1987.

Dormont D, Assouline E, Gelbert F, et al: MRI study of spinal arteriovenous malformations. *Neuroradiology* 14:351-364, 1987.

Dormont D, Gelbert F, Assouline E, et al: MR imaging of spinal cord arteriovenous malformations at 0.5T: study of 34 cases. *AJNR* 9:833-838, 1988.

El-Khoury GY, Whitten CG: Trauma to the upper thoracic spine: anatomy, biomechanics, and unique imaging features. *AJR* 160:95-102, 1993.

Elksnis SM, Hogg JP, Cunningham ME: MR imaging of spontaneous cord infarction. *J Comput Assist Tomogr* 15:228-232, 1991.

Ellis JH, Martel W, Lillie JH, Aisen AM: Magnetic resonance imaging of the normal craniovertebral junction. *Spine* 16:105-111, 1991.

Enzmann DR, O'Donohue J, Rubin JB, et al: CSF pulsations within non-neoplastic spinal cord cysts. *AJR* 149:149-157, 1987.

Falcone S, Quencer RM, Green BA, et al: Progressive posttraumatic myelomalacic myelopathy: imaging and clinical features. *AJNR* 15:747-754, 1994.

Fessler RG, Johnson DL, Brown FD, et al: Epidural lipomatosis in steroid-treated patients. *Spine* 17:183-188, 1992.

Fontaine S, Melanson D, Cosgrove R, Bertrand G: Cavernous hemangiomas of the spinal cord: MR imaging. *Radiology* 166:839-842, 1988.

Friedberg SR, Fellows T, Thomas CB, et al: Experience with symptomatic spinal epidural cysts. *Neurosurgery* 34:989-993, 1994.

Friedman DP, Flanders AE: Enhancement of gray matter in anterior spinal infarction. *AJNR* 13:983-985, 1992.

Friedman DP, Flanders AE, Tartaglino LM: Vascular neoplasms and malformations, ischemia, and hemorrhage affecting the spinal cord: MR imaging findings. *AJR* 162:685-692, 1994.

Gebarski SS, Maynard FW, Gabrielson TO, et al: Posttraumatic progressive myelopathy: clinical and radiologic correlation employing MR imaging, delayed CT-metrizamide myelography, and intraoperative sonography. *Radiology* 157:379-386, 1985.

Georgy BA, Chong B, Chamberlain M, et al: MR of the spine in Guillain-Barre syndrome. *AJNR* 15:300-301, 1994.

Goldberg AL, Rothfus WE, Deeb ZL, et al: The impact of magnetic resonance on the diagnostic evaluation of acute cervicothoracic spinal trauma. *Skeletal Radiol* 17:89-94, 1988.

Goyal RN, Russell NA, Benoit BG, Belanger JMEG: Intraspinal cysts: a classification and literature review. *Spine* 12:209-213, 1987.

Grabb PA, Pang D: Magnetic resonance imaging in the evaluation of spinal cord injury without radiographic abnormality in children. *Neurosurgery* 35:406-414, 1994.

Hackney DB, Asato R, Joseph PM, et al: Hemorrhage and edema in acute spinal cord compression: demonstration by MR imaging. *Radiology* 161:387-390, 1986.

Henderson FH, Crockard HA, Stevens JM: Spinal cord oedema due to venous stasis. *Neuroradiology* 35:312-315, 1993.

Hirono H, Yamadori A, Komiyama M, et al: MRI of spontaneous spinal cord infarction: serial changes in gadolinium-DTPA enhancement. *Neuroradiology* 34:95-97, 1992.

Isu T, Iwasaki Y, Akino M, et al: Magnetic resonance imaging in cases of spinal dural arteriovenous malformation. *Neurosurgery* 24:919-923, 1989.

Kalfas I, Wilberger J, Goldberg A, Prostko ER: Magnetic resonance imaging in acute spinal cord trauma. *Neurosurgery* 23:295-299, 1988.

Kendall BE, Stevens JM, Crockard HA: The spine in rheumatoid arthritis. *Riv di Neuroradiol* (Suppl2):23-28, 1992.

Kochan JP, Quencer RM: Imaging of cystic and cavitary lesions of the spinal cord and canal: the value of MR and intraoperative sonography. *Rad Clin North Am* 29:867-912, 1991.

Kulkarni MV, Boundurant FJ, Rose SL, Narayama PA: 1.5T MR imaging of acute spinal trauma. *Radiographics* 8:1059-1082, 1988.

Kulkarni MV, McArdle CB, Kopanicky D: Acute spinal cord injury: MR imaging at 1.5T. *Radiology* 164:837-843, 1987.

Kurata A, Miyasaka Y, Yoshida T, et al: Venous ischemia caused by dural arteriovenous malformation. Case report. *J Neurosurg* 80:552-555, 1994.

Larsson E-M, Desai P, Hardin CW, et al: Venous infarction of the spinal cord resulting from dural arteriovenous fistula: MR imaging findings. *AJNR* 12:739-743, 1991.

Larsson E-M, Holtas S, Zygmunt S: Pre- and postoperative MR imaging of the craniocervical junction in rheumatoid arthritis. *AJNR* 10:89-94, 1989.

Masaryk TJ, Ross JS, Modic MT, et al: Radiculomeningeal vascular malformations of the spine: MR imaging. *Radiology* 164:845-849, 1987.

Mascalchi M, Arnetoli G, Dal Pozzo G, et al: Spinal epidural angiolipoma: MR findings. *AJNR* 12:744-745, 1991.

Mathis JM, Wilson JT, Barnard JW, Zelenik ME: MR imaging of spinal cord avulsion. *AJNR* 9:1232-1233, 1988.

Mawad ME, Rivera V, Crawford S: Spinal cord ischemia after resection of thoracoabdominal aortic aneurysms: MR findings in 24 patients. *AJNR* 11:987-991, 1990.

Mikulis DJ, Ogilvy CS, McKee A, et al: Spinal cord infarction and fibrocartilagenous emboli. *AJNR* 13:155-160, 1992.

Miller SF, Glasier CM, Griebal ML, Boop FA: Brachial plexopathy in infants after traumatic delivery: evaluation with MR imaging. *Radiology* 189:481-484, 1993.

Minami S, Sagoh T, Nishimura K, et al: Spinal arteriovenous malformations: MR imaging. *Radiology* 169:109-116, 1988.

Mirvis SE, Geisler FH, Jelinek JJ, et al: Acute cervical spine trauma: evaluation with 1.5T MR imaging. *Radiology* 166:807-816, 1988.

Mirvis SE, Wolf AL: MRI of acute cervical spine trauma. *Applied Radiology* 15-22, December 1992.

Murphy MD, Batnitzky S, Bramble JM: Diagnostic imaging of spinal trauma. *Rad Clin North Am* 27:855-872, 1989.

Ogilvy CS, Louis DN, Ojemann RG: Intramedullary cavernous angiomas of the spinal cord: clinical presentation, pathological features, and surgical management. *Neurosurgery* 31:219-230, 1992.

Pagni CA, Canavero S: Spinal epidural angiolipoma: rare or unreported? *Neurosurg* 31:758-764, 1992.

Pathria MN, Petersilge CA: Spinal trauma. *Rad Clin N Am* 29:847-866, 1991.

Paulsen RD, Call GA, Murtagh FR: Prevalence and percutaneous drainage of cysts of the sacral nerve root sheath (Tarlov cysts). *AJNR* 15:293-297, 1994.

Petterson H, Larsson EM, Holtas S, et al: MR imaging of the cervical spine in rheumatoid arthritis. *AJNR* 9:573-577, 1988.

Popovich MJ, Taylor FC, Helmer E: MR imaging of birth-related brachial plexus avulsion. *AJNR* 10(Suppl):S98, 1989.

Preul MC, Leblanc R, Tampieri D, et al: Spinal angiolipomas. Report of three cases. *J Neurosurg* 78:280-286, 1993.

Quencer RM: The injured spinal cord: evaluation with magnetic resonance and intraoperative sonography. *Rad Clin North Am* 26:1025-1046, 1988.

Quencer RM, Sheldon JJ, Post MJD, et al: Magnetic resonance imaging of the chronically injured cervical spinal cord. *AJNR* 7:457-464, 1986.

Quint DJ, Boulos RS, Sanders WP, et al: Epidural lipomatosis. *Radiology* 169:485-495, 1988.

Rohrer DC, Burchiel KJ, Gruber DP: Intraspinal extradural meningeal cysts demonstrating ball-valve mechanism of formation. *J Neurosurg* 78:122-125, 1993.

Rothfus WE, Chedid MK, Deeb ZL, et al: MR imaging in the diagnosis of spontaneous spinal epidural hematomas. *J Comput Assist Tomogr* 11:851-854, 1987.

Ryken TC, Menezes AH: Cervicomedullary compression in achondroplasia. *J Neurosurg* 81:43-48, 1994.

Schweitzer ME, Hodler J, Cervilla V, Resnick D: Craniovertebral junction: normal anatomy with MR correlation. *AJR* 158:1087-1090, 1992.

Silberstein M, Tress BM, Hennessy O: Delayed neurologic deterioration in the patient with spinal trauma: role of MR imaging. *AJNR* 13:1373-1382, 1992.

Silberstein M, Tress BM, Hennessy O: Prediction of neurologic outcome in acute spinal cord injury: the role of CT and MR. *AJNR* 13:1597-1608, 1992.

Sklar E, Quencer RM, Green BA, et al: Acquired spinal subarachnoid cysts: evaluations with MR, CT myelography, and intraoperative sonography. *AJNR* 10:1097-1104, 1989.

Smoker WRK: Craniovertebral junction: normal anatomy, craniometry, and congenital anomalies. *Radiographics* 14:255-278, 1994.

Stern Y, Spiegelmann SM: Spinal intradural arachnoid cysts. *Neurochirurgie* 34:127-130, 1991.

Stevens JM, Olney JS, Kendall BE: Posttraumatic cystic and noncystic myelopathy. *Neuroradiology* 27:48-56, 1985.

Takahashi S, Yamada T, Ishii K, et al: MRI of anterior spinal artery syndrome of the cervical spinal cord. *Neuroradiology* 33:25-29, 1992.

Tarr RW, Drolshagen LF, Kerner TC, et al: MR imaging of recent spinal trauma. *J Comput Assist Tomogr* 11:412-417, 1987.

Terwey B, Becker H, Thron AK, Vahldiek G: Gadolinium-DTPA-enhanced MR imaging of spinal dural arteriovenous fistulas. *J Comput Assist Tomogr* 13:30-37, 1989.

Timms SR, Cure JK, Kurent JE: Subacute combined degeneration of the spinal cord: MR findings. *AJNR* 14:1224-1228, 1993.

Tomlinson FH, Rufenacht DA, Sundt TM Jr, et al: Arteriovenous fistulas of the brain and spinal cord. *J Neurosurg* 79:16-27, 1993.

Verstraete KLA, Martens F, Smeets P, et al: Traumatic lumbosacral nerve root meningoceles: the value of myelography, CT, and MRI in the assessment of nerve root continuity. *Neuroradiology* 31:425-429, 1989.

White KS, Ball WS, Prenger EC, et al: Evaluation of the craniocervical junction in Down syndrome: correlation of measurements obtained with radiography and MR imaging. *Radiology* 186:377-382, 1993.

Yuh WTC, March EE, Wang AK, et al: MR imaging of spinal cord and vertebral body infarction. *AJNR* 13:145-154, 1992.

CHAPTER 18

Syringomyelia and Congenital Abnormalities of the Spinal Canal

Case 1051A

15-year-old girl presenting with numbness and
weakness of the hands.
(sagittal, noncontrast scan; SE 550/20)

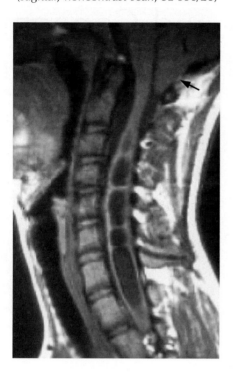

Case 1051B

Same patient.
(axial, noncontrast scan; SE 1000/20; C7 level)

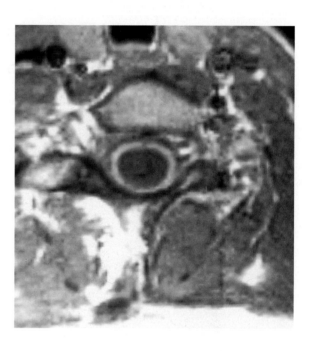

Purists describe dilatation of the ependymal-lined central canal of the spinal cord as "hydromyelia," reserving the term "syringomyelia" for acquired intramedullary cavities lined by glial reaction. In practice, the two terms are often interchanged, or combined as "syringohydromyelia." In view of common application, this chapter will use "syringomyelia" to include true "hydromyelia" as well as other types of intramedullary cysts.

The pathophysiology of congenital syringomyelia is not clearly established. Abnormal hydrodynamics within the spinal canal probably play a major role in syrinx formation. The most common anatomical correlate is crowding of tissue within the foramen magnum in the Chiari I and Chiari II hindbrain malformations (see Cases 712 to 715). Acquired anatomical distortions at the foramen magnum may also produce abnormalities of CSF dynamics and lead to syringomyelia (see for example Case 689).

Although syringomyelia in association with Chiari hindbrain malformations may be considered to be of congenital origin, affected patients often do not present until adolescence or adulthood. It is likely that enlargement of the cyst over many years precedes the onset of symptoms.

Intramedullary cysts are defined on T1-weighted scans as sharply marginated zones of low signal intensity. Intensity values within a syrinx may be slightly higher than those of subarachnoid CSF due to reduced signal loss from pulsation effects and/or mild elevation of protein. Cysts differing substantially in intensity from spinal fluid may be neoplastic and should be evaluated by contrast-enhanced studies.

The diameter of the cyst in Case 1051A varies from level to level, and the margins of the syrinx are mildly irregular. A septated, loculated, or "chain of lakes" morphology is common in syringomyelia. The compartments of the lesion usually communicate and are well decompressed by a single shunt. Conversely, postoperative recurrence of syringomyelia may involve only a few loculations of the original lesion.

Case 1051B illustrates the large, smoothly marginated central intramedullary cyst surrounded by a uniformly thin rim of compressed parenchyma.

Case 1052

55-year-old woman with a history of decompressive cervical laminectomy for a presumed spinal cord tumor.
(sagittal, noncontrast scan; SE 800/17)

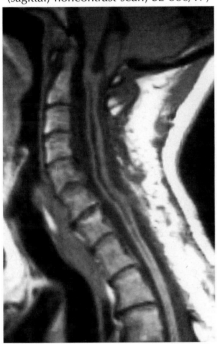

Case 1053

37-year-old man presenting with cervical myelopathy.
(axial, noncontrast scan; SE 800/17)

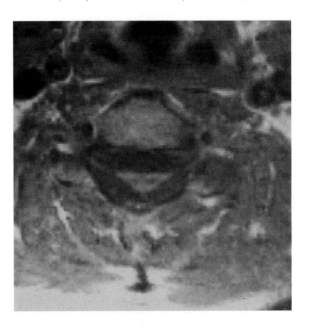

Some patients with syringomyelia present with collapsed cysts and atrophic spinal cords. Cord atrophy may be the result of prolonged compression from a previously distended syrinx or prior injury leading to both parenchymal damage and cavitation (see Cases 1017 and 1018).

In Case 1052, myelopathy with cord expansion had been thought to represent an intramedullary tumor when the patient was first evaluated as a young adult. Surgery at that time demonstrated benign syringomyelia. The follow-up scan above shows an abnormally thin cord with a collapsed central syrinx, associated with a Chiari hindbrain malformation.

Case 1053 illustrates an axial scan through an atrophic spinal cord containing small bilateral or "double-barrelled" cysts (compare to Case 1018). Anteroposterior narrowing of the cord is frequently seen in syringomyelia, while the transverse diameter is relatively preserved.

Compare the cross section of the spinal cord in Cases 1051B and 1053 to appreciate the potential variation in morphological presentation of syringomyelia. Between these extremes are some cases with normal cord dimensions and contour.

Other causes of cord atrophy include trauma, multiple sclerosis, ischemia, arteriovenous malformation, and amyotrophic lateral sclerosis.

Case 1054

51-year-old woman presenting with progressive quadriparesis.
(sagittal, noncontrast scan; SE 800/17)

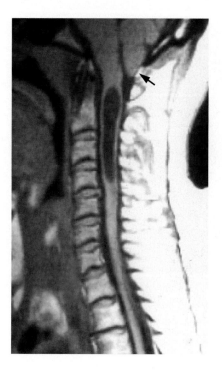

Case 1055

4-year-old girl with mild gait abnormality.
(coronal, noncontrast scan; SE 800/17)

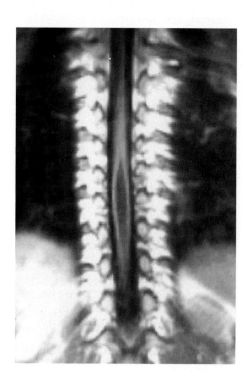

Syringomyelia often involves long segments of the spinal cord, as illustrated on the preceding pages. In other cases a benign, presumably congenital intramedullary cyst is quite localized.

Case 1054 demonstrates an expansile cyst involving the spinal cord from C2 to C4. The association of a Chiari I hindbrain malformation *(arrow)* suggests congenital origin of this localized syrinx. A contrast-enhanced scan was performed to exclude the alternative possibility of a cystic tumor (e.g., hemangioblastoma; compare to Case 138). No abnormal enhancement was present, and subsequent drainage of the cyst (with simultaneous decompression of the foramen magnum) led to dramatic clinical improvement.

The localized, slit-like mid thoracic cyst in Case 1055 resembles the appearance of diastematomyelia (see Cases 1083 and 1084; also compare to the astrocytoma in Case 936). Axial scans established the presence of a central syrinx (and the absence of cord division).

Tethering of the spinal cord was demonstrated in the lumbar region in Case 1055. Congenital abnormalities of the spinal cord are often multiple. The discovery of one congenital lesion should prompt a search for others.

Compare the central position and symmetrical morphology of the intramedullary cysts in the above cases to the eccentric, exophytic neuroepithelial cyst in Case 1029. Syringomyelia of congenital etiology (i.e., associated with Chiari hindbrain malformations, tethered cords, or spinal dysraphism) is usually central. Occasionally paired, parasagittal channels are seen. Unilaterally eccentric cysts are rarely of congenital origin.

Case 1056

3-year-old boy presenting with abnormal gait.
(sagittal, noncontrast scan; SE 500/20)

Case 1057

37-year-old woman presenting with back pain
and mild spasticity of the legs.
(sagittal, noncontrast scan; SE 600/19)

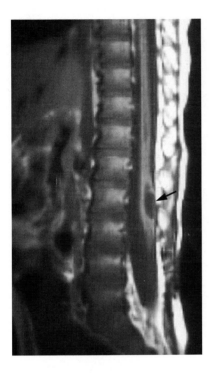

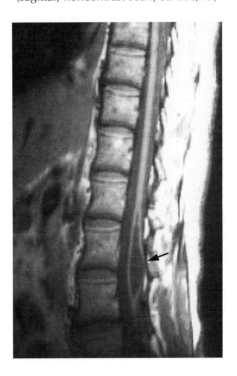

A common location for localized congenital syringomyelia is the caudal end of the central canal at the level of the conus medullaris. Focal dilatation of an intramedullary CSF chamber at this site has been termed a "terminal ventricle." Gross expansion of such terminal syrinxes may herniate through a defect in the posterior neural arch in patients with spinal dysraphism, forming a "myelocystocele."

In Case 1056, a mildly dilated central canal can be seen within the spinal cord at the thoracolumbar junction. The cord extends abnormally far caudally into the lumbar region, with the conus terminating at the L4 level. Within the low-lying conus is a focal cyst *(arrow)* representing a terminal expansion of the central canal.

The terminal cyst in Case 1057 is somewhat larger and more symmetrical than in Case 1056. Associated congenital abnormalities included abnormally low position of the conus medullaris and diastematomyelia in the thoracic region (not shown here). The presence of a "terminal ventricle" of any size is a clue to congenital malformation of the spinal cord, which may include additional lesions at other levels.

Case 1058

18-year-old man.
(sagittal, noncontrast scan; SE 800/17)

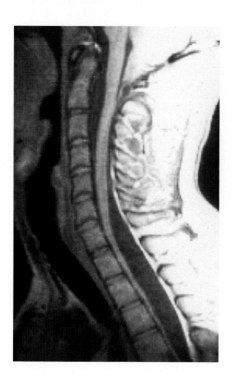

Case 1059

4-month-old boy.
(sagittal, noncontrast scan; SE 800/17)

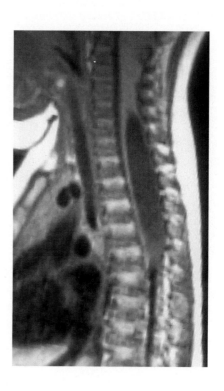

Congenital syringomyelia usually presents as a central intramedullary cyst. This morphology reflects dilatation of the central canal (i.e., "hydromyelia") in most cases.

Patients with Chiari II hindbrain malformations may demonstrate unusual, dorsally eccentric syringomyelia. In each of the above cases a large cyst fills the posterior portion of the spinal canal. The spinal cord parenchyma is compressed ventrally at the anterior margin of the cyst. No cord tissue is apparent at the posterior margin of the syrinx, in contrast to the cases illustrated previously in this chapter. As a result, the above scans could be assumed to represent arachnoid cysts (see Cases 1026 and 1027) or partial dorsal diastematomyelia (as has been described in some patients with Klippel-Feil syndrome and other congenital abnormalities).

However, axial images in Cases 1058 and 1059 demonstrated a thin rim of stretched parenchyma encircling the posterior margin of an eccentric intramedullary cyst (see Case 1061). This unusual morphology is part of the spectrum of cranial and spinal deformity seen in patients with Chiari II malformations.

DIFFERENTIAL DIAGNOSIS:
DORSAL CYST WITH CORD DEFORMITY

Case 1060

5-year-old girl presenting with neck pain.
(axial, noncontrast scan; SE 900/15; C3-4 level)

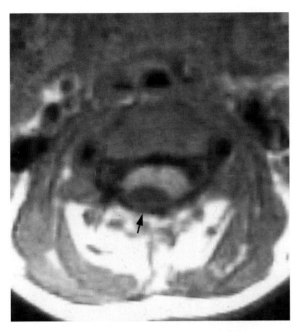

Arachnoid Cyst

Case 1061

3-year-old boy presenting with developmental
delay and leg spasticity.
(axial, noncontrast scan; SE 800/17; T2 level)

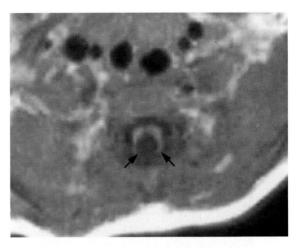

Eccentric Syrinx
(associated with Chiari II malformation)

Prominent CSF spaces along the dorsal surface of the spinal cord may represent several different pathologies. Arachnoid cysts frequently involve the posterior portion of the spinal canal, as discussed in Cases 1026 and 1027. Case 1060 illustrates an arachnoid cyst of the cervical canal *(arrow)*, causing secondary cord compression.

In Case 1061, a thin rim of cord tissue *(arrows)* surrounds the dorsal cyst, establishing it as intramedullary. This form of dorsally eccentric syringomyelia is occasionally encoun-

tered in patients with Chiari II hindbrain malformations, as discussed on the preceding page.

Another consideration in the differential diagnosis of these cases is "partial dorsal rachischisis" or "partial dorsal diastematomyelia." Failure of closure of the neural tube may result in a dorsal cleft within cord tissue. This congenital abnormality has been observed in patients with the Klippel-Feil syndrome.

Case 1062

6-year-old boy presenting with difficulty walking.
(sagittal, noncontrast scan; SE 800/15)

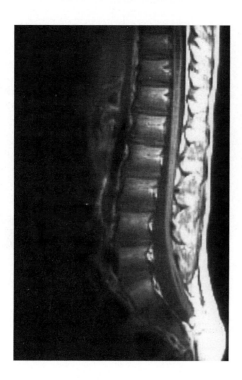

Case 1063

4-year-old girl with a history of myelomeningocele
repair at birth.
(sagittal, noncontrast scan; SE 550/20)

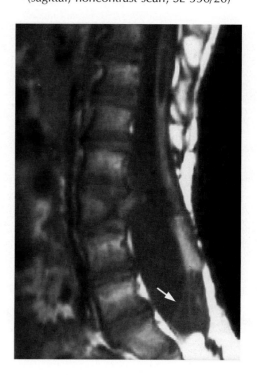

An abnormally low-lying spinal cord may be encountered as an isolated abnormality or in association with a complex malformation of the spinal canal. In the former circumstance, the cord may extend through the lumbar region to the termination of the thecal sac or be attached to a taut and/or thickened filum terminale at a midlumbar level. In other cases, the low-lying spinal cord may enter a lipomatous mass or a meningocele sac.

In Case 1062, the spinal cord extends inferiorly through the lumbar canal to terminate at the S2 level. Associated hypoplasia of the sacrum, sacral dysraphism, thoracic syringomyelia, and a small "terminal ventricle" are present.

On sagittal scans it may be difficult to distinguish between a stretched and thinned spinal cord and a thickened filum terminale within the lumbar spinal canal. Axial scans resolve this ambiguity by demonstrating nerve roots arising from spinal cord parenchyma (see Case 1064).

Case 1063 illustrates a low-lying spinal cord as part of a complex malformation. A large dysraphic defect and repaired myelomeningocele are present at the posterior margin of the spinal canal. The caudal sac is ectatic. Osseous abnormality involving the L3 vertebral body includes a posterior spur that was shown on axial images to represent diastematomyelia. A localized syrinx is present within the cord at the T10-T11 level. A band of low-lying neural tissue passes along the dorsal wall of the ectatic sac, appearing to be tethered posteriorly at the site of myelomeningocele repair. Nerve roots *(arrow)* extend caudally from this neural placode, identifying the more rostral tissue band as low-lying spinal cord rather than a thickened filum terminale.

Cases 1072, 1073, and 1094 present T2-weighted sagittal scans of tethered cords in association with lipomas and sacral agenesis.

Case 1064

8-year-old boy with a history of repaired myelomeningocele.
(axial, noncontrast scan; SE 1000/17; L3-4 level)

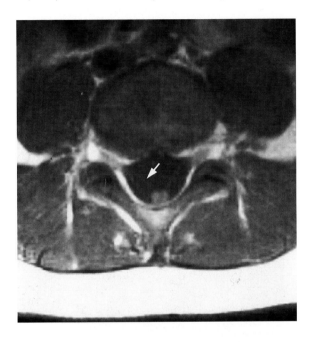

Case 1065

5-year-old girl with a dorsal soft tissue bulge at the lumbosacral junction.
(axial, noncontrast scan; SE 1000/20; S1-S2 level)

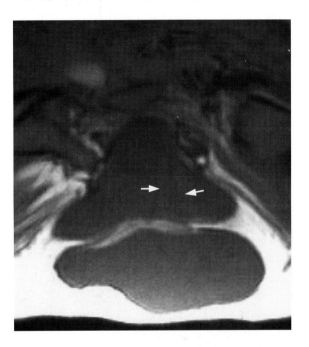

Axial scans confirm the nature of low-lying spinal cord parenchyma by demonstrating the presence of exiting nerve roots. By itself, the thick band of soft tissue within the dorsal subarachnoid space in Case 1064 is nonspecific; it could represent either a thick filum terminale or a thinned, low-lying spinal cord. (Clumping of intrathecal roots due to arachnoiditis may present a similar appearance; see Case 1005.) Visualization of emerging nerve roots *(arrow)* establishes the presence of spinal cord tissue at this level. Such documentation is important to identify the appropriate level for sectioning of the filum terminale to release a taut spinal cord.

Case 1065 is an axial view through the flat neural placode in a patient with a subcutaneous myelomeningocele. The plate of soft tissue traversing the meningocele sac represents the caudal portion of the spinal cord, which failed to close dorsally into a tube. Ventral and dorsal nerve roots *(arrows)* can be faintly seen extending anteriorly from the lateral margins of the placode. The dorsal nerve root usually arises at the edge of the unfolded neural plate, where it joins high intensity fat. This junction is therefore an important surgical landmark.

Case 1066

2-year-old girl.
(sagittal, noncontrast scan; SE 500/15)

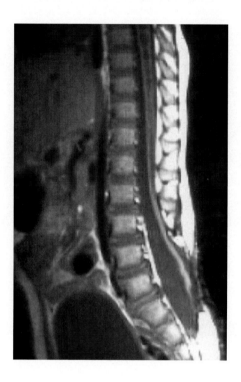

Case 1067

43-year-old woman presenting with worsening
paraparesis.
(sagittal, noncontrast scan; SE 600/17)

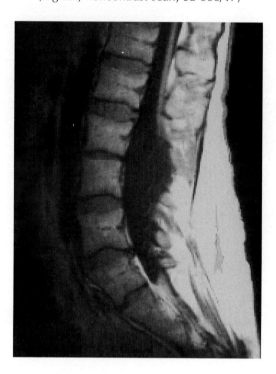

Tethering of a low-lying spinal cord in the lumbar region may occur dorsally as well as caudally. Dorsal tethering may be primary, due to failed dysjunction of cutaneous and neuroectoderm (see Cases 1089 and 1090). Secondary or acquired dorsal tethering of neural elements may develop due to the formation of adhesions after surgery to repair a myelomeningocele or release a caudally tethered cord. Progression of symptoms months or years after initially successful surgery raises the question of acquired postoperative tethering.

The usual dorsal position of neural tissue within a repaired myelomeningocele causes the spinal cord to drape across the last intact neural arch as it enters the meningocele sac. Such proximity does not by itself establish the presence of adhesions in this location. However, if the spinal cord appears tightly adherent to the dorsal dura, with abnormal angulation and/or absence of dorsal subarachnoid space, the possibility of acquired tethering should be considered. The clinical context is important in assessing the possibility of dorsal tethering in such cases.

In Case 1066, the low-lying cord deviates dorsally at it enters the area of dural ectasia and myelomeningocele repair. Dense adhesions were found at the previous operative site.

The neural tissue in Case 1067 is very closely applied to the posterior margin of the dural sac and meningocele. Dorsal adhesions frequently occur at the transition from the normal spinal canal to the dysraphic segment, as was true in this case.

Syringomyelia is present within the thoracic spinal cord in Case 1066.

Case 1068

1-year-old boy with a history of myelomeningocele
repair at birth.
(sagittal, noncontrast scan; SE 800/17)

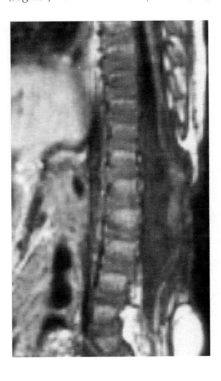

Case 1069

1-year-old girl with a history of myelomeningocele
repair at birth.
(sagittal, noncontrast scan; SE 800/17)

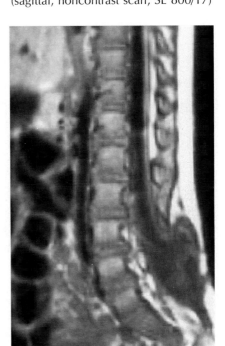

In each of the above cases, distorted neural elements within the lumbar sac are surrounded by tissue that is slightly higher in signal intensity and more heterogeneous than CSF. Subsequent surgery demonstrated intradural epidermoid masses.

Keratinizing epithelium may be incorporated within the spinal canal as a result of congenital malformation (failure of dysjunction of cutaneous and neuroectoderm) or as a consequence of surgery. Infolding of cutaneous tissue may occur during closure of a myelomeningocele defect in the neonatal period. Subsequent intraspinal proliferation of squamous epithelium can produce an enlarging epidermoid mass. Like acquired adhesions, this possibility is among diagnostic considerations in children (or adults) whose neurological function deteriorates some time after initial surgery.

The caudal portion of the thecal sac is characteristically ectatic in patients with congenital malformations of the spinal column and spinal cord. This patulous sac may demonstrate less CSF pulsatility than the more rostral subarachnoid space. As a result, there may be reduced signal loss and overall higher intensity within the caudal sac as compared to more superior portions of the spinal canal. This appearance may simulate the presence of epidermoid tissue with long T1 and T2 values.

Case 1070

9-year-old boy presenting with bladder dysfunction.
(sagittal, noncontrast scan; SE 600/15)

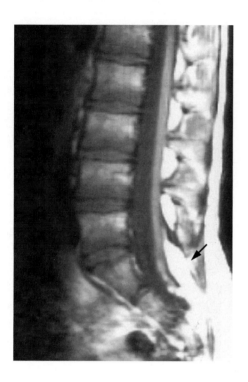

Case 1071

8-year-old girl presenting with a lipomatous
lumbosacral mass.
(sagittal, noncontrast scan; SE 1000/20)

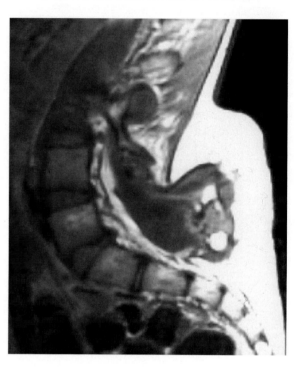

Lipomas at the caudal end of the dural sac commonly accompany tethering of the spinal cord and spinal dysraphism. Abnormal fatty tissue within the lumbosacral canal may be intradural, extradural, or both. Intradural lipomas are often continuous with dorsal subcutaneous fat through dysraphic defects in the posterior neural arch. Lipomatous tissue may ascend along the dorsal surface of the cord, infiltrate the filum terminale, or surround and compress the spinal cord and cauda equina.

The characteristically short T1 of lipid protons readily identifies intraspinal fatty tissue on short TR spin echo images. In Case 1070, high intensity lipomatous tissue surrounds the sacral termination of a tethered spinal cord. The intraspinal fat is most prominent along the dorsal surface of the low-lying cord, as is commonly the case. The lipoma extends dorsally through a dysraphic defect to blend with a localized mound of thickened subcutaneous fat. When a meningocele sac accompanies a lipoma through a spina bifida defect, the combined malformation is called a "lipomeningocele."

Case 1071 illustrates an occult lipomeningocele covered by a large mound of thickened subcutaneous fat. A complex mixture of lipomatous tissue and neural placode is present within the meningocele sac. The spinal cord enters the rostral pole of this heterogeneous mass. Associated scoliosis and exaggerated lumbosacral lordosis are present.

Case 1072

48-year-old man presenting with back pain.
(sagittal, noncontrast scan; SE 2800/90)

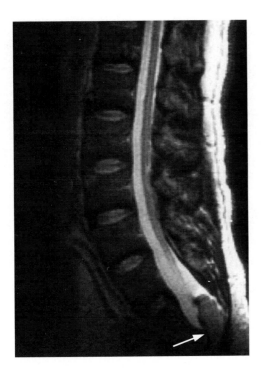

Case 1073

69-year-old woman presenting with progressive
gait abnormality.
(sagittal, noncontrast scan; SE 3400/90)

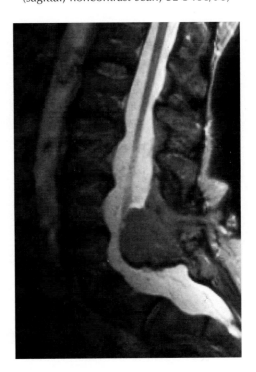

The signal intensity of spinal lipomas is characteristically low on T2-weighted images. The above examples are typical. (Compare to the appearance of the intracranial lipomas in Case 727.)

In Case 1072, a small lipoma *(arrow)* occupies the mildly ectatic caudal end of the lumbar subarachnoid space. A low-lying spinal cord extends through the lumbar region to terminate in the lipoma. (The junction of the cord and the lipoma was better seen on an adjacent section.)

Case 1073 illustrates the adult presentation of a congeni-tal spinal lesion (see Cases 1079 and 1080). A large, spherical, dorsally based lipoma occupies most of the ectatic spinal canal at the L4 level. Signal intensity within the mass is homogeneously low, and chemical shift artifact is present along its inferior and superior margins (see discussion of Cases 726 and 727). There appears to be communication between the intraspinal lipoma and dorsal subcutaneous tissues, suggesting dysraphism. The low-lying spinal cord is tightly stretched over the ventral margin of the intradural lipoma. Prominent scalloping of vertebral bodies indicates long-standing dural ectasia.

Case 1074

5-year-old boy presenting with urinary urgency
and incontinence.
(axial, noncontrast scan; SE 800/15; L4 level)

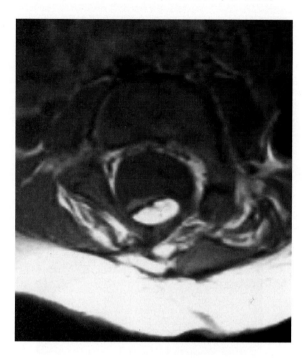

Case 1075

9-year-old boy presenting with increasing
leg spasticity.
(axial, noncontrast scan; SE 600/15; L5-S1 level)

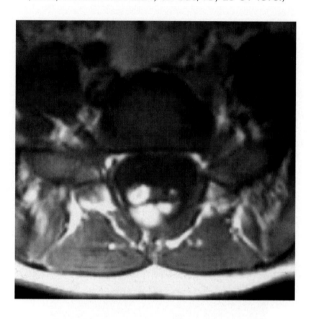

Axial views demonstrate the variable relationship of spinal lipomas to a low-lying spinal cord and/or neural placode. Lipomatous tissue is often applied to the dorsal aspect of the cord/placode, as illustrated in Case 1074. This characteristic appearance reflects premature dysjunction of neuroectoderm from cutaneous ectoderm, allowing mesenchymal cells to gain access to the posterior surface of the neural tube. In cases of spinal canal deformity with sub-

stantial rotation of the spinal cord (e.g., diastematomyelia; see Cases 1082 and 1086), the location of lipomatous tissue may help to identify the originally dorsal surface of neural tissue.

Case 1075 demonstrates a more complex and heterogeneous mixture of cord parenchyma and lipoma. Nodules of fatty tissue surround all but the ventral margin of the low-lying spinal cord.

Case 1076

4-month-old girl.
(axial, noncontrast scan; SE 800/15; L5 level)

Case 1077

3-year-old girl presenting with back pain.
(axial, noncontrast scan; SE 800/15; L3 level)

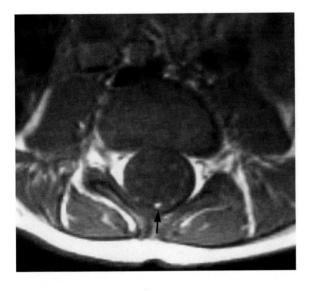

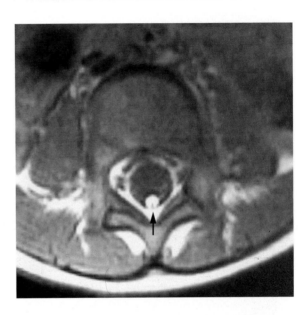

Fatty infiltration of the filum terminale may be an incidental finding, alone or in combination with other congenital abnormalities. In other cases, a lipoma involving the filum terminale is associated with symptomatic tethering of the spinal cord. Evidence of cord traction (i.e., a tight or stretched configuration with a low-lying conus medullaris) and clinical correlation are important in assessing the significance of filum fat.

Prominent T1-shortening highlights lipomatous infiltration of the filum terminale in each of the above cases. The amount of thickening of the filum correlates with the likelihood of significant cord tethering. A filum diameter of more than two or three millimeters is frequently symptomatic. The child in Case 1077 had a normally positioned conus medullaris and no evidence of neurological dysfunction, but she will be carefully followed as somatic growth continues.

It is important to emphasize that fatty infiltration of the filum terminale is not synonymous with thickening of the filum or tethering of the spinal cord. Pathologically thickened fila often contain no fat. Conversely, fat may be present within a filum of normal dimensions and without associated traction on the spinal cord (as in Case 1076).

Case 1078A

12-year-old boy presenting with progressive paresis
and bowel and bladder dysfunction five years after
shunting of a thoracic syrinx.
(sagittal, noncontrast scan; SE 600/15)

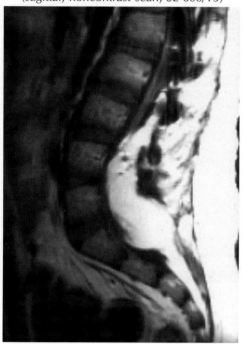

Case 1078B

Same patient.
(axial, noncontrast scan; SE 800/15; L5 level)

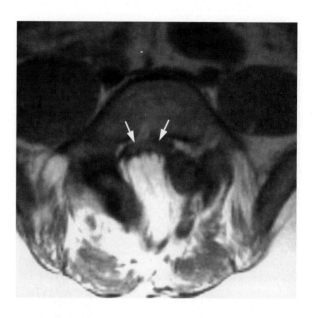

Serial MR studies of patients with intraspinal lipomas
have demonstrated interval growth in occasional cases.

Scans at the time of initial surgery in Case 1078 had identified a small lumbar lipoma accompanying the tethered spinal cord and syringomyelia. The bulky lipoma seen above
represented a substantial increase in size of the earlier lesion. The fatty mass is now large enough to compress the
low-lying spinal cord (*arrows;* Case 1078B) and cause recurrent symptoms.

Growth of an intraspinal lipoma is a rare cause of new
or recurrent symptoms in children after surgery for congenital cord lesions. More common etiologies include recurrence of syringomyelia, development of tethering adhesions, formation of an epidermoid mass, or increased tension on the spinal cord due to somatic growth.

Case 1078 emphasizes again that congenital malformations of the spinal canal are often multiple. When one is
found, others should be expected.

Case 1079

70-year-old woman presenting with back pain
and paraparesis after a fall.
(sagittal, noncontrast scan; SE 900/15)

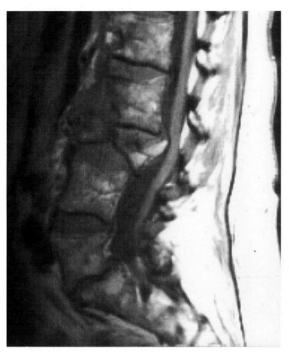

Tethered Cord

Case 1080

69-year-old woman presenting with progressive gait
abnormality.
(sagittal, noncontrast scan; SE 600/15)

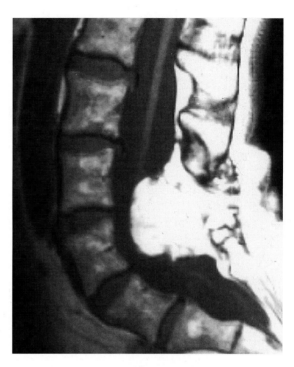

Lipoma
(Same patient as Case 1073)

Spinal cord malformations usually become symptomatic during childhood or adolescence, as growth of the spine increases the tension on tethered neural structures. Occasionally, adults present with symptoms arising from congenital lesions. The adult onset of dysfunction in such cases may be due to superimposed acquired pathology or time-related worsening of congenital abnormalities.

Case 1079 illustrates the former mechanism. A tethered spinal cord is present, extending through the lumbar region. This congenital abnormality had not caused symptoms until the fracture of L3 resulted in cord compression. Conversely, the compression fracture might have displaced

the cauda equina without neurological impairment in the absence of cord tethering.

The scan in Case 1080 is a T1-weighted view of the lipoma presented in Case 1073. Stretching of the spinal cord over the long-standing lipoma in this case has probably worsened gradually over decades, finally causing increasing symptoms and leading to evaluation. The ectatic dural sac with scalloping of vertebral bodies is a common finding in congenital malformations of the spinal canal.

Diastematomyelia (see Cases 1081-1086) may also present in adulthood, typically with gait abnormality or bowel and/or bladder dysfunction.

Case 1081

15-year-old girl scanned as a preoperative routine prior to scheduled surgery for scoliosis.
(sagittal, noncontrast scan; SE 550/20)

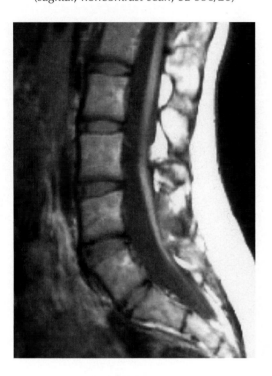

Case 1082

2-year-old boy with a history of myelomeningocele repair.
(sagittal, noncontrast scan; SE 500/20)

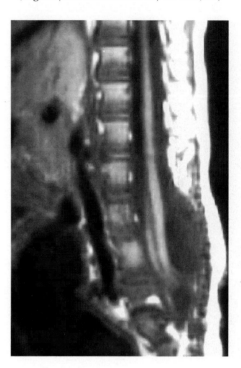

Diastematomyelia is a congenital malformation characterized by division of the spinal cord. In at least 50% of such cases the two hemicords are enclosed within a single arachnoidal and dural tube, with no apparent intervening septation. In the remaining cases, an osteocartilaginous septum divides the spinal canal. It has been recently proposed that this group of congenital abnormalities be categorized as split cord malformation (SCM) type I (separate dural tubes with an osteocartilaginous septation) and SCM type II (single dural tube with no rigid septation).

Sagittal scans are the least reliable views for the diagnosis and assessment of split cord malformations. The division between the two hemicords is usually sagittally oriented. As a result, sagittal scans may only partially image the dividing plane, resulting in negative studies or the false suggestion of syringomyelia. Poorly defined low signal intensity within the low-lying spinal cord at the L3 level in

Case 1081 represents the site of diastematomyelia which was clearly demonstrated on axial and coronal views.

Diastematomyelia is apparent on the sagittal scan in Case 1082 because intradural rotation causes one hemicord to project anterior to the other. Rotation of hemicords is a common component of split cord malformations, whether or not a septum is present. Case 1082 also demonstrates an ectatic dural sac in the lumbar region representing a repaired myelomeningocele.

As illustrated in these cases, diastematomyelia may be associated with abnormally low-lying spinal cords and the "tethered cord syndrome." Fibrous septation dividing the hemicords in type II SCM is often not apparent on preoperative imaging studies. However, such septae (and other fibroneurovascular bands) are usually present and can have the same tethering effect as the obvious bone spurs in type I SCM. Many surgeons now advocate exploration of all SCMs of either type to release tethering lesions.

DIFFERENTIAL DIAGNOSIS:
CSF-FILLED CLEFT WITHIN THE SPINAL CORD

Case 1083

3-year-old girl with difficulty learning to walk.
(coronal, noncontrast scan; SE 600/15)

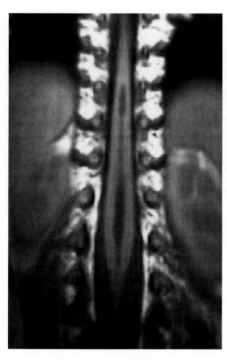

Diastematomyelia

Case 1084

9-month-old boy being evaluated for cutaneous
stigmata of lumbar dysraphism.
(coronal, noncontrast scan; SE 600/15)

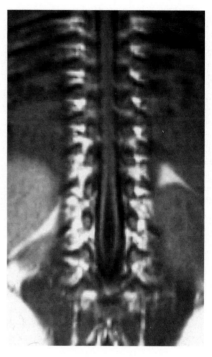

Syringomyelia

Coronal and axial scans are much more reliable than sagittal images for demonstration of split cord malformations. In Case 1083 the intramedullary cleft extends from the midthoracic region to the conus medullaris. No septation is apparent.

Syringomyelia (usually representing true hydromyelia) can present a similar appearance on coronal scans, as seen in Case 1084. Axial scans are necessary to determine whether central CSF on coronal images represents a cleft traversing the anteroposterior diameter of the spinal cord or an intramedullary cavity enclosed by cord parenchyma.

Both diastematomyelia and syringomyelia commonly occur in association with other malformations of the spinal canal, including tethering of the spinal cord and the various forms of spinal dysraphism.

About 90% of diastematomyelic hemicords reunite at a level below the split. A fibrous or osteocartilageneous septation passing between the hemicords represents an important potential cause of tethering in such cases.

DIASTEMATOMYELIA WITH RIGID SEPTUM (SPLIT CORD MALFORMATION TYPE I)

Case 1085

15-year-old girl being evaluated for scoliosis.
(axial, noncontrast scan; SE 1000/20; L3 level)

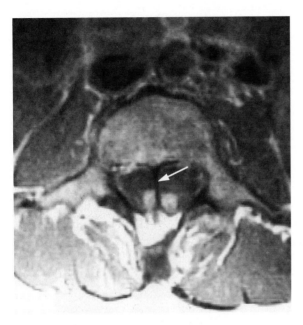

(Same patient as Case 1081)

Case 1086

16-year-old girl presenting with bowel
and bladder dysfunction.
(axial, noncontrast scan; SE 1000/20; L4 level)

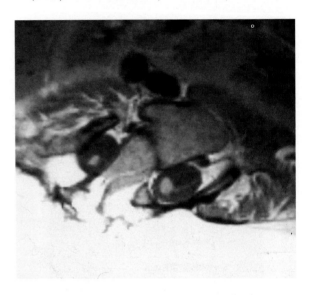

Axial views are the most reliable images for evaluating split cord malformations. Osteocartilaginous septa are well documented when present, and the size and morphology of the hemicords are clearly demonstrated.

Septations passing between the hemicords in diastematomyelia are variable in composition and morphology. Fibrous, cartilaginous, and osseous septa may be present. Bony partitions may be thin or thick, sagittal or oblique.

Case 1085 illustrates a thin plate of cortical bone in the midline *(arrow)*, bisecting the spinal canal. The low signal intensity of this structure is due to the low concentration of imageable hydrogen nuclei.

The septum in Case 1086 is a thick, obliquely oriented osseous structure containing cancellous bone. The two dural tubes are widely separated. Rotation of the hemicords within the dural sac(s) as seen in this case is a common component of split cord malformations, with or without intervening septations (compare to Case 1082).

The division of the dural sac and spinal cord in type I split cord malformations is approximately equal in about two thirds of cases.

DIASTEMATOMYELIA WITHOUT RIGID SEPTUM (SPLIT CORD MALFORMATION TYPE II)

Case 1087

4-year-old girl presenting with leg weakness
and numbness.
(axial, noncontrast scan; SE 1000/17; L2 level)

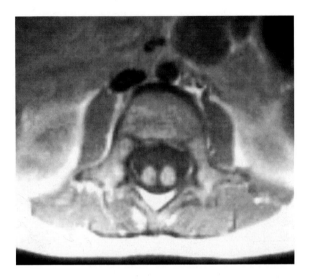

Case 1088

5-year-old girl presenting with constipation
and abnormal gait.
(axial, noncontrast scan; SE 1000/17; L2 level)

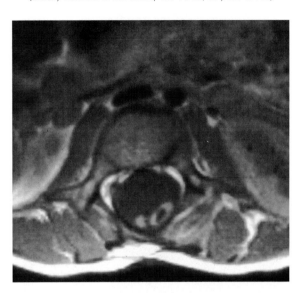

The above cases illustrate type II split cord malformations. Although division of cord parenchyma is apparent, there is no evidence of intervening osteocartilaginous septation or duplication of the dural tube.

As demonstrated here, the hemicords of diastematomyelia may be nearly equal in size or grossly asymmetrical. One or both hemicords may contain a syrinx (seen on the left in Case 1088) or be associated with a lipoma. The hemicords may be positioned side by side in the same coronal plane, as in Case 1087, or rotated with respect to each other, as in Case 1088.

In each of these cases the spinal cord extends abnormally far inferiorly within an ectatic dural sac. As discussed previously, diastematomyelia is usually associated with spinal cord tethering by adhesions even in the absence of mesodermal septations. Septae and adhesions associated with split cord malformations are often quite vascular and may be best seen on postcontrast scans.

DORSAL DERMAL SINUS SYNDROME

Case 1089A

50-year-old man presenting with back pain
and leg weakness.
(sagittal, noncontrast scan; SE 800/19)

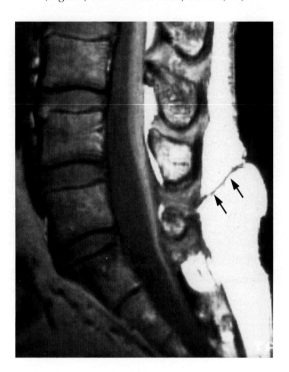

Case 1089B

Same patient.
(same image with different photography)

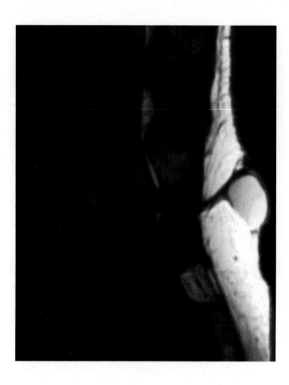

The "dorsal dermal sinus syndrome" includes a group of disorders caused by failed dysjunction of neuroectoderm from cutaneous ectoderm. In most cases, the persistent connection of the neural tube to the skin surface leads to the invagination of a dermal sinus. This tract extends from the skin of the back through subcutaneous tissues and between spinous processes to terminate at the dura or within the thecal sac. Intradural dermal sinus tracts may ascend for several levels along the spinal canal. Associated intradural dermoid or epidermoid tumors are present in about 50% of cases and may be either intramedullary or extramedullary.

Dorsal dermal sinus tracts are variably patent. Fibrous obliteration of the lumen of the tract may still be associated with symptomatic cord tethering. Patent dermal sinus tracts are a potential source of intradural infection and may present with isolated or recurrent meningitis.

Case 1089 is unusual in that failure of dysjunction has lead to eversion of neuroectoderm rather than inversion of cutaneous ectoderm. The dorsal subcutaneous mass at the L5 level, best seen in Case 1089B, proved to be a meningocele linked to the dura and the dorsal surface of the tethered spinal cord by a fibrous stalk. The angled course of the tethering stalk in this case (*arrows;* Case 1089A) is typical of a lumbar dorsal dermal sinus: the tract angles inferiorly as it extends anteriorly from the skin surface, reaches the interspinous region, and then angles superiorly as it passes into the spinal canal. Both the cutaneous origin and the dural or intradural termination of a dorsal dermal sinus tract are usually superior to the level where it enters the spinal canal.

Spinal dermoid cysts often have predominantly long T1 and T2 values resembling simpler arachnoid or parasitic cysts. Heterogeneity (especially T1-shortening) within a small portion of the lesion and/or the presence of an associated dermal sinus tract (which is found in about 20% of cases) are clues to the correct diagnosis.

Case 1090A

59-year-old man presenting with mild
cervical myelopathy.
(sagittal, noncontrast scan; SE 1000/17)

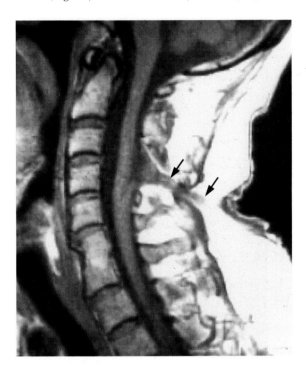

Case 1090B

Same patient.
(axial, noncontrast scan; SE 900/17; C4 level)

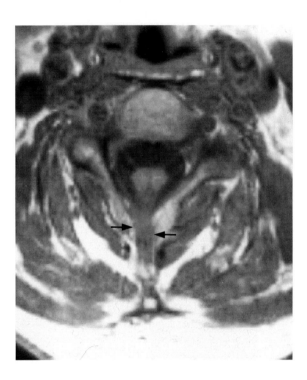

Manifestations of the dorsal dermal sinus syndrome are rare in the cervical region. When present, the lesions may demonstrate any of the various morphologies discussed on the preceding page.

Case 1090A demonstrates a band of fibrous tissue *(arrows)* connecting the dorsal surface of the spinal cord with a thickened and invaginated area of skin on the back of the neck. This tract represents a site of failed separation of neuroectoderm and cutaneous ectoderm ("non-dysjunction").

The lesion serves to tether the cervical spinal cord, as demonstrated in Case 1090B. The cord is pulled against the dorsal margin of the dural sac, and the posterior surface of the cord is tented.

Congenital fusion of the C6 and C7 vertebral bodies is present but unrelated to the dorsal dermal tract. (See Cases 1091 and 1092 for discussion of vertebral anomalies accompanying ventral adhesions of the neural tube.)

Case 1091

67-year-old man presenting with increasing difficulty walking and a fifty-year history of atrophic hands and arms.
(sagittal, noncontrast scan; SE 900/17)

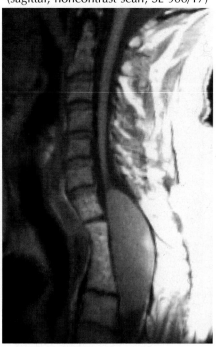

Case 1092

51-year-old man presenting with gradually worsening quadriparesis.
(sagittal, noncontrast scan; SE 500/20)

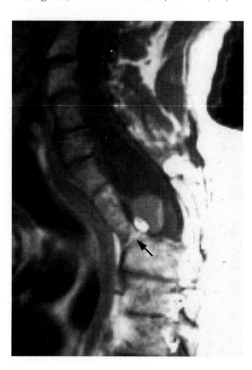

Neurenteric cysts represent one form of the "split notochord syndrome." This group of congenital disorders arises from abnormally persistent connection between embryonic endoderm and neuroectoderm. The presence of such midline ventral adhesions prevents normal induction and formation of the notochord, which typically "splits" around the area of endodermal/neuroectodermal connection. Aberrant notochordal development leads to vertebral anomalies at the affected level.

Like the dorsal dermal sinuses discussed on the preceding pages, ventral tracts between the embryonic endoderm and the spinal canal (or extending further to the dorsal surface of the embryo) may be variably patent. Enteric fistulae may communicate from the foregut to the spinal canal or the dorsal skin surface. Alternatively, localized cysts may form at any point along this potential tract, with fibrous obliteration or involution of adjacent segments. When such cysts occur within the spinal canal, they are termed "neurenteric" cysts.

Neurenteric cysts are most commonly found near the cervicothoracic junction. Adjacent vertebral anomalies are usually present, as in the above cases. The cysts are often intradural but extramedullary, although they may occur in epidural or intramedullary locations. They are frequently ventral and may become deeply embedded within the overlying spinal cord. Neurenteric cysts are typically unilocular, but irregular thickening of the wall is common. The signal intensity of the cyst content is variable.

The long-standing cyst in Case 1091 has caused expansion of the spinal canal and atrophy of the spinal cord. In Case 1092 a smaller cyst has become embedded in the ventral portion of the spinal cord, causing secondary syringomyelia superior to the lesion. A cleft in the spinal column is present at the anterior-inferior margin of the lesion (arrow), filled with high signal intensity that may reflect mucinous material of endodermal origin.

Case 1093

6-year-old girl presenting with bilateral leg weakness and a neurogenic bladder.
(sagittal, noncontrast scan; SE 550/20)

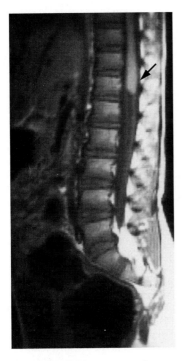

Caudal Regression Syndrome

Case 1094

13-year-old boy presenting with urinary incontinence.
(sagittal, noncontrast scan; SE 2800/90)

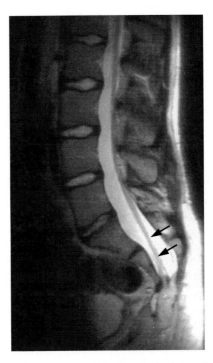

Sacral Agenesis and Tethered Cord

The syndrome of "caudal regression" includes a complex group of congenital malformations potentially involving the legs, genitourinary tract, gastrointestinal tract, and caudal spinal canal. Spinal manifestations include aplasia or hypoplasia of vertebrae and the terminal portion of the spinal cord. The syndrome occurs in about 1% of infants born to diabetic mothers, but only 15% of all caudal regression cases have this association.

Vertebral hypoplasia or aplasia may be limited to the sacrum. Such sacral agenesis may be partial or complete, unilateral (including "scimitar sacrum") or bilateral. In Case 1093, the sacrum is hypoplastic and a lipoma is present within the sacral canal. In more severe cases, multiple sacral, lumbar, and lower thoracic vertebrae may be absent.

A wedge-shaped or club-shaped deformity at the termination of an abnormally short spinal cord is characteristic of caudal regression syndrome. This morphology, illustrated in Case 1093, reflects greater hypoplasia of the ventral portion of the distal spinal cord than is present dorsally. There is often an associated clinical disparity in the level of

residual neurological function, with sensation preserved to lower anatomical levels than motor abilities.

Although the cord hypoplasia in caudal regression syndrome is static, patients may experience progressive symptoms due to bony or fibrous compression of the dural sac, which commonly occurs near the level of vertebral aplasia/hypoplasia. Surgery is indicated to relieve cord distortion and stabilize residual neurological function in such cases.

Sacral agenesis may alternatively be associated with tethering of the spinal cord. The distal segments of the sacrum are absent in Case 1094. Instead of demonstrating a truncated morphology, the conus medullaris is elongated. A thick band of intradural tissue *(arrows)* extends to the termination of the moderately ectatic sacral sac, with taut morphology indicating traction on the spinal cord. It is not possible to distinguish cord parenchyma from potentially thickened filum terminale on this sagittal scan (see discussion of Case 1064).

677

REFERENCES

Altman NR, Altman DH: MR imaging of spinal dysraphism. *AJNR* 8:533-538, 1987.

Armonda RA, Citrin CM, Foley KT, et al: Quantitative cine-mode magnetic resonance imaging of Chiari I malformations: an analysis of cerebrospinal fluid dynamics. *Neurosurgery* 35:214-224, 1994.

Banna M: Syringomyelia in association with posterior fossa cysts. *AJNR* 9:867-873, 1988.

Barkovich AJ, Edwards MSB, Cogen PH: MR evaluation of spinal dermal sinus tracts in children. *AJNR* 12:123-129, 1991.

Barkovich AJ, Raghavan N, Chuang S, Peck WW: The wedge-shaped cord terminus: a radiographic sign of caudal regression. *AJNR* 10:1223-1231, 1989.

Barkovich AJ, Sherman JL, Citrin CM, et al: MR of postoperative syringomyelia. *AJNR* 8:319, 1987.

Barnes P: Imaging in spinal dysraphism. *Contemp Diagn Radiol* 12:1, 1990.

Barnes PD, Lester PD, Yamanashi WS, et al: Magnetic resonance imaging in infants and children with spinal dysraphism. *AJNR* 7:465-472, 1986.

Brooks BS, Duvall ER, El Gammal T, et al: Neuroimaging features of neurenteric cysts: analysis of nine cases and review of the literature. *AJNR* 14:735-746, 1993.

Brophy JD, Sutton LN, Zimmerman RA, et al: Magnetic resonance imaging of lipomyelomeningocele and tethered cord. *Neurosurgery* 25:336-340, 1989.

Brunberg JA, Latchaw RE, Kanal E, et al: Magnetic resonance imaging of spinal dysraphism. *Rad Clin North Am* 26:181-205, 1988.

Byrd SE, Darling CF, McLone DG: Development disorders of the pediatric spine. *Rad Clin North Am* 29:711-752, 1991.

Caro PA, Marks HG, Keret D, et al: Intraspinal epidermoid tumors in children: problems in recognition and imaging techniques for diagnosis. *J Ped Orthopaed* 11:288-293, 1991.

Clifton AG, Stevens JM, Kendall BE: Idiopathic and Chiari-associated syringomyelia in adults: observation on cerebrospinal fluid pathway at the foramen magnum using static MRI. *Neuroaradiology* 33(suppl):167-169, 1991.

Davis PC, Hoffman JC Jr, Bell TI, et al: Spinal abnormalities in pediatric patients: MR imaging findings compared with clinical, myelographic, and surgical findings. *Radiology* 166:679-685, 1988.

Davis SW, Levy LM, LeBihan D, et al: Sacral meningeal cysts: evaluation with MR imaging. *Radiology* 187:445-448, 1993.

De Pena CA, Lee Y-Y, Van Tassel P, et al: MR appearance of acquired spinal epidermoid tumors. *AJNR* 10:597, 1989.

Han JS, Benson JE, Kaufman B, et al: Demonstration of diastematomyelia and associated abnormalities with MR imaging. *AJNR* 6:215-220, 1985.

Hoffman CH, Dietrich RB, Pais MJ, et al: The split notochord syndrome with dorsal enteric fistula. *AJNR* 14:622-628, 1993.

Isu T, Iwasaki Y, Akino M, Abe H: Hydromyelia associated with a Chiari I malformation in children and adults. *Neurosurgery* 26:591-597, 1990.

Kaffenberger DA, Heinz ER, Oakes JW, Boyko O: Meningocele Manque: Radiologic findings with clinical correlation. *AJNR* 13:1083-1088, 1992.

Kaplan JO, Quencer RM: The occult tethered conus syndrome in the adult. *Radiology* 137:387-391, 1980.

Kuharik MA, Edwards MK, Grossman CB: Magnetic resonance evaluation of pediatric spinal dysraphism. *Pediatr Neurosci* 12:213-218, 1985-1986.

Lee BCP, Zimmerman RD, Manning JJ, Deck MDF: MR imaging of syringomyelia and hydromyelia. *AJNR* 6:221-228, 1985.

Levy LM, DiChiro G, McCullough DC, et al: Fixed spinal cord: diagnosis with MR imaging. *Radiology* 169:773-778, 1988.

Merx JL, Bakker-Niezen SH, Thijssen HOM, Walder HAD: The tethered spinal cord syndrome: a correlation of radiological features and preoperative findings in 30 patients. *Neuroradiology* 31:63-70, 1989.

Milhorat TH, Johnson WD, Miller JI, et al: Surgical treatment of syringomyelia based on magnetic resonance imaging criteria. *Neurosurgery* 31:231-245, 1992.

Milhorat TH, Miller JI, Johnson WD, et al: Anatomical basis of syringomyelia occurring with hindbrain lesions. *Neurosurgery* 32:748-754, 1993.

Moufarrij NA, Palmer JM, Hahn JF, Weinstein MA: Correlation between magnetic resonance imaging and surgical findings in tethered spinal cord. *Neurosurgery* 25:341-346, 1989.

Muras I, Cioffi FA, Punzo A, Bernini FP: The occult intrasacral meningocele. *Neuroradiology* 33(suppl):492-494, 1991.

Naidich TP, Harwood-Nash DC: Diastematomyelia. Part I. Hemicords and meningeal sheaths. Single and double arachnoid and dural tubes. *AJNR* 4:633-636, 1983.

Naidich TP, McLone DG, Mutleur S: A new understanding of dorsal dysraphism with lipoma (lipomyeloschisis: radiological evaluation and surgical correction. *AJNR* 4:103-116, 1983.

Nelson MD Jr, Bracchi M, Naidich TP, McLone DG: The natural history of repaired myelomeningocele. *Radiographics* 8:695-706, 1988.

Nievelstein RAJ, Valk J, Smit LME, et al: MR of the caudal regression syndrome: embryologic implications. *AJNR* 15:1021-1029, 1994.

O'Connor JF, Cranley WR, McCarten KM, Radkowski MA: Radiographic manifestations of congenital anomalies of the spine. *Rad Clin North Am* 29:407-430, 1991.

Okumra R, Minami S, Asato R, Konishi J: Fatty filum terminale: assessment with MR imaging. *J Comput Assist Tomogr* 14:571-573, 1990.

Oldfield EH, Muraszko K, Shawker TH, Patronas NJ: Pathophysiology of syringomyelia associated with Chiari I malformation of the cerebellar tonsils. Implications for diagnosis and treatment. *J Neurosurg* 80:3-15, 1994.

Pang D: Sacral agenesis and caudal spinal cord malformations. *Neurosurgery* 32:755-779, 1993.

Pang D: Split cord malformation: Part II: clinical syndrome. *Neurosurgery* 31:481-500, 1992.

Pang D, Dias MS, Ahab-Barmada M: Split cord malformation: Part I: a unified theory of embryogenesis for double spinal cord malformations. *Neurosurgery* 31:451-480, 1992.

Pena CA, Lee Y-Y, Van Tassel P, et al: MR appearance of acquired epidermoid tumor. *AJNR* 10:597, 1989.

Pojunas K, Williams AL, Daniels DL, Haughton VM: Syringomyelia and hydromyelia: magnetic resonance evaluation. *Radiology* 153:679-683, 1984.

Raghavan N, Barkovich AJ, Edwards M, Norman D: MR imaging in the tethered spinal cord syndrome. *AJNR* 10:27-36, 1989.

Rogg JM, Benzil DL, Haas RL, Knuckey NW: Intramedullary abscess, an unusual manifestation of a dermal sinus. *AJNR* 14:1393-1396, 1993.

Samuelsson L, Bergstrom K, Thuomas K-A, et al: MR imaging of syringohydromyelia and Chiari malformations in myelomeningocele patients with scoliosis. *AJNR* 8:539, 1987.

Scatliff JH, Kendall BE, Kingsley DPE, et al: Closed spinal dysraphism: analysis of clinical, radiological and surgical findings in 104 consecutive patients. *AJNR* 10:269-277, 1989.

Sherman JL, Barkovich AJ, Citrin CM: The MR appearance of syringomyelia: new observations. *AJNR* 7:985-995, 1986.

Sherman JL, Citrin CM, Barkovich AJ: MR imaging of syringobulbia. *J Comput Assist Tomogr* 11:407-411, 1987.

Sigal R, Denys A, Halimi P, et al: Ventriculus terminalis of the conus medullaris: MR imaging in four patients with congenital dilatation. *AJNR* 12:733-738, 1991.

Slasky BS, Bydder GM, Niendorf HP, Young JR: MR imaging with gadolinium-DTPA in the differentiation of tumor, syrinx, and cyst of the spinal cord. *J Comput Assist Tomogr* 11:845-850, 1987.

Stovner W, Rinck P: Syringomyelia in Chiari malformations: relation to extent of cerebellar tissue herniation. *Neurosurgery* 31:913-917, 1992.

Terae S, Miyasaka K, Abe S, et al: Increased pulsative movement of the hindbrain in syringomyelia associated with the Chiari malformation: cine-MRI with presaturation bolus tracking. *Neuoradiology* 36:125-129, 1994.

Tortori-Donati P, Cama A, Rosa ML, et al: Occult spinal dysraphism: neuroradiological study. *Neuroradiology* 31:512-522, 1990.

Uchino A, Mori T, Ohno M: Thickened fatty filum terminale: MR imaging. *Neuroradiology* 33:331-333, 1991.

Warder DE, Oakes WJ: Tethered cord syndrome: the low-lying and normally positioned conus. *Neurosurgery* 34:597-600, 1994.

Wilberger JE Jr, Maroon J, Prostko R, et al: Magnetic resonance imaging and intraoperative neurosonography in syringomyelia. *Neurosurgery* 20:599-605, 1987.

Wilson DA, Prince JR: MR imaging determination of the location of the normal conus medullaris throughout childhood. *AJR* 152:1029, 1989.

Zimmerman RA, Bilaniuk LT, Bury EA: Magnetic resonance of the pediatric spine. *Magn Reson Q* 5:169-204, 1989.

Selected Pictoral Index

The following pages provide an abbreviated pictoral index to the cases in this volume. Topics have been selected to emphasize the various categories of pathology that may cause a particular MR appearance. An attempt has been made to minimize repetition of comparisons that are highlighted by "Differential Diagnoses" and/or chapter organization within the text.

The pictoral index is incomplete in several respects. Only one example of a given pathology is included on each page. Furthermore, the index is limited to the preceding case collection, which does not attempt to illustrate all manifestations of all disorders.

For these reasons, each index page represents an overview rather than a comprehensive "gamut." The cases listed will lead to adjacent cases, neighboring pages, and cross references that more fully discuss the general subject and the specific pathology.

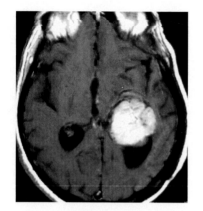

Meningioma
Case 64

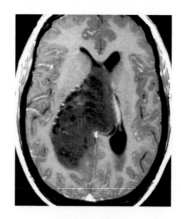

Astrocytoma
Case 113

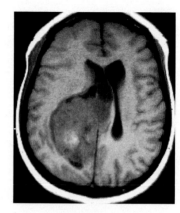

Oligodendroglioma
Case 114

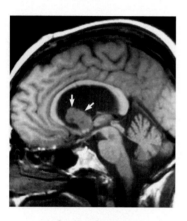

Subependymoma
Case 118

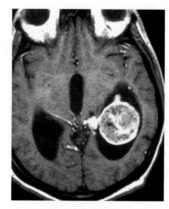

Dermoid Cyst
Case 287

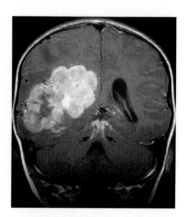

Choroid Plexus Carcinoma
Case 299

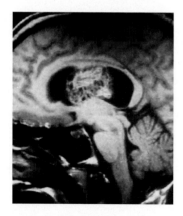

Central Neurocytoma
Case 308

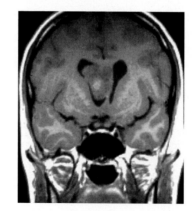

Ependymoma
Case 309

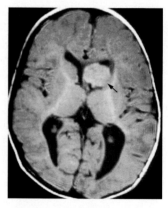

Giant Cell Astrocytoma
Case 756

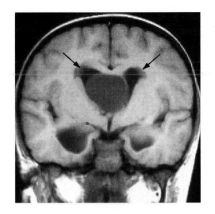

Cystic Astrocytoma
Case 103

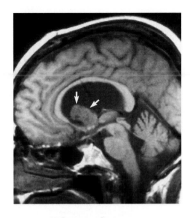

Subependymoma
Case 118

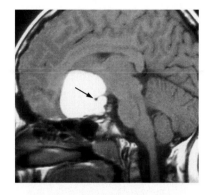

Craniopharyngioma
Case 228

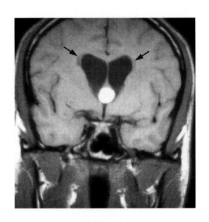

Colloid Cyst
Case 256

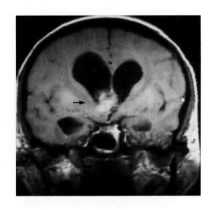

Meningioma
Case 267

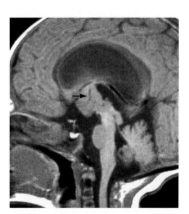

Choroid Plexus Papilloma
Case 302

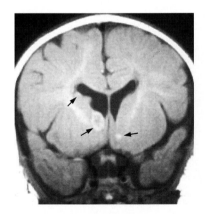

Tuberous Sclerosis
Case 750

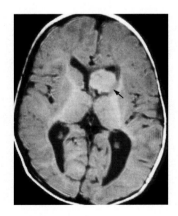

Giant Cell Astrocytoma
Case 756

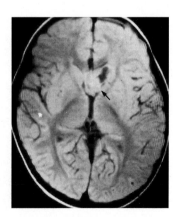

Septal Astrocytoma
Case 759

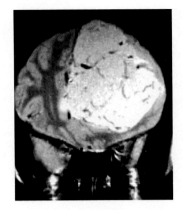

Meningioma
Case 40

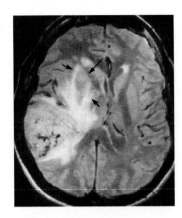

Glioblastoma Multiforme
Case 87

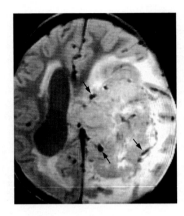

Malignant Ependymoma
Case 117

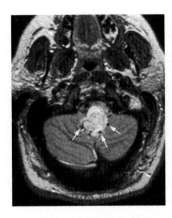

Hemangioblastoma
Case 137

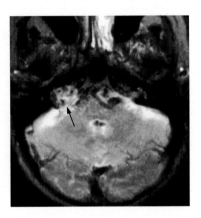

Glomus Tumor
Case 185

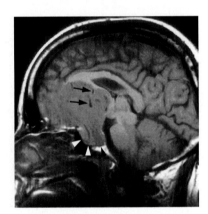

Pituitary Adenoma
Case 206

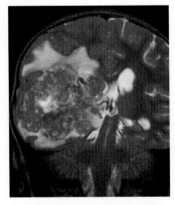

Choroid Plexus Carcinoma
Case 299

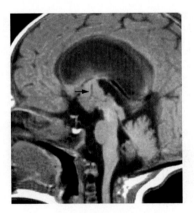

Choroid Plexus Papilloma
Case 302

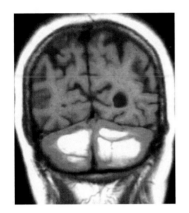

Metastasis
Case 9

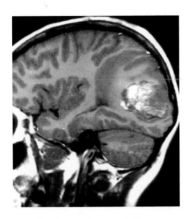

Glioblastoma Multiforme
Case 89

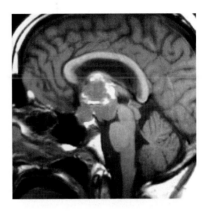

Germinoma
Case 238

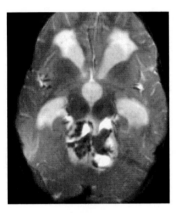

Teratoma
Case 276

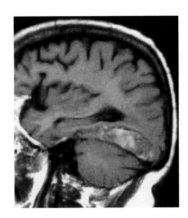

Infarction
Case 479

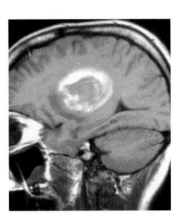

Spontaneous Hematoma
Case 557

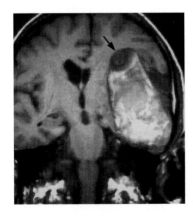

Thrombosed Aneurysm
Case 603

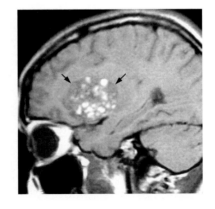

Thrombosed AVM
Case 615

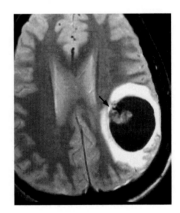

Ruptured AVM
Case 617

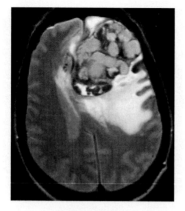

Metastasis
Case 10

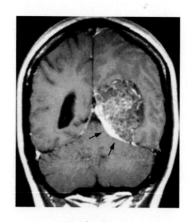

Meningioma
Case 53

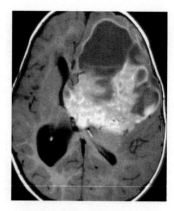

High Grade Astrocytoma
Case 98

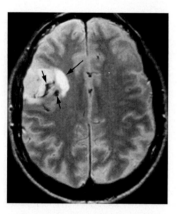

Oligodendroglioma
Case 112

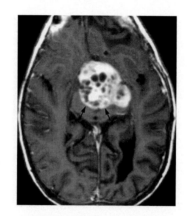

Hypothalamic Glioma
Case 247

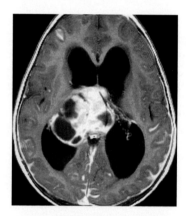

Pineoblastoma (PNET)
Case 280

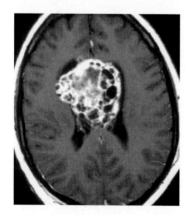

Teratoma
Case 283

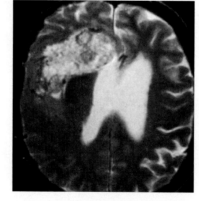

Dermoid Cyst
Case 288

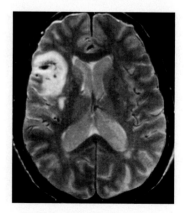

Hemorrhagic Infarct
Case 481

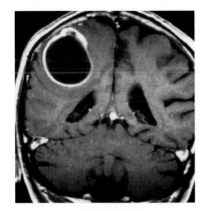

Metastasis
Case 15

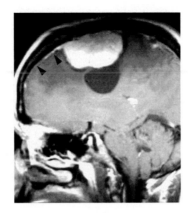

Meningioma
Case 52

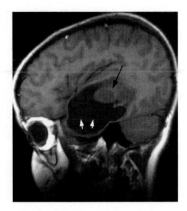

Anaplastic Astrocytoma
Case 85

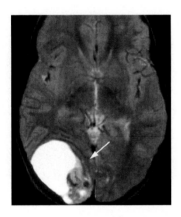

Ependymoma
Case 116

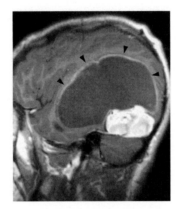

Pleomorphic Xanthoastrocytoma
Case 119

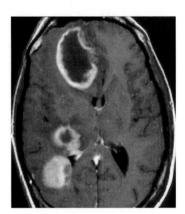

Primary CNS Lymphoma
Case 324

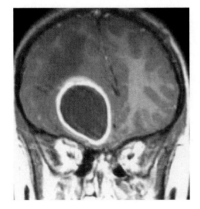

Abscess
Case 412

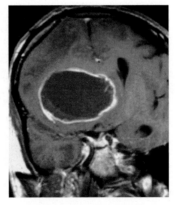

Glioblastoma Multiforme
Case 413

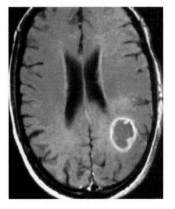

Toxoplasmosis
Case 421

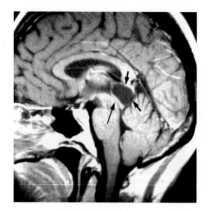

Pineal Cyst
Case 268

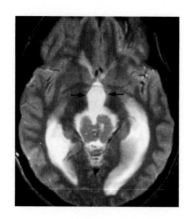

Germinoma
Case 272

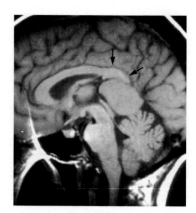

Meningioma
Case 274

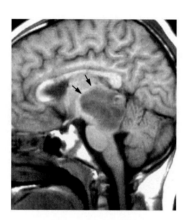

Pineoblastoma (PNET)
Case 279

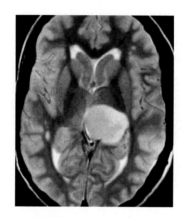

Diencephalic Glioma
Case 282

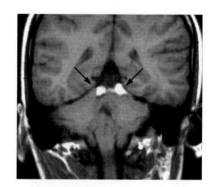

Lipoma
Case 290

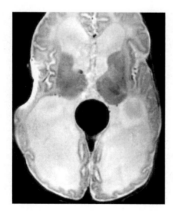

Vein of Galen Aneurysm
Case 611

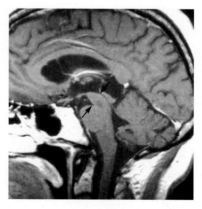

Arachnoid Cyst
Case 683

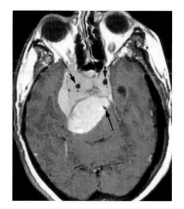

Meningioma
Case 60

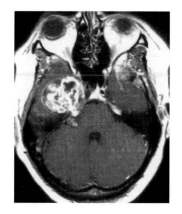

Trigeminal Schwannoma
Case 178

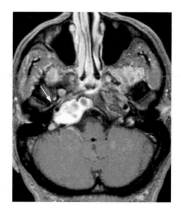

Chordoma
Case 195

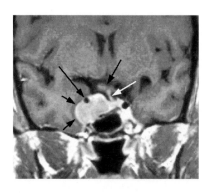

Pituitary Adenoma
Case 216

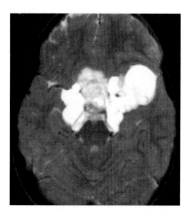

Hypothalamic Glioma
Case 245

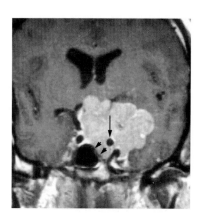

Craniopharyngioma
Case 249

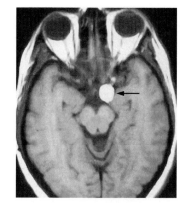

Dermoid Cyst
Case 286

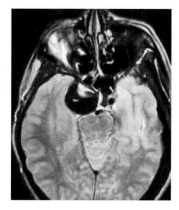

Aneurysm
Case 635

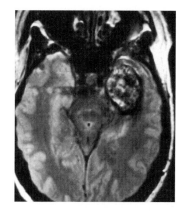

Cavernous Angioma
Case 636

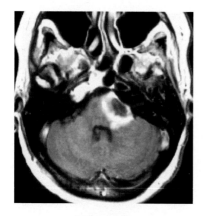

Metastasis
Case 21

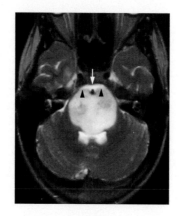

Glioma
Case 123

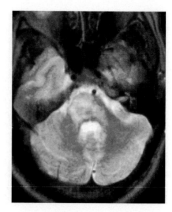

Multiple Sclerosis
Case 356

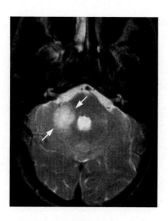

PML
Case 374

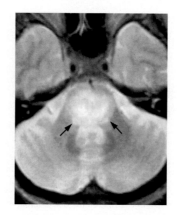

Central Pontine Myelinolysis
Case 375

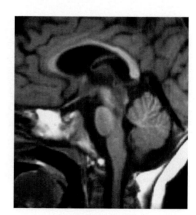

Leigh's Disease
Case 437

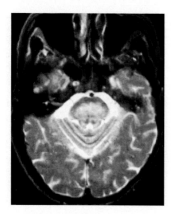

Ischemic Change
Case 518

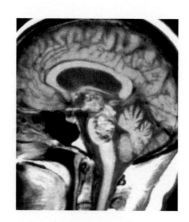

Cavernous Angioma
Case 637

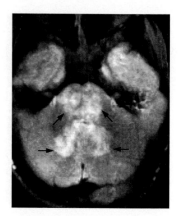

Neurofibromatosis
Case 766

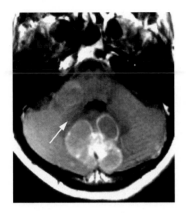

Metastatic Carcinoma
Case 22

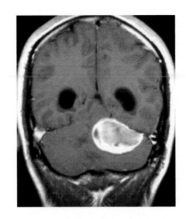

Hemangioblastoma
Case 142

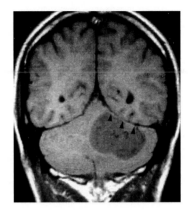

Medulloblastoma
Case 163

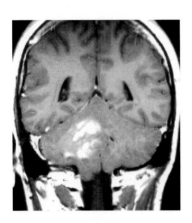

Astrocytoma
Case 164

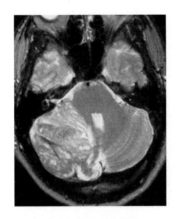

Lhermitte-Duclois
Case 165

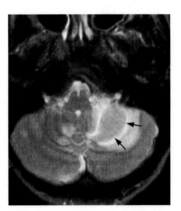

Primary CNS Lymphoma
Case 313

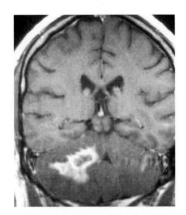

Radiation Necrosis
Case 449

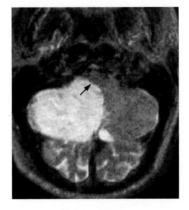

PICA Infarct
Case 530

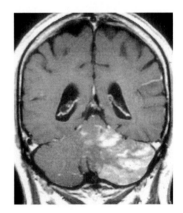

Dural AVM
Case 612

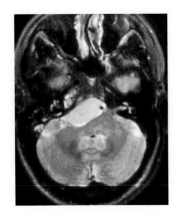

Meningioma
Case 38

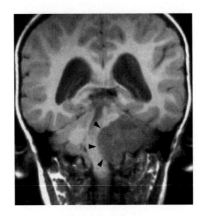

Ependymoma
Case 157

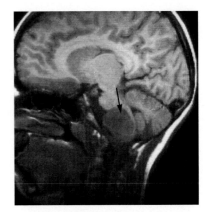

Exophytic Brainstem Glioma
Case 158

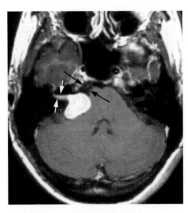

Acoustic Schwannoma
Case 170

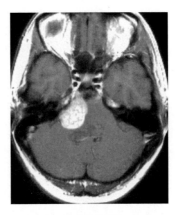

Metastasis
Case 173

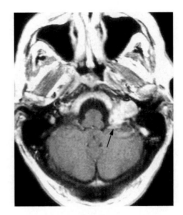

Glomus Tumor
Case 186

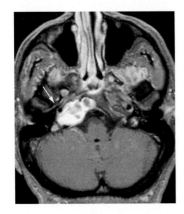

Chordoma
Case 195

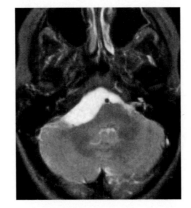

Epidermoid Cyst
Case 296

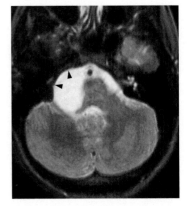

Arachnoid Cyst
Case 694

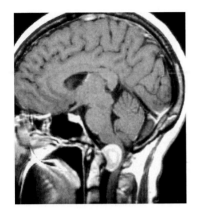

Meningioma
Case 63

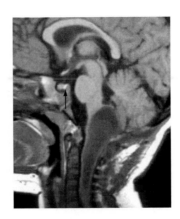

Astrocytoma
Case 126

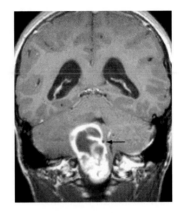

Hemangioblastoma
Case 139

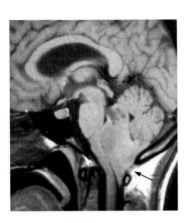

Ependymoma
Case 152

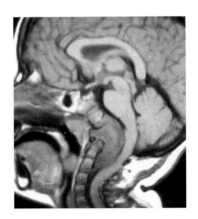

Chordoma
Case 194

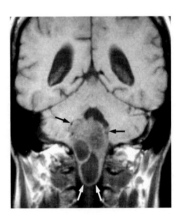

Choroid Plexus Papilloma
Case 303

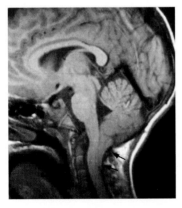

Chiari Malformation
Case 713

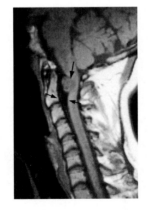

Schwannoma
Case 918

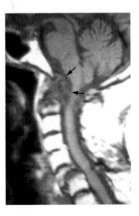

Pseudotumor (Arthritis)
Case 1044

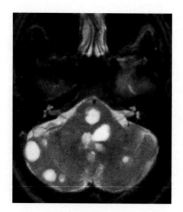

Metastases
Case 20

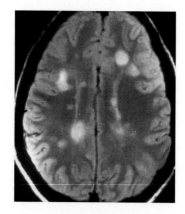

Multiple Sclerosis
Case 341

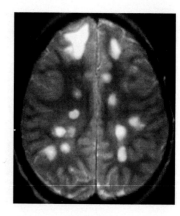

ADEM
Case 365

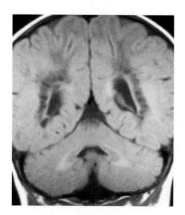

Canavan's Disease
Case 383

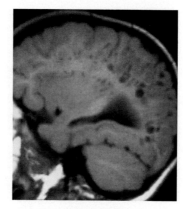

Hurler's Disease
Case 384

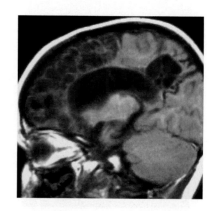

Multicystic Encephalomalacia
Case 702

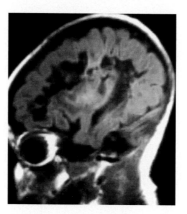

Periventricular Leukomalacia
Case 704

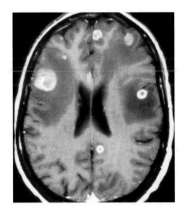

Metastases
Case 14

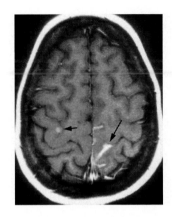

Meningeal Carcinomatosis
Case 31

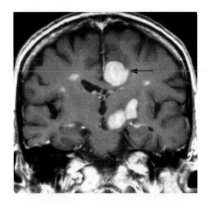

Primary CNS Lymphoma
Case 318

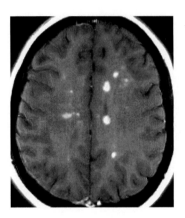

Multiple Sclerosis
Case 353

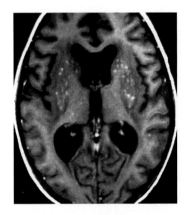

Encephalitis
Case 388-1

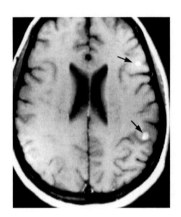

Tuberculosis
Case 424

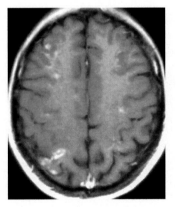

Watershed Infarcts
Case 490

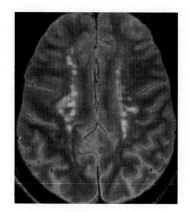

Multiple Sclerosis
Case 329

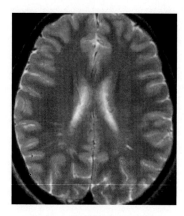

Prominent Perivascular Spaces
Case 334

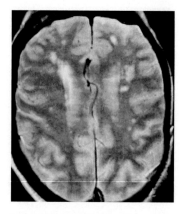

Systemic Lupus Erythematosis
Case 433

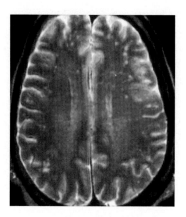

Lyme Disease
Case 435

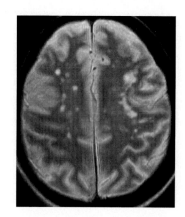

Sarcoidosis
Case 436

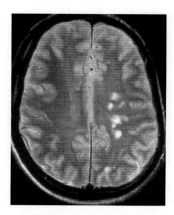

Watershed Infarction
Case 497

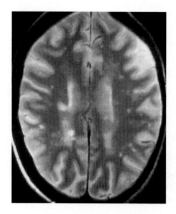

Small Vessel Infarcts
Case 512

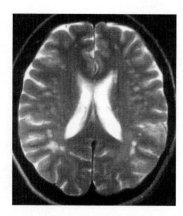

Diffuse Axonal Injury
Case 572

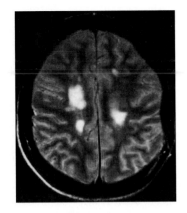

Multiple Sclerosis
Case 336

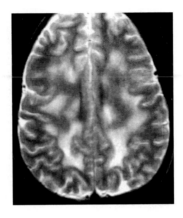

ADEM
Case 364

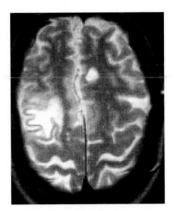

PML
Case 371

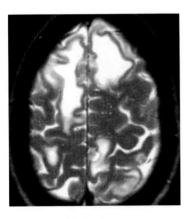

Metastases
Case 372

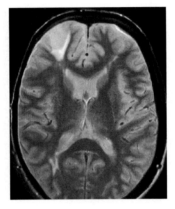

Infarcts
Case 502

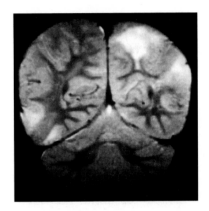

Tuberous Sclerosis
Case 762

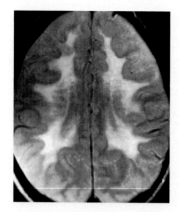

Metachromatic Leukodystrophy
Case 377

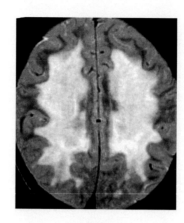

ADEM
Case 379

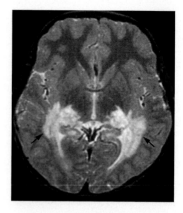

Adrenoleukodystrophy
Case 380

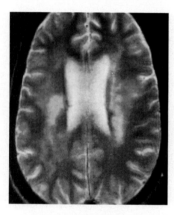

HIV Encephalitis
Case 426

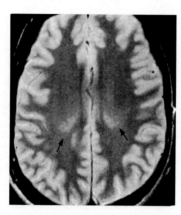

Amyotrophic Lateral Sclerosis
Case 428

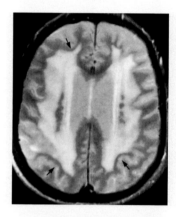

"Aging" White Matter
Case 515

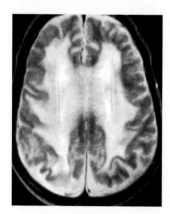

Post Radiation
Case 517

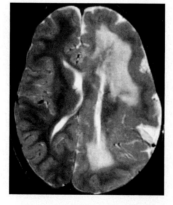

Unilateral Megalencephaly
Case 739

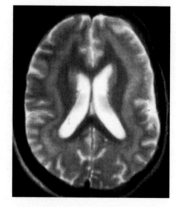

Band Heterotopia
Case 747

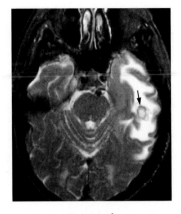

Metastasis
Case 4

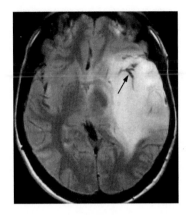

Astrocytoma
Case 81

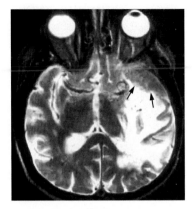

Sphenoid Wing Meningioma
Case 83

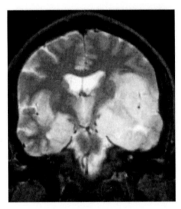

Gliomatosis Cerebri
Case 107

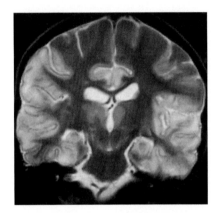

Viral Meningitis
Case 387

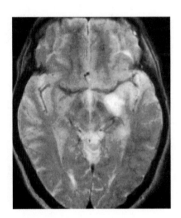

Herpes Encephalitis
Case 397

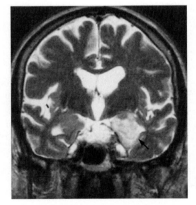

Limbic Encephalitis
Case 400

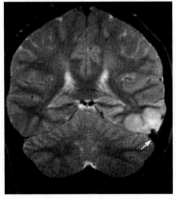

Transverse Sinus Thrombosis
Case 648

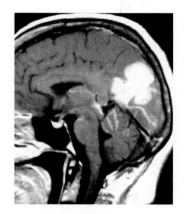

Leptomeningeal Carcinomatosis
Case 30

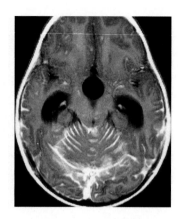

CSF Tumor Seeding
Case 161

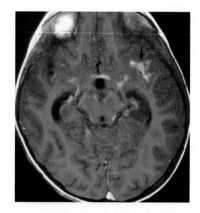

Tuberculous Meningitis
Case 386

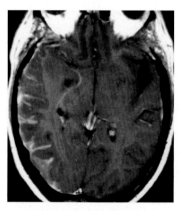

Systemic Lymphoma
Case 386-1

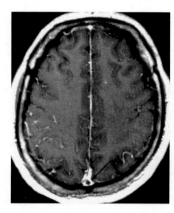

Superior Sagittal Thrombosis
Case 386-2

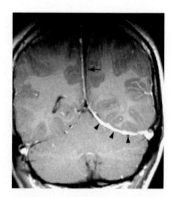

Subdural Empyema
Case 393

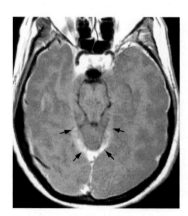

Intracranial Hypotension
Case 463

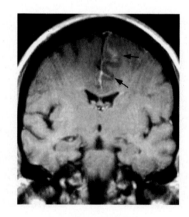

Acute Infarction
Case 484

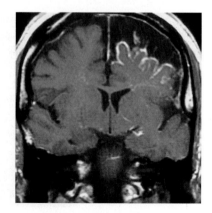

Sturge Weber Syndrome
Case 770

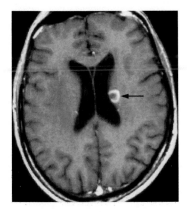

Metastatic Carcinoma
Case 19

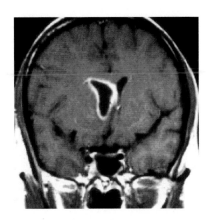

Primary CNS Lymphoma
Case 319

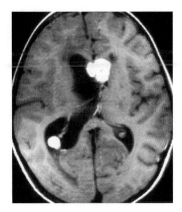

CSF Tumor Seeding
Case 322

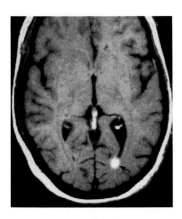

Multiple Sclerosis
Case 351

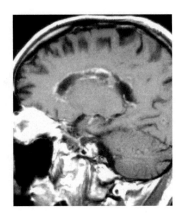

Ventriculitis
Case 389

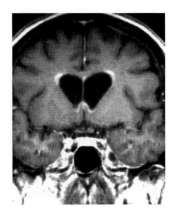

Metastatic Lymphoma
Case 390

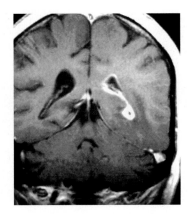

Subependymal Tumor Spread
Case 391

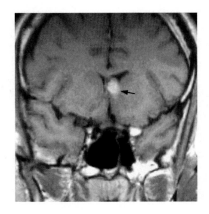

Tuberous Sclerosis
Case 757

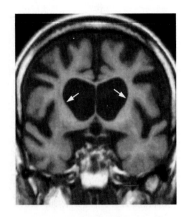

Huntington's Disease
Case 456

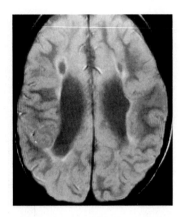

Periventricular Leukomalacia
Case 500

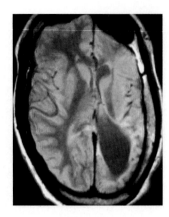

Old Infarct
Case 541

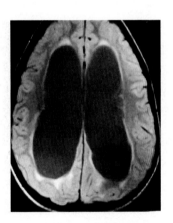

Hydrocephalus
Case 650

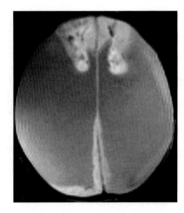

Hydranencephaly
Case 654

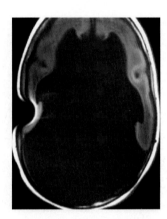

Holoprosencephaly
Case 655

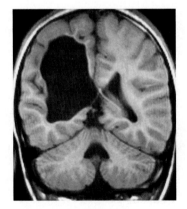

Porencephaly
Case 697

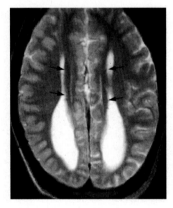

Colpocephaly
Case 722

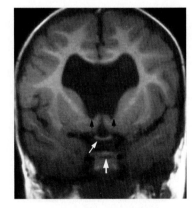

Septo-Optic Dysplasia
Case 728

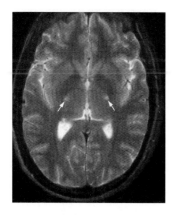

Amyotrophic Lateral Sclerosis
Case 428

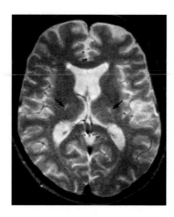

Extrapontine Myelinolysis
Case 430

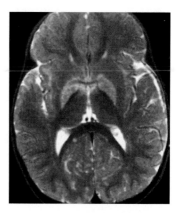

Leigh's Disease
Case 439

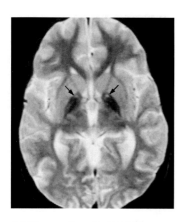

Hallervorden-Spatz Disease
Case 444

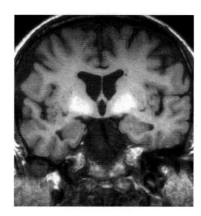

Chronic Hepatic Disease
Case 446

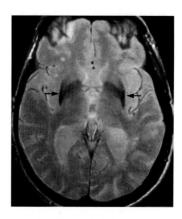

Parkinson's Disease
Case 454

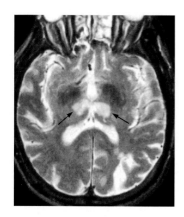

Basilar Artery Ischemia
Case 538

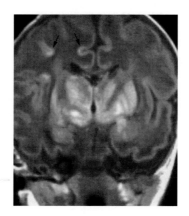

Anoxia
Case 552

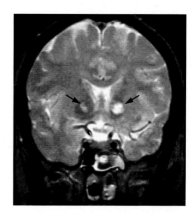

Carbon Monoxide Poisoning
Case 554

INTRAMEDULLARY EDEMA

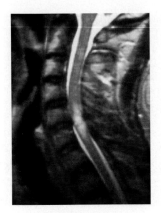

Astrocytoma
Case 938

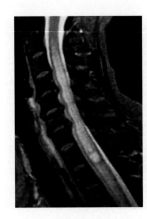

Metastasis
Case 961

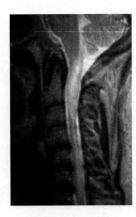

Multiple Sclerosis
Case 986

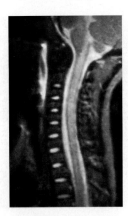

Transverse Myelitis
Case 989

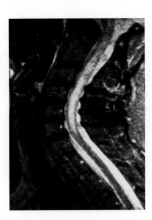

Radiation Myelitis
Case 997

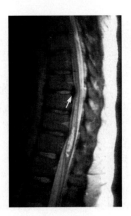

Infarction
Case 1032

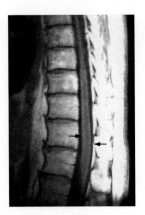

Dural AV Fistula
Case 1037

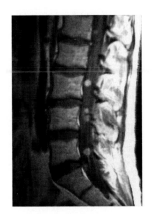

Metastatic Carcinoma
Case 910

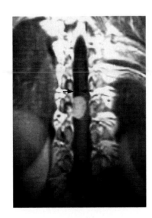

Meningioma
Case 915

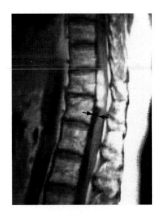

Schwannoma
Case 922

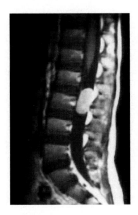

Ependymoma of the Filum
Case 949

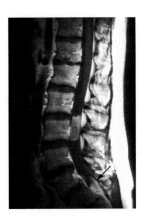

"Drop" Metastasis
Case 951

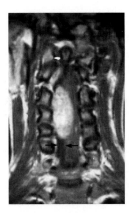

Exophytic Cord Ependymoma
Case 953

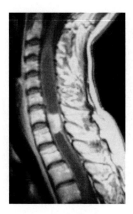

Ependymoma
Case 948

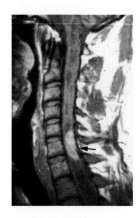

Hemangioblastoma
Case 957

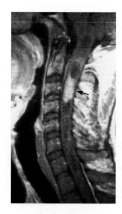

Astrocytoma
Case 958

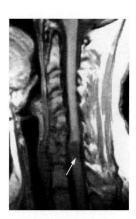

Cystic Myelomalacia
Case 1015

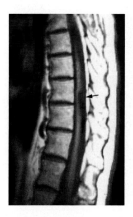

Arachnoid Cyst
Case 1026

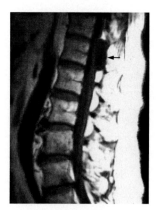

Meningeal Cyst
Case 1028

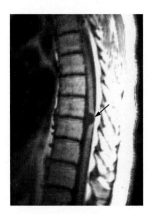

Neuroepithelial Cyst
Case 1029

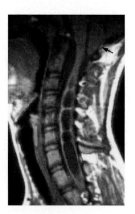

Syringomyelia
Case 1051

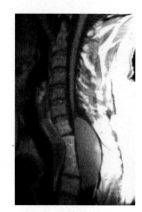

Neurenteric Cyst
Case 1091

INDEX

Myelomeningocele—cont'd
  repair of, dorsal tethering of neural tissue after, 662
Myxopapillary ependymomas, 586, 588, 590

N

Nasoethmoidal encephaloceles, 118, 119
Nasopharyngeal carcinoma
  clival meningioma differentiated from, 118
  metastatic carcinoma of colon differentiated from, 119
Necrosis of brain tissue, radiation, 277
Nerve root(s)
  compression of, from spondylolisthesis, 531
  intradural enhancing, differential diagnosis of, 569
  thick, differential diagnosis of, 565, 621
Nerve(s)
  cranial
    fourth, schwannoma of, 105
    hypoglossal, schwannoma of, 105
    multiple, masses of, differential diagnosis, 107
    third, enhancing mass involving, differential
        diagnosis, 106
    trigeminal, schwannomas of, 104
  spinal, extradural thickening of, differential diagnosis,
      578
Neurenteric cysts, 676
Neuritis, optic, 489, 490
Neuroblastoma, 559
  lumbosacral, 580
  olfactory, 127, 189
Neurocytomas, central, 190
Neuroectodermal tumor, primitive, 594
Neuroepithelial cysts, 436-437
Neurofibromas, spinal, 576
Neurofibromatosis, 468, 469
  tupe 1, 468, 469
  type 2
    bilateral acoustic neuromas in, 99
    multiple meningiomas with, 37
    multiple schwannomas with, 107
Neurohypophysis, "ectopic," 137
Neuromas, see Schwannomas
Neuronal migration disorders, see specific type, e.g.,
        Lissencephaly, Pachygyria, Polymicrogyria,
        Heteropia, Schizencephaly
Neuropathy, cranial, vascular tortuosity causing, 393
Nodules, multiple superficial enhancing, differential
        diagnosis of, 263

O

Occipital cyst, extracranial, in infant, differential diagnosis
        of, 473
Occipital encephaloceles, 472
Occlusive vascular disease, MR angiography in, 337
Ocular masses, primary, 496
Odontoid process, "high-riding," 647
Olfactory neuroblastoma, 127, 189
Oligodendrogliomas, 64, 65

Olivopontocerebellar degeneration, 284
Ophthalmopathy, thyroid, 498
Optic chiasm, enlarged, differential diagnosis of, 489
Optic nerve
  glioma(s) of, 482, 483, 484, 485
    contrast enhancement of, 485
    differential diagnosis of, 488, 489
    on T1-weighted images, 482, 483
    on T2-weighted images, 484
  thickening of, differential diagnosis of, 488
Optic nerve sheath meningiomas, 486-488
  contrast enhancement of, 487
  differential diagnosis of, 488
Optic neuritis, 489, 490
Orbit
  benign mixed tumor of lacrimal gland involving, 494
  dermoid cyst of, 494
  effects of sinus disease on, 501
  hemangiomas of, 492
  lymphangiomas of, 493
  masses of, in children, 495
  metastases to, 497
  pseudotumor of, 499
  trauma to, 500
  vascular malformation of, 491-493
Osseous deformity of cervical canal, 543
Ossification of posterior longitudinal ligament, 542
Osteomyelitis, 600-607
  contrast enhancement of, 606
  differential diagnosis of, 604-605, 607
  spinal deformity due to, 602
  on T1-weighted images, 600
  on T2-weighted images, 601

P

Pachygyria
  on T1-weighted images, 450
  on T2-weighted images, 451
Papillomas, choroid plexus
  in fourth ventricle, 186, 187
  in third ventricle, 186
Parasagittal chordomas, 117
Parasellar mass containing blood products, differential
        diagnosis of, 390
Parasellar meningioma, 26, 27, 34, 52
Parasellar region
  dermoid cyst of, 176, 177
  Tolosa-Hunt syndrome in, 154
Paraspinal masses of neural origin, 579
Paraspinal "small blue cell" tumors, 561
Parkinson's disease, 280
Patent aneurysms, 366
Pericallosal artery aneurysm, 366
Perineural cyst, 639
Perivascular spaces, prominent, 207, 233
Periventricular heterotopic gray matter, 460